INDIVIDUAL SUPPORT

Ageing

WENDY MORTON • NICOLE DAWSON • LISA TAFFE

INDIVIDUAL SUPPORT

Ageing

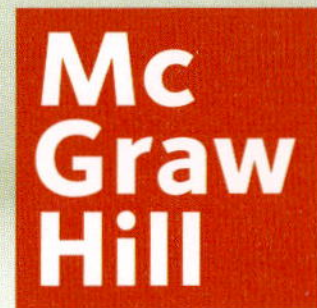

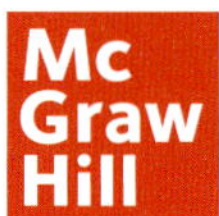

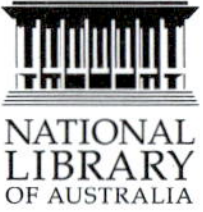

A catalogue record for this book is available from the National Library of Australia

Authors: Wendy Morton, Nicole Dawson, Lisa Taffe
Title: *Individual Support: Ageing*
ISBN: 9781743767252 (paperback)

Published in Australia by
McGraw-Hill (Australia) Pty Ltd,
Level 33, 680 George Street, Sydney NSW 2000
Publisher: Matthew Coxhill
Production editor: Caroline Hunter
Copyeditor: Robyn Flemming
Permissions editor: Debbie Gallagher, Legend Images
Indexer: Kerryn Burgess
Interior design: Simon Rattray, Squirt Creative
Cover design: Simon Rattray, Squirt Creative
Cover image: Getty Images/Maskot
Images in Chapter 15: Alan Laver
Typeset by Straive, India
Printed in Singapore by Markono Print Media Pte Ltd

CONTENTS IN BRIEF

CONTENTS

CHAPTER 4 COMMUNICATING IN THE WORKPLACE 76

CHAPTER 5 RESPECTING DIVERSITY 103

PART 2 GENERAL CARE 131

CHAPTER 6 PROVIDING CARE AND SUPPORT 132

PART 4 HEALTH 383

PREFACE

Individual Support: Ageing has been expressly researched and developed for the training package qualification CHC33021 Certificate III in Individual Support. The text is inclusive of the most recent events in aged care reform, including the Royal Commission, and incorporates clear information regarding new and impending changes to aged care legislation and the aged care sector in general.

The core units of CHC33021 Certificate III in Individual Support are addressed, as are the Ageing specialisation units of competency. The remaining seven elective units of competency were selected to provide a broad platform of information that facilitates the development of knowledge across important aspects of working in aged care, including palliative care, assisting with medications and identifying potential abuse.

The text is targeted at entry-level care workers and provides comprehensive material that forms the foundation of best practice in aged care. Learning is supported by Industry in focus boxes, Workplace scenarios and Practice points that highlight issues in the workplace and provide specific information that can be applied in the work setting.

Underpinning all seventeen chapters of this text is the philosophy of person-centred care. Person-centred care seeks to place the person, their values, their perspective and their environment as the focus of care in the face of diminishing capacity and the challenge to maintain independence and dignity. It incorporates the needs of carers and families as equal stakeholders in the provision of services.

Individual Support: Ageing is a valuable resource that aims to empower learners as they face working in an industry that requires skills, knowledge and attitudes reflecting the care that is needed to make a difference in the lives of our older, vulnerable population.

We wish you all the best with your studies!

Wendy Morton
Nicole Dawson
Lisa Taffe
September 2022

ABOUT THE AUTHORS

NICOLE DAWSON DipAppSci, GradCertGerontol, Cert IV TAE, Cert IV OccHealthSafety

Nicole is a proud Kamilaroi woman who was raised on Awabakal country. As a Registered Nurse with more than 30 years' experience, Nicole has worked in many roles that support older people. In her early career Nicole worked as an RN and later as a Nurse Unit Manager and After-Hours Manager, managing an aged care facility with more than 360 residents. Nicole also worked as an Emergency Department RN for HNE Health, prior to accepting the position of Aged Services Emergency Team (ASET) RN.

Today, Nicole is a trainer and assessor within the aged care and disability sectors, and a clinical educator within the health sector. As the director of her own company, Nicole's primary work is the research and development of accredited and non-accredited course content related to aged care, disability support and clinical care. Nicole's special interests include wound care, counselling and teaching.

WENDY MORTON BA, DipEd (Nursing), GradCertGerontol, Cert IV TAE, MEd (Adult)

Wendy is a Registered Nurse with long-standing experience in aged care and acute care. Wendy currently works for TAFE NSW as a Head Teacher of Community Services and has been teaching health and aged care for more than 25 years. She is currently enrolled in a Master of Gerontology at Charles Sturt University and is a member of the Australian Association of Gerontology. Wendy has worked for the NSW Education Standards Authority and in other areas of TAFE NSW, writing and reviewing curriculum, learning resources and assessments, as well as contributing to and reviewing publications relating to aged care and disability.

Wendy has a special interest in the application of person-centred care and in enhancing the role of the care worker through education and training, particularly considering the increasing complexity of care needs among the older population and growing community expectations regarding quality care.

LISA TAFFE BHSc, DipAppSc, DipTAE, GradDipEmergN, GradDipMid, GradDipVET

Lisa is a Registered Nurse with more than 30 years' experience, including as a midwife and emergency nurse, and has further qualifications in sports science, geriatric care, trauma and teaching. Commencing with TAFE NSW 20 years ago, Lisa took on the Head Teacher role in 2011, and now looks after Health, Aged Care, Nursing and First Aid for the Macksville, Coffs Harbour, Grafton, Maclean and Trenayr campuses.

Lisa balances work with TAFE and NSW Health with being a mother of five and a commitment to her local community. This includes being a volunteer ambulance officer (first responder) and actively supporting a range of local sporting groups.

ACKNOWLEDGEMENTS

The development of this edition would not have been possible without the help and encouragement of our colleagues in vocational education and training and in industry.

McGraw Hill and the authors would also like to thank the following for their valuable contributions to the writing of this book: Claire Clifford, Sara Leslie, Wendy Reilly and Rebecca Webber.

In addition, thanks to the following for their contributions to the photographs included in this text:

- Avril Bowd, Kurrajong Community Nursing Home
- Melissa Howe, Sanjeev Kumar, Elizabeth Lee, Norman Lee, Robert McIlwaine and Roslyn McIlwaine.

TEXT AT A GLANCE

Learning objectives ▼

These points help orient you to what is covered in the chapter.

LEARNING OBJECTIVES

2.1 Identify and respond to legal requirements
2.2 Identify and meet ethical responsibilities
2.3 Contribute to workplace improvements

Introduction ▼

Each chapter begins with an Introduction to provide a big picture overview and identify the key concepts to be covered in the text.

INTRODUCTION

THIS CHAPTER LOOKS AT THE SYNDROME OF DEMENTIA, and at the skills and knowledge required to provide person-centred care and support to people living with dementia by following an established individualised plan. Working with people living with dementia requires discretion and judgement. A care worker is supervised, either directly or indirectly, in this role, which they may carry out in the context of a residential aged care facility (RACF), a community or a family home.

This chapter introduces the condition of dementia, its related complications, and strategies to use when caring for and supporting those with dementia, their families and carers. There are various types of dementia with differing signs and symptoms, age of onset, severity and longevity. This chapter addresses the most common types and the recommended care strategies and support mechanisms available to implement person-centred holistic care.

Industry in focus ▼

At the start of each chapter the Industry in focus box introduces relevant news, developments and controversies linking the chapter topic to the aged care sector.

INDUSTRY IN FOCUS

The basis of person-centred care: Personhood, relationships and the environment

The Australian health-care system is consistently faced with challenges as the population ages and lives longer. The progressive, degenerative neurological health condition known as dementia is particularly challenging and requires patience and understanding along with a caring, supportive, individualised approach known as the person-centred approach.

With a person-centred approach and individualised care planning, caring for someone with dementia can be very rewarding and fulfilling. The concept of personhood in relation to dementia, introduced by Kitwood (1997), has allowed for the relationship between individuality and person-centred care to develop and be applied holistically and thoroughly while developing relationships and considering environments and how they can be adapted or modified during care and support.

According to Kitwood, **personhood** focuses on the status of being a person with individual physical, mental, cognitive, social, emotional, religious, cultural and financial characteristics, likes, dislikes, needs and wants. It is natural to assume that one's personhood determines the types of relationships and environments we encounter during our lifetime. Relationships are formed in a variety of ways and for various reasons, often sustaining or diminishing personhood, which is particularly important in caring for someone with dementia. Environments in which we socialise, learn, function and live also play a role in determining our individual personhood and its characteristics. Therefore, the basis of person-centred care is the link between personhood, relationships and environment.

Practice points ▼

These real-world practice tips provide additional pointers to help you apply your learning.

PRACTICE POINT

Working outside of your scope of practice is a breach of your duty of care and can place the older person at risk of harm from your actions, even if those actions are well intended. Remember: you are accountable for your actions in the workplace.

Workplace scenarios ▼

These mini case studies scattered throughout each chapter apply the content in an imagined real-world scenario.

WORKPLACE SCENARIO

Finding the balance between focusing on tasks and focusing on the individual

It is a busy morning shift at the RACF and Zac is already behind with his routine because his colleague has called in sick and a replacement care worker hasn't arrived yet. Zac needs to help Myrtle, a resident, to get out of bed and to shower before breakfast. Myrtle is quite independent but needs some minimal help and supervision because she is at risk of falling due to her frailty. Zac realises he doesn't have time to give to Myrtle before breakfast unless he takes over the tasks that she can do by herself. He decides to explain the situation to Myrtle and to give her the option of having breakfast in bed and a shower after breakfast, when he has more time. Myrtle is quite thrilled to have breakfast in bed. Zac assists her to use the toilet and to get back into bed, ready for breakfast. He is able to give Myrtle the time she needs after breakfast, by which time the staff replacement has arrived.

Check your understanding ▼

Questions at the end of each major section give you the opportunity to test your knowledge and reinforce learning of the chapter content.

CHECK YOUR UNDERSTANDING

1. What is the role of the Aged Care Quality and Safety Commission?
2. What does duty of care mean in the context of working as a care worker?
3. Explain dignity of risk.
4. List four employee responsibilities when working as a care worker.
5. What is the difference between a policy and a procedure?

Summary ▼

The chapter summary provides a quick review of the key learning objectives.

SUMMARY

- Ageism is a form of discrimination that treats a person unfairly based on chronological or perceived age. It is a contributing factor to the stereotype that portrays older people as asexual beings who have nothing to contribute to society in general. Far from reality, ageism and the myths that accompany stereotypical attitudes of older people can have a negative and destructive impact on the wellbeing and self-esteem of an older person, leading to depression and other forms of mental ill-health.
- All people have the right to autonomy and positive self-esteem. The care worker can empower older people to feel secure and confident by respecting their identity and empowering their self-motivation and strengths for self-care.
- The care worker can support healthy ageing in many ways, but especially by identifying and reporting variations in the older person's physical, emotional and psychological wellbeing.

Glossary ▼

At the back of the book is a glossary of the main terms from each chapter.

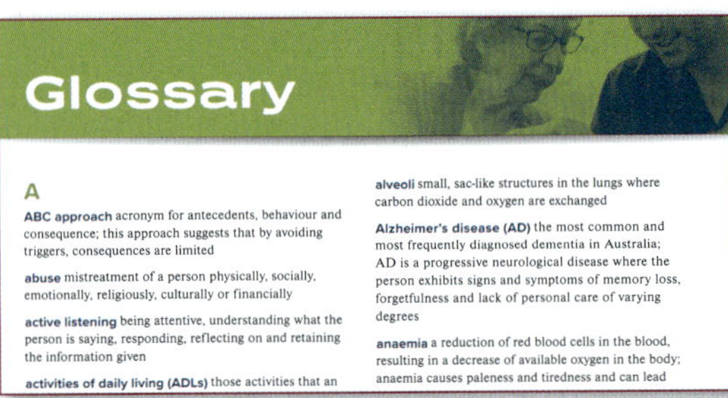
Glossary

A

ABC approach acronym for antecedents, behaviour and consequence; this approach suggests that by avoiding triggers, consequences are limited

abuse mistreatment of a person physically, socially, emotionally, religiously, culturally or financially

active listening being attentive, understanding what the person is saying, responding, reflecting on and retaining the information given

activities of daily living (ADLs) those activities that an

alveoli small, sac-like structures in the lungs where carbon dioxide and oxygen are exchanged

Alzheimer's disease (AD) the most common and most frequently diagnosed dementia in Australia; AD is a progressive neurological disease where the person exhibits signs and symptoms of memory loss, forgetfulness and lack of personal care of varying degrees

anaemia a reduction of red blood cells in the blood, resulting in a decrease of available oxygen in the body; anaemia causes paleness and tiredness and can lead

Review questions ▼

Review questions at the end of each chapter act as a revision and checkpoint for each chapter's skills, knowledge and understanding.

REVIEW QUESTIONS

2.1 Outline the purpose of the Aged Care Quality Standards in the aged care industry.

2.2 **(a)** What is meant by the term "restrictive practices"? Provide an example to support your answer.

(b) Why are restrictive practices of concern in aged care?

2.3 List examples of events that apply under the Serious Incidents Response Scheme.

2.4 What is the role of a support worker and supervisors in reporting such events?

2.5 In the workplace, what do each of the following terms mean? Provide an example for each term.

(a) Responsible.

(b) Accountable

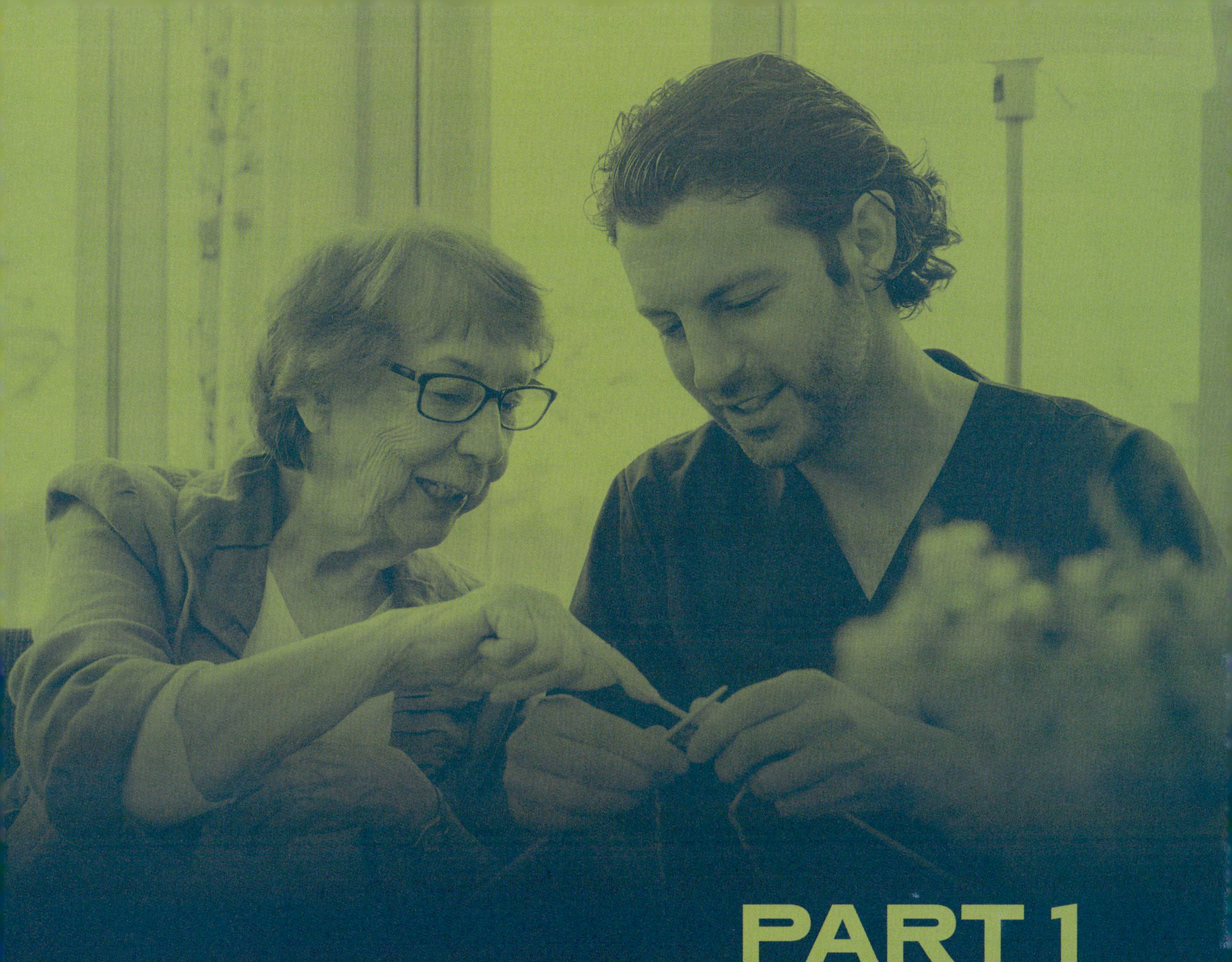

PART 1
Working in aged care

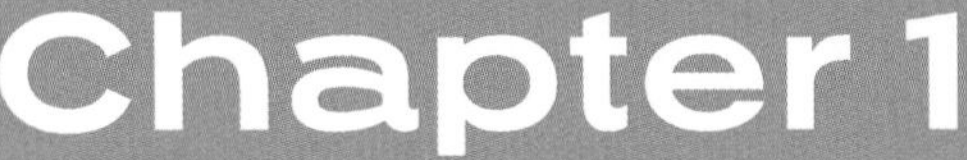

Chapter 1

Working in aged care

LEARNING OBJECTIVES

1.1 Understand aged care in Australia

1.2 Interpret the care worker role

1.3 Understand organisational requirements

1.4 Work in an aged care context

INTRODUCTION

WELCOME TO WORKING IN AGED CARE! Working with older people is a rewarding job that enables a deeper understanding of the older population on both a generational and an individual level. The aged care industry is diverse and offers many types of service delivery to older people, including residential, transitional and home care.

Older people have unique and sometimes complex issues that come with ageing, and the ability to provide support for them requires specific skills and knowledge. As you navigate the industry as an aged care worker (**care worker**), you will build your own skills and knowledge base over time. This chapter provides an overview of some of the key information that you need to know to work in aged care, including how aged care is structured in Australia and the requirements of the care worker role. Important concepts such as duty of care, compliance, and working legally and ethically are also discussed in this chapter. It is important to remember that care workers are an important and valued part of a multidisciplinary team within the aged care service, and while it may be daunting to be starting work in aged care for the first time, information is always available for you to access to support you in your new role.

INDUSTRY IN FOCUS

A contemporary view of aged care

Aged care services in Australia are continually changing to meet the needs of the aged and ageing population over time. The demand for quality aged care services is projected to increase as Australians live longer and reproduce less. Advances in medical technology and processes have seen older Australians remain living at home independently for longer periods of time, and the demand for in-home aged care services is expected to increase over the next three decades.

Historically, aged care services in Australia were provided in nursing homes or hostels that were owned by the Commonwealth government. These homes were staffed by nurses, doctors and other health professionals, and the medical model of care was practised. Much like in a hospital, people living in the facilities were called patients and were treated according to their medical diagnosis. While the care was delivered in an empathetic way, it was also institutionalised in its task-based practice.

Today, aged care services in Australia focus on models of care that are fundamentally person focused. Service delivery revolves around the concepts of autonomy and self-determination, and the legislation relating to aged care services endorses this approach to care.

The rights-based approach to care promotes the rights of the people receiving aged care services and is legally represented by the *Aged Care Act 1997,* the Australian Consumer Law, the National Aged Care Advocacy Program (NACAP), the Charter of Aged Care Rights, the Aged Care Quality Standards, the United Nations Charter of Human Rights and the United Nations Principles for Older Persons (1991). Rights-based approaches to care facilitate informed decision making for older people receiving services and ensure that advocacy and support is available to them and their carer.

Diversity is recognised within aged care services as a vital component of individuality and wellbeing. Under the Department of Health, the Aged Care Sector Committee created a projected vision for the future of aged care in the short, medium and long term called the Aged Care Roadmap. One of the important outcomes of the roadmap is the Diversity Framework, which developed three separate action plans for the aged care sector to support diversity for the lesbian, gay, bisexual, transgender, questioning, intersex and asexual (LGBTQIA+), culturally and linguistically diverse (CALD) and Aboriginal and Torres Strait Islander communities.

Another example of rights-based aged care services is subsidised community care programs. Older people who are eligible for a government-subsidised program, such as a home care package, have the choice about who will provide the services within their package. This is consumer-directed choice, and while it supports the right of older people to choose an organisation to work for them, it also encourages a transparent and ethical market for home care providers to facilitate service delivery.

Current aged care services are required to demonstrate compliance within the regulatory framework of the industry. Part of working in a compliant manner includes the implementation of evidence-based practice, or best practice. This means that the services provided by an aged care service organisation must be based on information that is factual and deemed correct within the industry. Evidence-based practice is validated by research and is supported by scientific data and practice.

The Royal Commission into Aged Care Quality and Safety was established on 8 October 2018 to determine if the quality of care of aged care services was meeting the requirements of those receiving the services. The outcomes of the Royal Commission highlighted glaringly distressing problems with Australia's current aged care system, and 148 recommendations were made for its reform. These recommendations will take time to be addressed and endorsed; however, aged care in Australia is certainly undergoing changes yet again.

Person-centred care and rights-based approaches to service delivery are here to stay. The focus of service delivery is one that facilitates choice, goal setting and achievement, and the wellbeing of all people receiving aged care services.

Getty Images/E+/xavierarnau

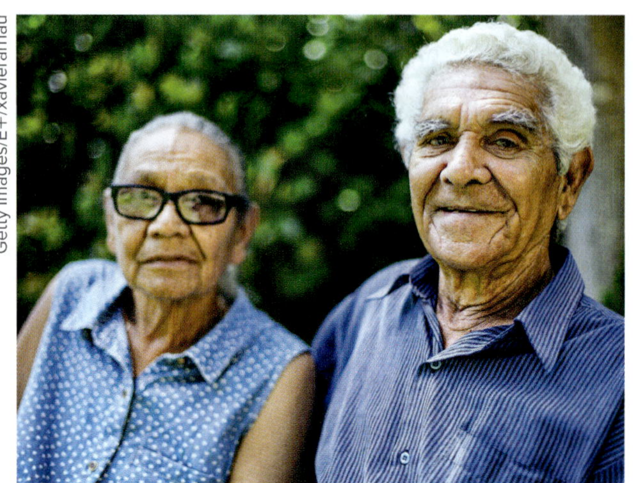

Australia's population is ageing and the challenge is to ensure that the country's aged care system can cope with the increased demand for services

1.1 UNDERSTANDING AGED CARE IN AUSTRALIA

Australia's population is ageing due to lower birth rates and an increased life expectancy. By 2061, the aged population is expected to account for around 23 per cent of the population (Liotta 2021). That might seem a long time away; however, the challenge is to ensure that Australia's aged care system can cope with the demand for aged care services from such a large cohort of people. The structure of aged care has shifted to include an emphasis on in-home support to prevent premature admission into residential aged care facilities and to promote autonomy and independence. The aged care system in Australia will undergo many transitions over the next three or four decades to ensure our ageing population can be supported effectively.

1.1.1 The structure of aged care services in Australia

MY AGED CARE

The Commonwealth government has developed a portal of information about aged care in Australia. The My Aged Care website is a digital platform that provides easy-to-understand and accessible information about aged care services. The platform details the types of services available for older Australians, the eligibility processes for accessing them, assistance with identifying an organisation (provider) to provide the services, and the associated fees and costs.

In Australia, the Commonwealth government is primarily responsible for aged care services. Under the Department of Health and Aged Care, the government provides a majority of the funding for aged care and oversees the compliance framework that regulates the different service types within the aged care system.

Government-subsidised aged care services include:

- residential aged care facilities
- home care
- respite care
- flexible care.

RESIDENTIAL AGED CARE FACILITIES

Residential aged care facilities (RACFs) (also known as nursing homes) provide support for people who can no longer live independently in their own home. RACFs provide permanent residential accommodation, care, and respite (or short-term) accommodation and care. The types of services that are offered in an RACF include:

- personal care, such as showering, continence care and skin care
- meals and nutritional support
- nursing and clinical care
- allied health support, such as physiotherapy and speech therapy
- laundry, cleaning and maintenance services
- other services, such as hairdressing and entertainment.

Staff who are employed at RACFs include registered nurses, enrolled nurses, team leaders, care workers, managers, administration staff, cleaners, kitchen workers, activities officers and maintenance workers. Other workers, such as physiotherapists and dietitians, may be contracted to work at the organisation on certain days of the week.

ACUTE CARE IN RESIDENTIAL AGED CARE FACILITIES

Unfortunately, there are times when the person residing in an RACF will require acute care. Acute care is care that supports an emergency or a potentially life-threatening event, such as a stroke or a diabetic emergency. RACFs provide clinical and nursing care; however, they don't provide emergency and acute care. The Aged Care Emergency (ACE) service provides information to RACFs to ensure that optimal acute care interventions are implemented, and to prevent older people being sent to hospital via ambulance unnecessarily. In the event a resident becomes very unwell, the registered nurse (RN) from the facility can contact an RN from the ACE service to determine the appropriate course of action for the resident.

PRACTICE POINT

Care workers spend the most time with people who live in residential aged care facilities and therefore they will often be the first to notice when someone is very unwell. Always trust your observations and concerns about a person and report them to the RN or the supervisor immediately. Your ability to recognise when something isn't right about someone is invaluable to their wellbeing.

HOME CARE

As a result of Australia's projected ageing population, the availability of services for older people has broadened. They now have access to more service types under government-funded programs. Providing support to an older person at home promotes the longevity of their abilities and independence and prevents premature admission to an RACF.

The **Commonwealth Home Support Programme (CHSP)** provides support to people at home with activities of daily living (ADLs) that include meal provision, domestic activities (such as cleaning), general home maintenance, home modification, transport, and some nursing and allied health services. In-home respite can also be accessed through the CHSP. A home assessment is required to determine the suitability of a person to access services under the CHSP and this assessment will be conducted by a Regional Assessment Service (RAS).

The CHSP is not appropriate for many older people who have higher care needs. This type of high-care support is available through the government-subsidised **Home Care Packages (HCP) Program**, which offers four levels of home care packages, based on level of need for support. Assessment for eligibility for a package is necessary. Once approved, the person selects an organisation to provide their care.

Services offered under a care package depend on the level of package the person has been approved for and include personal care, home and yard maintenance, clinical and nursing care, domestic support, allied health support, social support, and support with conditions such as incontinence.

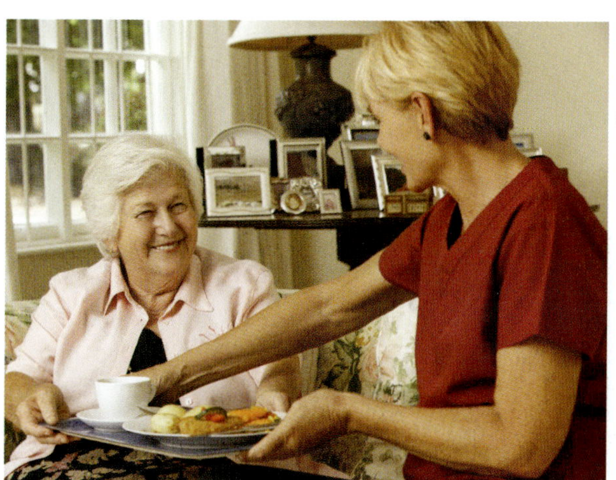

Shutterstock

Providing at-home support promotes independence

RESPITE CARE

The word "respite" means to take a break. Respite care is designed to provide support for a brief time so that the person and their **carer** can do things independently. Respite can be provided for hours, days or weeks, depending on the person's needs and their eligibility for some types of respite. Respite can be planned, or it can be organised in an emergency situation.

People who have been deemed eligible for respite by the **Aged Care Assessment Team (ACAT)**, a government-funded assessment service, can access respite services at Commonwealth-funded RACFs for up to 63 days in each financial year, and for an additional 21 days in exceptional circumstances. While at the facility, the person will be able to access the same services as the long-term residents.

Respite can occur through the CHSP and HCP programs when a person requires someone to be with them in their home for a short time (such as when the carer has to leave for an appointment). A care worker will visit the person and stay with them until the carer returns. This is known as flexible respite.

Many older people who receive home care packages will attend a day centre, which is a form of respite. The organisation that manages the day centre will collect the person from their home and return them at the end of the day. While at the day centre, the person has an opportunity to mix with other people and to participate in activities, meals and entertainments. This type of respite is referred to as community respite.

Cottage respite is respite that is usually overnight, such as for a weekend, which is taken at a community cottage-style facility or in the home of a host family.

FLEXIBLE CARE

The government also funds other care services for older people who don't meet the criteria for residential care or home care. Flexible care includes the following:

- *Transitional care:* Support, including rehabilitative care, is provided to older people when they leave hospital for a period of up 12 weeks. This care is funded jointly by the Commonwealth and state/territory governments.
- *Short-term restorative care (STRC):* This package of services, which is provided for up to eight weeks, is designed to assist older people who have experienced an event that has reduced their ability to function independently. Services may include allied health services such as occupational therapy, nursing services and personal care. The aim of STRC is to "restore" or "re-able" the person's functional capabilities with their activities of daily living to support them to stay at home independently.
- *Multi-Purpose Services (MPS):* There are countless rural communities, towns and council areas that don't have a hospital, an RACF or other vital services, because of their remoteness. MPS aims to address this void, to enable older people to receive care within their own community. People who receive support from the MPS are required to be assessed by the ACAT to determine their eligibility. The majority of MPS programs are government run.
- *National Aboriginal and Torres Strait Islander Flexible Aged Care (NATSIFAC):* Under this program, government grants are awarded to organisations that can provide culturally appropriate aged care services specifically to Indigenous Australians.

1.1.2 Funding

Aged care services are primarily funded by the Commonwealth government through subsidies and grants. Some aged care programs are funded jointly by the Commonwealth, state and territory governments.

A residential aged care facility (the provider) can apply for government grants of money for use in improving the RACF and care outcomes for service users. Most of the funding for RACFs comes from the older person using the service and from Commonwealth government subsidies. Residents of an RACF pay fees for the services they use, with the amount they pay determined by a government income and assets test prior to admission. People with higher means will pay an accommodation fee as agreed with the facility.

Prior to being admitted as a short-term or long-term resident in an RACF, the individual must be assessed by the ACAT to ensure they are eligible for such a placement, by determining the level of care support they need.

On admission, and annually thereafter, the person will be assessed by the facility to determine the amount of subsidised care they require. The government pays money to the provider to support the provision of care to the person. The more needs the person has, the higher the subsidy. In October 2022, the **Australian National Aged Care Classification (AN-ACC)** replaced the former Aged Care Funding Instrument (ACFI) method of assessing the needs of an older person in the context of the government funding they receive. Assessments under the AN-ACC are conducted by contracted organisations, rather than by staff of aged care service providers.

The CHSP is also funded. Organisations that offer these services receive funding by means of a government grant, and the people who receive the services also pay a small fee that is agreed with the organisation.

The HCP program is subsidised by the government using the **consumer-directed care** model. This means that when a person is assessed by ACAT as being eligible for a home care package, they choose the organisation they want to provide the support within their package. Once selected, the organisation is subsidised by the government. A person who receives an HCP is also required to pay a fee for service. A new Support at Home Program is due to commence in July 2023 and will combine all current home care models into one, integrating a single assessment process. The new program is a major overhaul of current processes and programs.

1.1.3 Support practices

PERSON-CENTRED APPROACHES

Older people are their own experts, and as such they have the right to autonomy within their service delivery. The person-centred approach to providing support to an older person is intended to ensure that the person is at the centre of all decision-making processes about their care. In the instance that an older person receiving services doesn't have capacity to make decisions, their substitute decision maker is consulted. People with impaired capacity are still supported to be autonomous and to exercise choice to the extent they're able.

Every individual has the right to exercise self-determination and to make decisions about their care provision and the way they choose to live their life. The Aged Care Quality Standards fully endorse these concepts, and all providers of government-funded aged care services must be able to demonstrate how they support the autonomy of the people who use their services.

Treating people with dignity and respect is the foundation of excellent service provision and is extended to cultural and diverse populations within the service. Concepts such as ageism, stigma and paternalism are destructive and damaging, and have no place in aged care in Australia.

Ageism is the term used to describe discrimination against a person based on their chronological age. Ageism, like all forms of discrimination, can have a negative impact on a person's wellbeing. It occurs when a person is treated differently because of their age (or perceived age). The discrimination may be obvious, such as someone making statements like "old people shouldn't drive" and "older people don't need intimacy". These stereotypes and attitudes are damaging to the wellbeing of the older person, as they can add to a sense of hopelessness and futility, which can develop into depression.

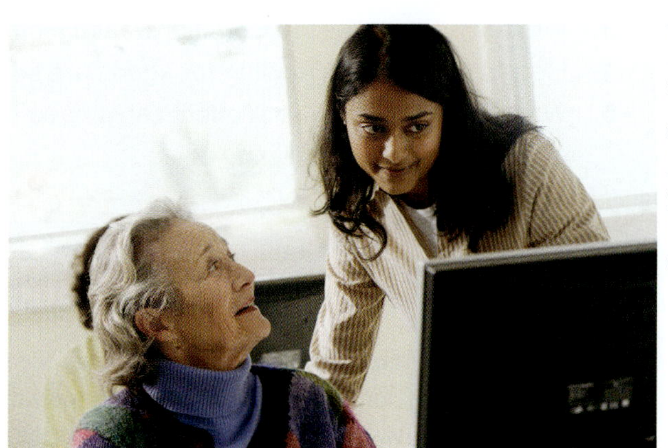

Stewart Cohen/Pam Ostrow/Blend Images/Alamy Stock Photo

Treating people with dignity and respect is the foundation of excellent service provision

Paternalism means that a person uses their position to restrict the needs and wants of another person. This practice may be well intended; however, it is potentially damaging. For example, a care worker might intervene and not allow someone to have an extra serving of dessert, because they feel it could harm the person's health. While the care worker means well, the older person may feel they are being treated condescendingly.

Individuality and all its expressions are essential for a person's wellbeing and self-determination, and the older population are not exempt from this concept. Care workers can apply a person-centred approach to the care and support they provide to older people in every aspect of their job role. Communication that reflects dignity, respect and choice will nurture rapport and trust between the older person receiving services and the care worker. This can only have positive outcomes for the person's wellbeing and sense of self.

WORKPLACE SCENARIO

Accessing aged care services

Rakesh (78) lives with his husband, Phil, in their own home. Rakesh has struggled with his physical health over the past couple of years, as he has emphysema. Phil, also an older man, seemed physically well until he suffered a stroke five months ago that has left him with a cognitive injury. Phil now tends to repeat himself a lot and forgets that he can no longer do things like drive the car. Rakesh loves his husband very much but finds he is exhausted from caring for him and needs a break.

When their niece visits them for dinner one evening, she notices how tired they both look. She mentions the My Aged Care website, which has information about how Phil could be assessed for eligibility for respite services. Rakesh isn't in favour of Phil staying in an aged care facility, even if only for a few weeks; however, he likes the idea of day respite. Rakesh feels that if Phil could access respite at a day centre for one day a week, he would really enjoy the social interaction and Rakesh could take a break. Rakesh and Phil decide they will investigate My Aged Care together.

CHECK YOUR UNDERSTANDING

1. What is the purpose of the My Aged Care portal?
2. List three government-funded aged care service types.
3. What services does the Commonwealth Home Support Programme (CHSP) provide?
4. How is government funding for aged care services sourced?
5. What is ageism, and what effect can it have on an older person?

1.2 INTERPRETING THE CARE WORKER ROLE

The role of an aged care worker can be applied in a diverse context of care delivery for older people, within community and health services. Working with older people requires an understanding of the aged care system in Australia, the models of care that are applied in aged care services, and the legal and ethical requirements of the job role.

Job requirements for care workers include the safe and respectful provision of personal support such as showering, dressing, continence care, grooming, and other supports that help the person with ADLs. Supporting the older person's **psychosocial** needs to meet their goals, and to stay connected with their network of friends and family, is also an important aspect of your role of promoting and maintaining their wellbeing.

To work effectively in aged care, the care worker must be capable of working collaboratively with other members of the care team. Excellent communication skills are important to ensure the continuum of service that ensures older people have all their support needs met. Legislation, industry regulation, and organisational policies and procedures all exist to support the care worker in the role of providing safe care and support services to older people.

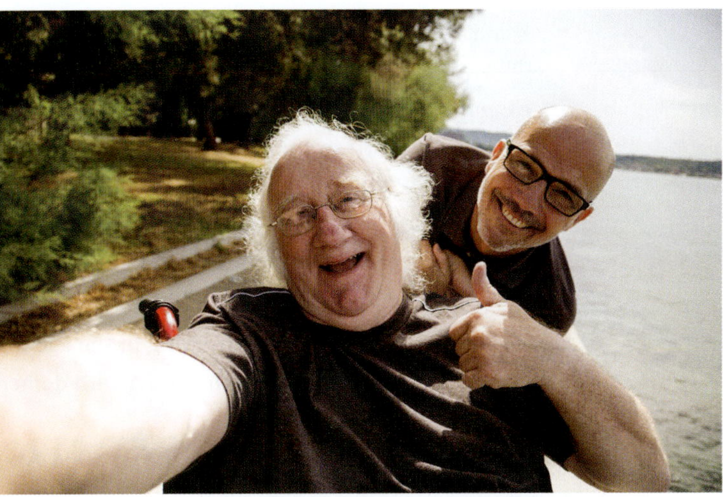

EyeEm/Alamy Stock Photo

Care workers need excellent communication skills to ensure that older people have all their support needs met

1.2.1 The requirements of the job role

JOB DESCRIPTION

A job description, also known as a position description, is a written account of the tasks, responsibilities and organisational expectations of a job role or position. The job description is helpful when a person applies for the role of care worker so that they can determine if they meet the criteria for the role. An individual's suitability for a role as care worker in an aged care context will be determined by how well they can meet the criteria within a job description.

A job description for an aged care worker may include the following sections.

- *Job title:* For example, care worker (also sometimes known as personal support worker, community worker, etc.).
- *Job summary:* This section is a brief summary of the nature of the job. It includes information about the workplace that is often reflective of the organisation's values and mission statement. The summary states the type of person the organisation is looking for by providing succinct information about the role and the employee attributes that it deems necessary for the role.
- *Job responsibilities:* This section usually lists specific tasks and responsibilities of the job role. Responsibilities include:
    - provides support to residents with personal care and activities of daily living according to the care plan
    - works within the compliance framework of the organisation by adhering to all policies and procedures of the organisation
    - communicates respectfully at all times with all residents and staff
    - contributes to workplace safety
    - reports all incidences and hazards immediately
    - seeks clarification from team leader or RN when work instructions are unclear
    - ensures confidentiality of all resident information, records and documentation.

- *Worker qualifications and skills:* This section states the requirements that the organisation expects the care worker to have, and may include the following:

  Essential:
  - Certificate III in Individual Support: Ageing (or working towards)
  - a positive attitude to working with older people
  - ability to work in a culturally and socially diverse environment
  - effective verbal and written communication skills.

  Desirable:
  - two years' experience of working in the aged care sector
  - experience of working with people with dementia
  - current driver's licence
  - competence in qualification HLTHPS006 Assist Client with Medication.

The format of job descriptions varies between organisations, and information about the role may be provided at different opportunities. Some job descriptions are extremely detailed, which enables care workers to understand the scope of practice they will work within; while others are brief and rely on other documents, such as duty or task sheets, to identify the tasks the care worker can and cannot perform.

A professionally written job description also includes information about the physical requirements of the role, such as an estimation of the duration of continuous work within a typical shift, the requirements for musculoskeletal flexibility and dexterity, and the expected level of mobility of a care worker.

PROVIDING INDIVIDUAL SUPPORT

The term "individual support" refers to the identified interventions necessary to support a person with their needs. The person's needs can be identified from a collaborative process of formal and informal assessments that gather information about the person. This information identifies the needs they require support with. The person's needs, and the interventions to support them, are developed into a **care plan** in consultation with the person. The care plan provides care workers and health professionals with the information they need to provide support to the person.

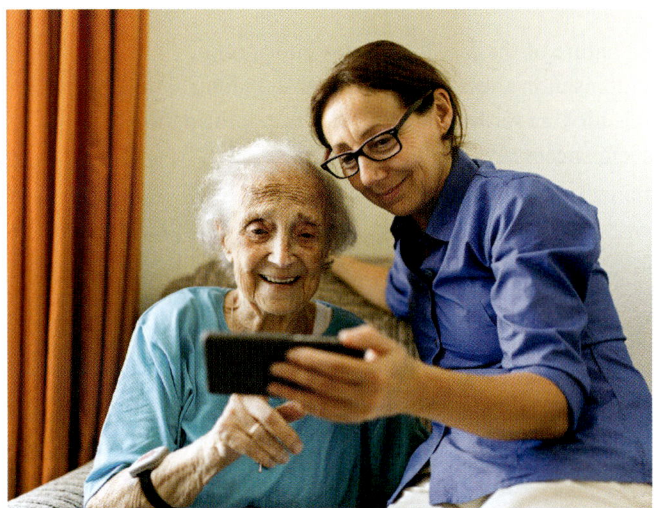

Getty Images/E+/FredFroese

The type of support required will be based on the person's specific individual needs

In the event you are unsure of what you can and cannot do as part of your scope of practice as a care worker, it is your responsibility to ask for clarification from the RN or supervisor.

Individual support is more than assisting an older person with their shower or with mobility. Every individual has needs within specific health areas or domains that include physical, psychological, social, sexual, cultural and spiritual needs. Individuals who have identified needs in one or more of these domains of health and wellbeing may require support from care workers and other health workers. The type of support required will be based on the person's specific individual needs, as reflected in their care plan. Table 1.1 provides examples of support that a care worker may provide to an older person in the context of individualised support. Keep in mind that the support provided can address several needs simultaneously.

TABLE 1.1 Domains of health and wellbeing

Health and wellbeing domain	Type of support
Physical	Providing physical assistance with hygiene and personal care, including: • showering/bathing • toileting and continence • grooming (hair, shaving, makeup, etc.) • skin care • nail care. Providing mobility support, including: • repositioning • assisting with mobility aids such as walkers. Assisting with oral care, such as: • teeth cleaning • denture care.
Psychological	• Showing empathy and understanding to the older person. • Implementing care plan interventions that support hope and recovery around mental health issues such as depression. • Monitoring and documenting behaviour charts. • Promoting principles of self-determination, inclusivity and enablement. • Providing sleep support.
Social	• Organising activities for the person. • Organising outings for the person. • Promoting family and friend connections. • Organising phone or FaceTime conversations for the person and their support network.
Sexual	Supporting the activities that the person identifies with regarding sexuality, such as: • helping to select clothing and accessories • assisting with hairstyles and grooming • advocating for the person's rights to intimacy and sex • providing support and being non-judgemental of individual sexual orientation and preferences.
Cultural	A culture is any group that shares similar values or beliefs. Cultural support may include: • organising travel to places of worship or to cultural events • planning celebration activities for the person or group of people • ensuring that meals are appropriate for religious and ethnic groups • advocating for the human right to belong to a culture or religion.
Spiritual	Spirituality is personal and not always related to religion. Support may include anything that the person requires to meet their spiritual needs, such as prayer time, room décor, clothing, creativity, access to nature.

LEGAL AND ETHICAL RESPONSIBILITIES

To work in the aged care industry, all care workers are required to act in a legal and ethical manner. Legal responsibilities are those that are bound by laws, while ethical responsibilities are those that are bound by the expectations of an industry and of society in general. Responsibilities often have both legal and ethical involvement.

LEGAL RESPONSIBILITIES

As a care worker, you can ensure you meet your legal obligations as determined by your role by following the policies and procedures of the organisation you work for. Your legal responsibilities include, but are not limited to, reporting your concerns of abuse of older people, following duty of care requirements, and ensuring confidentiality and privacy of the older person's information.

Policies and procedures are developed in alignment with legislation and ensure that the law is implemented in all work practices. A **policy** is a document that tells you what is to occur and why, while **procedures** tell you how it will occur. Policies and procedures will exist for all activities and practices that occur in the workplace and cover aspects of the role including safety management, human resource management, privacy and confidentiality, and complaints management. If you are unsure about an aspect of the job role, the policies and procedures of the workplace can provide valuable and accurate information to support you to work legally.

PRACTICE POINT

The workplace will have many policies and procedures in place to support you to work legally and ethically. When you commence a new job with an organisation, it is best practice to locate the policies and procedures so you can access them readily when you need information from them. Over time, it is a good idea to familiarise yourself with the policies and procedures that are often required for the care worker role.

ETHICAL RESPONSIBILITIES

The term "ethical responsibilities" refers to your obligation to work in a reasonable manner, in alignment with the expected behaviours of the organisation. Working ethically means doing the right thing by your colleagues, the older people you support and those people's families. This may have different meanings among the more than 250,000 care workers in Australia and therefore ethical obligations are set out in a document called the code of conduct. The code states in specific detail the behaviours and actions that are expected by an organisation or industry.

Many health professionals, including doctors and nurses, are registered to practise with the Australian Health Practitioner Regulation Agency (AHPRA). Registration ensures individual accountability for practising ethically, in alliance with the health professional's specific code of conduct.

Care workers in Australia are unregistered and unlicensed, making it difficult for individual accountability to be monitored. In 2017, the Commonwealth government launched the National Code of Conduct for Health Care Workers (the National Code). This document provides a minimum set of standards of conduct and practice for care workers and other practitioners who are unlicensed or unregistered. Disciplinary action can be taken in the event a worker is found to put a person at serious risk of harm by not practising the standards within the code, which relates to the overall requirement to work ethically and safely, including working within your scope of practice, obtaining consent and preventing exploitation of clients. (More detailed information about the National Code can be found at www.coaghealthcouncil.gov.au/NationalCodeOfConductForHealthCareWorkers.)

1.2.2 Scope of practice

Scope of practice refers to the tasks and responsibilities of a particular qualification or job role. All health workers have a scope of practice that is defined by the type of work they are qualified to do. A registered nurse and a doctor both have roles that support the health and wellbeing of people; however, they have quite different scopes of practice. As licensed health professionals, the work that nurses and doctors do is regulated by the AHPRA, which stipulates the standards that define the scope of practice for health professionals.

Care workers are not licensed workers in Australia; however, as a care worker you also have a scope of practice that is unique to your role in supporting older people at work. Your scope of practice includes working within the relevant qualification you are working towards or have completed, such as the Certificate III in Individual Support. Other ways you can work within your scope of practice include performing the tasks and expected responsibilities as defined in your job description, following delegation and instructions from the RN and, most importantly, following the policies and procedures of the organisation you work for.

There will be times when you are unsure of the tasks and processes you can implement that are within your scope of practice, and this is the time to seek clarification from the RN or supervisor. To work outside of your scope of practice is a breach of your duty of care and may result in harm to the person you support, yourself and others.

1.2.3 Role boundaries

The role of the aged care worker involves tasks and procedures that may include personal and psychosocial support of older people, assisting people with nutritional needs, documentation and reporting, and some clinical tasks. While the scope of practice of care workers is more diverse than these examples, it is important to realise that several roles may be involved with the one task. As an example, a care worker may be supported to perform basic wound care; however, the RN will perform complex wound care when necessary to the same wound. If the wound becomes infected, it is the doctor's role to examine and order antibiotics, not the role of the RN.

This example illustrates the role boundaries that exist among health workers, each with their own scope of practice. Working within your scope of practice and respecting work role boundaries are important aspects of risk minimisation and ensuring the safety of the older people receiving support.

WORKPLACE SCENARIO

What do you do when you are asked to do something beyond your scope of practice?

Ray is a care worker who works night shift in a residential aged care facility. Tonight, Mrs Baxter is very unwell, and the RN has left a message for the doctor to call him back regarding some medication for her. When the doctor calls back, the RN is on his break and Ray answers the call. The doctor tries to give Ray a phone order for the medication. Ray explains politely to the doctor that it isn't in his scope of practice to accept the phone order for medication. However, he will locate the RN for him, he says.

CHECK YOUR UNDERSTANDING

1. What do you do if you don't understand the information in the care plan?
2. List three examples of assisting a person with their physical support needs.
3. What is meant by the term "ethical responsibilities"?
4. Why are role boundaries important?
5. What are two examples of workplace conditions?

1.3 UNDERSTANDING ORGANISATIONAL REQUIREMENTS

A legal and human rights framework is essential for the quality and safe care of older people and ensures that service delivery is consistent with the ideals of ethical and rights-based support. The role of the care worker in aged care services is to ensure that the rights of older people are upheld and that any breach of their rights is reported to the appropriate person immediately.

The legal framework in aged care exists to protect the rights of older people. Care workers can ensure their accountability with their legal requirements when they work within the boundaries of organisational policies and procedures.

Working in aged care requires workers to understand the policies, procedures and processes that provide them with guidance for safe and supportive practices within the industry, and the significant role that safeguarding the organisation has in the bigger picture of quality and safe service provision of aged care.

1.3.1 Rights and their relevance in aged care

HUMAN RIGHTS

All of us have fundamental human rights that we have come to expect in today's society. The events of World War II left the world reeling at the ability of humans to inflict unspeakable atrocities on other humans. As a result, in December of 1948, the United Nations General Assembly in Paris proclaimed the *Universal Declaration of Human Rights* (see Figure 1.1).

The Declaration sets out the human rights that are universally protected and has set the benchmark for other treaties for rights of particular populations, such as the United Nations Principles for Older Persons and the Principles for the Protection of Persons with Mental Illness and the Improvement of Mental Health Care.

Human rights apply to us all, and this also includes older people who receive aged care services. All aged care workers ensure that they uphold the human rights of older people in all that they do within their role. These rights include the right to:

- choose one's religion, gender and sexual orientation, and to practise one's culture
- make choices and to have equal access and opportunities
- be treated with respect and dignity
- have one's autonomy supported at all times
- be safe and not be exploited or discriminated against.

FIGURE 1.1 Universal Declaration of Human Rights

RIGHTS OF WOMEN
RIGHTS OF OLDER PERSONS
SELF-DETERMINATION
INDIGENOUS PEOPLES AND MINORITIES
RIGHTS OF PERSONS WITH DISABILITIES
RIGHTS TO WORK IN FAIR CONDITIONS
PREVENTION OF DISCRIMINATION
RIGHTS OF THE CHILD
RIGHTS OF JUSTICE

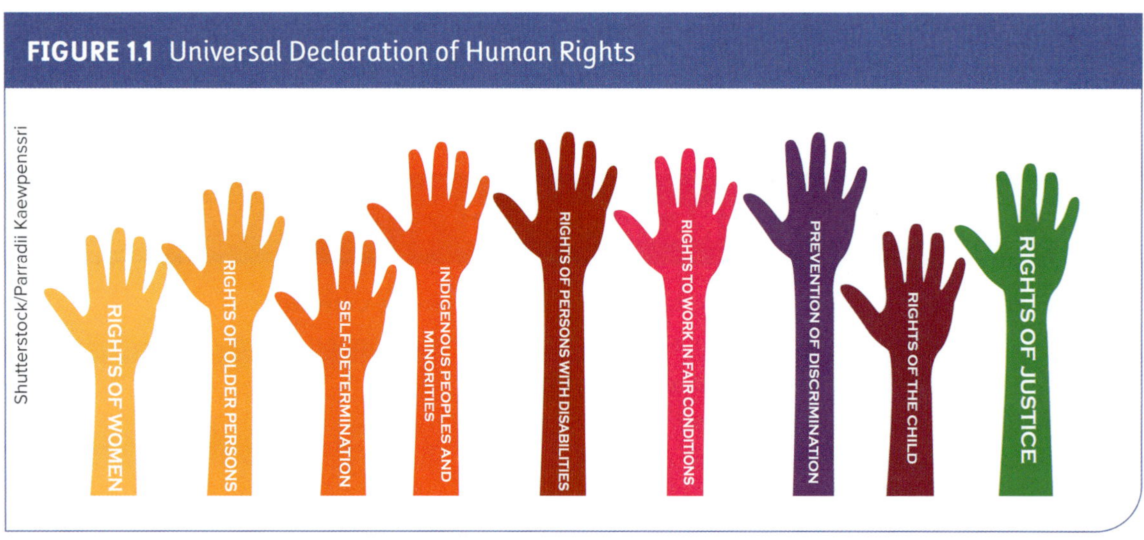

Shutterstock/Parradii Kaewpenssri

We all have our own beliefs and sets of values, and therefore we have our own attitudes and opinions. This is true to the nature of being an individual, as these beliefs and values are unique to us and have developed over time, influenced by our life events, our culture and our society. We can share values and beliefs with others, such as a religious or cultural belief; however, we are all affected differently because we all experience the effects of these values and beliefs differently. It is essential that workers in aged care remain non-judgemental when they are working with older people. Older people are all individuals, too, and each person has their own life story.

As a care worker, your values and beliefs may be vastly different from those of the older people you support, and that is to be expected. It is not acceptable to judge older people based on your own beliefs, and it is certainly not acceptable to impose on older people your opinions on their beliefs. When a care worker judges an older person, they are not only breaching their duty of care as a worker but are also negatively impacting the older person's psychological wellbeing.

It is also unacceptable to attempt to coerce the older person to change the way they think or want things done, simply because you don't agree with them. There may be times when the values and beliefs of a worker and the older person they are supporting are diametrically opposed and, as a result, the worker may feel they cannot provide support to that person. In this circumstance, the worker is obligated to discuss their options with their RN or supervisor to find a solution (e.g. the worker may be allocated to work with a different person).

Challenging the basic human rights of an older person has no place in aged care services. The abuse of the rights of older people was the catalyst for the Royal Commission into Aged Care Quality and Safety, which was established on 8 October 2018. The eight Aged Care Quality Standards that were introduced into aged care in 2019 also place an emphasis of the rights of service users (consumers). The Quality Standards are discussed in detail in Chapter 2.

LEGAL RIGHTS

Older people who receive aged care services have the same civil and legal rights as the rest of the population, and there are several legislative instruments that support these rights.

COMPLAINTS

Care recipients, and their carer or family, can make complaints about the services they are provided. Complaints can be made from within the service provider's policy framework, which aims to ensure open disclosure of incidents where the provider is at fault and facilitates complaint resolution through grievance procedures. In the event the complaint isn't resolved, the older person has the right to advocacy services to support them with a resolution.

Older people who receive government-funded care services can also submit a complaint with the Aged Care Quality and Safety Commission (the Commission) or with state or territory government agencies, such as the Queensland Health Ombudsman and the NSW Ombudsman.

Australia has legislation in place to protect people from different forms of discrimination. While it does not have a human rights Act, other laws prohibit the infringement of rights of older people. They include the *Age Discrimination Act 2004,* the *Disability Discrimination Act 1992,* the *Racial Discrimination Act 1975* and the *Sex Discrimination Act 1984.*

The Commission also extends protection of the rights of older people who receive government-funded aged care services through the auditing and compliance requirements of all aged care service providers. Some examples of the mechanisms that support the rights of older people include the **Serious Incident Response Scheme (SIRS)** (for the mandatory notification of reportable incidents of abuse), the National Quality Indicator Program (which requires all providers of care services to report three times a year on incidents such as pressure injuries, falls and the use of **restrictive practices**) and the Charter of Aged Care Rights.

The Aged Care Quality Standards also support older people who are receiving care from a government-funded service to make a complaint. Standard 6, "Feedback and Complaints", supports the individual, their family, friends, carers and others to make a complaint in a safe and respected environment. All providers of services must demonstrate that they are compliant with this standard in order to pass an audit by the Commission or to gain accreditation or re-accreditation.

CHARTER OF AGED CARE RIGHTS

The Charter of Aged Care Rights (the Charter) is a document that states the rights of all people receiving government-funded aged care services. All providers of such services are required to provide a signed copy of the Charter to all service users. The rights apply to all government-funded care recipients regardless of the type of service they receive. The Charter of Aged Care Rights is available for download from the Aged Care Quality and Safety Commission website (www.agedcarequality.gov.au/consumers/consumer-rights) and is illustrated in Figure 1.2.

Another safeguarding body in the aged care industry is the Older Persons Advocacy Network (OPAN), which is an organisation that upholds the rights of older people with advocacy and other programs that determine how best to address the evolving issues in aged care. OPAN is funded by the Commonwealth government to deliver the National Aged Care Advocacy Program, which offers confidential advocacy support at no cost to older people and their carers. Approved aged care providers can also access NACAP for information on their obligations around the rights of people who use their service.

OPAN delivers NACAP through nine state and territory organisations. These organisations are all members of OPAN and ensure that advocacy services are available for older people throughout Australia.

PROFESSIONAL CONDUCT

As an employee, you are a representative of the organisation you work for and so the manner in which you conduct yourself at work is expected to be professional at all times. The values of an organisation are those that contribute to its achieving its overall goals. These values reflect the expected conduct of employees, such as respect, compassion, integrity and fairness. They are reminders to employees of how to conduct themselves at work.

FIGURE 1.2 Charter of Aged Care Rights

I have the right to:

1. safe and high quality care and services
2. be treated with dignity and respect
3. have my identity, culture and diversity valued and supported
4. live without abuse and neglect
5. be informed about my care and services in a way I understand
6. access all information about myself, including information about my rights, care and services
7. have control over and make choices about my care, and personal and social life, including where the choices involve personal risk
8. have control over, and make decisions about, the personal aspects of my daily life, financial affairs and possessions
9. my independence
10. be listened to and understood
11. have a person of my choice, including an aged care advocate, support me or speak on my behalf
12. complain free from reprisal, and to have my complaints dealt with fairly and promptly
13. personal privacy and to have my personal information protected
14. exercise my rights without it adversely affecting the way I am treated.

Source: Aged Care Act 1997, Schedule 1—Charter of Aged Care Rights. CC BY 4.0 https://creativecommons.org/licenses/by/4.0/.

Aged care services may also have their own code of conduct that is aligned with the organisation's values. This code will set out the types of behaviours that the organisation expects you to work within and will include aspects of care service delivery such as treating people with respect and ensuring their autonomy and dignity, reporting concerns related to a person who is receiving support, reporting breaches of care, working in a diverse workplace, and the use of social media relevant to the organisation. The code of conduct is introduced to all new employees, and the organisation will require you to formally acknowledge that you agree to work under the terms in the code, usually via a signed agreement.

While you are bound to work under the code of conduct of your organisation, you are also bound to work under the National Code of Conduct for Health Care Workers.

1.3.2 Working as part of a team

There are several work roles within aged care services, and all work closely together as one interdisciplinary team. An interdisciplinary team is a team of workers and health professionals with different qualifications and expertise. Each team member brings a unique set of skills and knowledge to the provision of care and support to older people who are receiving aged care services.

It is essential that the interdisciplinary team functions as one cohesive support network to ensure a continuum of care for the older person. Effective communication is the essential component of teamwork. Effective communication enables each member of the team, and most importantly the older person and their carer or family, to understand the older person's needs and goals and what interventions are necessary to achieve them. Mutual respect among the team is also paramount in order to achieve optimal wellbeing outcomes for the older person. Table 1.2 sets out specific roles and responsibilities of the interdisciplinary team members for aged care.

The interdisciplinary team fundamentally provides a **holistic** approach to the person-centred care of the older person, encompassing all aspects of care and support for them. Effective communication within the team will ensure the older person has access to the recommendations of health professionals and, therefore, positive outcomes for their wellbeing.

There will be occasions when the care worker will be delegated tasks by the registered nurse, who is able to do so if they are confident that the care worker can perform the task. The RN can delegate tasks according to the delegation rules stated by the Nurses and Midwives Board of Australia. Some of these tasks may involve written instructions from other health professionals that have contributed to the development of the person's care plan, such as limb exercises, basic wound care, or monitoring the effectiveness of recommended equipment as prescribed by the occupational therapist. In the event you don't feel comfortable with a delegation, you have the right to request more information and training before accepting the task.

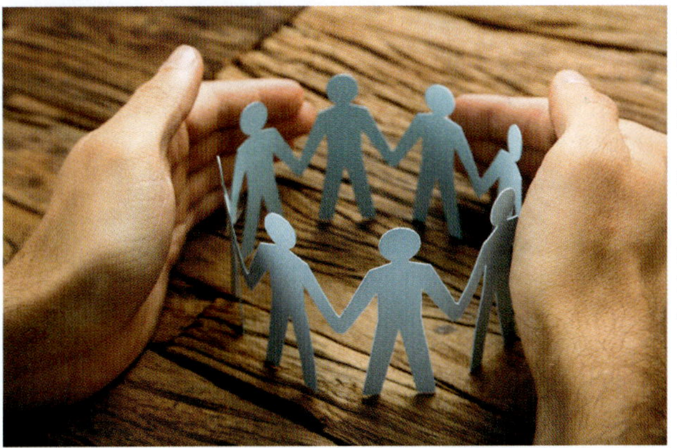

Andriy Popov / Alamy Stock Photo

The interdisciplinary team should function as a cohesive support network to ensure a continuum of care for the older person

1.3.3 Technology in the workplace

Technology in the workplace is an important aspect of the continuum of care for older people who use the aged care service. Technology allows workers and other team members to communicate effectively using digital platforms such as computer software and mobile phones, and to transmit and store infinite amounts of documentation and client-related records. Passcode or login requirements offer another safety mechanism for the protection of personal data about the older person and support the legal obligation of workers to uphold the privacy of the person.

TABLE 1.2 Role of interdisciplinary team members

Roles	Responsibilities (examples)
The older person	Provide information to the team about needs and goals
Care worker	• Provide support according to the person's care plan • Report to the RN or supervisor • Document according to policy
Team leader/ supervisor	• Provide support and instruction to team of care workers • Assist with care work • Participate in team meetings and case conferencing • Assist the RN with formal assessments • Documentation
Enrolled nurse	• Supervise a team of workers • Provide clinical support • Liaise with doctors • Documentation
Registered nurse	• Make clinical judgements about care support • Liaise with doctors and other medical professionals • Complete and interpret assessments • Provide instruction and delegation to other team members • Documentation and reporting • Manage meetings and case conferencing • Medications and clinical management
Doctor	• Attends clinical consultation with the person • Provides instruction to RN • Prescribes medication and treatments for the person • Refers the person to other practitioners
Physiotherapist	• Assesses mobility and movement • Assesses the need for mobility aids and exercises • Documentation • Rehabilitation interventions
Speech pathologist	• Provides assessment, interventions and instructions for swallowing impairment, such as meal and fluid modification • Assesses and provides instruction for speech therapy after medical events such as stroke • Liaises with the person and their family
Dietitian	• Provides assessment and instruction about the nutritional and hydration needs of older people • Provides instruction for feeding regimes for people with feeding tubes • Liaises with the person and their family
Occupational therapist	• Assesses the person's abilities to attend to ADLs and facilitates rehabilitation and restorative therapy with the use of adaptive equipment and processes • Liaises with the person and their family
Medical specialists	• Provide consultation and treatment as per their field of expertise

The workplace also uses technology for other communication purposes, such as email, intranet and staff rostering. Many reports are completed via a computer-based platform that is linked to other industry organisations such as the Aged Care Quality and Safety Commission to ensure that data collection for compliance purposes is provided and that information of concern, such as abuse, is reported immediately.

Technology is used in the workplace to monitor and record clinical observations such as urinalysis and blood pressure. Medication charts are also inclusive of a digital medication chart system.

Organisations are increasingly using digital technology to document and communicate information about the person using the service. Care workers also use the technology employed by their organisation in performing their role.

WORKPLACE SCENARIO

The importance of professional conduct

Mrs Ryan is having coffee at a busy café when she notices two care workers from the organisation that provides in-home care to her father, Tim Clarke, who has dementia. The workers are wearing their work uniforms and are chatting loudly. Mrs Ryan overhears one of the workers say, "I like most of my people, but that Mr Clarke does my head in. He just wants to follow me everywhere when I'm there and he smells like pee all the time!" The other worker laughs loudly and replies: "Yeah, Timmy does stink a bit. And his wife Mavis is a real whinger. She never looks happy." Mrs Ryan approaches the workers and, visibly upset, tells them she is disgusted to hear them talking about her parents in public in this way. She will speak to the manager of their organisation about their behaviour, she says, and intends to lodge a formal complaint with the Aged Care Quality and Safety Commissioner.

CHECK YOUR UNDERSTANDING

1. What is the Charter of Aged Care Rights?
2. What is OPAN, and how does it support older people who receive government-funded aged care services?
3. What is the name of the code that ensures the accountability of care workers?
4. There are several work roles within aged care services and all work closely together as one interdisciplinary team. Name four of these roles.
5. Why is technology important in the workplace?

1.4 WORKING IN AN AGED CARE CONTEXT

The skills and knowledge required to work within an aged care context develop over time, with experience. New concepts become familiar and new care workers become confident in their role. Some aspects of working in the aged care domain are specific to the job and having an awareness of them is important for working safely. This section will look at the principal aspects of working in an aged care context, and at how they apply to the role of a care worker.

1.4.1 Individualised planning

Individualised planning is the process of working collaboratively with the older person and other health professionals to determine the support the person requires to meet their goals. An individualised plan (also known as a service plan or a care plan) is a document that describes how care services and other support can be provided to the person according to their needs and preferences.

A process of information gathering is the first phase of the development of the individualised plan. This information is obtained from both formal and informal assessment processes, and always with prior informed consent from the person. A formal assessment is when a validated assessment tool (such as a falls risk assessment tool) is used and involves asking the person a series of questions. Some formal assessments are based on a score system to assist in determining the severity of signs and symptoms, which can then guide planning. It is the role of the registered nurse to facilitate formal assessments, although enrolled nurses and team leaders may also be delegated by the RN to complete this task.

Informal assessment processes are those that don't use validated tools but are based on observations and information provided by the person, the RN or the care worker. Clinical observations may include noticeable changes in the person's general condition, such as mobility changes, increased incontinence, a persistent cough, behaviour changes, and so on. It is important that as a care worker you report all concerns you have about the person to the RN or supervisor, because this information is valuable in providing timely support for the person. Information that is collected during the planning phase is used to identify the person's specific needs. This is an important and irreplaceable role within the context of the development and monitoring phases of the individualised plan.

The next phase of planning development is to determine strategies and interventions that can provide the necessary support for the person. This may include discussions with them about their preferences and what has or hasn't worked for them previously. Some needs may be newly identified and will require referral to other health professionals. For example, assessment processes and discussion with a person may reveal they are depressed and will require referral to their doctor or a psychologist, in addition to the support within the care plan. Any type of support that is documented in a care plan must be monitored for effectiveness and reviewed on a regular basis.

The purpose of the individualised plan is to provide a go-to document that explains the type and frequency of care support for an individual in a format that all workers understand. This ensures a continuum of care for the person, regardless of the worker who provides it. If, at any point, you are unsure about how to provide support safely and in a way that is preferred by the person, refer to the individualised plan for clarification. The plan should reflect the needs of the person at any given time; hence, it is a fluid document that changes as the person's needs change.

1.4.2 Person-centred communication

Communication is the process of sending and receiving information between people or groups. When providing support to older people, it is essential that you use person-centred communication techniques. Communication needs to be used effectively to ensure positive outcomes for the people you support and the people you work with. Effective communication involves using appropriate verbal and non-verbal methods to exchange information.

VERBAL COMMUNICATION

Effective verbal communication involves:

- using normal volume of voice when speaking
- using normal tone of voice (tones that are stern or melodious can sound patronising)
- speaking clearly and at normal speed
- not using jargon or terms the person doesn't understand.

NON-VERBAL COMMUNICATION

Effective non-verbal communication involves:

- sitting at eye level with the person so they can see your face
- using open body language (don't cross your arms)
- using appropriate facial expressions in the context of the conversation
- ensuring appropriate use of eye contact
- using gestures to demonstrate you are engaged in the conversation (such as nodding your head).

In the context of person-centred communication with older people, the care worker needs to consider the person's communication needs. One way to do this is to read the person's care plan to determine if they have specific communication requirements. Table 1.3 illustrates specific communication techniques for person-centred communication where a barrier to communication exists.

TABLE 1.3 Addressing communication barriers

Communication barrier	Do	Don't
The person is hearing impaired	• Ensure you check the care plan • Introduce yourself and show the person your identification badge if you have one • Face the person; they may lip-read • Ensure the environment isn't noisy • Ensure hearing aids are in place and working • Say the person's name • Speak clearly and slowly • Expect to repeat what you say • Always use communication devices if the person has one • Keep your hands away from your face when talking	• Speak to the person as you approach them • Yell or speak excessively loudly • Attempt to have a conversation in a noisy room • Exaggerate words or sounds • Use complex and long sentences • Rush communication
The person is visually impaired	• Ensure you check the care plan • Gently touch the person to gain their attention • Introduce yourself by name and position • Introduce others by name and position if present • Ensure the environment has sufficient lighting • Check the person is wearing prescription glasses and they are clean • Speak clearly and at normal volume and speed • Be as descriptive as possible in conversation content	• Yell or speak excessively loudly • Attempt to speak to the person from behind • Leave the room without ending the conversation and telling the person you are leaving • Use visually descriptive words such as "look" and "seeing"
The person has a cognitive impairment such as dementia	• Ensure you check the care plan • Understand any triggers the person may experience that cause them distress • Avoid sensory overwhelm of the person; ensure the environment isn't too bright or noisy • Sit at eye level with the person • Engage in eye contact if possible • Speak at normal tone and volume • Speak clearly and slowly • Repeat if necessary • Use open body language and positive facial expressions • Use gestures to assist the person to interpret the message • Follow the person's cues, such as head nodding and facial expression • Make more than one attempt to communicate; come back to the person a few minutes later	• Use long and complex sentences • Include more than one instruction in a sentence (e.g. "Please stand up and take off your cardigan") • Raise your voice or talk loudly • Talk rapidly • Talk to the person from another room or in the doorway • Rush the person • Argue with the person • Get frustrated with the person and walk away • Use a tone that is condescending or patronising

(Continues)

TABLE 1.3 Addressing communication barriers (continued)

Communication barrier	Do	Don't
The person speaks a different language	• Ensure you check the care plan • Build trust through compassion • Use picture and word boards if appropriate • Use translation apps such as Google Translate if policy allows • Learn and use key words and phrases, supported with gestures • Ensure body language is respectful and relevant • Determine if there is a staff member on shift who can interpret • Use a registered translator/ interpreter for all communications relevant to sensitive information	• Yell at the person or speak excessively loudly • Overemphasise gestures • Use a tone that is condescending or patronising • Display frustration

Communication barriers reflect the need to ensure that person-centred communication skills are implemented when interacting with older people. However, the values of respect, autonomy and dignity must be the fabric of all communications with all people you support.

1.4.3 Recording and maintaining information

An important part of your role as a care worker in aged care is information management. Documentation is essential for maintaining a continuum of care and support services for the person using the service. It occurs both in RACFs and within in-home care services. The following are examples of documentation.

- The person's *care plan* (individualised plan).
- ***Progress notes*** *or case notes:* a record of daily or incidental occurrences.
- *Handover reports:* a shift-to-shift update of specific information about the person.
- *Incident reports:* a record of an incident that caused, or almost caused, harm to a person(s).
- *Checklists:* a list of specific tasks such as validated assessments.
- *Referral forms:* a summary of relevant information about a person when they are referred to an agency or health professional.
- *Hospital transfer form:* a summary of relevant information about a person when they are transferred from the RACF to hospital.

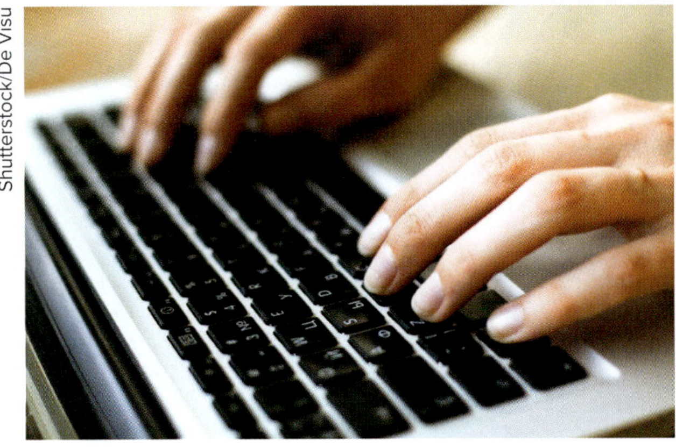

Shutterstock/De Visu

Documentation is essential for maintaining a continuum of care

RECORDING INFORMATION

Information can be recorded in written format or electronically. Any information you document about a person must be factual and concise. All documentation can be used in a court of law; therefore, it should be recorded in a way that states the facts, is clear and legible, and is current and correct. Although important, you are not required to document your opinion.

Any written documentation must be recorded in pen, not pencil, and be dated and timed. After completing documentation, you must sign your name. When you place your signature against documentation, you are taking accountability for what you have written.

Electronic documentation will require a passcode or other unique identification method to document in a person's file. The code may substitute your signature in some instances; therefore, it is best practice to keep it private and not to share it with another staff member.

Some organisations will implement software that is specifically designed for aged care record requirements, and you will be educated in the workplace on how these programs work.

All staff who work in aged care are bound by privacy and confidentiality laws. Personal and sensitive information is protected by the *Privacy Act 1988* and the Australian Privacy Principles. Each state and territory also has its own laws about privacy. The legal obligation of care workers surrounding the privacy and confidentiality of older people's information in the workplace extends to the safe storage of records and other documentation types.

The storage of records in any aged care service must ensure that the person's information is kept secure. Paper-based records and documents should be kept in a locked cabinet or dedicated records room, and electronic records and forms of documentation must be passcode protected. As a care worker, you can ensure the privacy of the people you support by always logging out of the electronic file before walking away and by not sharing your passcode. When using paper-based documentation, always date and sign what you have written and store the file securely. Don't leave folders or files open for others to read. The workplace will have policies and procedures to guide you on correct documentation procedures and the privacy and storage of records.

WORKPLACE SCENARIO

The role of the care worker in individualised planning

Yolanda is an experienced home care worker who has been providing personal support to Mr Walker in his home for the past few weeks. Today is a hot day, and when Mr Walker asks for some ice to put in his drink, Yolanda notices that the freezer is full of unhealthy frozen food. Mr Walker tells Yolanda that he really enjoys salads and fresh food; however, the pain in his wrists from arthritis makes it difficult for him to prepare meals that involve cutting, peeling and dicing. Yolanda reads his care plan and sees that it indicates Mr Walker is independent with meal preparation. She informs her supervisor that Mr Walker's situation has changed and that the care plan requires updating. Yolanda organises a time for the supervisor to visit Mr Walker to reassess his nutritional needs.

CHECK YOUR UNDERSTANDING

1. What is an individualised plan?
2. What are two factors to consider when using verbal communication?
3. List three ways to use effective non-verbal communication.
4. Why is documentation important in aged care services?
5. How can a care worker maintain the privacy and confidentiality of the person's records and documentation?

SUMMARY

- Aged care services in Australia are primarily funded by the Commonwealth government.
- The core focus of care service delivery is a person-centred and rights-based philosophy.
- Legislation and regulation of aged care providers aims to ensure quality service delivery.
- Care workers have legal and ethical responsibilities when working with older people in aged care services.
- Working within scope of practice is an important requirement for the care worker role.
- The key to working legally and ethically is to follow policies and procedures and always to ask for clarification if in doubt about work practices and processes.

REVIEW QUESTIONS

1.1 What is a job description?

1.2 Outline the difference between a policy manual and a procedure manual.

1.3 List four attributes of effective teams.

1.4 **(a)** Outline the steps in the development of an individualised plan.

(b) What is the role of the care worker in the development of the individualised plan?

BIBLIOGRAPHY

Australian Government, Department of Health, *About the Multi-Purpose Services (MPS) Program*, https://www.health.gov.au/initiatives-and-programs/multi-purpose-services-mps-program/about-the-multi-purpose-services-mps-program, accessed 29 November 2021.

Australian Government, Department of Health, *Minimising the Use of Restrictive Practices*, https://www.agedcarequality.gov.au/minimising-restrictive-practices, accessed 29 November 2021.

Australian Government, Department of Health, *Quality Standards*, https://www.agedcarequality.gov.au/providers/standards, accessed 29 November 2021.

Australian Government, Department of Health, *Serious Incident Response Scheme*, https://www.agedcarequality.gov.au/sirs, accessed 27 November 2021.

Liotta, M., "Ageing population and per-person health costs to rise", *News GP*, June 2021, https://www1.ra,cgp.org.au/newsgp/professional/ageing-population-and-per-person-health-costs-to-r, accessed 18 November 2021.

United Nations, *Universal Declaration of Human Rights*, https://www.un.org/en/about-us/universal-declaration-of-human-rights, accessed 12 November 2021.

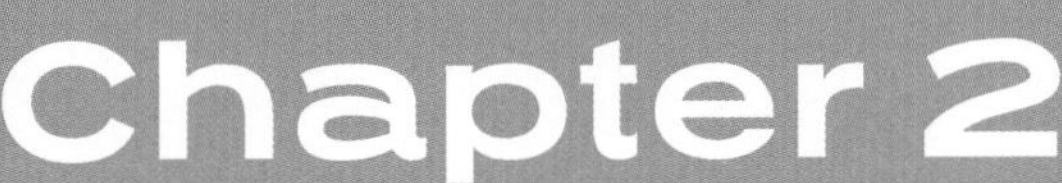

Chapter 2

Working legally and ethically

LEARNING OBJECTIVES

2.1 Identify and respond to legal requirements

2.2 Identify and meet ethical responsibilities

2.3 Contribute to workplace improvements

INTRODUCTION

WORKING LEGALLY AND ETHICALLY is essential for maintaining a safe and fair work environment that promotes and facilitates empowered and autonomous support for older people who require aged care services. The aged care services industry is bound by legislation, regulations and ethical guidance with regard to how aged care services are provided. As a care worker, it is not possible to know all the laws that apply to aged care services, as many of them differ between Australia's states and territories. However, it is important that you understand the basic legislation and ethics that underpin the role of a care worker.

INDUSTRY IN FOCUS

The Royal Commission into Aged Care Quality and Safety

Australia's aged care system has been struggling under a fabric of confusing legislation, regulation, funding issues and outdated models of care. In October 2018, the Royal Commission into Aged Care Quality and Safety (the Royal Commission) was established. Leading up to this date, incidences of the abuse and neglect of older people receiving aged care services in Australia made headlines in the news, exposing the conditions that some older people were experiencing within their aged care service. The aim of the Royal Commission was to review the current status of the aged care system in Australia and to deliver a report to the Commonwealth government stating its findings and recommendations.

The Royal Commission consulted with the public, aged care services users and their carers and families, aged care organisations, allied health professionals, aged care industry experts and peak bodies, and government departments. In October 2019, an interim report was delivered to the government, followed in 2020 by a special COVID-19 report. In February 2021, the Royal Commission delivered its final report to the Commonwealth. This report detailed 148 recommendations for the reform of aged care in Australia.

Some of the key recommendations referred to a rights-based system, financial sustainability and funding, a new Aged Care Act, and the implementation of governmental and independent advisory bodies. The Royal Commission also recommended an overhaul of the Aged Care Quality Standards and of the Aged Care Quality and Safety Commission. The recommendations may not all be actioned by the Commonwealth; however, many of them are fundamental catalysts for the Five Pillars of Aged Care Reform that the government is rolling out over the next several years. Australia's aged care system has commenced a transition into a system that will be worthy of providing aged care services to our most vulnerable members of society.

2.1 IDENTIFYING AND RESPONDING TO LEGAL REQUIREMENTS

2.1.1 The Australian legal system

A country's legal system is essential for maintaining a safe society. Australia's legal system is based on the English Westminster system, whereby a parliament of elected members debates and decides on legislation that applies to all states and territories. In this democratic system the head of state (the Monarch) is different from the head of government (the Prime Minister). Each state and territory also has its own parliament that enacts legislation based on Commonwealth laws. Table 2.1 describes some of the types of law within the Australian legal system.

2.1.2 The legal requirements of the work role

LEGISLATION THAT APPLIES TO THE AGED CARE SECTOR

THE AGED CARE ACT

The aged care system in Australia is governed by several laws, including the *Aged Care Act 1997* (the Act), which oversees government-funded aged care services. The Act covers the **compliance** of aged care services and regulates the industry's fees, subsidies and funding. It also regulates the quality of care that recipients of aged care services will receive, along with how their rights will be protected.

TABLE 2.1 Types of law within the Australian legal system

Type of law	Description
Common law	Common law in Australia is a legal framework that is born of decision making that is determined by judges. Common law applies to everyone and does not exempt some people, such as may occur in other types of law. The outcomes of judicial cases and decisions by judges are used as precedents for ongoing common law requirements. An example of common law is the law relating to theft.
Parliamentary law	Laws are made in parliament when a majority vote by politicians of the Senate and the House of Representatives enables a bill to be passed. A bill is a request to change or create a law that has been presented by a government minister or other members of parliament. The governor general makes the final determination on whether a bill can become law. An example of parliamentary law is the *Aged Care Act 1997* (Cth).
Criminal law	Criminal law in Australia relates to laws that are intended to regulate the behaviour or conduct of people and organisations to ensure the safety and wellbeing of society. Examples of breaching criminal law include the manufacture and sale of illicit drugs.
Customary law	Customary law is the set of rules and expectations that exist within an Indigenous community. Customary law includes practices and beliefs that are intended to maintain a cohesiveness of expected behaviour and conduct within a community. An example of customary law is Indigenous law.
The law of torts	Torts are part of civil law whereby one person or organisation causes a wrongdoing to another. Torts include negligence, false imprisonment and defamation. A person or organisation can sue for damages when they are a claimant in a tort.

The Aged Care Act is endorsed within a quality framework that involves other legislation and Commonwealth regulatory bodies. The framework ensures that specific principles are implemented in a compliant manner by approved providers of aged care services. An approved provider is an organisation that receives government funding, such as residential aged care facilities and community care services. These principles include the Accountability Principles 2014, the Quality of Care Principles 2014 and the User Rights Principles 2014. Another important piece of legislation relevant to aged care is the *Aged Care Quality and Safety Commission Act 2018*. This Act is essential for ensuring that all providers of aged care services are compliant with the Aged Care Quality Standards and other regulatory requirements.

As an outcome of the Royal Commission into Aged Care Quality and Safety, the *Aged Care Act 1997* is expected to be replaced on 1 July 2023. The new Act will complement the reform of aged care services in Australia.

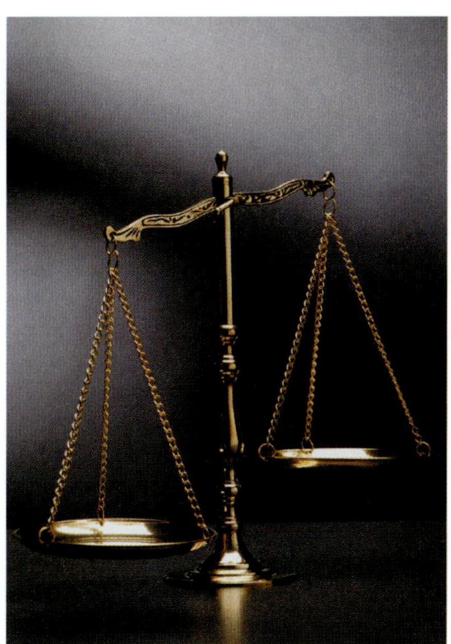

Design Pics/Kelly Redinger

The aged care system in Australia is governed by several laws

THE AGED CARE QUALITY AND SAFETY COMMISSION

The role of the Aged Care Quality and Safety Commission (the Commission) is to regulate government-funded aged care services in Australia, thereby protecting the safety and wellbeing of service users. The Commission's responsibilities and powers include:

- ensuring service providers are compliant with the Aged Care Quality Standards through a process of **auditing**
- receiving and investigating, where appropriate, all notifiable incidents as they relate to the Serious Incident Response Scheme

- receiving complaints from consumers and providers
- imposing **sanctions** on the business undertakings of approved providers
- assessing, accrediting and monitoring services
- conducting home care investigations.

AGED CARE QUALITY STANDARDS

Another regulatory function of the Commission is to enforce the Aged Care Quality Standards (the Quality Standards) within residential aged care and home care services. The eight standards were implemented in July 2019 and are designed to ensure that organisations meet compliance with quality and safe care for people who receive support from them (see Figure 2.1). The eight standards are:

1. consumer dignity and choice
2. ongoing assessment and planning with consumers
3. personal care and clinical care
4. services and supports for daily living
5. organisation's service environment
6. feedback and complaints
7. human resources
8. organisational governance.

Each standard is represented in three ways:

- a statement of outcome for the consumer (resident)
- a statement of expectation for the organisation
- organisational requirements to demonstrate that the standard has been met.

PRACTICE POINT

During an audit, a representative from the Aged Care Quality and Safety Commission may ask you about the Quality Standards and how you apply them in your job role. It is best practice to understand the Quality Standards and how they apply in your work practices, to ensure both excellent service delivery and a confident response to the accreditor's question!

ACCREDITATION AND AUDITING

As part of compliance processes, the Aged Care Quality and Safety Commission periodically audits aged care facilities to ensure the Quality Standards are met. Each organisation must provide evidence that these standards are implemented within their governance processes.

The Quality Standards are the foundation on which government-funded organisations are assessed for accreditation. All residential aged care facilities must be accredited by the Commission under the Aged Care Quality and Safety Commission Rules 2018 (the Rules) every three years or if an issue of concern is raised. Accreditation with the Commission ensures that the facility is providing the level of safe and quality care that the community expects.

Failure to meet this mandatory compliance may result in remedial processes or the revocation of government funding until the failure-to-comply issues have been remedied. Compliance with the Quality Standards can be demonstrated in the practices and procedures that an organisation undertakes.

The Commission also provides quality reviews of home care services to determine if the Quality Standards are being implemented. Not all of the Standards apply to home care services, and the Commission has a

FIGURE 2.1 The eight Aged Care Quality Standards

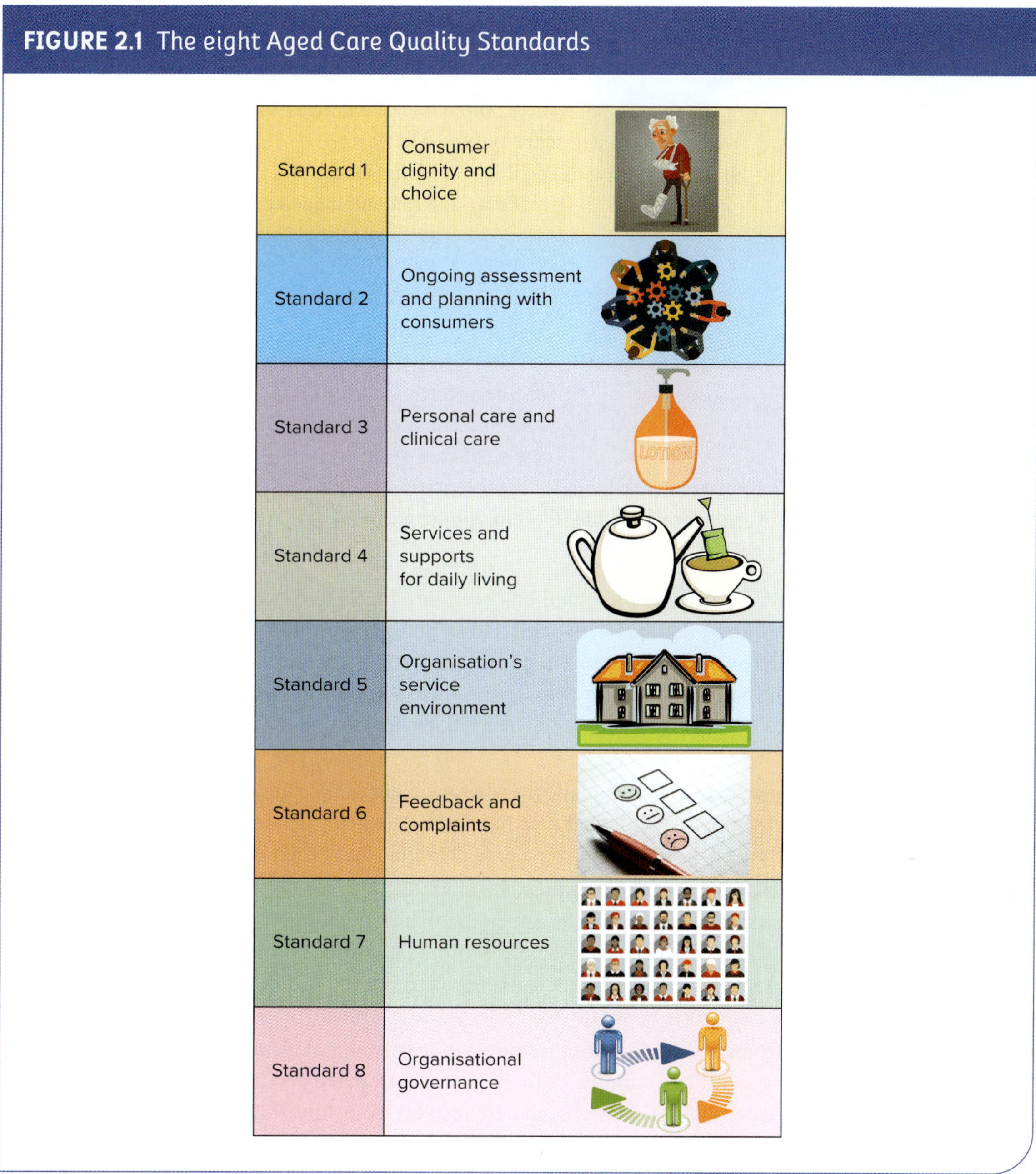

Source: Adapted from Australian Government, MyAgedCare, Aged Care Quality Standards, https://www.myagedcare.gov.au/aged-care-quality-standards. Images from top to bottom: Shutterstock/Pretty Vectors, Oxy_gen, © McGraw-Hill Education, Shutterstock/vectorisland, Vector, Tero Vesalainen, Aelitta, danleap/iStock/Getty Images.

guide for services to assist them with the quality review, taking into consideration the Standards that do and don't apply across the diversity of service types.

AGED CARE LEGISLATIVE REFORM

The aged care system in Australia is changing, due largely to the findings and recommendations of the Royal Commission into Aged Care Quality and Safety and to the fact that Australia's ageing population is increasing, placing a greater demand on the supply of aged care services.

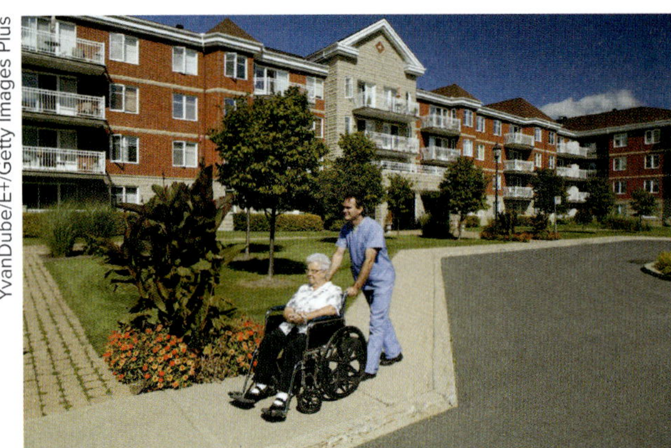
YvanDube/E+/Getty Images Plus

Aged care facilities are audited periodically to ensure the Quality Standards are met

As a result of the Royal Commission, the Australian government has developed five pillars of reform that will be delivered across a five-year period. These five pillars incorporate major changes and transitions of the aged care system. They are:

Pillar 1: Home care
Pillar 2: Residential aged care services and sustainability
Pillar 3: Residential aged care quality and safety
Pillar 4: Workforce
Pillar 5: Governance.

The Royal Commission made 148 recommendations for the reform of aged care in Australia, based on its findings. These recommendations focus heavily on how a new aged care system is governed, including a new Aged Care Act, an Aged Care Commission that includes representation over many facets of aged care systems including an Aboriginal and Torres Strait Islander Commissioner and other legislative reforms. The proposed aged care legislative reforms are as follows:

- The National Aged Care Advisory Council has been developed to represent the diverse needs of older Australians and their families with regard to the implementation of aged care reforms. The council is required to provide advice to the government about the expectations that older people and their families have about aged care services in Australia under the new reforms. It reports to the Minister for Health and Aged Care and the Minister for Senior Australians and Aged Care Services.
- The Aged Care Engagement Hub is a platform whereby older people and their families can become involved in the processes of aged care reform in Australia. Others who can utilise the hub to participate include aged care workers, aged care providers and other aged care organisations.
- The Home Care Packages Program was introduced in 2021 to ensure that home care providers are reviewed to minimise fraud, to monitor the allocation of subsidies and to remove unfair costs that may be incurred in a home care package service delivery. This process is transparent and guided by the Home Care Packages Assurance Framework, legislated by the *Aged Care and Other Legislation Amendment (Royal Commission Response No. 1) Act 2021.*
- The Independent Health and Aged Care Pricing Authority is an independent body that provides costing studies that assist the Commonwealth government to make decisions about annual funding for residential aged care (and residential aged care respite) from July 2023. Costing information can help to regulate funding in aged care and enable a transparent approach to funding sustainability in the aged care sector.
- In October 2022, the Australian National Aged Care Classification (AN-ACC) funding model will replace the Aged Care Funding Instrument as the assessment process that enables targeted subsidised care for people receiving residential aged care services.

THE NATIONAL DISABILITY INSURANCE SCHEME

The National Disability Insurance Scheme (NDIS) is an Australian government funding scheme that supports the needs of people with a serious or permanent disability. People with disability can apply for funding to the NDIS through an assessment process that indicates how much money the government will provide to them to access the support they need. An NDIS provider is an organisation that assists the person to access their specific supports, which may include physical support, social support, personal support and other aspects of living.

Some young people with disability may live in a residential aged care facility (RACF), even though they are not elderly, because they have needs that require assistance that cannot be provided at home. Young people who live in an RACF may have NDIS funding that supports them to access services that the facility cannot provide. For example, a person may have a disability support worker visit them at the RACF to take them out for coffee or to accompany them to a cinema. The person with disability chooses how their funding is used and which disability support organisation they want to provide their supports.

TORTS

DUTY OF CARE

All care workers have a duty of care to the older people they provide support to. The term "duty of care" means that a worker must do everything reasonably practicable to prevent foreseeable harm to those in their care. Care workers can uphold duty of care by:

- following policies and procedures
- working within scope of practice
- following the person's care plan
- asking the person for their consent
- asking the registered nurse (RN) or the supervisor for clarification about anything they don't understand
- reporting concerns about the person
- documenting according to workplace requirements
- reporting the actions or omissions of others that breach duty of care.

Breaching duty of care through an action, or by an omission, can result in harm to the person. In serious cases, a breach of duty of care can result in neglect, which may lead to litigation. Remember that all workers are accountable for the decisions they make around the provision of care. While it is not possible to prevent all harm from occurring to the people you support, it is important to ask yourself what reasonable steps you can take to keep people safe.

DIGNITY OF RISK

All individuals have the right to make their own decisions about their life and to take risks, and this includes older individuals. The term "dignity of risk" refers to recognising that the people you support have the right to take risks when making decisions about their lives. While there is a need to balance duty of care requirements with dignity of risk, all older people have the right to take risks. According to the Quality Standards, dignity of risk is one of the seven concepts that make up the foundation standard that is Standard 1, "Consumer Dignity and Choice".

Service providers are expected to support the older person to understand the risks that may be associated with the choices they make, and then to support the person to manage the risk. All organisations are expected to problem solve with the person (or the person's decision maker) to manage such risks in a way that is least restrictive to the person's autonomy.

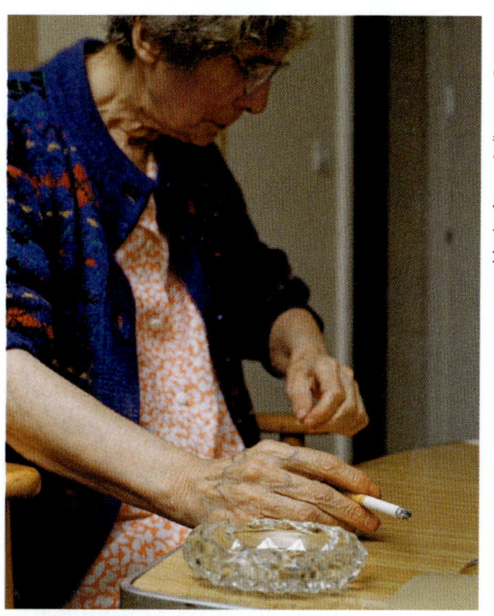

Haris Artemis/Image Source

Older people have the right to make their own decisions about their life, which includes taking risks

CONSENT

Consent is an agreement by a person to permit something or to participate in something. Consent is obtained frequently when working in aged care.

The person requiring support, or their carer, family member or significant other, is approached by the service for consent regarding various aspects of service delivery.

Consent may be obtained for factors involved with the service agreement, such as sharing information about the person, deducting fees from their financial institution, administering their medications and photographing them. Consent may be obtained at the start point of service delivery and will be requested many times during service delivery as the person's needs change. Valid consent must be informed and must never be coerced or obtained through deceptive methods. In Australia, laws about consent and decision making exist to protect vulnerable people from harm and exploitation.

A key concept in consent is "capacity". Having capacity means that a person understands information and can apply it in making a decision. Incapacity can be transient or permanent. In Australia, all adults are deemed to have capacity unless stated otherwise by a relevant medical practitioner or psychologist.

A person needs to have the capacity to understand information in order to give or refuse their consent. In the event the person lacks capacity (due to a cognitive issue), their substitute decision maker will grant or decline consent on their behalf. A substitute decision maker may be a carer, family member or public guardian; however, this varies between the different states and territories in Australia.

Consent may be of different types:

- *Informed consent:* Specific and factual information is provided to the person about the reason their consent is being sought. This allows them to understand the possible consequences of giving consent to the request, such as the risks and benefits, before either declining or granting their consent. Information given to the person must not be influenced by the opinion of the person giving it, as this is a coercive approach to obtaining consent. Informed consent can be withdrawn by the person at any time.
- *Verbal consent:* Consent may be given verbally, usually for minor activities or treatments such as support with personal care. For example: "Would you like me to help you with your shower now?" is a question that requests consent that the person can give or decline.
- *Implied consent:* This type of consent can apply to tasks that may occur frequently, or to minor activities or treatments where the person's action indicates their consent (such as when they offer their dentures to a care worker to be cleaned, or hold out their hand for some hand lotion).
- *Written consent:* Written consent is required for important processes such as a medical procedure where risk is elevated, or where medications are used as a restrictive practice (a chemical restraint).

It is essential that you obtain consent from the person before you attend to their support needs. Asking for permission to do something provides the person with the opportunity to pose questions, request more information or refuse your request. Don't take a refusal personally; there are many reasons why a person might refuse your request. Your role is to try to determine why they refused and to seek support from the appropriate person. For example, the person may refuse your request to get them out of bed for a shower. On further discussion, you learn they are feeling unwell and want to stay in bed. Your role is to ensure their comfort and to report your findings to the RN or supervisor immediately. It is important to document refusals according to the policy of the organisation, as frequent refusals may indicate the person has unmet needs that can be addressed.

Keep in mind that asking for consent is showing respect for the autonomy of the person you support and helps to build rapport between you and them.

CONFIDENTIALITY, PRIVACY AND DISCLOSURE

There are legal and ethical obligations surrounding confidentiality and privacy in the context of how a person's information is managed within the aged care service. Privacy legislation such as the *Privacy Act 1988* (Cth) and the Australian Privacy Principles provide direction on the expectations of aged care services regarding the policies, procedures and protocols they should have in place about confidentiality, privacy and disclosure.

Confidentiality means to protect and to keep private information. Confidentiality is an important component of privacy, and care workers can maintain confidentiality by preventing the older person's information from being accessed by others. An example of confidentiality in aged care is the use of electronic passcodes to access documentation and personal files. When a care worker signs out of a person's file in the electronic documentation system, they are effectively maintaining that person's confidentiality.

Privacy can refer to both privacy of information and personal privacy, both of which are key aspects of providing safe aged care services. Privacy of information is essential to ensure the older person has a sense of trust and safety within the context of their service provision. Sensitive health and medical information about the older person is often required to be obtained during assessment procedures, and this must be managed according to legislative requirements.

The term "disclosure" means to share someone's information. Disclosure of private, personal or sensitive information can only occur in particular circumstances according to the policies and procedures of the organisation. Those circumstances may include:

- when consent to share information is obtained from the person or their decision maker
- in an emergency situation that requires disclosure of information to medical or health personnel
- if information is requested by police or is subpoenaed by a court of law in Australia.

Information about a person might be referred to as being available only on a "need-to-know" basis. Care workers must always maintain the confidentiality of private information about people who require support, according to workplace policy.

GUARDIANSHIP, POWER OF ATTORNEY AND ENDURING POWER OF ATTORNEY

There are times that an older person is unable to make informed decisions that impact their finances, health or wellbeing. These times may be temporary or may progress to a permanent state of incapacity to manage decision making safely. There are also times when an older person may wish for someone to make decisions on their behalf, even though they don't lack capacity. They may have nominated another person to make decisions on their behalf when they still had capacity, or their family or a public trustee may have assigned this responsibility to another person. Table 2.2 describes key terms that are relevant to safe decision making on behalf of the older person.

2.1.3 An employee's responsibilities and rights

RESPONSIBILITIES

As an employee, you have responsibilities and rights that are bound in legal and ethical obligations. Aged care organisations are heavily regulated and are expected to demonstrate how compliance and other regulatory requirements are being met. Care workers have a responsibility to meet these requirements. They include:

- following the policies and procedures of their organisation
- representing the values, vision and mission of their organisation
- working within professional boundaries and scope of practice
- reporting concerns about legal and ethical breaches by others
- working in a professional manner and abiding by code of conduct expectations
- participating in work-related activities such as hazard identification, reporting and documentation processes
- ensuring that the rights of older people are upheld during service delivery at all times.

TABLE 2.2 Key terms relevant to safe decision making on behalf of the older person

Term	Definition
Power of attorney	A general power of attorney is a legally binding document that provides consent for the person to appoint an individual to manage their financial and legal affairs while the person still has capacity. For example, a nominated individual can manage a person's finances while they are travelling overseas.
Enduring power of attorney	This legally binding document provides consent for the person to appoint an individual to manage their financial and legal affairs, including at a time when the person doesn't have capacity to make their own decisions.
Private guardian	When the person doesn't have capacity to nominate an enduring guardian, a private guardian may be appointed by the Guardianship Division of the NSW Civil and Administrative Tribunal. A private guardian may be the person's carer, friend or family member. The private guardian makes decisions on behalf of the person related to their medical, health and lifestyle needs.
Enduring guardian	An enduring guardian is an individual nominated by the person, when they have capacity to do so, who can legally make decisions on their behalf about their medical, health and lifestyle needs. An enduring guardianship can be revoked by the Guardianship Division of the NSW Civil and Administrative Tribunal or the NSW Supreme Court.
Public guardian	When a person doesn't have capacity to nominate an enduring guardian and they don't have family or friends who can fulfil this role, a public official called a public guardian is appointed by the Guardianship Division of the NSW Civil and Administrative Tribunal to manage their lifestyle, health and medical decisions.
NSW Civil and Administrative Tribunal (NCAT)	The NCAT provides tribunal support for aspects of society. It has a Guardianship Division that supports the needs of people who cannot make their own decisions about matters that place them in a vulnerable position, such as financial, medical/health and lifestyle decisions.

Employee rights in the workplace include:

- a safe working environment
- a work environment free of abuse and judgement
- the right to consultation
- fair treatment and equal opportunities
- accessible work-related equipment such as personal protective equipment
- fair work conditions and fair pay.

Rights and responsibilities of employees are essential for the development of a workplace culture that is cohesive and productive, and just and equitable. Under the *Fair Work Act 2009* (Cth), an industrial tribunal called the Fair Work Commission provides information and support for both employers and employees regarding workplace rights and responsibilities.

THE NATIONAL AGED CARE MANDATORY QUALITY INDICATOR PROGRAM

The National Aged Care Mandatory Quality Indicator Program (the QI Program) is a government program that collects information from residential aged care facilities every three months to monitor trends and quality in aged care services. The QI Program also provides information for providers of aged care services to enable them to monitor and improve the services they provide, and offers consumers and the community transparent access to information about aged care services. Figure 2.2 illustrates the areas that are required to be monitored by aged care facilities under the QI Program.

FIGURE 2.2 The five quality indicators of the QI Program

QI Program quality indicators

Pressure injuries

- Percentage of care recipients with pressure injuries, reported against six pressure injury stages.

Physical restraint

- Percentage of care recipients who were physically restrained.

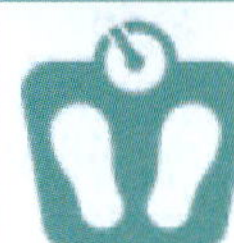

Unplanned weight loss

- Percentage of care recipients who experienced significant unplanned weight loss (5% or more).
- Percentage of care recipients who experienced consecutive unplanned weight loss.

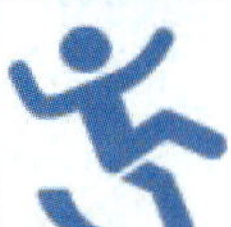

Falls and major injury

- Percentage of care recipients who experienced one or more falls.
- Percentage of care recipients who experienced one or more falls resulting in major injury.

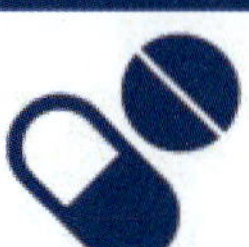

Medication management

- Percentage of care recipients who were prescribed nine or more medications.
- Percentage of care recipients who received antipsychotic medications.

Source: Australian Government, Department of Health, *National Aged Care Mandatory Quality Indicator Program Manual – 2.0 – Part A* (Final version) June 2019

THE SERIOUS INCIDENT RESPONSE SCHEME

Elder abuse occurs in both the community and residential aged care services, and often goes undetected. The insidious nature of abuse is not always obvious to others, and unfortunately older people are vulnerable to exploitation because they can be physically frail, cognitively impaired, or socially and geographically isolated. Most often the perpetrator of the abuse is someone the older person knows and who also has a position of power over them. People who are most likely to abuse older people include spouses, adult children of the person, carers and aged care staff.

Providers of and workers in residential aged care are required by law (i.e. it is mandatory) to report signs of abuse and allegations of abuse. Prior to April 2021, all workers within a residential aged care facility were required to report suspicions of unlawful sexual contact and unreasonable use of force against residents to the Aged Care Quality and Safety Commission. Current processes of reporting in RACFs include all forms of abuse, and the reporting mechanism is implemented under the Serious Incident Response Scheme (SIRS).

The SIRS initiative is aimed at identifying and managing incidents of abuse and preventing the reoccurrence of such incidents. The provider (facility) is required to have an incident management system in place that can identify, record, manage, resolve and report all serious incidents within the organisation. These incidents may be actual, suspected or alleged, and cover a broad range of incident types.

While some incidents will be managed within the facility, the facility has legal obligations to report serious incidents to the Commission. These incidents include:

- unreasonable use of force
- unlawful sexual contact or inappropriate sexual conduct
- neglect
- psychological or emotional abuse
- unexpected death
- stealing or financial coercion by a staff member
- inappropriate use of restrictive practices
- unexplained absence from care.

As a care worker, you have a legal obligation to report any suspicion you may have that a person is experiencing abuse. The signs may not always be obvious that a person has been or is experiencing abuse; however, there are some common indicators that can alert you that something is wrong. These may include changes in the way the person behaves, reluctance to undress or shower, change of behaviour around a particular visitor or staff member, and unexplained marks and bruising on their body.

Each organisation has a policy and procedure that states how to report concerns regarding abuse, and you will attend a mandatory annual training session on the topic.

At the time of writing, the reporting process for abuse in the home care sector was due to change in late 2022, to be aligned with the SIRS that currently exists for residential aged care facilities. Industry and public consultation for this change occurred between July and August 2021, after the Royal Commission into Aged Care Quality and Safety made its recommendations. Currently, if you work within in-home care services as a care worker, the reporting process is different until the changes commence.

Older people who live in their own homes may also be victims of abuse. The types of elder abuse that you need to report to your supervisor include physical abuse, sexual abuse, psychological or emotional abuse, financial abuse, and neglect. The reporting mechanism is different from that employed in RACFs. In the community, the focus for staff is to identify the person who is at risk of or is being abused, provide support for them (if they choose to accept it) and respond appropriately.

If the abuse is criminal, such as domestic violence or sexual abuse, the police may be notified. Seek support from your organisation and be aware of your workplace policy and procedures around elder abuse.

The person may be offered support, such as specialist assistance contact numbers, and if they consent, the police can be notified. If the person doesn't have capacity (e.g. if they have dementia) and they are at risk of harm, the organisation may report the abuse to the police. It is to be noted that if the alleged perpetrator is present and becomes threatening or has a weapon, the police *must* be notified. Always consider your own safety.

Home and community care organisations can be guided by the NSW Interagency Protocol document titled "Preventing and Responding to Abuse of Older People (Elder Abuse)", published in June 2018. This document provides information on how to respond to abuse in the home care setting and offers a framework for organisations' responses to abuse.

Regardless of the type of abuse, your role is to report your suspicions of abuse to your supervisor and to follow their instructions. Always document incidents according to your organisation's procedures for documentation.

THE USE OF RESTRICTIVE PRACTICES

A restrictive practice in the context of aged care services is any practice or action that restricts the freedom of movement or rights of the older person receiving care. As a result of legislative updates of the *Aged Care Act 1997* and the Quality of Care Principles 2014, from July 2021 all providers of government-funded aged care services have to meet specific compliance criteria to address the use of restrictive practices. The Aged Care Quality and Safety Commission defines restrictive practices as including chemical restraint, environmental restraint, mechanical restraint, physical restraint and seclusion.

Restrictive practices have historically been implemented to manage or control a person's behaviour in the context of preventing harm as a result of that behaviour, such as aggression. As a result of the Royal Commission, the new legislative changes require organisations to have a behaviour support plan in place for people who experience behaviours of concern; to apply, monitor and document behaviour supports; and to ensure that any form of restrictive practice is used only as a last resort after all other avenues of intervention have been unsuccessful. The obtaining of relevant consent is another aspect of the use of restrictive practices that has been reviewed and changed under the updated legislation. Government-funded aged care services can be issued notices of non-compliance from the Commission if they don't meet the required changes to the use of restrictive practices and may even be presented with civil penalties.

More information on restrictive practices in aged care services can be found at https://www.agedcarequality.gov.au/sites/default/files/media/overview-of-restrictive-practices_0.pdf.

WORKPLACE HEALTH AND SAFETY

Risk management is a constant consideration for the care worker. The nature of the job involves potential risk in many environments, from the RACF or the person's home, to the day centre or even an outing to the shops. Hazards are those things that can cause harm, and the risk of harm can be minor or even catastrophic for older people.

Commonwealth work health and safety legislation is ingrained within the policies and procedures of aged care services, and ongoing education and professional development will involve risk management. The risk management framework within an aged care service involves identifying potential hazards, implementing measures to eliminate or control the hazard, and reporting the hazard and associated risks according to the organisational policies and procedures.

Risk management can be applied by care workers when planning for activities, assisting the person with medications, working within their home and planning an outing for them. Risks can be modified or minimised with an approach of "foreseeable harm" in mind. Planning may involve risk minimisation strategies that can be implemented in the context of providing safe care, without impeding the person's dignity of risk.

POLICIES AND PROCEDURES

All providers of government-funded aged care services are required to embed legislation into the practices of the organisation. To continue to be compliant with legislation and to receive Commonwealth funding, aged care services must have policies and procedures in place to guide workers on how to work legally and ethically.

As noted in Chapter 1, a policy is a document that states *what* needs to occur and *why* it needs to occur. Organisational policies also contain information about the specific legislation and Quality Standards that apply to the policy. A procedure is a document that describes, often in a step-by-step sequence, *how* to do what the policy states. There may be several procedures for a single policy. Policies are often reviewed every 12 months; however, some may be reviewed less often. A policy will also be reviewed if a relevant change in legislation or industry practice occurs.

Always ask the RN or the supervisor for clarification if you are in doubt about any policy or procedure relevant to the work that you are required to engage in.

RIGHTS

INDUSTRIAL RELATIONS, TRADE UNIONS, AWARDS AND WORKING CONDITIONS

As an employee in the aged care sector, you have responsibilities, but you also have rights. Your rights as an employee are supported by laws, regulatory bodies and other organisations.

A union, or a trade union, is an organisation of workers who have the common goals of safe and fair work conditions. Unions have had a presence in Australia for many years and exist in most trades and industries, including health care. Workers can subscribe to be a member of a union that they feel represents

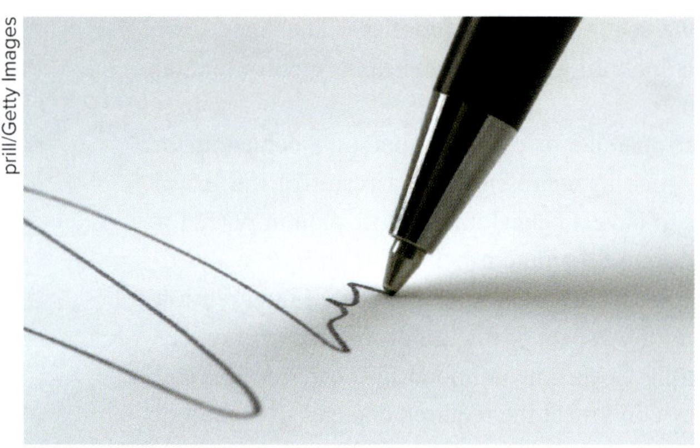

prill/Getty Images

An employment contract states the agreed terms and conditions of employment

their rights and roles in a proactive way. Unions can be beneficial in many ways, including by advocating for workers and supporting them when employers have breached workplace conditions.

Workplace conditions are those aspects of employment that reflect the rights and entitlements of a worker and include things like work hours, the frequency and duration of breaks, annual leave, maternity and parental leave, and access to an employee assistance program. An award is a legal document that states the conditions of employment and is specific to a distinct role within a profession or industry. An award will state rates of pay and other work conditions relevant to the role. Care workers who work in an RACF will potentially work under the Aged Care Award, and care workers who work in home care are employed under the Social, Community, Home Care and Disability Services Industry Award.

Casual work is work that is not fixed employment with an organisation. Work conditions differ between a casual worker and a permanent worker. A permanent worker has a workplace agreement or contract that states the minimum hours to be worked per pay period, and therefore has entitlements such as paid sick leave and paid annual leave. A casual worker can select how many hours they work and on what days or shift times they are available. Pay rates are slightly higher for casual workers because they have fewer workplace entitlements.

An award does not apply to a worker when the organisation they work for has an enterprise agreement in place. This type of agreement may be between an aged care service and the fair work commission or another industry entity and will state the employment conditions such as those covered in an award.

A contract or employment agreement is a document between an employer and a worker that states the agreed terms and conditions of employment. These documents may indicate whether the worker will be employed under an award or an enterprise agreement. The employer cannot provide workplace conditions less than the National Employment Standards which set out minimum work pay rates and conditions.

2.1.4 Recognising and reporting breaches of law

It is important that any breach in law is reported to management, or other aged care industry services such as regulatory bodies, to prevent harm from occurring to the person using the support, their carer and family. Harm may be potential, suspected, actual or historical in nature, and care workers have a duty of care to minimise foreseeable harm to those they support in the job role.

Recognising and reporting breaches of law is supported by different reporting mechanisms and processes, some internal to the workplace and some external to it. Reporting can take the form of a grievance or complaint, or it can be formal and follow a specific protocol.

INTERNAL MECHANISMS

The organisation's policies and procedures will provide guidance and instruction on how to make a report about a breach of law. Some of these policies will have specific requirements, such as:

- compulsory reporting under the Serious Incident Response Scheme
- mandatory reporting involving welfare of children in the workplace
- complaints
- responding to complaints
- grievance processes
- advocacy.

Care workers can seek clarification from the RN or supervisor regarding what actions to take to report a breach of a law that is recognised in the workplace.

EXTERNAL MECHANISMS

Outside of the aged care service, older people, their carer and their family can access organisations that can provide assistance regarding a breach of the law in the context of aged care services. These organisations can support the person with information about their rights, legal options and advocacy support, and include:

- the Aged Care Quality and Safety Commission (Any reports for suspected fraud can be made to the Commission, as well as other types of complaints.)
- My Aged Care
- the Older Persons Advocacy Network (OPAN)
- legal advisers such as solicitors
- the police.

Recognising and reporting breaches of law is an essential component of ensuring a safe environment for the older person, their carer and family, and the staff providing their services. All incidents of reporting must be documented according to the organisation's policies and procedures.

WORKPLACE SCENARIO

Restrictive practices

Carol is working as a team leader on the afternoon shift at the aged care facility in her community. She notices that Mr Jay is pacing up and down the corridor, mumbling angrily to himself. Day shift staff have reported that, earlier in the day, Mr Jay was attempting to leave the facility by waiting beside the door and pushing his way out when someone entered or exited. At these times, Mr Jay was able to be diverted with activities and staff conversation.

Carol checks on Mr Jay's behaviour support plan, which indicates that he is known to experience violent outbursts that require him to take a dose of antipsychotic medication to moderate his behaviour. Carol knows that this intervention is to be used as an absolute last resort and only after all other interventions in the behaviour support plan have been tried. She also knows that one intervention in particular is helpful in supporting Mr Jay to relax and in preventing his agitated mood from escalating into violence. This intervention involves modifying his environment.

Carol assists Mr Jay to his room, where she puts on his favourite Country music, lowers the lights to a safe level and sprays some lavender mist on the curtains. After making him a cup of tea and some snacks, she helps him into his armchair. Mr Jay is singing happily along with the music when Carol leaves the room, leaving the door unlocked. This intervention doesn't always work, but today it seems to have helped Mr Jay to settle and relax and has prevented him having to take medication.

CHECK YOUR UNDERSTANDING

1. What is the role of the Aged Care Quality and Safety Commission?
2. What does duty of care mean in the context of working as a care worker?
3. Explain dignity of risk.
4. List four employee responsibilities when working as a care worker.
5. What is the difference between a policy and a procedure?

2.2 IDENTIFYING AND MEETING ETHICAL RESPONSIBILITIES

Working ethically means to do the right thing by others and yourself in the workplace. It means being fair in one's dealings, having moral integrity, supporting the rights of others, and working in a way that is "good" and benefits your colleagues and the people you support.

2.2.1 Ethics and the organisation

An organisation's ethics are reflected in its values and are expressed in its vision, mission and purpose statements. These statements can be located on the organisation's website and in its promotional materials such as pamphlets and brochures. They are also often displayed prominently within the organisation's premises.

VALUES

As individuals, our values represent our principles and ethics. Organisations have values, too, and they represent the organisation's core ethics in terms of how it will function. The values of an organisation state what it stands for in regard to the types of services it provides. For example, value statements may contain words such as "trust", "dignity" and "respect". An organisation's values can be used to encourage employees to reflect on and be guided towards the behaviours that are expected of them and can help to define its purpose.

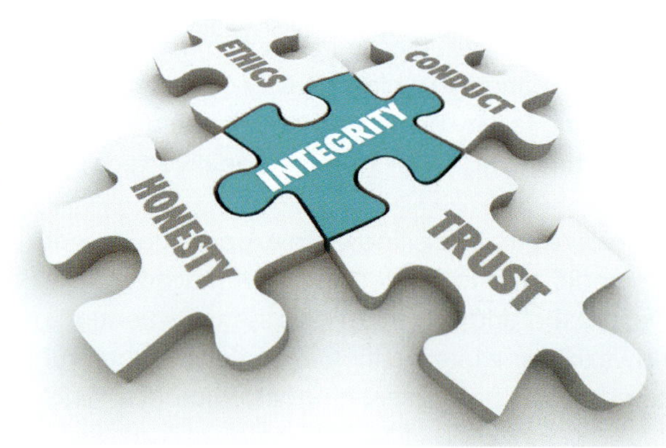

iQoncept/Shutterstock

An organisation's ethics are expressed in its vision and mission statements

VISION AND MISSION STATEMENTS

Along with values, most organisations have vision and mission statements that set out the direction the organisation wants to go in and the means by which it wants to get there.

A vision statement describes the organisation's "destination". Within aged care, a service's vision statement may include words or phrases such as "promote the autonomy of older people", "harmony and health", "responsive to the needs of the elderly", "respect diversity" and "empower communities".

A mission statement describes the purpose of an organisation. Mission statements explain the reason why the organisation has values and a vision statement. A mission statement for an aged care service may include words or phrases such as "provide", "promote", "stand with" and "facilitate".

PROMOTING AN ETHICAL ORGANISATIONAL CULTURE

An ethical organisational culture is one that recognises and respects opportunities for autonomy and self-determination of the people who receive services. It also demonstrates a workforce that is cohesive in its approach to working in a way that promotes dignity, transparent and inclusive problem solving and mutual respect.

An ethical organisational culture can be promoted by:

- employing staff who do the right thing all the time and thus act as role models for others
- having strong policies and procedures in the workplace
- promoting ethical work practices by investing in staff education
- having processes that support transparent and inclusive problem solving
- recognising staff who work ethically through promotions and other job role opportunities

- discouraging judgement of others and encouraging problem solving when values don't align
- ensuring that the organisation's work practices align with its values, vision and mission.

2.2.2 Ethics and the care worker

"Accountability" describes the position of taking responsibility for our own decisions and actions and for the outcomes that are associated with them. All health-care workers, including aged care workers, are accountable for their actions in the workplace. Different roles within the aged care system are regulated by different industry boards and other bodies; however, unlicensed workers such as care workers are bound to practise under the National Code of Conduct for Health Care Workers, which holds each individual care worker accountable for their actions in their job role.

The accountability of care workers is guided and supported by legislation, policies and procedures, and ongoing professional development. Working within your scope of practice also ensures accountability of the work you engage in; however, you are also accountable for incidents that occur if you choose to work outside of your scope of practice.

PRACTICE POINT

Working outside of your scope of practice is a breach of your duty of care and can place the older person at risk of harm from your actions, even if those actions are well intended. Remember: you are accountable for your actions in the workplace.

2.2.3 Identifying potential ethical issues and dilemmas

Part of working ethically includes recognising when an issue or situation involves ethical components. Ethical issues can quickly become complex when they are not identified or managed correctly. Self-awareness of ethical obligations is key to preventing ethical dilemmas before they arise.

PERSONAL CONFLICT

Personal conflict occurs when two or more people cause a disruption in the workplace due to a dispute between or among them. This situation often results in efforts by the organisation to provide mediation processes to the parties in an effort to negotiate and problem solve to resolve the conflict; however, many instances of personal conflict may result in disciplinary action.

Personal conflict in the workplace can also occur when a worker is put in a position where their own values and beliefs are compromised or challenged. For example, a care worker may be asked to provide personal care for a person whose religious views are diametrically opposed to those of the care worker. In this instance, the care worker has the right to approach their supervisor, who should make every attempt to modify the situation–for example, by providing the person with a different care worker.

CONFLICT OF INTEREST

Conflict of interest in the role of care worker can take different forms and can create an environment that is ethically challenged. A conflict of interest occurs when an individual has a personal or private interest in a specific aspect of the workplace. The job role should not have personal aspects attached to it that may be perceived as benefiting the social domain of the worker. The following are examples of personal conflict within the job role.

- The worker refers an older person or their family to a business the worker is linked to.
- A worker provides care to a member of their own family within the role of paid care worker.
- Promotions are prioritised for relatives or friends.

- A personal relationship is established with a family member of the older person who uses aged care services.
- A complaint is dealt with differently because the person is a friend.

Conflict of interest in the workplace has the capacity to evolve into a complex legal issue.

2.2.4 Recognising and responding to unethical conduct

REPORTING

As a care worker, you should always report any unethical behaviour of those you work with or for. Unethical behaviour will almost always affect another person or group of people, and calling it out can create a platform for change. Always consult the organisational policies and procedures that relate to making a report, such as those about grievance procedures and complaint management processes.

It can also be helpful to discuss your concerns with the RN or supervisor, and it is acceptable to organise a private meeting with management if necessary.

When reporting unethical conduct, you should be sure that your report is made in good faith and is accurate. You will need to know who was involved and who else was present. Facts are important, so be sure that you state what the unethical incident was, and what (if anything) you have done to address the issue. You may have approached the individual involved. Keep in mind that policies and procedures will direct you in how to make the report and to whom.

MINIMISING THE POTENTIAL FOR UNETHICAL CONDUCT

Many workers don't realise their behaviour is unethical and may approach their work practices with the same attitude every day. The potential for unethical conduct in the workplace may be minimised by:

- ensuring that all staff are given a copy of the organisation's code of conduct at commencement of employment, which they are expected to sign
- ensuring that all employees are provided with training and education about the code of conduct at commencement of employment and annually thereafter
- reminding staff about the national code of conduct through media such as posters in the staff room, messages on payslips and other means of communication.

Working legally and ethically involves working with a sense of doing the right thing and asking for clarification when necessary. Working within the scope of practice, following policies and procedures, and ensuring you attend mandatory education are all ways you can work safely in aged care and provide support that is person-centred, ethical, and within the boundaries of legislation and regulations.

WORKPLACE SCENARIO

Conflict of interest

Marnie is a supervisor within a home care organisation that provides support to older people living in their own home. Recently, several clients have requested assistance with lawn mowing, as they can no longer mow their lawn independently and don't have family to help them. Marnie knows that the clients should be given information about local lawn care contractors so they can select one of their choosing, taking into consideration the extra costs and the contractor's availability. Instead, Marnie provides the care workers with business cards for her husband's lawn mowing business. One of the workers, Anne, refuses to take the card and tells Marnie that she has a conflict of interest and is working unethically. Marnie realises her error of judgement and returns to following policy and procedures regarding referring clients to independent contractors for lawn care.

CHECK YOUR UNDERSTANDING

1. What does the term "values" mean in relation to an organisation?
2. List three ways in which an ethical culture can be promoted in the workplace.
3. What is meant by the term "accountability"?
4. Describe how personal conflict occurs in the workplace.
5. Describe one way that unethical conduct can be minimised in the workplace.

2.3 CONTRIBUTING TO WORKPLACE IMPROVEMENTS

The way we work is constantly changing and evolving, and the impending reforms in the aged care sector will see many changes in the way our work is carried out. Work practices should be constantly reviewed because this will ensure that they will continually improve, ultimately leading to the best possible service delivery for older people and the best possible work environment for care staff.

2.3.1 Continuous improvement

The term "continuous improvement" describes the practices and processes that constantly review the way things are done in order to learn from them or improve them. Also known as quality improvement, these processes enable us to learn from incidents that didn't work effectively in order to prevent them from reoccurring, and to monitor workplace practices to determine if they are occurring in the best possible way. Risk minimisation is a key factor in continuous improvement initiatives and incidents, with safety being one of the ultimate goals. Other goals of continuous improvement include environmental, community and financial sustainability. All aged care services strive to provide their services in a manner that reflects the needs of the community and supports the financial viability of the service. The underlying factor of continuous improvement in all aged care services is optimal outcomes for consumers of their services, and the regulatory and compliance requirements of aged care services are therefore heavily focused on the transparency and reflective aspects of continuous improvement processes.

2.3.2 The benefits of improving work practices

The following are some of the benefits of continuous improvement in the workplace.

- *Transparency:* Continuous improvement assists in developing an open and honest relationship between the organisation and those who use its services.
- *Safety:* Risks are minimised through learning from and reflecting on incidents.
- *Accountability:* Care staff acknowledge that processes and practices can be improved.
- *Cohesion:* Care staff, older people, their carers and families can work together to identify issues and problem solve to improve outcomes.
- *Legal obligations are met:* All aged care providers are required to have a Plan for Continuous Improvement (PCI), as a legal obligation under the Aged Care Quality and Safety Commission's regulations, that is in alignment with the Quality Standards.

In the context of aged care services, a stakeholder is an individual or an organisation that has an interest in the person's care services and their outcomes. All aspects of a continuous improvement plan must be monitored and evaluated for effectiveness, and this can occur when the organisation consults with stakeholders such as staff, service users and their carers and families, visiting contractors, and external organisations and agencies.

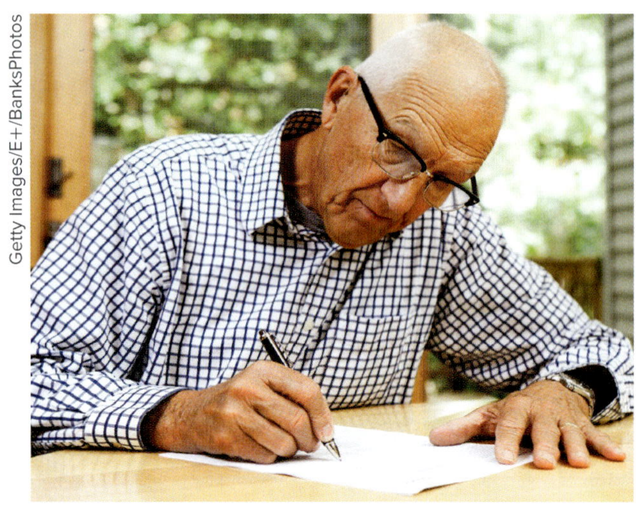
Getty Images/E+/BanksPhotos

Consultation may occur through feedback surveys and questionnaires

2.3.3 Consultation and feedback

Consultation means communicating with another person about a particular issue or to seek advice. Consultation can occur between individuals and between organisations. The purpose of consultation is to share information and ideas that can provide valuable feedback about processes and practices. Consultation is essential for continuous improvement processes.

The older person and their carer and family are an important part of consultation processes that aim to improve aspects of service delivery. Consultation may occur through meetings, feedback surveys and questionnaires, and other methods of communication, to determine levels of satisfaction regarding services or to problem solve.

Employees are also part of consultation processes within an organisation, as the work health and safety legislation expects all organisations to consult with employees about risk minimisation in the workplace. Not all employee consultation is related to safety; it may occur for other reasons that are relevant to continuous improvement processes. This may include asking employees for feedback about practices or impending changes to processes, and staff appraisals. Staff appraisals are also known as performance appraisals and usually occur yearly. The purpose of a performance appraisal is to provide an opportunity for staff to reflect on and provide feedback about the way they do their job. Organisations can provide constructive, not critical, feedback to staff and work with them to determine ways to support them to make changes or improvements to practices. Performance appraisals are part of a continuous improvement plan, and they provide an opportunity for consultation between the organisation and the individual staff member to determine what support can be offered to the staff member to improve or maintain their practices.

2.3.4 Contributing to the team

TEAMWORK

Teamwork is essential for the workplace to meet goals and deliver excellence in service delivery. Aged care services incorporate the skills and knowledge of a multidisciplinary team in order to deliver effective consumer outcomes and meet the regulatory requirements of the industry.

Working as part of a team includes:

- working within scope of practice
- showing respect for the roles of others in the team
- working collaboratively
- participating in and contributing to the team planning and goal-setting processes
- working in alignment with the values of the team
- working legally and ethically at all times.

Teams have a common goal, and all team members play an important role in safe and effective service delivery, ensuring a continuum of care to the older person.

PROFESSIONAL DEVELOPMENT

Professional development is ongoing once you have obtained your qualification. The nature of the health and aged care industries is continually evolving and changing, based on the applications of modern technologies and new information to current best practices and models of care. Working in the aged care sector will require you to take part in yearly and ongoing training and development events.

As part of the safety and compliance framework of the aged care sector, employees are required to undertake further education on an annual basis. This education is aimed at ensuring that workplace practices, and individuals receiving care support, are safe. The topics covered include work health and safety training (specifically, manual handling and infection control), reporting of suspicions of abuse of older people, fire safety and food safety.

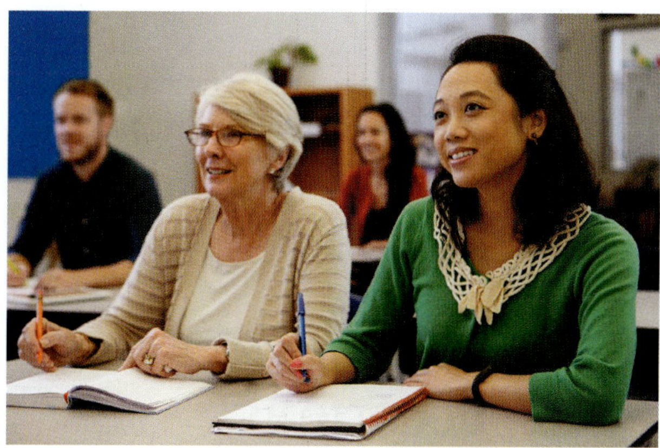

iStock/Getty Images Plus/monkeybusinessimages

Employees are required to undertake further education on an annual basis

Professional development also includes education and training that is scheduled at any time as part of an education calendar. This education may be around new equipment, changes to policies and procedures, or specific topics that are relevant to providing support (e.g. understanding delirium, supporting people at end of life, etc.).

Ongoing training and development are essential to ensure a modern and well-informed workforce in the aged care sector that results in positive health and wellbeing outcomes for older people receiving services.

WORKPLACE SCENARIO

Performance appraisals and professional development

Roman loves his job in aged care and has a great working relationship with his colleagues. During his performance appraisal this week, his manager acknowledges how well Roman works with older people and mentions that his colleagues always speak highly of him. However, he also observes that Roman seems awkward when working in the dementia wing of the organisation and asks him what his thoughts are about this.

Roman explains that he is uncomfortable when working with people with dementia, because he feels unsure of how to communicate with them. He says that he wants to do something about this. Roman's manager suggests that the organisation pay for Roman to enrol in a dementia-specific course that could help him to interact more confidently with people with dementia. Roman says he would be very interested in enrolling in such a course.

CHECK YOUR UNDERSTANDING

1. What is continuous improvement?
2. What is a performance appraisal?
3. What are three ways to work as part of a team?
4. What are two benefits of continuous improvement in the workplace?

SUMMARY

- Regulation of aged care services is overseen by the Commonwealth government and state and territory governments.
- Current legislation related to aged care services is complex. The new aged care reforms will create new legislation to support a rights-based aged care system, according to the recommendations of the Royal Commission.
- Care workers have a responsibility to work legally and ethically. They are supported to do so by policies and procedures, job descriptions, codes of conduct and consultation in the workplace.

REVIEW QUESTIONS

2.1 Outline the purpose of the Aged Care Quality Standards in the aged care industry.

2.2 **(a)** What is meant by the term "restrictive practices"? Provide an example to support your answer.

(b) Why are restrictive practices of concern in aged care?

2.3 List examples of events that apply under the Serious Incidents Response Scheme.

2.4 What is the role of a support worker and supervisors in reporting such events?

2.5 In the workplace, what do each of the following terms mean? Provide an example for each term.

(a) Responsible.

(b) Accountable

BIBLIOGRAPHY

Aged Care Quality and Safety Commission, *Charter of Aged Care Rights*, updated 6 May 2022, www.agedcarequality.gov.au/consumers/consumer-rights, accessed 22 June 2022.

Australian Government, myagedcare, *Legal Information, n.d.*, https://www.myagedcare.gov.au/legal-information, accessed 10 December 2021.

Australian Government, Department of Health, *National Aged Care Mandatory Quality Indicator Program Manual–2.0–Part A* (Final version), June 2019, https://www.health.gov.au/resources/publications/national-aged-care-mandatory-quality-indicator-program-manual-20-part-a, accessed March 2022.

Australian Government, Department of Health, *Five Pillars over 5 Years: A Snapshot of the Australian Government's Aged Care Reforms*, infographic, 11 May 2021, https://www.health.gov.au/initiatives-and-programs/aged-care-reforms/five-pillars-to-support-aged-care-reform, accessed March 2022.

Fair Work Commission, https://www.fwc.gov.au, accessed 17 July 2020.

Office of the Royal Commission into Aged Care Quality and Safety, *Background Paper 4: Restrictive Practices in Residential Aged Care in Australia*, 3 May 2019, https://agedcare.royalcommission.gov.au/search?query=restrictive+practices, accessed 20 December 2021.

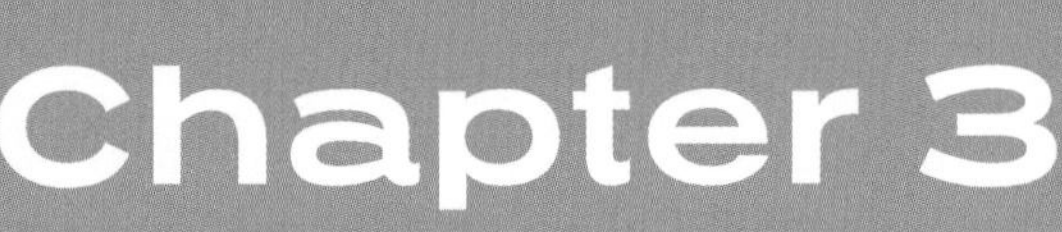

Chapter 3

Working safely

LEARNING OBJECTIVES

3.1 Follow safe work practices for direct care support

3.2 Follow safe work practices for manual handling

3.3 Follow safe work practices for infection control

3.4 Contribute to safe work practices in the workplace

3.5 Reflect on safe work practices

INTRODUCTION

CARE WORKERS WORKING IN AGED CARE SERVICES work with a range of people with various levels of mobility, cognition and dependency, and experience a variety of hazardous and unpredictable situations and settings. These may include challenging behaviours, wet floors, dangerous substances, unguarded equipment and stress.

Workers and persons conducting a business or undertaking, often the employer, have an important role in maintaining safety and security in the workplace and must adhere to legal and industry requirements. Current legislation seeks to ensure workplace health and safety (WHS) through the development of safe work habits, policies and procedures, and by upholding a **duty of care** to protect the health, safety and wellbeing of workers, persons being cared for and others in the workplace.

This chapter examines the importance, principles and management of WHS and provides guidelines for identifying and reporting common hazards and risks, and implementing safe work practices, to ensure a healthy, safe and productive work life.

INDUSTRY IN FOCUS

Working safely: Everyone's responsibility

Even though health and safety guidelines constantly change, the principles underlying workplace health and safety remain consistent: both employers and employees are legally accountable and ethically responsible for protecting the welfare, health and safety of themselves and others in the workplace, including visitors and contractors. Safe Work Australia is the national body responsible for the development and evaluation of the model WHS laws that are made up of the Work Health and Safety Act, regulations and codes of practice as they pertain to specific industries (such as aged care) and activities in those industries (such as manual handling). Each state and territory is responsible for the regulation of these laws in its jurisdiction, including inspecting workplaces regarding compliance and potential breaches, and for giving advice.

Whenever legislation, regulations and work practices change, it is the responsibility of organisations to update their policies and procedures and to provide training. All changes should be made in consultation with staff and follow processes for hazard identification and risk management and be regularly evaluated using a continuous improvement model. Such consultation requires a dialogue between managers and care staff and provides the opportunity for people to come together to manage risks in the workplace. Consultation and collaboration will include such issues as:

- how risk management is undertaken
- suggested changes that affect the health and safety of everyone in the workplace
- procedural decisions
- the adequacy of facilities and equipment.

Consultation processes may involve the establishment of work groups or a committee, the nomination of representatives from various parts of the organisation, and the implementation of meetings. Meetings should occur every three months and at any other time when requested by at least half of the committee—for example, when there are successive outbreaks of gastroenteritis over a period of, say, four months. The committee may make recommendations about areas for improvement, such as hand hygiene audits, and may review statistics and evaluate existing measures to ensure the health and safety of everyone in the workplace. It is necessary, though, to remember that WHS does not simply rest with a committee; it is *everyone's* responsibility.

3.1 FOLLOWING SAFE WORK PRACTICES FOR DIRECT CARE SUPPORT

Workplace accidents and injuries are costly and can lead to a loss of working time. Workers and employers must be aware of their responsibilities, both as an individual and as a team member, in maintaining safety within the work environment.

3.1.1 Work health and safety legislation

The aim of **work health and safety legislation** is to prevent and protect people from injury, illness and disease, and to ensure safety and wellbeing for all. Legislation is in place at both the state and national level to guide and assist employers and employees to comply with specific standards and requirements that contribute to protecting and maintaining safety and wellbeing in the workplace. While the *Aged Care Act 1997* and the Aged Care Quality Standards outline service provider responsibilities in relation to WHS, it is the Commonwealth *Work Health and Safety Act 2011* (the WHS Act) that clearly outlines the duty of care that both the employer and employees have to protect the health, safety and wellbeing of all people at or near the workplace. This may include visitors, contractors, cleaners, gardeners and volunteers.

Safe Work Australia is the statutory body responsible for the overall development of national WHS policy; however, each state and territory has its own WHS legislation, regulations, codes of practice and standards. Each state is also responsible for enforcing its WHS laws and investigating workplace incidents.

It is important for a worker to be aware of the legislation relevant to the state in which they work.

REGULATIONS

Regulations outline the mandatory requirements of the WHS Act. They provide guidelines on how to manage responsibilities and risks associated with the work being performed and the overall management of WHS in the workplace. Of particular importance to care workers are the regulations associated with identifying and managing hazards, personal protective equipment (PPE) and hazardous manual tasks.

Regulations assist in protecting a care worker's psychological and physical safety and wellbeing from:

- poor manual handling practice
- infection transmission
- trips, slips, falls and sprains
- faulty equipment
- workplace or occupational stress
- increased and unreasonable workloads
- repetitive tasks
- workplace violence and bullying.

CODES OF PRACTICE

Codes of practice complement the WHS Act and regulations and offer a practical, detailed guide on how to comply with legal obligations. Codes of practice don't replace the legislation in place. Relevant codes of practice for the care industry relate to hazardous manual tasks, first aid, managing WHS risks, managing the risk of falls, and WHS **consultation**.

EMPLOYER AND EMPLOYEE RIGHTS AND RESPONSIBILITIES

While WHS is the responsibility of everyone in the workplace, the actual roles of the employer and the employee do differ in some ways. The employer must provide the systems and framework that allow the employee with the requisite knowledge and resources to safely perform their role.

A PERSON CONDUCTING A BUSINESS OR UNDERTAKING

An employer, also known as the **person conducting a business or undertaking (PCBU)**, has a duty of care under the WHS Act to have systems and processes in place that protect and maintain the health, safety and wellbeing of all persons. This includes preventing, minimising and eliminating hazards and risks in order to reduce accidents, injuries, illnesses and diseases in the workplace. The WHS Act also has provisions ensuring that PCBUs have meaningful, scheduled and planned collaborative and open consultations with staff relating to WHS issues. The PCBU has the overall responsibility of ensuring that the workplace and its employees are following WHS laws and practices and may face prosecution for failing to do so.

As an employee, you have a duty of care not only to yourself, but also to your colleagues, clients or residents, to comply with your WHS responsibilities. Table 3.1 lists some of these responsibilities. Further responsibilities are outlined in the WHS Act.

TABLE 3.1 Employer and employee responsibilities

PCBU (employer) responsibilities	Employee responsibilities
Provide safe work systems	Follow the workplace's safe work systems
Provide a safe work environment	Identify and report an unsafe environment
Provide adequate and appropriate PPE	Wear PPE as intended
Provide adequate, regular and appropriate training and education	Attend the training and education provided
Develop accessible policies and procedures	Follow policies and procedures
Provide personal hygiene facilities (e.g. toilets, change-rooms, lockers)	Use the facilities supplied appropriately
Ensure emergency procedures are in place	Be aware of all emergency procedure responses
Ensure compliance with requirements of the WHS legislation	Follow compliance requirements
Notify and record details of workplace incidents	Report and record details of incidents and near misses

The WHS Act also outlines the rights of both the PCBU and its employees. As a care worker, you have the right to:

- be shown how to work safely
- be trained in how to use equipment safely
- use appropriate PPE
- ask questions if you feel unsure or unsafe about a task or procedure
- refuse work you think is unsafe
- be consulted on WHS matters
- receive workers compensation and fair pay
- work in a workplace that is free of bullying and harassment.

A PCBU has the right to expect that you, as a care worker, will perform your role reasonably and in accordance with the workplace's WHS policies and procedures. If not, it has the right to dismiss you.

3.1.2 Work health and safety policies and procedures

All workplaces are required to have WHS policies and procedures. The policies outline what will be done to ensure a safe workplace and describe the organisation's responsibilities in terms of the safety and health of its employees. Procedures describe and detail how to meet the policy objectives. All care workers should receive training in WHS procedures at the beginning of their employment, regularly review them in team meetings, and complete refresher training on an annual basis or as procedures, equipment or the work environment change.

WHS policies and procedures include important information regarding:

- hazard identification and control systems
- manual handling
- infection control
- personal protective clothing and equipment
- standard precautions

- handling hazardous/dangerous materials and goods
- completing safety data sheets
- emergency procedures and general safety precautions, including the location of first-aid equipment
- staff development and training programs
- waste management
- WHS personnel.

Policies and procedures are of key importance for all care workers and should be:

- easily accessible by all workers at all times
- easy to read, understand and interpret
- regularly reviewed and updated annually, or when legislation changes, or when an issue or concern is raised about a policy or procedure
- easily implemented.

Workers should be informed of all changes and be provided with additional training or education if required. Changes to WHS documentation and information should be made in consultation and collaboration with workers and follow risk management processes.

3.1.3 Hazard identification and risk management

A **hazard** is something with the potential to cause harm to a place, person or environment; while a **risk** is the likelihood and level of severity of an injury, illness or disease as a result of exposure to the hazard. **Hazard identification** is the process of identifying actual and potential hazards and is key to providing a safe workplace. All personal support workers should receive extensive training in the hazard identification process, as they encounter hazards and issues that can only be experienced by the hands-on nature of the work they do. However, the responsibility for identifying hazards lies with everyone. Hazard identification is a continuous process that should be incorporated into everyday practice.

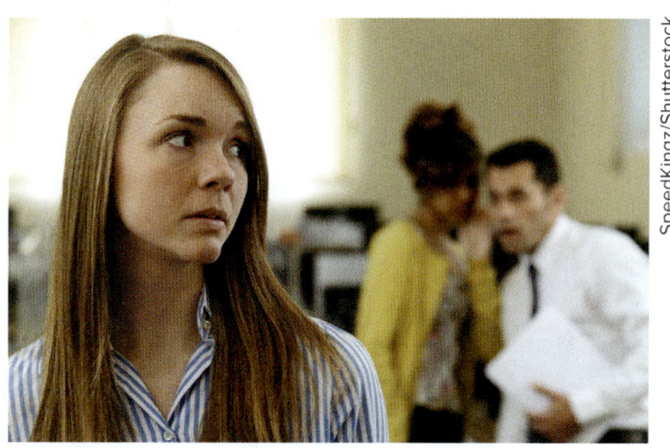

SpeedKingz/Shutterstock

Hazards can include conflict with colleagues, bullying and harassment

COMMON HAZARDS AND RISKS IN THE AGED CARE WORKPLACE

The types of hazards and risks most likely identified in aged care, home and community care, and disability service environments are outlined in Table 3.2.

The types of hazards you encounter will depend on the environment you work in and the clients you work with. Residential care and home and community care will present a variety of differing environmental hazards due to the different nature of a facility and a home. The client-related hazards will also differ depending on the client's needs and impairments. Care workers should be aware of all the potential hazards in whichever workplace they perform their role.

RISK MANAGEMENT

Identifying hazards is the first step in risk management. **Risk management** is a four-step process of managing a risk. Figure 3.1 shows a visual representation of the process of identifying, assessing, controlling, and reviewing and monitoring risks.

TABLE 3.2 Common hazards and risks in the aged care workplace

Type of hazard	Workplace example	Risk
Physical	Lifting, supporting and moving clients/equipment	Musculoskeletal injury and slips, trips and falls
Psychological	Conflicts with colleagues, bullying and harassment, death of client	Work-related stress, grief and loss, mental health issues
Occupational violence	Aggressive behaviour from client or family member	Psychological or physical harm
Biological	Exposure to bodily fluids and infectious aerosol particles	Transmission of disease, such as influenza and COVID-19
Chemical	Exposure to chemical/cleaning agents	Eye, nose and throat damage, skin irritation
Ergonomic	Poor design of facilities/homes/centres	Awkward postures leading to musculoskeletal strain or injury

FIGURE 3.1 The four-step risk management process

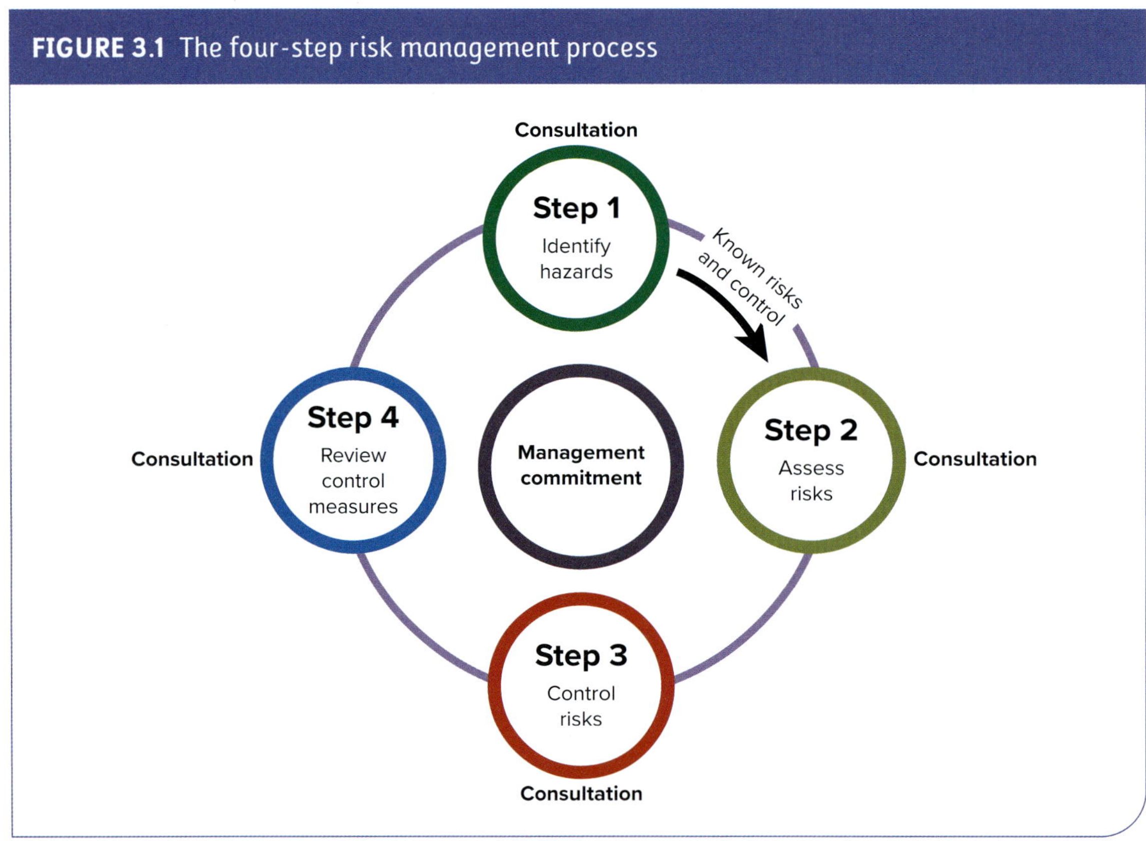

1. Actual and potential hazards are identifiable in a range of practical ways, from using our senses (observation, smell and hearing) to completing inspections, or during verbal handovers with colleagues.
2. Assessing requires determining the likelihood of harm and potential consequence or severity of the result if the hazard is not managed. Risks should be assessed using a risk matrix, which assists in prioritising the risks from low to high. The matrix will be explored further later in this chapter.

3. Once a hazard has been identified and assessed, strategies are required to limit, minimise or eliminate any harm arising (or potentially arising) from it. The hierarchy of control is the most effective system for controlling or reducing an identified risk.
4. Outcomes of the risk management actions implemented are reviewed and monitored to determine the success of the strategies, or whether further action or training is required in order to keep the risk level low or non-existent. Evaluation also forms part of the continuous improvement process.

Workers will experience various hazards and associated risks within their work roles. They also have a legal and ethical responsibility to carry out their work in a way that is not harmful to their own or others' health, safety and wellbeing. It is critical for a worker to maintain workplace safety by identifying workplace hazards and implementing risk management processes to minimise or eliminate risk.

STEP 1: IDENTIFYING HAZARDS IN THE WORKPLACE

Each organisation and service is required to have specific processes in place for identifying hazards. Hazard identification should be carried out on a regular basis, but also in the event of:

- new work practices or equipment being implemented
- new venues/facilities being used
- changes being made to work practices
- new clients being taken on
- an increase in incidents or near misses.

Processes in many organisations include inspecting the workplace, staff consultation, and a review of data such as safety audits, incident reports, and accident or near-miss reports.

- *Workplace inspections:* A PCBU is responsible for regularly inspecting the workplace and observing work practices, equipment and the general condition of the facility or service. Workplace inspections are conducted to detect faults with equipment, infrastructure, processes and resources. Inspections conducted regularly and consistently will detect hazards in a timely manner, before they deteriorate further and increase the likelihood of risk occurring. Workplace inspections may be undertaken by managers, supervisors and WHS safety committee members using observational skills and formal checklists. In the home and community care setting, individuals' homes become an employee's workplace and workplace inspections must therefore be carried out prior to or on the first home visit. A formal checklist will be used to identify the hazards room by room and in the home's external surroundings. Once inspections are completed the data will be reviewed, the hazards assessed for risk and an action plan formulated.
- *Safety audits:* Safety audits are essential to ensure early detection and monitoring of hazards and risks. Such audits range from handwashing procedures to equipment audits to detect faults or malfunctions. Regular formal and informal audits by safety representatives allow for honest, reliable, accurate and unbiased data to be collected and interpreted. Once the data is collated, interpreted and considered, significant changes can occur, including changes in policies and procedures, with the aim to limit, minimise and/or exclude risk and increase health, safety and wellbeing.
- *Staff consultation:* PCBUs are obliged under the *WHS Act 2011* to consult with staff on matters related to workplace health and safety. Hazard

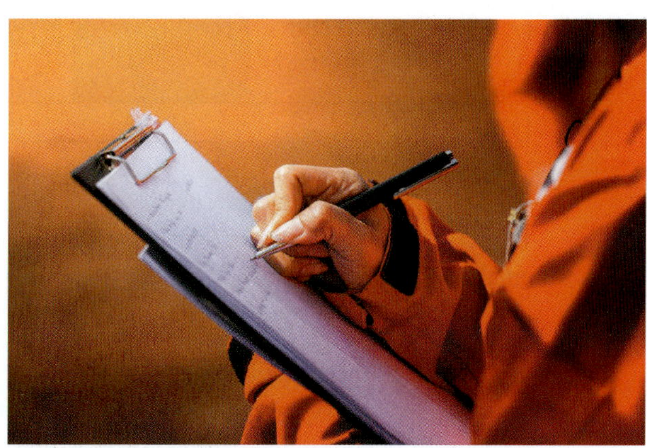

Thank you for your assistant/iStock/Getty Images Plus

Safety audits are essential to manage hazards and risks

identification can be discussed formally in regular staff meetings, in "toolbox talks" or with the workplace's WHS committee, and informally while on the floor or in the break room. Staff also should feel comfortable enough to approach team leaders or management to verbally report hazards and then submit the appropriate documentation.

- *Data reviews:* Information from safety audits, incident/accident and near-miss reports, complaints and sick leave records should be reviewed to identify if any common hazards are identified or if patterns identify the existence of potential hazards. Safety data sheets and equipment instruction manuals can also be consulted to identify possible hazards. The data is then used to develop strategies to minimise the risk associated with the actual or potential hazard.

STEP 2: RISK ASSESSMENT

The risk assessment of any hazard considers two key measurements:

- The *level* of risk–the likelihood of any injury, illness or possible death arising from the hazard.
- The *consequence* of the risk–the possible extent of harm arising from the risk, which could be simple or complex.

Risks associated with a hazard are typically assessed using a risk matrix (Figure 3.2) and can be classed as follows:

- *Low/minor:* situations where there is a limited chance of someone being injured.
- *Medium/moderate:* situations where there is a chance of someone being hurt.
- *High/major:* situations where it is likely that someone will be hurt.

The rating given to the hazard will determine if the hazard needs to be dealt with immediately or can be addressed at a later date.

FIGURE 3.2 Risk matrix example

	Likelihood				
Consequence	Rare	Unlikely	Possible	Likely	Almost certain
Minor: potential first aid	Low	Low	Low	Medium	Medium
Moderate: potential medical treatment for injury or illness	Low	Low	Medium	Medium	High
Major: potential serious injury or fatality	Low	Medium	Medium	High	High

Risk assessments should be conducted on any new activity, client or equipment, and be documented on the appropriate organisational tool. A risk assessment document should not only outline how severe the risk might be, but also what action should be taken to control the risk and the urgency of controlling it.

STEP 3: RISK CONTROL

Risk control is the most important step in the risk management process. The WHS Act and industry best practice endorse the **hierarchy of control** as the most effective strategy for managing and controlling risk (see Figure 3.3). The means of controlling risk are ranked from the highest to lowest levels of protection and reliability.

FIGURE 3.3 Hierarchy of control

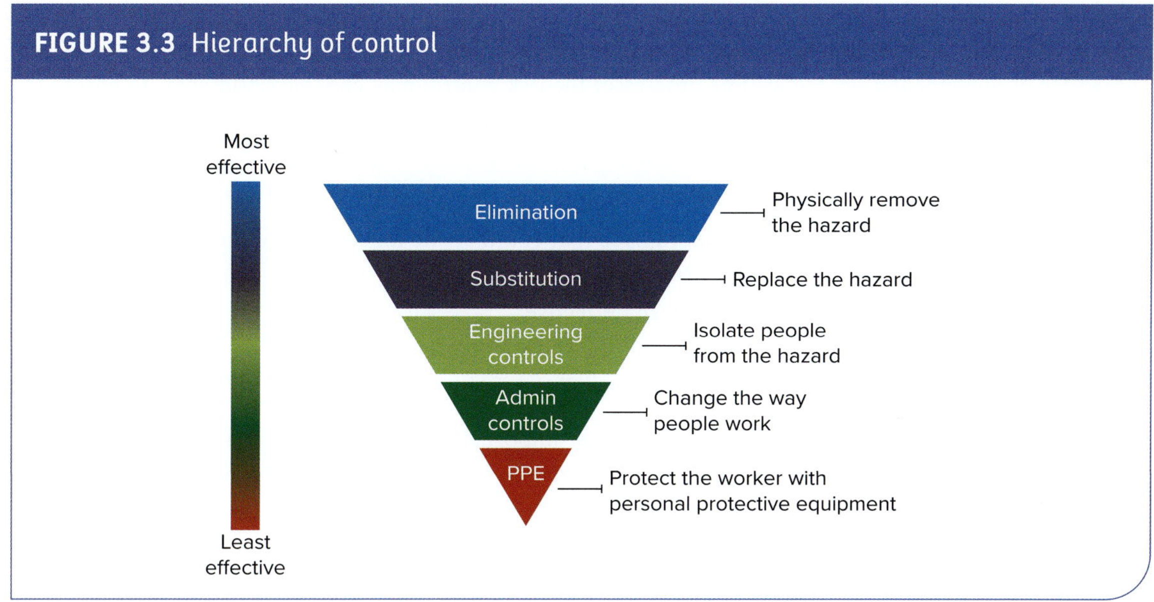

Source: Adapted from https://www.pinnacol.com/knowledge-center/hierarchy-of-controls-explained-workplace-safety

The WHS Act states that elimination of risk is the required first step if it is "reasonably practicable" to do so. Reasonably practicable in relation to WHS is what could be done at the time and with the appropriate knowledge to ensure health and safety. At times, risk control needs to be implemented immediately when the hazard is identified to ensure that no one comes to harm, with longer-term action implemented afterwards to ensure the ongoing safety of employees and clients.

The PCBU or WHS committee will consider the likelihood of hazards and risks occurring and the degree of harm that could result and then make a knowledge- or evidence-based decision on how to control the risk.

When the risks are physical or equipment-related, elimination can be the most practical measure. However, when risks are structural or related to human behaviour or condition, the emphasis may be placed on minimising the risk.

Risk control actions will be made known to all employees who may be at risk of a documented hazard. Employees should be alerted via team meetings, updated policies and procedures, or specific training related to the risk control implemented.

PRACTICE POINT

We are all accountable for risk management in the workplace. In the event you notice anything that could be dangerous for any person, you must do something about it in a timely manner. For example, if there is a water or urine spill on the floor (the hazard), the older person may slip in it and fall (risk) and injure themselves (which can be catastrophic). The following actions are required:

1. Modify the risk by placing a "wet floor" sign by the spill. This will alert people to the hazard.
2. Access appropriate equipment and mop up the spill. This action will further modify the risk.
3. Leave the sign in place until the floor is dry. This action further modifies the risk until the dry floor eliminates it.
4. Report and document the hazard if it is a result of a leaking tap or something of that nature.

STEP 4: REVIEWING AND MONITORING

Once a risk control has been implemented, it must be evaluated as to its success. It may have been successful at the time of implementation, but as time progresses the risk control may become unsuitable. To ensure the continued health and safety of employees and the workplace, the PCBU must ensure regular reviews of all implemented risk control methods.

WHS regulations also require risk controls to be reviewed in the following instances:

- before a change is introduced in a workplace that could create a new or different risk that the current control method won't manage effectively
- when data shows the control measure isn't effective
- when new hazards or risks are identified
- when requested by a health and safety representative or committee.

Risk management is a continuous cycle of utmost importance in an industry dealing with vulnerable people and physically and emotionally high-risk work. All employees, whatever their position, have an active role to play in identifying, controlling and evaluating the risks in the organisation.

COMMON RISK MANAGEMENT SOLUTIONS IN THE AGED CARE WORKPLACE

As stated earlier, common hazards and risks associated with aged care are physical and psychological. Musculoskeletal injuries and mental health issues can be minimised with good risk controls, such as:

- safe handling and lifting techniques–for example, the manual lifting of clients should be eliminated with the provision of appropriate aids and equipment such as hoists, slide sheets and wheeled equipment
- current care plans that outline safe handling methods and equipment required
- a regular maintenance schedule of all equipment
- regular staff training on safe handling and equipment use
- policies and training on carrying objects safely
- policies and procedures that address workplace bullying and harassment
- access to and encouragement of the use of employee counselling and support services
- provision of PPE
- a well-maintained environment that is well lit and free of clutter and obstructions
- training in behaviour management and personal protective behaviours.

DISTRESSED BEHAVIOURS

Distressed behaviours are those behaviours that may cause stress or create a risk of harm to an individual or their surroundings. Care workers may experience a range of distressed behaviours from people in their care, as well as from family or visitors. It is essential for care workers to be able to interact with people and to know how to deal with these behaviours professionally and appropriately. Examples of behaviours that have potential to cause harm include:

- aggression
- agitation
- anxiety and distress
- sexual disinhibition.

On occasion, behaviours of concern may be demonstrated by colleagues and should be addressed according to workplace policies and procedures in conjunction with code of conduct guidelines.

Other distressed behaviours that present a risk to care workers may include:

- self-injury or self-harm by the older person
- refusal to follow treatment procedures for medical conditions
- absconding (running away)
- destruction of property.

When reporting, responding to and recording any client risk factors, including distressed behaviours, care workers should always follow their organisation's policies and procedures. They should also:

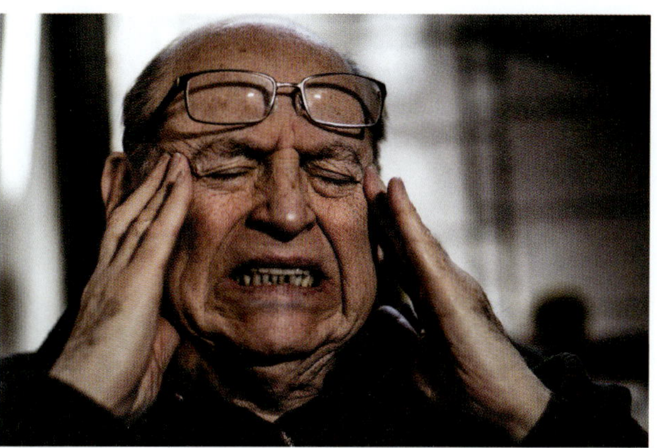

Care workers should be able to deal with distressed behaviours in a professional and appropriate manner

Steve Prezant/Getty Images

- follow any strategies outlined in a documented behaviour management plan
- complete an incident report and make notes in the care plan or other documentation of relevance to the organisation
- focus on the behaviours and not on the person displaying the behaviours
- maintain a professional approach and treat the individual with dignity
- listen to what is being said
- acknowledge any threats to self-harm or to harm other people or property
- inform the person of their legal obligation to report any types of risks to the appropriate authority, including health professionals.

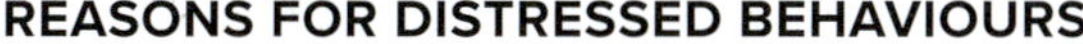

REASONS FOR DISTRESSED BEHAVIOURS

Distressed behaviours may exist or develop for various reasons and can be triggered or caused by environmental, psychological and medical factors. Behaviours are often a means of communication, especially in people with dementia, brain injury or developmental disability. Some behaviours may be linked to stress, anxiety, substance abuse, medications, pain or discomfort, and to medical conditions such as brain tumours, delirium, hormone imbalance or urinary tract infections. It is important to consider that such behaviours may be occurring as a result of the inability to communicate fear, anger or frustration, confusion, disorientation and fatigue.

Distressed behaviours are challenging for the affected person as well as family, visitors, bystanders and staff. It is extremely important that an initial assessment of the situation occurs before intervention to ensure safety for all is maintained, and to identify any triggers, escalators or preventative strategies. Having a clear understanding of what can trigger a behaviour, and how to prevent escalation of the behaviour, can lead to minimisation of harm and risk to the person, the care worker and the community. A planned and coordinated approach to the behaviour will always elicit the most favourable outcome.

3.1.4 Reporting

HAZARDS AND RISKS

Reporting hazards and risks is key to maintaining a safe workplace and plays an important role in preventive action. The first step in reporting existing or potential hazards will usually be to contact your supervisor, team leader or manager. Depending on the nature and urgency of the risk, you may also need to contact a health professional such as a doctor or the emergency services.

The existing or potential hazards will also need to be documented using the appropriate process, forms and/or electronic platform. This report should be provided to the registered nurse (RN), the supervisor

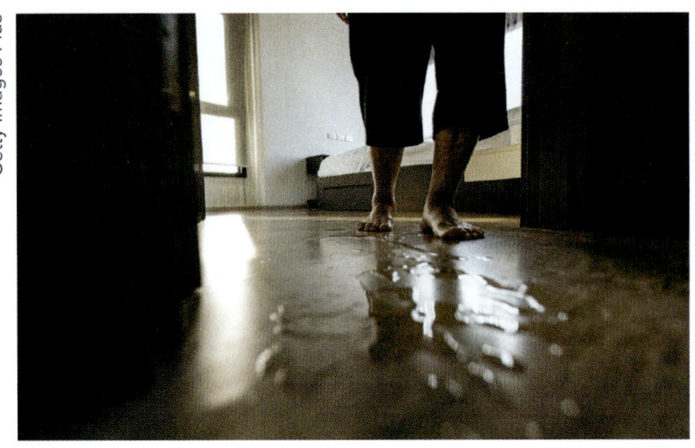
Satjawat Boontanataweepol/iStock/ Getty Images Plus

To maintain a safe workplace any hazards, such as a liquid spill on the floor, should be reported immediately

and/or the manager and the WHS representative as soon as possible. However, there will be times when accidents or incidents occur as a result of hazards that could not have been planned for or avoided.

INCIDENTS AND ACCIDENTS

Care workers, by law, need to report and record all incidents and injuries in the workplace according to regulations and the organisational practice. Incidents and accidents need to be reported to the facility or service within 24 hours of them occurring. The facility or service is then obliged by law to report any accidents resulting in major injury or death to their state WHS authority. All injuries or illnesses must be recorded in an injury register.

Information provided in the incident or accident reports will be used to identify how to prevent the incident or injury from reoccurring, whether a new risk has arisen that needs controls applied, and if further training is required or a review of a procedure is needed.

The key incident reporting categories are as follows:

- *Near-miss reporting:* A near miss is when an incident occurs, but no accident or injury results. Reporting the incident means the organisation has an obligation to remove and control the hazard. A record must be kept by the employer, and these records can be used to continuously improve workplace processes and to prevent the incident reoccurring. Reporting a near miss forms part of the professional approach to safety and open disclosure.
- *Accident reports:* Reporting accidents is a legal and ethical requirement but also assists with research, continuous improvement, policy reform and changes in the way we perform our roles. Accident reports also help to identify, eliminate and manage risks and hazards. Accidents occurring at work should be reported immediately to a supervisor and authorities, whether they appear severe or minor. Minor injuries could be sprains and strains, cuts, or any other injury that may not involve having to take time off work. It is best practice to record the injury, even if it seems minor, in the event it develops into something more serious in the future.

  Major injuries/incidents are those that could lead to significant time off work and medical treatment, permanent disability or even death. In this instance, the state WHS regulator will need to be contacted immediately and certain actions taken to assist in an investigation.

  Investigating how and why an accident occurred leads to better prevention in the future. Minor accidents can be investigated internally. This is another process in place, especially in residential aged care facilities (RACFs), home and community care and disability services, which leads to the identification and management of hazards and risks. Investigating accidents forms part of continuous improvement and the prevention of further same or similar accidents and ensures that PCBUs and employees are responsible and accountable for care.
- *Damage reports:* Any damage done to equipment or property of the client, care worker or service needs to be recorded in an incident report. Damaged equipment must also be tagged and logged in maintenance logs to ensure it doesn't present a risk to others.
- *Medication errors:* Missed medication, incorrect medication or dosage given, or client refusal all need to be recorded in an incident report and be verbally reported to the RN or supervisor, according to organisational practices.

When completing any incident or accident reporting, it is important to:

- be objective–state the facts, not feelings
- be clear–easy to read and understand
- be correct–make sure all details are accurate

- be concise–only include necessary information (who, what, where and when)
- complete all sections of the report.

An example of an incident form can be found at https://www.safework.nsw.gov.au/safety-starts-here/easywhs/reporting/template. Reports and records should be kept securely in the office or electronically, where workers and management can access them subject to approval, for as long as legally deemed necessary.

3.1.5 Workplace injuries

Due to the close physical nature and type of tasks carried out by care workers, the risk of injury can be high. When a worker is injured at work, there are certain responsibilities and actions they and their employer must take. Injured workers are required to:

- seek immediate assistance, first aid and/or medical treatment
- document and report the injury or illness as soon as practical. If you are unable to do this yourself due to injury, it can be completed on your behalf by another person
- complete a workers compensation claim if necessary
- provide a medical certificate, or a fit-to-work or return-to-work certificate, issued by a treating doctor (according to the situation)
- comply with the treatment ordered by the treating doctor
- comply with the return-to-work program
- cooperate with all involved in the management of the situation
- arrange for all expenses associated with the injury or illness to be paid by the relevant insurance company, which may involve providing receipts and invoices
- ensure the PCBU and insurance company have all the necessary contact and payment details.

Your employer must:

- provide first aid
- record the injury in the incident and injury register
- inform their state regulator if the injury is deemed serious
- inform the organisation's insurer
- assist the worker to apply for workers compensation if required
- have a documented return-to-work program
- provide suitable employment while the worker recovers at work or returns to work.

WORKERS COMPENSATION AND INJURY MANAGEMENT

If an effective and committed WHS system is in place, fewer workers will experience work-related injury, illness, death or disability. Workers compensation and injury management laws in Australia reinforce the essential need to have a current and continuous workers compensation insurance policy and a strategy in place for the injured worker to return to work. The WHS Act includes guidance and recommendation for workers compensation and injury management schemes. Workers compensation in Australia is a "no fault" scheme, meaning that an injured person has no obligation to prove negligence of the PCBU. Injury management can form part of workers compensation or can be an independent management strategy without workers compensation being enforced. Workers compensation often involves a monetary component where the injured worker's income is paid in the form of income replacement payments, medical expenses payments, reimbursed hospital stay costs or, sometimes, lump sum payments. Should a death occur during the course of work, payments may be payable to a family member on behalf of the deceased worker. Under workers compensation, formal return-to-work programs exist whereby the injured worker is encouraged and supported to return to work when able without pressure to return too quickly. Injury management can include returning to work on reduced duties, taking on a different role temporarily, and modification of equipment and work environments.

For further workers compensation and injury management information, refer to the WHS Act.

PENALTIES FOR BREACHES OF WHS LEGISLATION AND REGULATIONS

Each state's regulator has set financial or other penalties (including prison terms) for breaches of the WHS Act by employers and individuals. A breach is considered to be:

- any action that places a person at risk of illness, injury or death
- a failure to take action to prevent or avoid a situation that is risky
- a failure to comply with regulatory requirements.

Most of the WHS Acts of the states and territories outline breaches as category 1, 2 or 3.

- *Category 1:* Gross negligence or reckless conduct that exposes a person to risk of death or serious injury.
- *Category 2:* Failure to comply with health and safety duty that exposes a person to risk of death, serious injury or illness.
- *Category 3:* Failure to comply with health and safety duty.

There are also the perceived penalties of defamation and loss of reputation that a breach or infringement of the WHS Act can have for an individual or business.

WORKPLACE SCENARIO

Distressed behaviours and safety

Ian has multi-infarct dementia (vascular dementia) and is prone to anxiety and mood swings. He has been assessed as having "sundowning" and can become particularly anxious at around 5 pm when, it has been identified, he used to return home from work. He now regularly attends a program that provides activities for people who exhibit agitation in the late afternoon and/or early evening, and this calm, purposeful environment supports Ian to be "himself".

One day, however, Ian becomes extremely agitated. He starts to yell, bangs his fist on a table, runs his fingers through his hair repeatedly and grinds his teeth. To reassure him, one of the care workers, Ellie, places her hand on his arm and speaks quietly, but he pushes her away and she almost falls. At this point, her colleague Will intervenes and advises Ellie to stay calm and to fetch their supervisor, Mary. When Mary arrives, Ian is somewhat settled but still appears anxious. Mary suggests that when Ian feels calmer, he be taken to his room where he will be assessed for pain or discomfort and other possible triggers for his behaviour.

Mary advises Ellie and Will that they need to be safe, and that the following protective measures are necessary should anyone behave in this way again:

- Stay calm.
- Move quietly and in a non-threatening manner.
- Remain at a safe distance from the person.
- Call for assistance.
- Don't confront the person.
- Don't invade their personal space.
- Don't turn your back towards the person.
- Try to maintain positive body language.
- Remain near an exit.

Mary reminds Ellie and Will that their safety is most important. If situations arise that cannot be managed, they should leave and seek help, she says.

CHECK YOUR UNDERSTANDING

1. Brainstorm a list of hazards you may encounter in the workplace.
2. What possible risks might a care worker encounter in the workplace?
3. How do you report a hazard?
4. What is the hierarchy of control?
5. What reporting obligations do you have as a care worker?

3.2 FOLLOWING SAFE WORK PRACTICES FOR MANUAL HANDLING

Manual handling is a regular requirement of the care worker's everyday role; therefore, it is essential for workers to have an effective understanding and awareness of manual handling procedures. **Manual handling** refers to the action of using your body to move people or objects. Specific actions include twisting, carrying, reaching, bending, pushing and pulling. Some typical manual handling tasks required of the care worker include assisting a person to get in or out of bed or to sit or stand from a chair, assisting in showering, pushing a wheelchair and making a bed. If workers don't use specific techniques, skills, knowledge and/or equipment, they may sustain injuries that could be temporary or permanent. For example, they may be injured during a lift or when transferring a person because:

- the equipment was an incorrect choice for the person's weight
- the person didn't have the strength to assist
- the worker didn't use the correct equipment
- the worker didn't use the correct technique.

If risks are identified, information on the methods and equipment a worker should use when performing manual handling tasks should be outlined in a person's care plan.

3.2.1 Safe manual handling in the aged care workplace

HAZARDOUS MANUAL TASKS

A hazardous manual task is any task that involves:

- sustained awkward posture
- repetitive movements
- repeated, sustained or high force
- handling of people
- unstable, unbalanced or hard-to-hold loads.

Continuous exposure to hazardous manual tasks puts care workers at risk of musculoskeletal injury if good techniques and equipment aren't used. Table 3.3 outlines the common manual handling tasks that place the body at risk.

TABLE 3.3 Common hazardous manual tasks/manual handling hazards in the workplace

Hazardous manual task	Manual handling task	Risk
Lifting	Transferring individuals	Back injury; shoulder, arm or neck strain from repeated load lifting
Twisting	Transferring, assisting to walk, moving loads	Back injury, sprain or strain of abdominal muscles from twisting the body when moving heavy or unpredictable weights/loads
Repetitive movements	Showering, vacuuming, cleaning surfaces	Muscle strain or fatigue from short repetitive movements
Bending	Bed making, cleaning, assisting a person to dress	Back, neck or knee strain from repeated bending
Reaching	Bed making, putting things on shelves, cleaning showers/ baths	Back, neck or shoulder strain due to reaching away from the body or lifting and moving items that are a long way from the body
Pushing and pulling	Moving wheelchairs, trolleys or beds	Back, stomach or arm strain if load is heavy or awkward or equipment is poorly maintained
Awkward sustained posture	Showering, cleaning and grooming tasks	Muscle strain or nerve compression

As hazardous manual tasks can lead to injuries that may have a long-term impact on a care worker, workplaces emphasise the importance of following manual handling policies and procedures which have been written in line with the National Code of Practice for Manual Handling.

NATIONAL CODE OF PRACTICE FOR MANUAL HANDLING

The National Code of Practice for Manual Handling (the Code) has the purpose of providing practical, realistic and achievable advice on how to meet the requirements of the National Standard for Manual Handling in order to reduce workplace injuries and for the identification, assessment and control of risks arising from manual handling activities in workplaces.

The Code works on the general principles of reducing risk by using work design and equipment to:

- minimise the lifting and lowering forces exerted in manual handling
- avoid the need for bending, twisting and reaching movements
- reduce pushing, pulling, carrying and holding.

The Code provides templates and questions for the employer and their staff to work through to determine the best means available to reduce the risk of the manual handling task. Just like standard hazard identification in the workplace, manual handling uses risk assessment and risk control measures.

3.2.2 Managing manual handling tasks

As mentioned earlier in the chapter, hazard identification is a process of identifying any foreseeable hazards before an accident or injury occurs. It is most important to identify manual handling hazards as soon as possible to prevent the occurrence and reoccurrence of manual handling issues.

A risk assessment of all manual handling tasks or activities is essential in preventing injury, disability or death. Risk assessment should be conducted prior to a new work practice being introduced and when an injury has occurred due to a manual handling task. A risk assessment of a manual handling activity such as mobilising a person should include assessing the person's ability to mobilise, risk of falling, and ability to comprehend what is being requested of them. When conducting a risk assessment, the PCBU or WHS committee and those actually performing the tasks should assess the following areas:

- actions and movements undertaken when performing the role
- workplace/station design and environment
- posture and position
- duration and frequency of manual handling
- weights, loads and forces
- age, skills and experience of the personal care worker.

Hazardous manual handling activities are a major cause of injury in personal support work and therefore the care worker must be familiar with control measures in place that will increase safety and minimise injury. The aim of control measures is to eliminate the risk of injury by:

- developing and implementing policies and procedures
- encouraging the use of equipment such as mechanical hoists and mobility aids
- maintaining equipment in good order, ensuring servicing of equipment is regular and thorough
- educating and training staff in the use of equipment and work practices
- encouraging individuals to do as much as possible for themselves safely
- working effectively as a team
- managing time effectively and not rushing or taking short cuts.

Other aspects of the hierarchy of control can also be used to decrease the risk involved in manual handling tasks. Care workers should be given the opportunity to trial the control measures and provide their feedback before the control is implemented permanently.

Workers must apply control measures to avoid hazards and to work safely. In most cases, control measures are well known and can be applied to many situations. These should be outlined as follows:

- in the older person's care plan
- in workplace policies and procedures manuals
- at training sessions.

Employers should regularly review the risk controls in place and provide annual refresher training in manual handling training to ensure staff are up to date with current practices.

BODY MECHANICS

Safe manual handling is based on an understanding of body mechanics and correct techniques for manual handling. Body mechanics refers to the interactive relationship between the musculoskeletal and nervous systems to efficiently maintain balance and posture while performing manual handling activities. The musculoskeletal system is the primary system at risk when performing manual handling activities; therefore, the following techniques and body mechanics are recommended:

- Maintain a wide base of support, with feet apart to the width of the shoulders, to distribute weight evenly.
- Keep the centre of gravity low by bending at the knees, not the hips.
- Keep loads as close to the body as possible so as not to reach and stretch, putting pressure on muscles, ligaments and tendons. Keeping the load close also helps in maintaining balance.
- Brace the abdominal muscles.
- Avoid bending, stretching and twisting.
- Use both arms and legs.
- Use the legs and leg muscles, not your back.
- Avoid any sudden or jerky movements.

FIGURE 3.4 Safe lifting techniques

BEND YOUR KNEES AND SQUAT
USE MUSCLES IN LEGS AND ARMS, NOT YOUR BACK
KEEP ITEMS CLOSE TO YOUR BODY

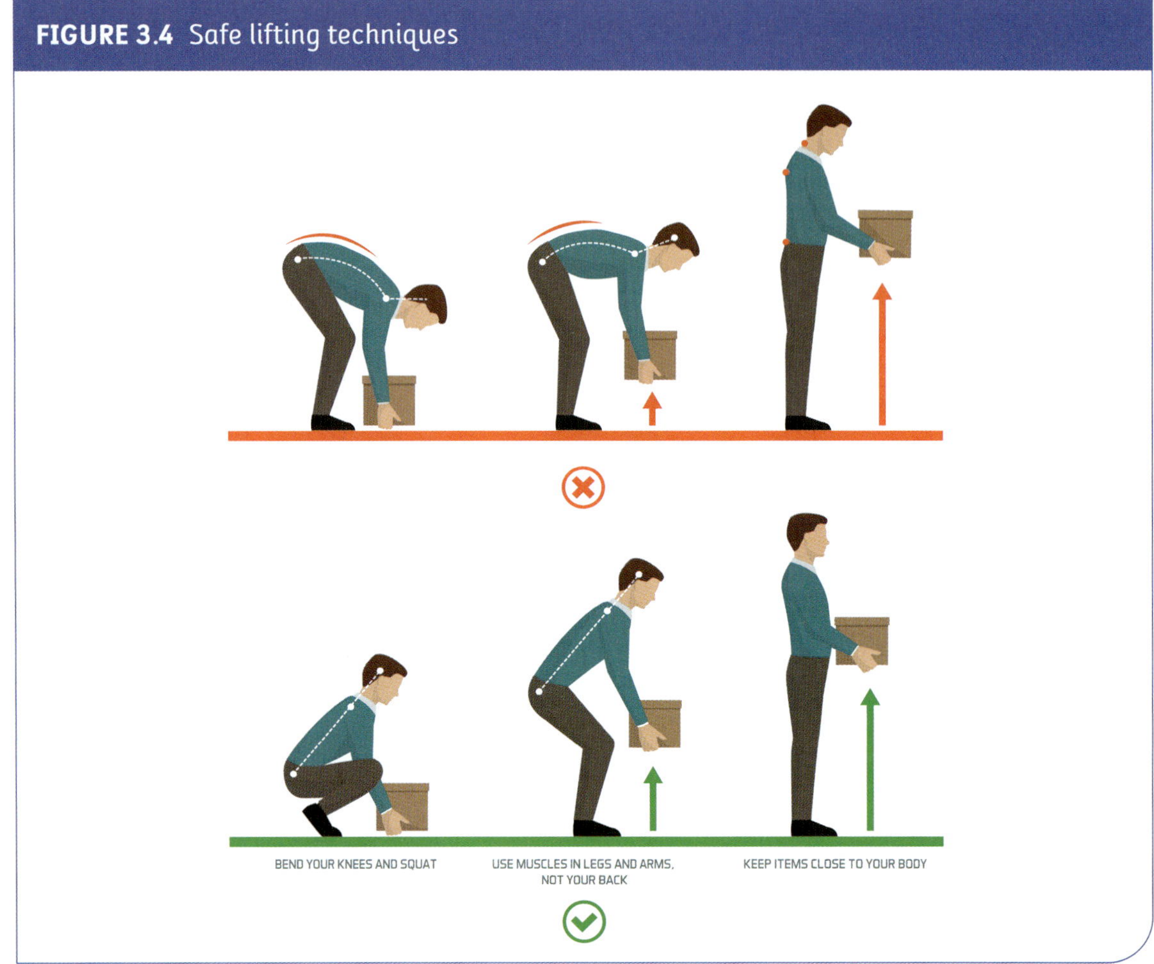

Source: elenabsl/Shutterstock.com

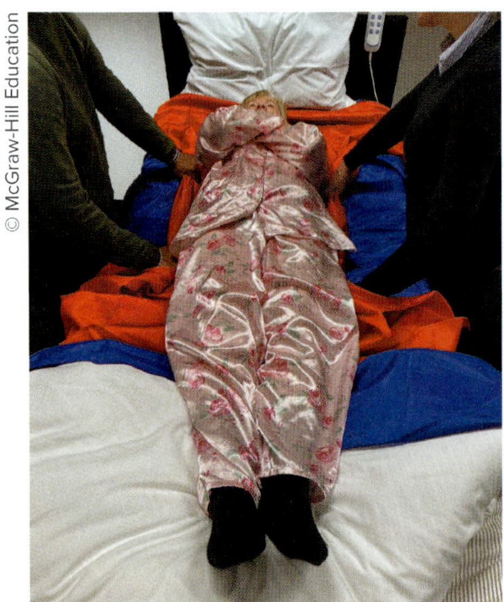

Manual handling equipment includes slide sheets, as shown here

- Push, rather than pull, whenever possible.
- Have feet facing the direction in which you are moving.

A prime example of the above recommendations can be seen in Figure 3.4 when applied to safe lifting techniques.

To prevent wear and tear on the body and to extend the working life of a personal care worker, it is imperative to avoid placing their back and joints at risk. The implementation of manual handling equipment and practices aims to preserve, protect and reduce the likelihood of injury.

MANUAL HANDLING EQUIPMENT

Before performing any manual task or activity, it is essential to risk assess the situation and decide whether an aid or specific piece of equipment could be used to make the task safer for all concerned. Manual handling equipment can vary from a small trolley to a large hoist. Other equipment includes items such as wheelchairs, slide sheets, walking belts, and mobility aids such as walking sticks and rails. It is the PCBU's responsibility to ensure that employees using such equipment are trained, instructed and skilled in its use. Manufacturers of the equipment and aids have the responsibility to provide easy-to-follow instructions and care and maintenance requirements. The employee has the responsibility to NOT use the aid or equipment if they have not received training or instruction. The employee also has the responsibility to use the equipment or aid as intended and not inappropriately. Any damage or performance issues must be reported immediately.

MANUAL HANDLING PROCEDURE

Safe manual handling procedures should be clearly documented in a manual handling policy, or in a separate guide that is accessible to all employers. Depending on the organisation or facility, procedures could include lifting and transferring people, assisting with showering and bathing, completing domestic assistance tasks, and feeding and transporting people. Procedural instructions should be easy to read and are best accompanied by visuals to ensure complete comprehension. Best practice for facilities or services would be access to a video library that contains short clips on how to perform all manual handling tasks safely. Staff should continue to receive training on manual handling procedures on an annual basis so that the PCBU and the personal care workers themselves are aware that they are safely carrying out manual handling tasks according to procedures.

WORKPLACE SCENARIO

Safe manual handling

Kim, a care worker, is about to attend to Selin's personal care, and it becomes apparent he requires assistance from a colleague to help Selin out of bed and into a commode chair for showering. Kim is aware that other care staff are busy, and he chooses to move Selin himself. Selin, who is obese and has difficulty supporting her own weight, reminds Kim that he needs to get a mobility belt and position the commode chair adjacent to the bed, so that she doesn't have to move very far. However, Kim can't locate the belt and decides to go ahead without it.

Kim assists Selin to sit up and moves her legs over the side of the bed; however, when he attempts to support her as she stands, they both fall onto the bed. Selin is very upset, and Kim is extremely apologetic. He makes Selin comfortable and goes and asks his colleague Harry for help. Harry brings the mobility belt. Before they enter Selin's unit, they discuss what they will do:

- Harry anticipates that Selin will have difficulty standing and that both he and Kim will use the belt to support her. If Selin is reluctant, they will use the standing lifter that is available in the equipment room.
- They both check the environment for hazards, including assessing that there is enough room for the procedure and that the belt and the commode chair are the correct size for Selin.
- Harry then explains the procedure to Selin. He outlines what he and Kim will do and what is expected of Selin. They obtain her consent to proceed.

When the procedure is accomplished, Kim takes Selin to the shower. He asks Harry to return in 30 minutes to assist with transferring Selin to a wheelchair so that she can attend the morning activities in the lounge area. Later that day, Kim and Harry discuss what happened and Kim confirms he will ask for assistance in the future as this "near miss" could have resulted in injuries to both Selin and himself.

Harry also reminds him to report the incident to their supervisor, Chin.

CHECK YOUR UNDERSTANDING

1. Name common hazardous manual tasks in the workplace.
2. How can hazardous manual tasks be managed?
3. Describe body mechanics and why it is important in manual handling.
4. You are to assist a client from the bed to a shower chair, but their hoist is one you are unfamiliar with. What action should you take?
5. Identify three control measures that could eliminate or reduce the risk of manual handling injuries.

3.3 FOLLOWING SAFE WORK PRACTICES FOR INFECTION CONTROL

Exposure to infection can be high for care workers. The spread of infection is a hazard that presents a risk both to personal care workers and to clients. Exposure to bodily fluids and the possible inhalation of infectious aerosol droplets are the two greatest infection control risks faced by care workers.

Like all other hazards, risk controls are developed to ensure the risk is eliminated or minimised as much as possible. Infection control procedures centre on minimising the transfer of disease through the implementation of standard precautions. Standard precautions are the basic means of preventing the spread of infection via hand washing, the use of PPE, safe disposal of waste, and regular cleaning and the safe handling of laundry and linen. Employees should have access to a wide range of PPE, well-stocked handwashing facilities and hand sanitiser.

When infectious and transmissible diseases such as influenza, gastroenteritis or COVID-19 are present in the workplace, additional precautions are implemented as standard precautions may not be adequate to prevent transmission.

All risks of infection MUST be reported. In the event you are unwell, you must stay away from the workplace until you are free of symptoms.

Infection control is covered in greater detail in Chapter 16.

3.4 CONTRIBUTING TO SAFE WORK PRACTICES IN THE WORKPLACE

Safe work practices are essential to ensure the health, safety and wellbeing of everyone in the workplace. Safe work practices are guided by an organisation's policies and procedures, and best practice guidelines, as informed by evidence-based research and findings. Organisations develop safe operating procedures or safe work procedures to accompany equipment and resources in conjunction with manufacturers' recommendations.

Manual handling and infection control, in particular, require safe operating procedures. The care worker is required to contribute to safe workplace practices in a variety of situations, especially those that impact on others, by:

- understanding and complying with safety signs and symbols
- raising WHS issues or concerns with the designated persons and according to organisational procedures
- participating in workplace safety meetings, inspections and consultative activities
- contributing to the development and implementation of safe workplace policies and procedures.

3.4.1 WHS responsibilities

SAFETY SIGNS AND SYMBOLS

The display of safety signs and symbols assists in keeping the workplace safe by providing quick visual references in regard to the location of key emergency equipment, what PPE is required for particular areas or tasks, and the locations of specific hazards such as chemicals and biological waste (see Figure 3.5).

It is important that care workers know the meaning of each sign and follow the directions they provide.

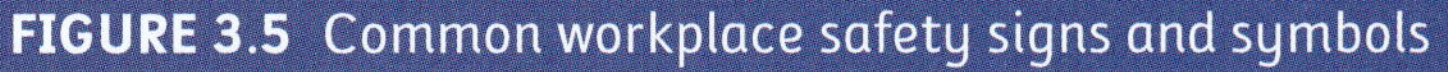

FIGURE 3.5 Common workplace safety signs and symbols

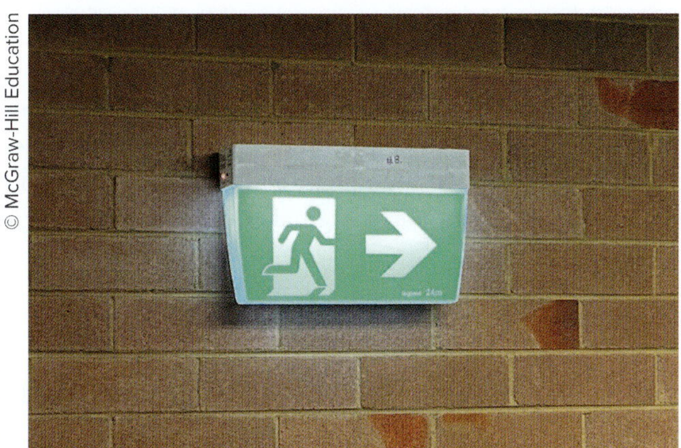

(a) Emergency exit

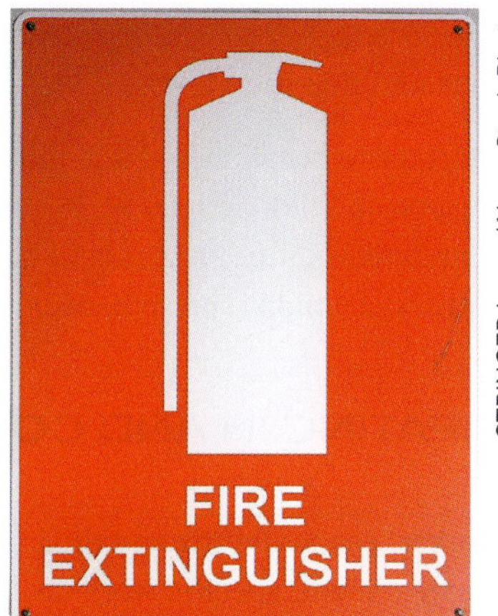

(b) Fire extinguisher location

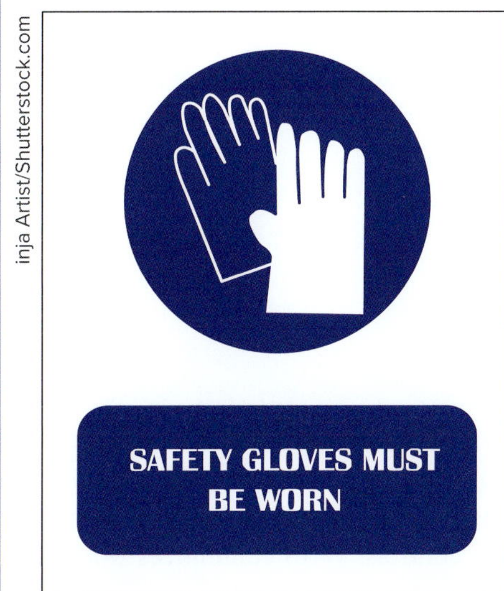

(c) PPE required in the area

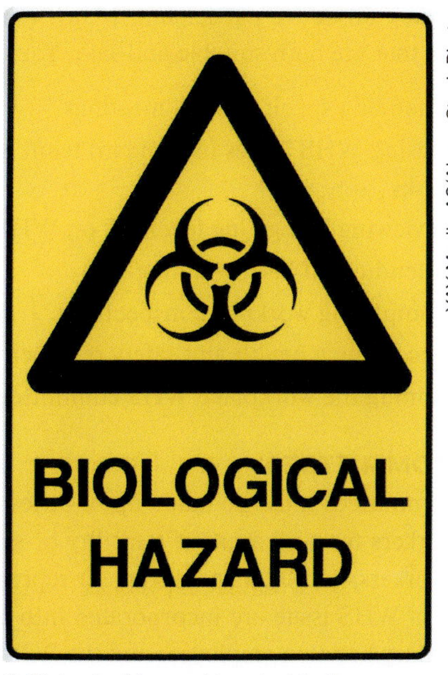

(d) Biological hazard located in the area

RAISING WHS ISSUES OR CONCERNS

Under the duty of care principle, care workers should raise any WHS concerns they come across. Reporting and sharing information concerning WHS plays a large part in protecting the health and safety both of the older people receiving services and of colleagues. Workers can do the following to raise WHS issues:

- *Write a report:* Write about the hazard in the communication book or on a hazard identification form. The report should be factual and easy to understand.
- *Raise or report the issues with the appropriate person:* Ask your WHS representative, nominee or WHS committee chairperson, or your manager, for advice on what to do.
- *Put alert tags on faulty equipment:* Attach alert tags or signs to let everyone know there is a problem with the equipment and that it is not to be used.
- *Complete a hazard identification form:* Pass this form onto the WHS representative, supervisor or manager in order for the hazardous equipment to be repaired or removed.
- *Notify all workers at handover:* Advise all workers replacing a shift about any identified hazards.
- *Telephone a supervisor:* Inform a supervisor of a hazard or risk as soon as possible if it is of a serious and urgent nature.

It is important to remember that contractors, suppliers and manufacturers of equipment and goods also have WHS responsibilities. Serious WHS concerns that are not acted on, or where there is a delay in correction, control or elimination of the risk, should be escalated and reported to appropriate authorities (e.g. the police, Safe Work Australia, union representative, WHS hotline or the Aged Care Safety and Quality Commission).

PARTICIPATING IN AND CONTRIBUTING TO WORK HEALTH AND SAFETY

As a care worker, you are at the frontline in identifying and feeling the impact of any WHS issues related to your work environment, specific work tasks or the people you provide services to. Under the WHS Act, the employer must consult with you and your fellow care workers about any WHS issues that may have an effect on your day-to-day role.

By being an active participant in any WHS consultation activities, you can be involved in developing solutions that are both suitable and safe. You can participate by:

- attending specific WHS meetings
- raising WHS issues in standard team meetings and making suggestions on improving procedures or tasks
- reviewing and giving feedback on WHS policies and procedures
- attending all WHS training
- completing workplace inspections
- becoming a health and safety representative
- joining the workplace WHS committee.

WHS COMMITTEES

WHS committees must be made up of at least 50 per cent workers. An effective committee will be made up of workers from all areas of a facility or service, such as catering, maintenance, care workers and allied health workers, as well as management representation. This assists in ensuring that the perspectives of all areas on a WHS issue are incorporated into any practices and risk controls. WHS committees work as an intermediary between employees and the PCBU and assist in developing procedures and reviews, identifying trends through the use of WHS data and conducting consultative activities.

HEALTH AND SAFETY REPRESENTATIVES

A **health and safety representative (HSR)** is a person who has been nominated by the workplace to be their representative to management in relation to WHS issues. An HSR must complete specific training in order to conduct this role. Workers can approach the HSR to raise issues of concern, to request their assistance in reporting concerns to management, and when seeking the latest WHS information concerning legislation or job roles. As a member of any WHS committee, the HSR will conduct workplace inspections and risk assessments and be involved in any incident or accident investigations.

WHS RESPONSIBILITIES OF THE EMPLOYER/PCBU

Aside from the responsibilities outlined earlier in the chapter, the employer has other obligations to ensure the safety of all involved in the organisation. For instance, the employer must consult all employees in relation to the following WHS matters:

- changes to and reviews of policies and procedures
- changes to work practices
- risk assessments and risk controls to be implemented
- any new WHS legislative changes.

The PCBU also has the responsibility and legal requirement to ensure that all employees are suitably qualified and skilled to carry out their job role and the responsibilities assigned to them. This includes checking and verifying qualifications and referees.

Safety and security checks are also the responsibility of the PCBU and form part of the protection for vulnerable persons such as the elderly and people with a disability. Police checks (commonly known as Australian Federal Police Checks or National Police Checks) and checking a person's immunisation status form part of the sector's recruitment process.

PCBUs are also legally required to develop and establish emergency procedures for a variety of events both internal and external. Such events include fires, floods and bomb threats, and medical emergencies such as heart attack, seizures and the like. Organisational responsibilities encompass:

- policy and procedure development and implementation
- staff education and training in the event of an emergency
- maintenance of equipment and resources
- supply of emergency equipment
- supply of first-aid assistance
- appropriate signage in appropriate places
- training exercises and drills
- developing and implementing a smoking/non-smoking policy
- designation of appropriate, accessible evacuation points.

3.4.2 Emergency procedures

While fires, chemical exposure, natural disasters or bomb threats may occur rarely, all care workers must know and be prepared for their role in the event of such an incident or emergency. Your main role will be to assist people to safety while also safeguarding yourself. Understanding emergency procedures and attending all workplace drills are critical in developing and maintaining this knowledge.

It is essential, wherever you are working, to be aware of the location of exits and safety evacuation points, fire extinguishers and blankets, and first-aid kits. This is also true if your workplace is a client's home in the community.

It is also important to know how to handle possible threats to your personal safety due to client or visitor behaviour or when working at night. Care workers can prepare for possible incidents by:

- being aware of any behavioural support triggers and strategies
- knowing the location of exit points
- being aware of and alert to changes in surroundings or individual behaviour
- keeping their mobile phone or personal duress alarm on their person at all times
- parking in well-lit areas as close as possible to the client's home in the community
- carrying a torch
- calling in arrival and departure if working at night in the community.

WORKPLACE SCENARIO

Practising emergency procedures and responsibility for security

Care managers Mal and Nic conduct sessions to practise emergency procedures four times a year, as well as at staff induction. All staff are required to attend the sessions, which are conducted to cover all shifts. Attendance is recorded for compliance purposes. In these sessions, staff:

- identify emergency evacuation routes and assembly points
- nominate the care managers to maintain current lists of people who require assistance to evacuate and what assistance they require
- nominate an evacuation coordinator for each shift—usually the fire warden
- nominate a staff member who can administer first aid
- provide training in the use of fire equipment and how to evacuate people who are immobile, frail and/or cognitively impaired
- discuss problem-solving scenarios and identify what documentation is required in the event of an emergency
- undertake an evacuation of the whole facility, including visitors.

The fire warden also explains their responsibilities, which include:

- controlling litter and other fire hazards
- organising the safe storage of hazardous chemicals and oxygen
- regularly monitoring fire doors, equipment and alarms
- providing evacuation plans that are detailed, clear, accessible and in languages that reflect the diversity of the workplace.

Nic reminds care staff they are responsible for the security of the facility and for the people who live there. He explains that these responsibilities include:

- locking the doors at dusk
- being aware of visitors and contractors entering and leaving the building
- ensuring that visitors and contractors log in and log out
- maintaining their national police check.

CHECK YOUR UNDERSTANDING

1. What actions should you take to contribute to the safety of the workplace?
2. How could the PCBU consult and collaborate with employees?
3. Why is it important for the PCBU to perform police and working with children checks?
4. What types of emergency incidents might a care worker be exposed to?
5. List four steps to take to protect your personal safety at work.

3.5 REFLECTING ON BEING SAFE AT WORK

Reflection is the art and skill of analysing and constructively reviewing a situation with the aim of gaining insights and making judgements about it. It is often used to learn and improve practices. Being safe at work requires care workers to reflect on current practices, knowledge and behaviours, as well as on their own stress levels. Debriefing is a process that adds value to reflection and assists in continuously making improvements to safety at work.

3.5.1 Maintaining current safe work practices

There are many strategies available for maintaining WHS currency in order to remain safe in the workplace. PCBUs develop policies and procedures, encourage education and development, and provide regular training for all employees as a way of remaining current and safe. Maintaining up-to-date skills and knowledge is essential for the safety of everyone in the workplace and is the responsibility both of the PCBU and of the employees themselves.

It is best practice for resources, equipment, and policies and procedures to be regularly reviewed and updated as a way of staying current and ensuring safe work practices. This means that the PCBU has a responsibility to supply access to the latest equipment and resources, as well as to provide staff with access to instruction and training in the use of such equipment.

Workplaces also implement mandatory training for staff, including hand hygiene, bullying and harassment training, manual handling and protective behaviour strategies. Continued professional development is a recommendation from the most recent Royal Commission into Aged Care.

It is anticipated that continued professional development points for care workers will be introduced. This essentially means that care workers will be required to attend a set number of hours, or to accrue a set number of points, of professional development, as occurs for other health-care professionals, in order to remain current in the industry.

3.5.2 Managing stress and fatigue

Care workers in the aged care industry can face significant stress due to the physical and emotional demands of their work, the pressure to achieve set tasks in minimal time frames, and the fatigue associated with staff shortages or conflicts.

Stressful work situations also include:

- when work becomes too difficult or problems remain unresolved
- when life feels unbalanced because of worrying about work all the time
- when people feel they cannot do a good job at work because of restrictive time frames
- dealing with loss and grief when a client dies
- lack of job security.

Such situations can make people feel worried, angry and/or anxious. These feelings are often called stress. Workers can also feel stressed about their own family problems or health problems, as well as about work or money. Stress of any type can impact on the safe performance of work and therefore needs to be addressed.

Signs and symptoms of stress and fatigue can include, but are not limited to, the following:

- feeling fatigued most of the time
- having difficulty getting organised
- often feeling angry and/or depressed
- having difficulty concentrating
- being unable to relax or sit quietly
- having difficulty sleeping.

If a worker is stressed, they may experience:

- an increase in their heart rate
- decreased blood flow to their digestive organs
- fast and shallow breathing
- tense muscles.

Each time a worker feels stress, there is an effect on the body—and this effect is cumulative. The body has no time to recover and repair when stress is ongoing or when the period between stressful situations is too short.

Burnout is a phenomenon that occurs when a worker has been exposed to unacceptably high levels of stress for a prolonged period of time. When a care worker is continuously in a stressed state or at the burn-out stage, they are more susceptible to injury.

PERSONAL MANAGEMENT STRATEGIES

Strategies for managing stress include:

- eating a healthy diet, getting enough sleep and exercising regularly
- learning relaxation techniques that suit you
- talking to a trusted family member or work colleague/supervisor
- seeking professional help through your workplace's employee assistance program (EAP), which is a confidential counselling service that offers support and assistance to those who have work-related issues that are impacting on their work safety, overall performance and wellbeing
- taking time off, if necessary
- participating in interests or hobbies outside of work.

ORGANISATIONAL STRESS MANAGEMENT ASSISTANCE

An RN, supervisor or team leader can assist a care worker who is feeling stressed or overwhelmed, by:

- referring the employee to the EAP
- providing debriefing with a professional as soon as possible after an incident of a serious nature
- allowing the employee time off to recover appropriately from a serious incident
- reallocating the employee's duties for a period of time if required
- acknowledging the impact of staff shortages and rostering work accordingly
- ensuring a fatigue management program is established, implemented and maintained
- having an open-door policy for employees and actively listening to their assessment of the causes of their stress.

The health, safety and wellbeing of all people in the workplace is supported when management, workers and the persons being cared for are committed to promoting a culture of safety through regular and consistent consultation, collaboration and risk management processes. Organisations that place a strong emphasis on workplace health and safety are of value to the overall health and wellbeing of personal care workers.

WORKPLACE SCENARIO

Managing stress and fatigue

During a recent period of lockdown, care worker Huong was asked to work longer shifts. As her team leader, Ceza, was on leave, Huong took on responsibilities she knew were beyond her scope of practice. Despite being contracted to work a 42-hour fortnight, in one month Huong had worked 200 hours and felt exhausted.

When Ceza returned, Huong spoke to her and explained she felt stressed, exhausted and on the verge of burnout. She was experiencing headaches, poor sleep, indigestion and irritability, she said, and felt her performance at work had suffered because of the increased expectations. Ceza acknowledged it was a difficult period and said that management was looking at initiatives to help staff manage their stress and fatigue.

Over the following month, Huong reached out to Ellie, who had been working at the facility for much longer than Huong. Ellie asked Huong if she would like to meet regularly for a coffee or to go for a walk after work, as they lived close to one another and shared a ride when they were rostered on at the same time. Ceza also organised regular debriefing sessions, where staff could discuss events or issues in private and work together with the more senior staff to solve problems.

At a staff meeting, the care manager, Nori, acknowledged that it had been a very stressful period and thanked the staff for their hard work and commitment. He also outlined changes to rostering and said senior management were examining the possibility of engaging more team leaders to manage the increasingly complex needs of the people in their care. He also reminded staff to practise self-care and to seek assistance, if needed, by visiting their GP or by accessing the organisation's new employee assistance program.

CHECK YOUR UNDERSTANDING

1. How can you maintain currency and safe work practices?
2. What are the main causes of stress in the aged care workplace?
3. Identify the possible impact of unmanaged stress.
4. How can you manage stress?
5. What organisational systems should be in place to assist you to look after your emotional health and wellbeing?

SUMMARY

- All PCBUs and workers have a responsibility to ensure the safety and wellbeing of anyone entering a workplace, including contractors, visitors, cleaners, builders, etc.
- WHS laws are in place to help prevent injury and illness and to promote holistic safety and wellbeing.
- National WHS laws guide and protect PCBUs and workers across state borders, while state and local regulatory bodies also provide guidance via policies and procedures and codes of practice.
- Workers contribute to prevention and promotion by:
  - identifying and reporting hazards
  - implementing policies and procedures
  - attending training and education
  - evaluating and reviewing processes and systems.
- Manual handling injuries can be prevented by implementing safe manual handling strategies and using assistive equipment.
- Infection transmission can be reduced through the use of standard and additional precautions.
- Following safe work practices such as obeying safety signs, following correct emergency procedures and contributing to the development of overall safety of the workplace benefits employers, care workers and clients.
- Stress is a possible consequence of working in the aged care industry. The use of both personal and organisational strategies will help to minimise the impact of stress on the individual.

REVIEW QUESTIONS

3.1 **(a)** What is the hierarchy of control?
(b) How does the hierarchy of control assist the care worker with manual handling tasks?
3.2 List common hazards and risks in aged care.
3.3 What is the role of a workplace health and safety committee?
3.4 Outline why restrictive practices are a safety issue in aged care.
3.5 Why is professional development important?

BIBLIOGRAPHY

Aged Care Quality and Safety Commission, *Continuous Improvement*, 24 December 2019, https://www.agedcarequality.gov.au/providers/assessment-processes/continuous-improvement, accessed 24 April 2022.

Australian Ageing Agenda, *Stressbuster: Top Tips for Aged Care Staff to Deal with Job Stress*, 9 October 2015, a www.australianageingagenda.com.au, accessed 14 March 2022.

Australian Government, *Work Health and Safety Act 2011*, https://www.legislation.gov.au, accessed 4 March 2022.

Comcare, *Workplace Health and Safety Management System*, 30 November 2020, https://www.comcare.gov.au/safe-healthy-work/healthy-workplace/whs-system, accessed 14 March 2022.

NSW State Insurance Regulatory Authority, *When a Worker is Injured: A Workers Compensation Guide for Employers*, 2015, https://www.sira.nsw.gov.au/resources-library, accessed 13 March 2022.

Royal Commission into Aged Care Quality and Safety, *Final Report: List of Recommendations*, 1 March 2021, https://agedcare.royalcommission.gov.au/publications/final-report-list-recommendations, accessed 15 March 2022.

Safework Australia, *How to Determine What is Reasonably Practicable to Meet a Health and Safety Duty*, 19 November 2020, https://www.safeworkaustralia.gov.au/resources-and-publications, accessed 4 March 2022.

Safework Australia, *Managing Risks*, 23 February 2022, https://www.safeworkaustralia.gov.au/, accessed 4 March 2022.

Safework Australia, *Model Work Health and Safety Bill*, 9 December 2019, https://www.safeworkaustralia.gov.au/, accessed 8 March 2022.

Safework Australia, *National Code of Practice for Manual Handling*, https://www.safeworkaustralia.gov.au/, accessed 14 March 2022.

Safework Australia, *Top Tips for Doing Safety Inspection in Your Workplace*, June 2017, https://www.safeworkaustralia.gov.au/resources-and-publications, accessed 11 March 2022.

Safework NSW, *Code of Practice Hazardous Manual Tasks*, August 2019, https://www.safework.nsw.gov.au/, accessed 8 March 2022.

WorkSafe Queensland, *Penalties*, 14 September 2020, https://www.worksafe.qld.gov.au/, accessed 14 March 2022.

WorkSafe Tasmania, *Penalties*, 24 February 2020, https://www.worksafe.tas.gov.au/, accessed 11 March 2022.

WorkSafe Victoria, *Aged Care Safety Basics*, 29 October 2019, https://www.worksafe.vic.gov.au/aged-care-safety-basics

WorkSafe Victoria, *Hazardous Manual Handling Health and Safety Guide*, 3 March 2020, https://www.worksafe.vic.gov.au/, accessed 11 March 2022.

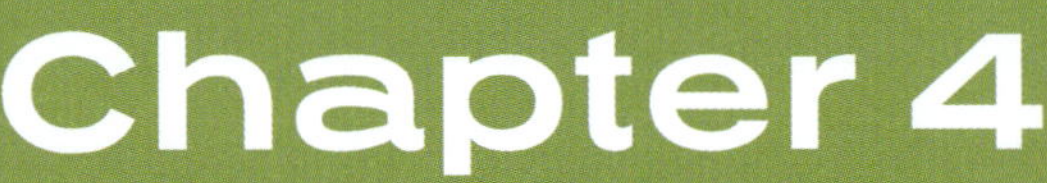

Chapter 4

Communicating in the workplace

LEARNING OBJECTIVES

4.1 Communicate effectively

4.2 Collaborate with colleagues

4.3 Understand constraints on communication

4.4 Complete workplace documentation and correspondence

4.5 Contribute to continuous improvement

INTRODUCTION

THE PROCESS OF SENDING AND RECEIVING a message is called **communication**. It involves interaction between participants. People use many ways to communicate, both verbal (sharing information via speech using words) and non-verbal (body language, gestures, pictures, props and sign language).

Effective communication skills that we will be exploring in this chapter include:

- active listening
- verbal and non-verbal communication
- building a trusting relationship
- being clear
- showing empathy
- asking questions
- clarifying and paraphrasing
- providing and accepting feedback.

INDUSTRY IN FOCUS

Effective communication to enhance care

Aged care services require communication that is effective, clear, easy to understand and tailored to the needs of the older people requiring support and their carers/family members. Communication will also be necessary between other services and workers in the industry, so it needs to be professional.

When working with people accessing services there will be constraints on communication, especially if the person has dementia or other cognitive issues. Anything that affects the brain, whether through disease or injury, will impact on the way the person processes information. For example, they may need:

- time to process information given to them
- clarification of the message
- information to be provided in different ways or in more than one way (verbally and in written form).

Some causes of damage to the brain include:

- a stroke or an accident that has resulted in an acquired brain injury (ABI)
- effects of medication
- metabolic issues
- delirium from an illness such as a urinary tract infection (UTI)
- other ailments such as Alzheimer's (the most common cause).

Dementia is a disease of the brain that will continue to destroy brain cells and eventually lead to end of life. It cannot be cured. Other illnesses or diseases may be resolved with the correct treatment. Dementia affects the way a person thinks, their memory, behaviour and social interaction, and eventually their physical health.

It is the right of all people accessing services to clearly understand the information presented to them, and it is the responsibility of all workers to assist those people to understand it.

Organisational policies and procedures, legislation and best-practice guidelines outline the requirements of all workers when communicating with older people and their family members, colleagues, health professionals and other services.

4.1 COMMUNICATING EFFECTIVELY

Effective communication is at the core of all work in community services. Without it, the needs of the older person who requires support won't be met. Workers in community services have a duty to ensure that older people understand their rights in regard to which services are available to them. Ineffective communication can lead to the older person feeling inadequate, disempowered and helpless. When communicating, our language and words should be inclusive, person centred, and show empathy and compassion.

4.1.1 Types, modes and models of communication

TYPES OF COMMUNICATION

Verbal communication is about using language, written and spoken, to get a message across. It can be formal or informal. It is important to remember the following when communicating verbally.

- Grammar is the way verbal communication is structured. It needs to be accurate and familiar for the person listening, to assist them to understand what is being communicated.
- Speed affects comprehension. The older person may miss some words and context if the person who is trying to communicate with them speaks too quickly. People with cognitive delays may become frustrated and may not understand instructions.
- Mispronouncing words can also change their meaning.

Non-verbal communication is the unspoken part of communication. Reading body language is crucial to understanding a message. Non-verbal cues can also be misinterpreted. Work in aged care services requires an understanding of body language and the meanings of certain movements or gestures. For example:

- *Body movements and posture:* The way we move our bodies may indicate whether we are feeling nervous, excited or anxious. A simple shrug of the shoulders can communicate: "I don't know."
- *Facial expressions:* Our face can convey surprise, happiness, anger, fear, sadness and disgust.
- *Eye contact:* We can show empathy or concern even if we are not engaged in a conversation. Be aware that direct eye contact may not be appropriate in some cultures or settings.
- *Appearance:* Our appearance can indicate our professionalism, self-identity and feelings. For example, dressing professionally for an interview will make a favourable impression on the interviewer.
- *Sign language:* Sign language is a non-verbal language that persons who are deaf use to communicate. Key word signing uses manual signs derived from Auslan (Australia's sign language), and gestures along with speech, to support communication. Children and adults with communication difficulties can be taught to use the signs to better communicate their needs.
- *Personal space:* The space around us is personal to us. The meanings we attach to personal space are usually culturally determined. For example, if a person steps back from someone who is verbally aggressive, this can convey that they don't want to participate in the conversation. Alternatively, standing very close to someone may indicate feelings of intimacy.

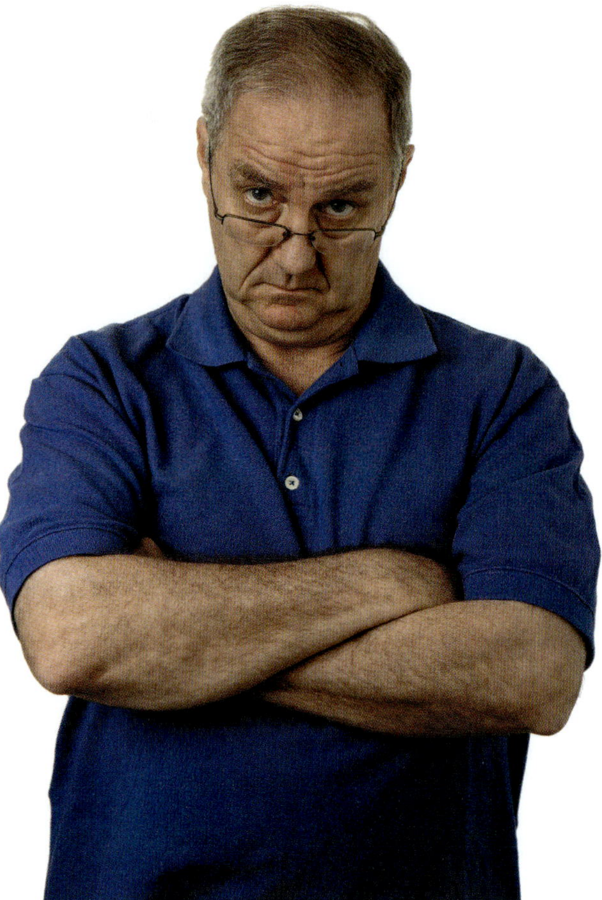

Our facial expressions and body language can indicate our emotions

Written communication may be used for many reasons. It can follow after verbal instructions or messages to reinforce their meaning. Written communication and documentation is a legal requirement in community services and is guided by legislation, regulations, principles, policies and procedures. This written work needs to be specific, clear, concise and in a language that is familiar to the reader.

MODES OF COMMUNICATION

The term "communication modes" refers to how information is transferred, received and interpreted. For instance, it can be communicated via emails, letters, webinars or training sessions, and can be in paper or digital form. The different modes include the following:

- *Interpersonal communication:* communication that takes place between two people. It can be formal or informal, verbal or non-verbal.
- *Interpretive communication:* communication such as when students study and interpret what they learn about a topic by reading written information, listening to audio-recordings or looking at images.
- *Presentational communication:* a facilitator presents a topic that the audience then needs to understand. It is not a two-way form of communication, but the audience does have an opportunity to ask questions at the end of the presentation.

MODELS OF COMMUNICATION

Over the years, scholars have developed several models of communication that explain how communication evolves. The following are the three most well-known of these models.

- *Linear model:* Here, communication is in one direction only (e.g. when we watch a YouTube instructional video). A message is sent and received, but there is no feedback.
- *Interactive model:* Here, a message is sent and received, and feedback is given back to the person who sent the message, and so on, back and forth.
- *Transactional model:* Here, information is sent and received simultaneously. We are sending information at the same time as the other person is sending information. We are always encoding and decoding information at the same time, through all forms of communication, verbal and non-verbal.

4.1.2 Communication techniques

Active listening is showing someone that the listener is actually listening to them and is actively involved in the conversation. It can influence the relationships between colleagues and with older people, their families and other stakeholders. This builds trust, shows respect and can empower others. It is about being attentive, understanding what the person is saying, and responding to, reflecting on and retaining the information given.

Active listening involves the following techniques:

- *Paying attention:* for example, making eye contact, nodding, leaning a little closer to the person, asking open-ended questions to get a better idea of what they are saying ("Tell me about . . .").
- *Reflective listening:* listening intently, reflecting on what has been said, then repeating it back to the sender in your own words.
- *Summarising:* making a summary of the key points in the message and sending those back to the **sender** of the original message. This can show the person sending the message that the **receiver** has understood the content.
- *Paraphrasing:* rephrasing what the message sender has said while maintaining the same meaning in the message. Paraphrasing is a shorter version of the original message.

It is very important in any interaction that workers clarify the meaning of instructions with the appropriate people if they don't understand something. If instructions are misunderstood by a person performing a role, this can lead to physical or psychological harm of themself or others.

The way information is responded to, whether verbal or non-verbal, and the actions taken afterwards, must always be positive and respectful and uphold the person's human rights.

4.1.3 Factors that can influence communication

LANGUAGE

For people to be able to communicate and understand each other, they need to speak the same language. If the older person requiring support doesn't speak the language of the support worker, the worker has a **duty of care** to assist them to understand. Communication should be tailored to the needs of the older person. For example, the worker could:

- learn some words in the older person's language
- use gestures and props—for example, hold up a cup to ask if they would like a cup of tea
- use an interpreter or a family member if appropriate.

CULTURE

Australia is a very multicultural country, with over 300 languages spoken.

- One in five people (21 per cent) speak a non-English language at home.
- English is not the first language for 15 per cent of Australians (3.5 million people).
- English is not spoken at home by 0.5 per cent of Australians (117,000 people).

The 2016 Census of Population and Housing showed that more than a quarter (26 per cent) of Australia's population (6,163,667 people) were born overseas, up from 25 per cent in 2011. Of the overseas-born population, nearly one in five (18 per cent) had arrived since the start of 2012.

The ten most reported countries of birth for those born overseas were (ABS 2017):

- England (14.7 per cent)
- New Zealand (8.4 per cent)
- China (8.3 per cent)
- India (7.4 per cent)
- Philippines (3.8 per cent)
- Vietnam (3.6 per cent)
- Italy (2.8 per cent)
- South Africa (2.6 per cent)
- Malaysia (2.2 per cent)
- Scotland (1.9 per cent).

Every culture has its own norms, customs and values that influence communication. It is the responsibility of the worker to understand these when working with older people.

The following factors can influence communication.

- *Past trauma:* for example, a previous experience where the communication wasn't successful and psychosocial harm occurred.
- *Body language:* especially the use of or lack of eye contact or touch.
- *Gender-appropriate services:* for example, when women can only be cared for by other women.
- *Family dynamics:* for example, when there are hierarchies in families from different cultures that need to be considered in determining who to talk to about the older person's care.

Culturally aware communication includes:

- establishing trust
- not making assumptions
- allowing time for the person to respond
- choosing an appropriate setting in which to communicate

- treating each person as an individual
- being an active listener
- using a cultural interpreter.

RELIGION

A person's religion can play a large part in the way they communicate in a multicultural society. Many religions have beliefs, rules, norms and values, just like cultures do. There may be topics of conversation that are taboo in some settings or between genders. Workers should be aware of body language that may be offensive to followers of some religions. Touch can be taboo, too, so placing a hand on someone's shoulder or arm in a comforting gesture may actually cause the person distress. Being aware of others' beliefs, rules, norms and values will build a relationship of trust. Always seek support from the person or consult their care plan or a supervisor if there is any confusion around the services to be provided.

EMOTIONAL STATE

A person's emotional state can also influence their ability to communicate. Emotions can transfer from one person to another. Have you ever walked into a room where someone was very sad? Did that make you feel sad? Alternatively, if someone is always positive and upbeat while at work, that can also affect the way others feel. Having a positive attitude when supporting older people can lift their mood and empower them to think positively about ageing and the support they are receiving.

The older person's feelings and moods should be considered at the time of service. They may not hear what is being said to them or want to listen if they are feeling down. As care workers, we need also to understand that the older person requiring support may be experiencing grief. They may be grieving for the loss of:

- a partner/husband/wife
- their independence
- their home (after moving into residential care)
- friends and social connections
- mobility and their ability to do things they used to do
- their memory.

These are major lifestyle transitions that can influence emotions and, ultimately, the ability to communicate effectively with others. Colleagues and other people that workers interact with may also be experiencing emotions that aren't obvious, so the worker should consider this when communicating with them.

DISABILITY AND AGE

When communicating with someone with a disability, it is vitally important to understand that they are a person first and their disability doesn't define them. Many people with disabilities find it difficult to communicate for many reasons. Factors that can influence communication include:

- sensory impairments
- past trauma/bad experiences
- cognitive abilities
- access to aids and equipment to support communication
- attitudes of others
- access to services.

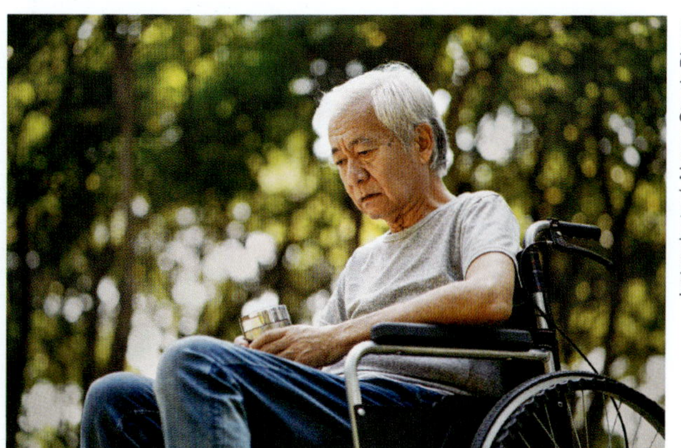

imtmphoto / Alamy Stock Photo

A person's emotional state can influence their ability to communicate

As with disability, the ageing process can leave the person with impairments of the senses and other body systems. Older people may not want to admit that they need support, so they often won't tell workers or services what they need. Losing one's independence can be very difficult for the person.

HEALTH

Health and wellbeing can influence the way a person communicates, or their understanding of what others are saying. Health factors that can influence communication can include:

- medication (not taking it, or taking too much)
- time of day (the older person may get tired at the end of the day, so supports may need to be done earlier in the day)
- the person's disease or illness
- poor physical health
- pain and discomfort.

4.1.4 Communication styles

Every person will have their own style of communication. Understanding each person's style will assist you to build relationships and support cohesion in teams. Following are some of the communication styles workers may experience in the working environment.

ASSERTIVE COMMUNICATION STYLE

Assertive communication is about being firm but fair. The assertive communicator has confidence in their subject and can articulate their needs well. They also know how to actively listen and to compromise. Assertive communicators are objective and don't let emotions cloud their judgement. They will hear everyone out and are focused on finding a solution without comprising their own wants, ideas or values.

AGGRESSIVE COMMUNICATION STYLE

The aggressive communicator is argumentative, intimidating and sometimes hostile. Like the assertive communicator they are confident, but they don't listen to others' views and will dismiss any attempt to sway their opinion. They will also use aggressive body language such as hand gestures, getting in people's personal space and using dismissive facial expressions. This style doesn't mean that they aren't good at their job or aren't knowledgeable about a subject, but the way they communicate will often put others off, which can lead to an environment of bullying and contempt.

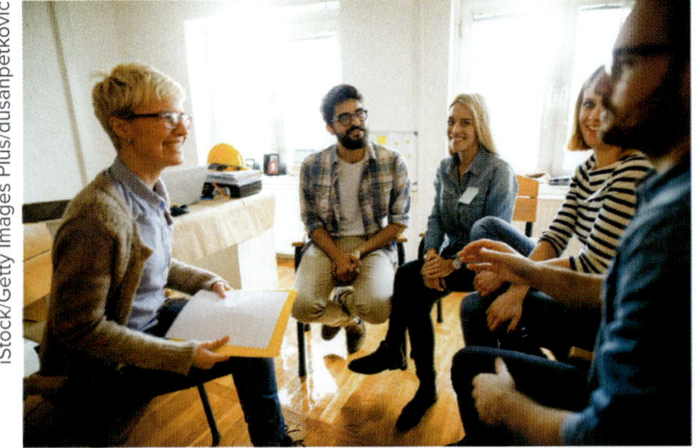

iStock/Getty Images Plus/dusanpetkovic

Understanding individual communication styles helps support cohesion in teams

PASSIVE OR SUBMISSIVE COMMUNICATION STYLE

Passive communicators are submissive, easygoing and like to please people. They will let assertive or aggressive communicators take the lead and will stay out of their way. The passive communicator can be seen as a "walkover", which doesn't support an inclusive environment, especially in teams. They struggle to communicate their own wants and needs and, because of this, they may be overlooked. They often let people have their way, which is not effectively communicating their needs.

PASSIVE-AGGRESSIVE COMMUNICATION STYLE

The passive-aggressive communication style is a combination of two very different styles. Passive-aggressive communicators won't come right out and say they dislike or don't agree with something; instead, they operate in the background. They can be toxic in the team environment, as they may work behind the scenes to get what they want instead of being upfront with their dissatisfactions. In time, this can spread throughout the team unit and no one ends up getting what they need.

MANIPULATIVE COMMUNICATION STYLE

Manipulative communicators are often hard to detect. They know what they want and how to get it, but they are not truthful about their wants, needs or feelings. They will trick others into thinking something completely different until they get what they want, often at the other's expense.

4.1.5 Communicating service information

Effective communication is always required when providing **service information**. Communication occurs between the older person, their family or carer, other services, colleagues and health professionals. As everyone may be from different backgrounds and have different communication needs, the communication process will always need to be respectful and professional. Everyone involved in the care team needs to understand how to communicate important information about services.

INFORMATION ABOUT SERVICES

Information about services can be detailed, with technical information that may not be understood by everyone. Employees may need clarification regarding their employment contract, so they know their role and responsibilities. Older people may need the information read to them or explained. Information can be misinterpreted, so it is vitally important to ensure that the message receiver understands it.

Consider the following:

- Is there a clear purpose to this information? What does the person need to know?
- Is there too much information? Can it be reduced without losing anything important?
- Is the information correct and factual?
- Does it make sense?
- Is the correct mode, model and style of communication being used?

Examples of service information can include:

- policies and procedures
- employment contracts
- service contracts
- care plans
- audit outcomes
- budgets
- funding
- codes of conduct.

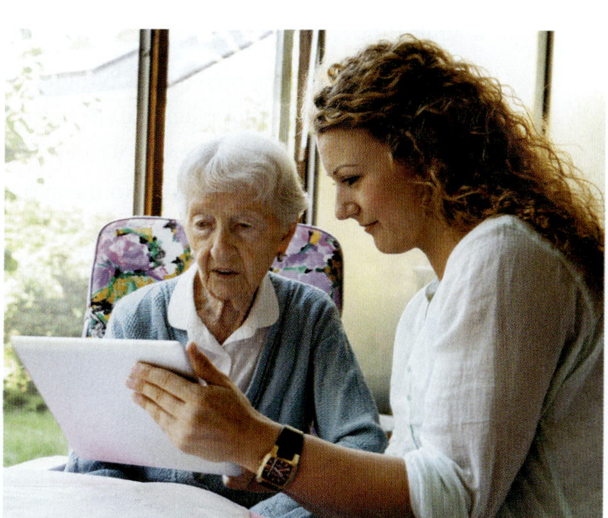

Getty Images/E+/SilviaJansen

Sharing information can take many forms

TAILORING COMMUNICATION TO MEET INDIVIDUAL NEEDS

Each individual, whether an older person, a colleague or another stakeholder, will have different communication needs. Be aware of those needs and communicate with them in a way they understand.

Consider the following factors:

- *Method of delivery:* Does the person need the information to be explained verbally, to be provided in written form or to be demonstrated, or all of these?
- *Content:* Is the content relevant and engaging? Is it easily understood? Is it in the correct language?
- *Frequency:* Will the person require a repeat of the information, or is once enough?

EXCHANGING INFORMATION

The aged care industry provides services to older people to enable them to live independently in their own home or in a residential aged care facility (RACF). Older people are assessed for the right services to meet their needs, and the government will fund these services depending on the level of support the person requires.

Information sharing is an important aspect of care. The information gathered assists services to provide the best support possible for the older person. The information being shared should be clear, and it should be shared in a timely manner. If not, the older person may miss out on vital information and services.

There will be times when information needs to be shared with other services. Often, one service won't have the resources or capacity to support all aspects of the older person's needs. Referrals may then be needed to other services. An example of this would be an older person who needs support to maintain their home, which a home care service can provide, but they also need the support of a physiotherapist for their mobility. If this need is identified, a referral will be made to a physiotherapist, or the service may take the older person to their doctor to get a referral.

Other information that may need to be shared includes:

- incident reports
- individual plans
- information about the older person's needs
- contact details
- next of kin.

CONFIDENTIALITY OF PERSONAL INFORMATION

The individual or their representative must give consent before any information is exchanged. Organisations will have a particular consent form relating to the information to be shared. Australian legislation protects the personal information of people accessing services. This legislation is reflected in the organisation's policies and procedures.

Guidelines include:

- Don't share personal details of older people you support with colleagues who are not in the care team or with other clients of the organisation.
- Always get consent–verbal, written or implied, depending on the information and circumstances.
- Follow procedures relating to the gathering, storing and disclosure of information.
- Keep written information locked in a cabinet and limit access to it.
- Ensure computers and smartphones are password protected.

4.1.6 Legal and ethical responsibilities

Legal and ethical frameworks guide workers in their professional practice and protect the rights of everyone accessing services, including:

- clients and family members
- all staff
- contractors

- volunteers
- health professionals.

Your organisation will have specific policies around communication that you need to be aware of. These can include policies relating to:

- privacy and confidentiality
- duty of care
- dignity of risk
- complaints and grievances
- documentation standards and protocols
- **communication hierarchy** (who must report to whom)
- work health and safety (WHS).

You should become familiar with, and comply with, your legal and ethical responsibilities outlined in the organisation's policies, procedures and code of conduct/ethics.

Policies outline *what* workers need to do to meet their legal and ethical responsibilities, while procedures outline *how* to perform their duties. Codes of conduct or ethics outline the expected behaviours when working.

Legal and ethical frameworks within organisations are developed from Australia's legislation, regulations, codes of practice, industry standards and industry codes of ethics (e.g. Australian Community Workers Code of Ethics). Human rights and the relevant United Nations declarations and conventions underpin our legislation and constitution. If breached, consequences can include employee dismissal, government sanctions placed on the organisation, prosecution and fines.

WORKPLACE SCENARIO

Active listening for person-centred care

Ed, the nurse practitioner, discusses the possibility of running a trial "buddy system" in the facility where he works with the care manager, Souha. The aim would be to deepen relationships between staff and the people they support, facilitating communication and broadening the existing culture of caring. Coupled with this is a plan to extend continuity of care, requiring new and existing staff to commit to a minimum of three days per week in one area.

Manu, a care worker, requests that he be buddied with Akeem. Akeem (90) has Alzheimer's disease and Manu has established a good relationship with Akeem and his family since he came to the facility, so Ed agrees. The trial requires staff to spend specific time with their "person" every time they're at work, focusing on communication and engagement. Ed shows Manu and the other staff various memory aids such as picture-based memory books that can be used as prompts or cues during conversations. Ed encourages the staff to think of communication as a partnership and explains how to create a supportive environment in those moments of conversation.

Akeem's family are asked if they would like to work on a memory book with Akeem and Manu, and they make time to go through pictures and words that are meaningful to Akeem and themselves.

At the end of the trial, Ed suggests that this approach be permanently adopted, and that interested staff attend discussion groups to learn better communication techniques, problem solving and how to extend the cueing system to include various interests personally relevant to the people they support, such as gardens, pets and foods.

CHECK YOUR UNDERSTANDING

1. What skills are needed by aged care workers to effectively communicate with older people accessing aged care services?
2. Describe active listening.
3. What factors can influence the way an older person communicates?
4. Describe the assertive communication style.
5. What should an aged care worker do to keep a client's information confidential?

4.2 COLLABORATING WITH COLLEAGUES

Teamwork is required in all services, both internally and externally. Direct support with older people involves working with colleagues, the older person, their family, managers and other services in the community service sector.

Older people requiring support may need to access more than one service, so understanding how the sector functions and how to access other services will assist a worker and service to provide quality care that meets all the person's needs.

There are protocols regarding communication between other services that must be followed. Some services will need referrals from a health professional to access them; others may require a booking by the older person themselves or may be happy with a verbal handover.

4.2.1 Communication protocols and lines of authority

Communication protocols are instructions that need to be followed when communicating internally within your organisation and externally with other people and services. These instructions will include who care workers must communicate with and the process for contacting the person or service.

Internally, within organisations, there are lines of authority when communicating and protocols to follow. An understanding of the organisation's structure from the head of the organisation down is required. This is so that information can be communicated up and down the line of authority to the appropriate person for decision making and the resolution of issues in a cost-effective way.

Knowing who is who in the organisation will save time and resources. As an example: If a care worker is unsure of a work instruction relating to an older person's care, that worker would contact their direct supervisor, not the CEO of the company.

4.2.2 Work instructions

Work instructions are those instructions relating to the tasks to be performed. These instructions may be written in a person's care plan, the care worker's job description, and the organisation's policies and procedures. If instructions are provided verbally, they should be followed up with written instructions so they can be reviewed by the person carrying out the tasks.

Some instructions and tasks will have a time frame for completion. Once this time frame has been agreed upon, it must be adhered to. There may be other tasks that cannot occur until the original task or instruction has been completed, and so on. There will be a flow-on effect that can have consequences for the quality care of the older person and the organisation.

CLARIFYING WORK INSTRUCTIONS

When receiving any instructions, it is important to listen actively and to clarify the meaning if you are unsure. Don't interrupt; ask questions when appropriate; and don't assume understanding. Clarification may be required about:

- what needs to be done
- when it needs to be done
- how it should be done
- what resources are required
- priority of tasks.

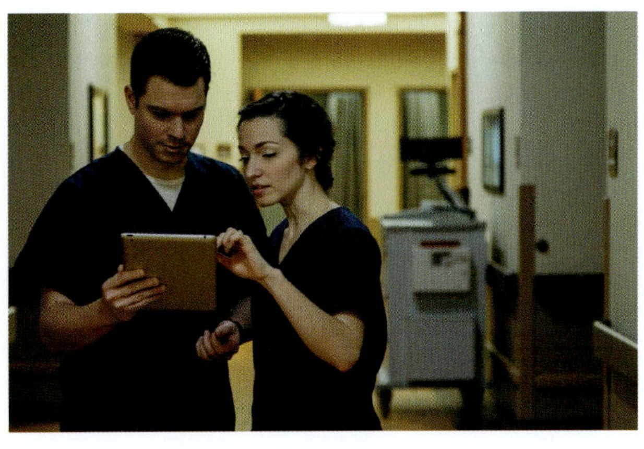

Getty Images/Andersen Ross Photography Inc

Clarify the meaning of work instructions if you are unsure

If an aged care worker doesn't understand the instructions given and doesn't clarify with the registered nurse (RN) or the supervisor, they will have breached their duty of care and the older person receiving support and the worker may be harmed. For example, a worker who isn't sure how to use a piece of manual handling equipment uses it anyway. The client falls, the worker tries to stop them from falling, and both the worker and the older person are injured.

4.2.3 Industry terminology

In aged care, industry terminology is used that relates directly to the sector and to the support to be provided to the older person. **Industry terminology** is the particular words, phrases and acronyms that are used and understood by a particular industry. They will be found within the organisation's correspondence, on medical charts and in other information produced within the sector. These terms will also be used by the people working in services. The organisation and other services will have a glossary of acronyms and terms used in the aged care sector.

The following terminology is used in aged care.

- *ACAT:* aged care assessment team.
- *Personal care:* assistance provided to a person to support personal hygiene.
- *CDC:* consumer-directed care (where the consumer directs their services).
- *IP:* individual plan/care plan.
- *RACF:* residential aged care facility.

If unsure of the meaning of industry terminology, you can ask your supervisor, consult the organisation's glossary, or access government websites or My Aged Care. Always clarify the meaning of industry terminology. It will be used in verbal, written and digital communication.

WORKPLACE SCENARIO

Social media in the workplace

When Ronny started work as a care worker in a facility, the team leader, Jing, outlined their social media policy, stating that the use of mobile phones is confined to break times and that at no time should personal information about colleagues or people receiving support be shared.

Ronny enjoyed his work and enrolled in a course to achieve a qualification in aged care. During the course, he developed a close relationship with another student, Hakim, who works for another facility

(Continues)

close by. They often discussed their work and shared stories, but Hakim was careful not to use the names of people he supports or provide information that would breach any person's confidentiality.

After class one day, Hakim saw that Ronny had posted photos on Instagram of someone he supported who had died that day. Ronny had used their name, identifying them in a photo, and included photos of their room and belongings. Ronny had also commented on Facebook about how they had died and how their family would soon be arguing about his will. Hakim was disturbed and uncomfortable and rang the facility where Ronny worked to report the incident. Jing spoke to Ronny immediately and stated that these actions might compromise his future career. Ronny was dismissed, having breached policy and engaged in unethical behaviour. Jing also contacted the family and advised them to contact a lawyer.

Later that month, Ronny received a letter stating that he was being sued by the person's family for defamation.

CHECK YOUR UNDERSTANDING

1. Why is it important to collaborate and communicate with colleagues?
2. What are lines of authority?
3. What are work instructions?
4. Why is it important to clarify work instructions?
5. Why is it important to understand industry terminology?

4.3 ADDRESSING CONSTRAINTS ON COMMUNICATION

4.3.1 Understand the causes of constraints

If the **messages** sent are not received the way the sender intended, misunderstandings can occur. These misunderstandings can cause difficult situations and sometimes conflict. Therefore, it is very important to check that the receiver has understood the message.

Constraints, or barriers, can include, but are not limited to:

- cognitive abilities of the older person, including dementia
- poor comprehension if English is spoken as a second language
- physical barriers, including stress, sensory issues and environmental noise
- organisational culture
- conflicting information
- cultural differences
- emotional factors
- jargon
- values, beliefs and attitudes.

All communication should be respectful, clear and empathetic. Understanding constraints on communication and learning how best to respond in any given situation will assist a successful outcome.

COGNITIVE DIFFICULTIES, INCLUDING DEMENTIA

A person with dementia or other cognitive issues is still an individual, and all communication needs to take their individual differences into account. Losing the ability to communicate is extremely frustrating for the person with reduced cognitive abilities. Aged care workers need to consult with the older person's family members or carers to find out the best way to communicate with the person.

Tips:

- Maintain the person's dignity by talking to them as an adult, not a child.
- Speak clearly, in a gentle tone of voice. A person's ability to hear high tones decreases with age.
- Use the person's preferred name frequently.
- When you greet the person, help them by reminding them who you are—for example: "Hello, Jean. It's Carol here."
- Keep your sentences short and simple. Never overload the person with too much information at one time. Be patient and allow them time to process and comprehend.
- Talk about what you are doing when providing care.
- The concept of "don't" is often difficult for people with dementia to understand, so try to phrase things in a positive way.
- When chatting with the person, try to be on the same eye level as them.
- Use body language—gestures, facial expressions and visual demonstration—to convey meaning.
- Use touch to gain the person's attention and convey your feelings (if this is appropriate for the person).
- Assess whether the person has special needs such as hearing or visual impairment that you should take into consideration.

Getty Images/Morsa Images

All communication should be respectful, clear and empathetic

ENGLISH AS A SECOND LANGUAGE AND CULTURAL CONSIDERATIONS

Australia is a very multicultural country, and there are many people accessing aged care services who don't speak or comprehend English. Many aged care workers also speak languages other than English, so communication can be misunderstood. Colleagues, older people and their families have a right to inclusion and to be free from discrimination. Access and equity are a social justice principle that all workers should follow to protect the rights of individuals. For instance, if an older person doesn't speak or understand English and all the organisation's documentation is written in English, then translation and interpreter services must be provided so that the person understands the written material. If these services aren't provided or the family isn't consulted (if they speak and understand English), then the person cannot utilise the services and isn't able to make an informed decision. This is discrimination.

Tips:

- Speak slowly, but not so slowly as to sound patronising.
- Pronounce words correctly.
- Be aware of body language and tone of voice.
- Be culturally aware and understand the protocols of communication.
- Learn some words in the person's first language.
- Access translation and interpreting services.

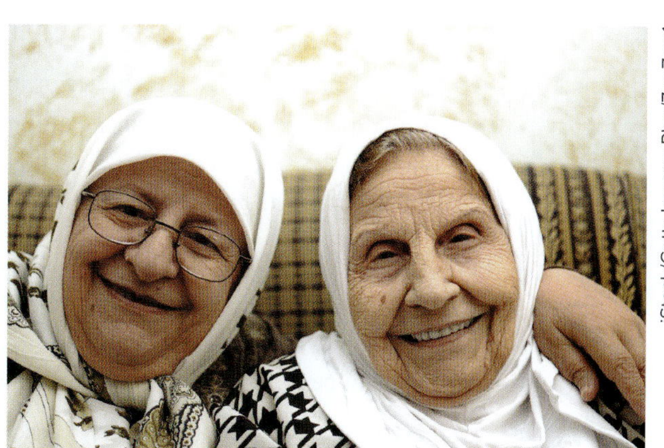

iStock/Getty Images Plus/ZouZou1

It is important to be culturally aware and to understand the protocols of communication

TRANSLATORS AND INTERPRETERS

There are legal and ethical guidelines that relate to translation and using an interpreter. Translation is about written information and translating one language to another. Interpreters deal with a spoken language or sign language and relay it back in another language in real time.

In community services where an older person doesn't speak or understand English, families may act as an interpreter for the person needing support. This can be seen as a conflict of interest, as family members may not be able to be impartial. The family may believe they have their loved one's best interests at heart, but their interpretation of what the person needs may be very different from what the person might want. If this situation occurs, it needs to be reported to the organisation, which has a duty of care to make sure the older person's information is correct by getting the assistance of a qualified professional interpreter.

PHYSICAL CONSTRAINTS

Physical barriers to communication are those factors in the environment that prevent effective communication. Barriers that physically get between the sender and receiver of a message can include:

- poor phone connection
- poor internet connection
- noise
- workplace design
- time and distance.

SENSORY CONSTRAINTS

Having a vision impairment will prevent a person from receiving a message as they may not be able to see body language or other non-verbal communication. Follow these guidelines when communicating with a person with vision impairment:

- Introduce yourself when entering a room.
- Always let the person know what is happening.
- If there is a group of people, announce who is speaking.
- Let the person know who is entering and leaving the room.

Depending on the severity of their hearing impairment, the person may not be able to hear words or the speaker's tone of voice. They won't be able to hear warnings of danger, such as a fire alarm. Follow these guidelines when communicating with a person with a hearing impairment:

- Always face the person.
- Speak clearly. Not everyone with a hearing impairment is completely deaf.
- Use written communication.
- Utilise a sign language interpreter or learn Auslan (Australian sign language).
- If the older person has a hearing aid, make sure it is turned on and that the batteries are charged and not flat.
- Speak a little louder than normal, but never shout.

STRESS AND EMOTIONAL CONSTRAINTS

Stress or poor emotional wellbeing can affect the way a person reacts. If we are angry, we may misinterpret what the sender of a message is saying and react hastily and illogically. If we are sad, we may not actively listen, as we will be focusing on what is making us sad. In such cases:

- leave the conversation and come back when the emotion has settled
- use relaxation techniques
- use self-reflection techniques
- admit your error and apologise if you are wrong about something.

ORGANISATIONAL CULTURE

All workplaces have their own culture. They all have their own set of norms, values and principles shared among the people who work there. Individual workers will also have attitudes and beliefs about how they should communicate or that influence their communication. Some internal cultures can be toxic, and workers may experience bullying. To have a culture that is psychologically safe:

- have leaders with an open-door policy
- encourage open and honest communication in teams
- ensure job satisfaction and that staff aren't overworked
- ensure that all employees agree with the organisation's mission and vision and have the same values.

CONFLICTING INFORMATION

If an older person is receiving conflicting information from many sources or from the person they are communicating with, they may become quite confused. Service information can be confusing as it is! To prevent this from happening, workers should always:

- be prepared
- ensure that the information they are providing is correct
- clarify the person's understanding
- provide the information in different forms—verbal, and backed up in writing
- communicate in the person's preferred way.

VALUES, BELIEFS AND ATTITUDES

Everyone has their own values, beliefs and attitudes. They make up who we are and can influence the way we communicate. In the workplace, care workers should be aware of their own values, beliefs and attitudes, and recognise that people from different backgrounds, or of a different gender or age, may think very differently from them. They should respect these differences and not try to impose their own values, beliefs and attitudes on others, as this might influence the other person's decision making.

4.3.2 Identify and report complicated or difficult situations

Misunderstandings and conflicts are best identified as soon as possible. No one likes conflict. For older people, barriers to communication can cause them to experience frustration and stress and may even make them withdraw from people and from performing activities of daily living.

Misunderstandings and conflicts between colleagues can be stressful and can affect the team dynamic. They can also affect service provision and should be dealt with promptly. Competing interpersonal, financial and organisational priorities can also lead to complicated or difficult situations within organisations.

If a complicated situation arises, it should be reported to a supervisor for assistance with finding a resolution before it leads to conflict or violence. Supervisors and managers will have the skills, knowledge and procedures to assist. There are policies and procedures in all community service organisations to assist with **conflict resolution**. Organisations may also have training in these policies and procedures for all staff to attend, so that they understand the process.

Indicators that a complicated or difficult situation has arisen between colleagues include:

- Their body language is defensive (e.g. crossed arms, angry facial expression, avoidance of eye contact, clenched fists).
- They are speaking in raised voices or have adopted a belligerent tone.
- Their choice of words reflects heightened emotions.

Indicators of complicated and difficult situations within organisations include the following aspects of workplace culture:

- increased staff turnover
- uncooperative behaviour
- workplace bullying
- non-compliance with policies and procedures
- increased use of sick leave
- workers are underperforming
- increased reporting of grievances.

4.3.3 Resolve conflict situations

Conflict can occur for many different reasons and with anyone in the workplace. Communication is a powerful tool, and when used effectively it can assist us to avoid, defuse and resolve conflict. Conflict isn't always negative; managed well, it can assist with creativity and empower people towards a positive outcome. Poorly managed conflict, however, can cause psychological harm and ruin relationships in the workplace.

CONFLICT BETWEEN WORKERS

Conflict between workers needs to be dealt with as soon as possible. If it is not resolved quickly, the services the organisation provides will decrease in quality and staff may quit. It can also impact the organisation's resources and adversely affect the team.

Conflict can occur due to:

- conflicting values, beliefs and attitudes
- cultural or language barriers
- bullying and harassment
- lack of resources
- different personalities
- organisational culture
- mental illness.

There are conflict resolution and grievance procedures in all organisations that will guide workers in a conflict situation. Workers should do the following:

- Try to raise the issue with the person they are having difficulties with first. Often the other person doesn't realise there is a problem, and it can be resolved quite easily.
- Raise it with the other person as soon as they realise there is an issue.
- If this is not possible, seek the support of a supervisor who can assist with a resolution and provide mediation.
- If the issue is with a superior, go higher up the authority line.

During the conflict resolution process, workers should:

- manage their emotions and try to be objective
- admit their role in the problem, as no one is completely without fault

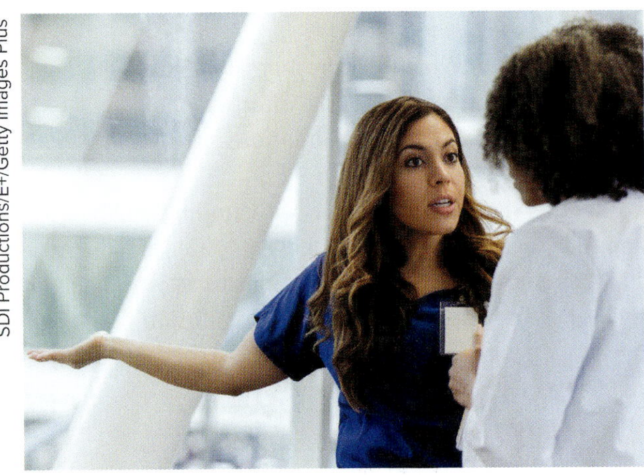

SDI Productions/E+/Getty Images Plus

Conflict between workers should be dealt with as soon as possible

- actively listen to what the person is saying and acknowledge their feelings
- use assertive language, not aggressive or passive language
- use "I" statements (e.g. "I feel", "I would like to"), as they focus on feelings without pointing the finger at the other person. "You" statements tend to come across as blaming the other person.

CONFLICTS WITH AN OLDER PERSON ACCESSING THE SERVICE

Conflicts with service users should never happen. The person accessing the service has the right to be free from conflict, and it is the worker's responsibility to keep their values, attitudes and beliefs in check and to support the person to resolve any issues early. An older person may have a complaint about the service, or someone in the service, and they should be assisted with the complaints process.

However, conflicts do occur, especially with people with cognitive decline. In such cases, workers should:

- understand the person's needs
- never argue with the person or say "no"
- remain calm
- use an even tone of voice
- use appropriate body language
- ask questions (but not too many) to try and find out what the person needs
- get assistance from another colleague or family member
- always respect the person's rights.

UNRESOLVED CONFLICT

Any unresolved conflict will also need to be reported to a supervisor. If left unresolved, it can be very overwhelming and can affect the worker's health, wellbeing and work performance. There are organisational policies and procedures for the supervision of employees.

The following is a typical process.

1. Refer to the RN or supervisor.
2. The RN or supervisor will hear each person's side of the story.
3. The RN or supervisor will then call a combined meeting.
4. Mediation is provided by the RN or supervisor. They are not there to tell people in conflict what to do. They will assist both people to come to their own solutions, so they are invested in the outcome. Being told what to do won't be taken well and the person will not be invested in the outcome.

If the RN or supervisor isn't able to mediate, the issue can be referred to a professional mediator who will start the process again by meeting each person separately before bringing them together to work on a resolution. If no resolution is possible, then disciplinary action may be required.

Sometimes people cannot agree on a resolution. The conflict will then be referred to the organisation, which will enforce a solution that is best for the organisation as a whole and will remind the workers that this must be complied with as part of their workplace responsibilities. If not, the issue will be dealt with accordingly through possible disciplinary action.

4.3.4 Collaboration versus confrontation

Confrontation usually occurs face to face but not always. It is when a person challenges another's ideas or actions. Confrontation can be managed within the organisation's policies and with the support of a manager so that it doesn't turn into a much bigger issue.

Collaboration is about working as a team to reach an agreed goal. It is about sharing ideas, valuing others' opinions and resolving issues together. Collaboration is needed when supporting older people and their family or carers so that they are always informed and happy with the services provided. Collaboration brings all stakeholders together with different knowledge and skills to provide support that is holistic.

4.3.5 Motivational interviewing versus a coercive approach

A **coercive approach** to dealing with conflict is about forcing someone to do what we want. This is bullying, which undermines the organisation's values and can cause psychological harm. It will damage relationships and lead to poor outcomes for older people accessing the service.

Motivational interviewing is a counselling method that motivates a person to make a change. Motivation is different for everyone, and motivational interviewing draws on a person's strengths and values their contributions, which boosts confidence and encourages the person to move towards change. Motivational interviewing involves:

- asking open-ended questions—this assists the person to talk so that the interviewer can learn more about them and their issue
- affirming—focusing and commenting on a person's strengths
- reflective listening—shows the person that you are invested in listening to them
- summarising—shows the person that they have been heard.

WORKPLACE SCENARIO

Addressing complaints

Alfons' father, Noah, has moved into a room near the office that the care staff use during night duty. Noah tells Alfons that when the staff start their shift and review what needs to be done during the night, he can often hear them making negative remarks about individuals and their families. He says that they discuss private matters such as financial arrangements and diagnoses and that they're often critical. Noah is upset about this and concerned that his personal information will be scrutinised and discussed.

Alfons is concerned too and tells Noah he'll speak to Maria, the care manager, but Noah is afraid that the complaint will not be well received and he will be victimised. Alfons acknowledges that it is difficult for Noah as he is dependent on the care staff, and he reassures him that this will not be the case—they have a right to voice their complaints and concerns without the threat of discrimination or victimisation.

Alfons requests to see Maria and tells her that Noah has a complaint they'd like to discuss. Maria suggests a time the following day, stating that she appreciates that it may be a difficult conversation but that resolving the issue will help to:

- improve the quality of care provided
- provide care staff with a better understanding of Noah's needs
- build positive relationships between Noah, Alfons and care staff.

During the meeting, Alfons encourages Noah to voice his concerns, which he does, adding that he believes such discussions among staff are unethical and undermine trust. Maria agrees and apologises, and thanks Noah and Alfons for bringing this to her attention. She also says that she appreciates the opportunity to handle the complaint quickly before it escalates and becomes more serious.

Maria reassures Noah that she will investigate his complaint by speaking to the staff, following up any further concerns that may come to light, and discussing what can be done to improve maintaining confidentiality and privacy during situations such as handover.

CHECK YOUR UNDERSTANDING

1. How do constraints on communication cause misunderstandings?
2. When communicating with a colleague, what are the signs that a person may not like what they are hearing?
3. How should aged care workers communicate with a person who has English as a second language and is of a different culture from their own?
4. Why is collaboration important when supporting older people?
5. What is motivational interviewing?

4.4 COMPLETING WORKPLACE DOCUMENTATION AND CORRESPONDENCE

Workplace documentation and correspondence is of high importance in an organisation, as it underpins quality service delivery, increases accountability and provides information needed for compliance with the industry standards.

Information must be accurate and up to date and adhere to legislative requirements. Organisations are accountable to older people accessing the service and their stakeholders, the government and funding bodies. All information contained in documentation should be factual, objective and unbiased. It should be completed on organisational templates and collect the correct information required for quality customer service.

4.4.1 Read and clarify workplace documents

Workers in aged care services have a duty of care to understand their role and responsibilities within the workplace. To do this they need to access, read and clarify workplace documents. These documents include:

- job description
- code of conduct
- policies and procedures
- equipment manuals
- meeting minutes
- emails
- memos
- care plans
- medication charts.

If the care worker is unsure of anything contained in any of the documentation, they must speak to the RN or supervisor for clarification. Failure to do this would be breaching their duty of care. Care workers will also need to read and clarify shift notes, communications between their team members and anything relating to the older people they support.

4.4.2 Complete documentation

There are standards set out in policies and procedures for the completion of workplace documentation. These standards are intended to guide employees in the correct way to document accurately and in accordance with

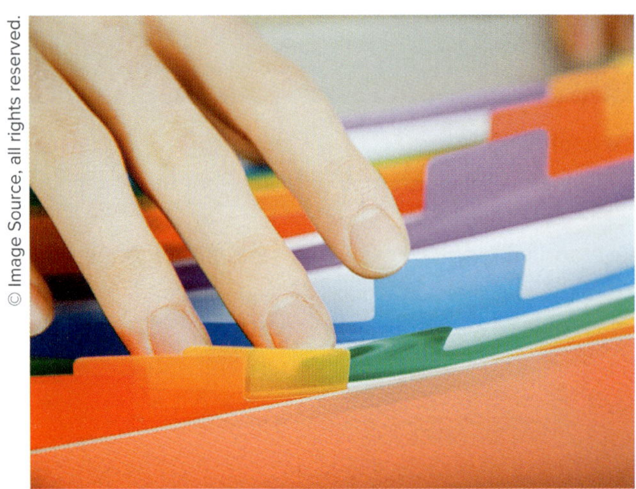

Documentation may be accessed by auditors and stakeholders, so it must be accurate

legislative requirements. Whether handwritten or in digital form, the standards need to be followed. Organisational documentation can be accessed by auditors, legal representatives and stakeholders, so it must be accurate.

Written standards:

- use the correct terminology
- are objective (without emotion)
- state only the facts
- are clear and concise
- include the time, date and a signature
- don't have any blank areas on the document that can be added to by others
- don't use jargon
- have correct spelling and grammar
- use only approved acronyms.

Digital documentation:

- uses approved fonts and font sizes
- uses correct file names when saving documents
- ensures the use of images or videos doesn't breach copyright laws
- uses version numbers when saving documents
- is formatted correctly
- follows archiving laws (how long the documentation is to be kept for).

USE CLEAR, ACCURATE AND OBJECTIVE LANGUAGE

Documentation that captures events on a day-to-day basis needs to be clear, accurate and objective. These are legal documents that contain information to prove that a worker has complied with the legislation and their duty of care responsibilities.

When documenting events in file notes or case notes and reports, the worker must use appropriate language that is objective, factual and non-biased. **Objective language** states the facts only and leaves out emotions and opinions. Subjective language is the opposite and doesn't provide the reader with accurate or sufficient information (see Table 4.1).

Aged care workers have a responsibility to write file notes, sometimes called case notes or progress notes. This documentation is vital and is often required for health professionals to see how the person is progressing. If the older person has dementia, the information can assist the care team to monitor and evaluate the strategies they are using to support the person (see Table 4.2).

TABLE 4.1 Examples of subjective and objective language

Subjective language	Objective language
Mary had a good day at her day centre today.	Mary was smiling and laughing throughout her stay at the day centre. When she arrived home, she said, "That was fun today."
John got cranky when I asked him to pick up his bag.	John stamped his feet and hit the wall when I asked him to pick up his bag.
Karen is unable to shower herself properly.	Karen needs assistance to wash and dry her back and feet.

TABLE 4.2 Example progress note

Date and time	Notes	Name and signature
17/03/2022 3 pm	Mary and care worker arrived home from the day centre today at 2 pm. Mary was smiling and laughing throughout the day at the day centre. She said, "That was fun today" when she arrived home. ------------------------	Care Worker *CW*

4.4.3 Digital media

The use of **digital media** in organisations has many benefits. It is important for administration, is cost effective, saves time and contributes to effective service delivery. Staff of aged care services will therefore need information technology (IT) skills. This can be quite overwhelming for care workers who have worked in the sector for many years and have only been accessing information in paper form.

There are protocols within all companies and organisations on the use of the following digital media when communicating.

WEBPAGES AND THE INTERNET

A company's webpage will also follow protocols and require a particular style guide to be used. It should contain clear, accurate and up-to-date information. People accessing the service can utilise the information on the webpage to see if it suits their needs.

While they are at work, employees can only visit webpages that relate to their work and that are credible (e.g. government websites). The internet is a valuable source of information to research other available services in the area that an older person might like to access. It can provide entertainment for an older person and assist with reducing isolation.

INTRANET

A company's intranet will contain many documents and programs that can assist with the completion of documentation. These include policies and procedures, templates and forms, portal access for employees, and WHS programs for recording hazards, risks and incidents. The intranet will be password protected and each employee will have their own password.

Employees need to know how to complete each document accurately. If they are unsure, they should seek assistance from a supervisor or the IT department

EMAILS

Emails are one of the most efficient ways of communicating in an organisation. Information can be sent and received in real time and can save the organisation resources. There are protocols for workers to follow when sending and receiving emails. These include:

- Each worker must have a company-approved signature with the correct information.
- Messages should have a clear subject line relating to the email content.
- Emails should not use emoticons, especially when sending externally.
- Always read an email carefully before replying to it.
- Check email content before sending.
- Salutations should be professional–for example: "Good morning/afternoon, John."
- Check that the message is being sent to the correct person.
- Use correct fonts and formatting.

SOCIAL MEDIA

Social media is used for promotional and marketing purposes and can be a valuable tool for sharing ideas and networking with others. Any platform will contain accurate information and should be in the preferred font and formats of the organisational brand.

As with all other digital media, there are protocols that workers must comply with. Employees should not mention where they work on their private social media platform. They must not add services users as friends. They should not talk about their work at all on their personal social network site, and they should not refer to their workplace in their personal profile. Any discussion about work on personal social media is a breach of privacy and will be dealt with according to privacy and confidentiality legislation.

PODCASTS AND VIDEOS

Podcasts and videos may be used to promote the organisation and its services. Podcasts are a series of episodes–in the form either of video, audio or radio. Videos can also be posted on websites to promote the organisation. These also follow organisational protocols relating to the use of digital media and must adhere to formatting and privacy guidelines and confidentiality policies and laws.

TABLETS, SMARTPHONES AND APPLICATIONS

These forms of digital media have changed the way organisations do business. Previously, everything was in written form and information was harder to access. Today, tablets and smartphones use applications to access information immediately. They are also a very useful tool for people with sensory issues, as they can be used as an electronic communication device to assist people to communicate with others.

These devices and applications should not be used by employees for personal use. They also should not be used to photograph services users without their written consent.

NEWSLETTERS

Organisations use newsletters to let older people accessing the service know about what is happening within the organisation. They can be delivered in paper or digital form and may be sent weekly or monthly. They may contain photos of events where services users were present, but consent will have been gained to use the images. These will also follow documentation protocols as they are promoting the organisation and its services.

WORKPLACE SCENARIO

Support documents

When care worker Siobhan arrives back at work after a week of leave, she checks the bowel charts and notices that two people, Bill and Yasmina, have not opened their bowels for several days. Knowing these individuals, she finds this strange and reports this information to Jim, the RN. Jim asks other staff if this is correct. Their colleague Ellie says she forgot to record Bill and Yasmina's bowel actions yesterday so Jim makes a note of this in their records, typing "bowel movements unrecorded on last 2 days" and reminds Ellie that this daily documentation is important.

Jim asks Siobhan to observe what Bill and Yasmina eat and drink during the afternoon and to report any signs of constipation. Later, Bill says he has pain in his stomach and after dinner Yasmina indicates she wants to use the bathroom.

Yasmina opens her bowels and Siobhan records this on the bowel chart immediately. She also reports Bill's stomach pain to Jim, who checks Bill's abdomen and assesses that he is constipated. Jim administers a suppository and Bill subsequently has a large bowel movement and says he has no more pain. Siobhan records this on the bowel chart.

Jim also records these events in the progress notes, explaining to Ellie that events and observations are recorded as soon as possible after they occur, and that bowel charting is a fundamental part of a care worker's responsibility.

CHECK YOUR UNDERSTANDING

1. List six workplace documents that the aged care worker must read.
2. List six standards for completing written documentation.
3. Describe the difference between subjective and objective language when completing documentation.
4. What organisational protocols exist for employees that relate to the use of personal social media?
5. List six organisational protocols that exist for sending emails.

4.5 CONTRIBUTING TO CONTINUOUS IMPROVEMENT

Continuous improvement is an ongoing process aimed at improving the quality of care delivered by services providing aged care support. It considers the needs of older people accessing services and may involve them in improvement processes. Improvements occur in a systematic way to improve quality over time. Organisations must also prove to auditors that they are continuously improving processes and services to meet funding requirements.

4.5.1 Improvements to work practices

Receiving and responding to **feedback** supports the improvement of work practices. If older people receiving services can give feedback and/or make a complaint, then services can only improve. Aged care workers are on the frontline and work very closely with older people and their family members or carers. As such, they have a unique opportunity to gather and pass on feedback to the organisation.

Aged care workers should also evaluate practices themselves and provide feedback on how a practice can possibly improve. They must complete hazard and incident reports that have identified a need to change a process or practice. Organisations can collect feedback in different ways—for example, through:

- customer surveys
- staff surveys
- complaints procedures
- staff appraisals
- internal and external audits.

Aged care workers should:

- explain and assist older people with feedback and complaints policies and procedures
- ensure privacy and confidentiality (collecting feedback requires trust)
- ensure that the older person knows how to complete forms or assist them to complete them
- allow time for the person to provide feedback
- follow up on any feedback to make sure that the client is happy or that the feedback has been received and acted on.

OBSERVING AND MONITORING

Aged care workers are observing older people when at work and are therefore in the best position to see if anything needs improving or changing regarding the support being provided. They can give feedback about organisational processes that may not be working for them and ideas on how to improve them.

4.5.2 Modelling change

Change needs to occur for continuous improvement. Work practices have changed over the decades; however, change is difficult for some people. It brings with it fear of the unknown and can cause genuine anxiety. It is important that changes are implemented gradually and positively. We have a responsibility to our colleagues and the people we provide services for to embrace change within our organisation and to be a role model for those who may be hesitant.

Just like the older people requiring support, getting out of our routines can be challenging. The implementation of change requires many factors, including:

- processes that are clear and easy to understand
- clear communication of the requirements
- training for all staff involved in the change
- continuous feedback and reflection
- a clear plan for implementation
- an appropriate time to implement the change
- monitoring and periodic review of the change to identify any risks
- a celebration once the change is established.

Be the change you want to see in the organisation and show others, through your actions, that change can be beneficial to everyone. Follow the new processes and give feedback.

4.5.3 Skills and knowledge development

To implement change and be a role model to others, a care worker may require further skills and knowledge. Care workers can seek support from their organisation about the professional development they will need in order to become "change champions".

Sometimes there may be gaps in a care worker's skills and knowledge. There will be some internal training available that needs to be completed to remain employed, but employees can also access external training to fill those gaps. Organisations will often pay for training, or there may be government funding available to complete accredited training. This will give the worker industry qualifications that are also required for employment. Aged care organisations will only employ people who have a minimum Certificate III in Individual Support.

PROFESSIONAL DEVELOPMENT

Professional development relevant to an aged care worker's role includes:

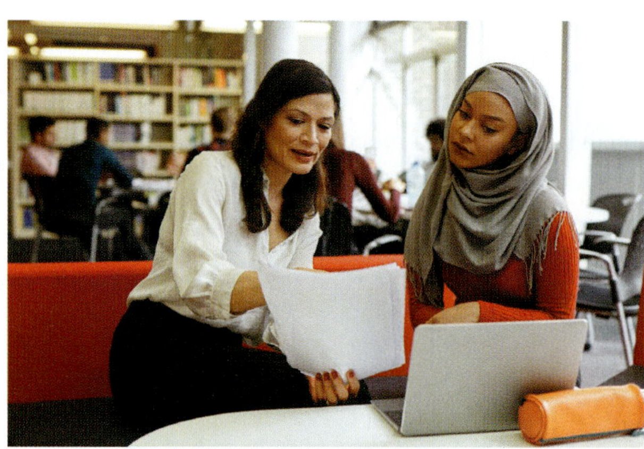

monkeybusinessimages/Getty Images

Professional development may be formal, including courses, or informal, such as self-paced online learning

- infection control
- manual handling
- documentation
- oral hygiene
- conflict resolution
- professional boundaries.

ACCREDITED TRAINING

Students can study a nationally recognised course and receive certification that qualifies them to work in their field. Course options include the Certificate III, Certificate IV and Diploma. There is also free training available in the sector, with courses provided by the government (e.g. training in infection control relating to COVID-19).

The University of Tasmania's free massive open online course (MOOC) on Dementia includes training in:

- preventing dementia
- understanding dementia
- understanding traumatic brain injury.

Gaps in skills and knowledge can be assessed in many ways. The care worker may recognise their own gaps, or they may come up in a performance review. Either way, the worker should be proactive regarding their professional development so that the support they provide to older people is based on best-practice guidelines and duty of care.

WORKPLACE SCENARIO

Professional development

After three months of working in the dementia-specific unit of a facility, care workers Anna and Houng discuss with Isla, the RN in charge of the unit, the possibility of learning more about dementia and how to support people with the condition, as well as their families.

Isla makes time to go through various courses she knows of, including the University of Tasmania's MOOC on Dementia. The course is free, and Isla suggests that it's a good place to start to understand the various types of dementia and how the condition progresses. They also discuss the possibility of joining an online learning platform that provides courses that run between 4 minutes and 2 hours and cover topics such as providing personal care for people with dementia, oral hygiene and supporting carers. Isla is pleased they both want to learn more and improve their skills.

Later, Isla discusses Anna and Huong's plans with the care manager. The manager asks Isla if they would like to apply for a training scholarship that would provide them a qualification at the next level and afford them both the opportunity to take on specific support for individuals in the unit, as well as roles as team leaders. Isla discusses this opportunity with Anna and Huong and they both agree that it will broaden their career options and enable them to provide better care support to people and families in their care.

Within six months, Anna has taken on a role as team leader in the dementia unit and Huong has moved into the community, working with people who have dementia in their own homes, as well as in a day care centre that provides respite for carers.

CHECK YOUR UNDERSTANDING

1. List four ways organisations collect feedback.
2. What factors are required when implementing changes to practices and processes within an organisation?
3. Who should a care worker seek support from if they recognise gaps in their skills and knowledge?
4. How can aged care workers assess whether they have gaps in their skills and knowledge?

SUMMARY

- Communication requires techniques that ensure an intended exchange of information between two or more parties is effective. Communication types, modes and models may differ, depending on the purpose of the communication. Care workers, as part of a care team, have legal and ethical responsibilities to communicate effectively within their role in aged care services.
- Collaborating with colleagues is important for a continuum of quality aged care service delivery to older people. Care workers must follow organisational protocols and lines of authority when communicating information in the workplace. Industry terminology is language that is used within a specific industry, and the aged care industry has its own terminology that sometimes overlaps with terminology used by the health system.
- It is important to address constraints on communication by determining what barriers are preventing a clear exchange and then collaboratively working towards a solution to optimise communication. Effective communication can be used to resolve complicated or difficult situations. Communication is essential for identifying and resolving areas of conflict.
- Completing workplace documentation and correspondence is an aspect of workplace communication that includes reading and clarifying documents, recording information in writing, and using digital media to communicate. Communication processes are also used for continuous improvement programs in the workplace.

REVIEW QUESTIONS

4.1 Identify some of the main skills required for effective communication.

4.2 Paraphrasing is an important aspect of communication. It indicates that the receiver has understood the sender's message. How do you paraphrase? Provide an example to support your answer.

4.3 How can resolving conflict result in a win–win situation?

4.4 Why are documentation and correspondence of great importance in an aged care organisation?

4.5 Identify professional development opportunities relevant to your work role.

BIBLIOGRAPHY

Australian Bureau of Statistics (ABS), *Cultural Diversity in Australia, 2016*, 2017, https://www.abs.gov.au/.

Australian Government, My Aged Care, https://www.myagedcare.gov.au/.

PRA Consulting, *5 Styles of Communication*, https://www.praconsulting.com.au/5-styles-of-communication/.

University of Tasmania, MOOC Dementia training, https://mooc.utas.edu.au/.

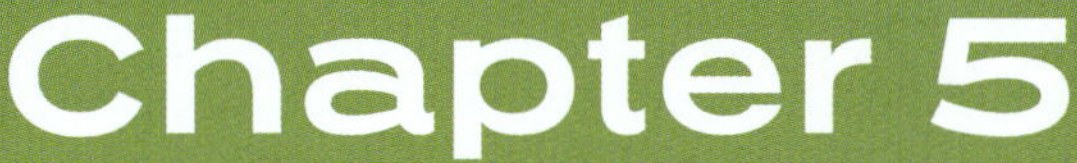

Respecting diversity

LEARNING OBJECTIVES

5.1 Reflect on culture and diversity
5.2 Understand ethical and legal factors
5.3 Recognise social and cultural competence and safety
5.4 Communicate with people from diverse backgrounds
5.5 Promote understanding across diverse groups

INTRODUCTION

REGARDLESS OF CULTURAL PERSPECTIVES AND BIASES, people are inherently different and unique. Everyone perceives things differently, thinks in different ways, has different priorities and arrives at different decisions in their own way. Each individual has personality traits leading them to display certain behaviours.

We all have personal values, beliefs, attitudes, and social and cultural perspectives that develop throughout the course of a lifetime. This could include holding different political views and having different social expectations from other people. People within our social networks (family, friends, fellow students, community members and spiritual connections) can contribute to our personal identity and to the ways in which we view other people and the world around us.

An essential skill in providing care and support is being able to understand how a person's culture may inform their values, beliefs and behaviours. Recognising that people are shaped by their cultural background can help us become culturally aware. Our cultural background influences the way we see the world around us, the way we relate to others, and the way we perceive ourselves. You don't need to be an expert in every culture to be culturally aware; it is your cultural awareness that helps you to explore cultural issues with those with whom you provide care and support.

INDUSTRY IN FOCUS

The Aged Care Diversity Framework

The **Aged Care Diversity Framework** embeds diversity in the design and delivery of aged care. It promotes safe, equitable and quality aged care to consumers, while enabling consumers and carers to be partners in this relationship.

The Diversity Framework supports an inclusive, respectful and person-centred aged care system. While some aged care service providers may choose to specialise in meeting specific needs of some groups, all elements of the aged care system and all aged care service providers should be able to accommodate consumers' diverse characteristics and life experiences.

The Diversity Framework encourages aged care providers to demonstrate continuous improvement in tailoring their services and delivering care that meets the diverse characteristics and life experiences of all clients.

Over 100,000 older people in Australia are from Aboriginal and Torres Strait Islander communities and over 36 per cent of older Australians were born outside of Australia. One in three older people were born in a non-English speaking country. More than one in ten people have diverse sexual orientation, gender identity or intersex characteristics, and almost 15,000 older Australians experience homelessness or are at risk of homelessness.

The Diversity Framework supports organisations to make informed choices, adopt systemic approaches to planning and implementation, and provide inclusive care and support. It supports a proactive and flexible system, and respectful and inclusive services, to meet the needs of the most vulnerable members of society (Australian Government, *Aged Care Diversity Framework*, n.d.).

5.1 REFLECTING ON CULTURE AND DIVERSITY

5.1.1 Culture

Culture refers to the set of customs, traditions, values, beliefs and views shared by members of a society or community, ethnic group or nation. Attitudes, beliefs, customs, language, arts, food preferences, family connections, expectations of the world, concepts of time, and so on, are all bound up in culture. A culture provides its members with rules for behaviour, and knowledge of what to believe and how to express their feelings. For many cultures, there is a predominant religion that is an important element in the lives of those people.

An essential skill in care and support is being able to understand how a person's culture may inform their values, beliefs and behaviours. Recognition that we are shaped by our cultural background will help us to become culturally aware. Our cultural background influences the way we see the world around us, the way we relate to others, and the way we perceive ourselves. You don't need to be an expert in each and every culture to be culturally aware; it is your cultural awareness that helps you to explore cultural issues with those to whom you provide care and support.

5.1.2 Diversity

Australia has an ever-increasing multicultural population, resulting in a wide diversity of people with social, cultural and spiritual differences. These differences are an essential part of a person's character. **Diversity** can be described as the inclusion of individuals regardless of differences in age, ethnicity, religion, gender, sexual orientation or disability. Valuing and respecting diversity across all areas of work can be demonstrated by supporting an inclusive environment that encompasses respect and acceptance of differences, and by working with a person's strengths and recognising people's individual differences.

When supporting diversity in the workplace, the skills of cultural awareness and cultural competence are required. It is important to acknowledge that political, socioeconomic and cultural diversity in Australia impacts on many different areas of work and life.

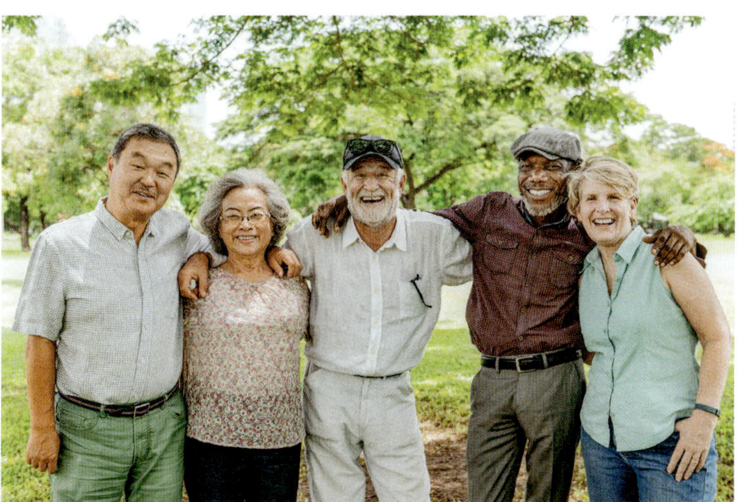

Rawpixel Ltd/Alamy Stock Photo

Our cultural background influences the way we see the world around us

TYPES OF DIVERSITY

As a care worker, you will come across a wide variety of diversity in the workplace. To be able to provide support to a person, a care worker needs to understand the following main types and characteristics of diversity.

- *Age.* Australia is an ageing society, which is reflected in the diversity of its population. Each generation has its own views and attitudes about the world around them that have been shaped by their life experiences and world events such as war and famine. The workforce of today spans several generations:
    - The Silent Generation (born before 1946)
    - Baby Boomers (born 1946–64)
    - Generation X (born 1965–81)
    - Generation Y (also known as the Millennials) (born 1982–96)
    - Generation Z (born 1997–2012). This generation has experienced high rates of psychological distress, loneliness, educational disruption, unemployment, housing stress and domestic violence, due to COVID-19 and the impact of the pandemic. Their social connectedness diminished during the pandemic, and it is recognised that not all effects from the pandemic are apparent as yet. As conditions such as the requirement to wear masks change, the effects of the pandemic may alter quickly and mental health and connectedness can improve (AIHW, 2021).
- *Ethnicity.* Australia is a diverse, multicultural country made up of people from over 200 different countries. Each of these ethnic groups has its own unique cultural diversity as a result of its history, personal experiences, and regional differences and associations. Additionally, there are intrinsic cultural differences arising from things such as class, gender roles, and city and rural environments.
- *Religion.* Defined as a planned and systematic collection of beliefs, cultural systems and worldviews that relate humanity to a specific way of being, religion crosses national, geographic and cultural boundaries, and generally focuses on individuals, families and communities. Religious institutions and rituals often play a significant role in catering to a person's social, psychological, cultural and spiritual needs.
- *Language.* The type of language spoken is a key indicator of belonging to a specific ethnic group. Having a commonly spoken language supports communication of values, beliefs and perceptions of a particular culture and participation in family, community and society. Most Australians speak English as their first language; however, a significant number of Australians speak languages other than English.

- *Sexual orientation and gender.* The term "sexual orientation" refers to the sex a person is attracted to, and "gender" refers to what the person identifies as or who they are. The acronym "LGBTQIA+" represents the words "lesbian, gay, bisexual, transgender/transexual, questioning, intersex and asexual". The "+" symbol represents the many other sexual orientations. "LGBTQIA+" is often used by the Australian government to describe a diverse group of people and populations.
- *Disability.* People with disability are an important part of diversity in Australia, and many share experiences and challenges in life similar to those that people without disability face. Disability can occur regardless of age, ethnicity, language, religion, socioeconomic background or sexual orientation.

INCLUSION

Inclusivity refers to non-exclusion—that is, the process of ensuring that people are not excluded on the grounds of gender, race, class, sexual preference, disability, religion, age, and so on. Marginalised groups are populations of people who are viewed as being different from society and are not accepted by society for that reason. Stereotyping of marginalised groups is a reality. In Australia, marginalised groups include:

- refugees
- people living with disability
- people who are disadvantaged economically
- those who have mental and emotional health issues
- Aboriginal and Torres Strait Islander people
- those for whom English is a second language
- people affected by domestic violence
- older people
- homeless people
- people with alcohol and drug problems.

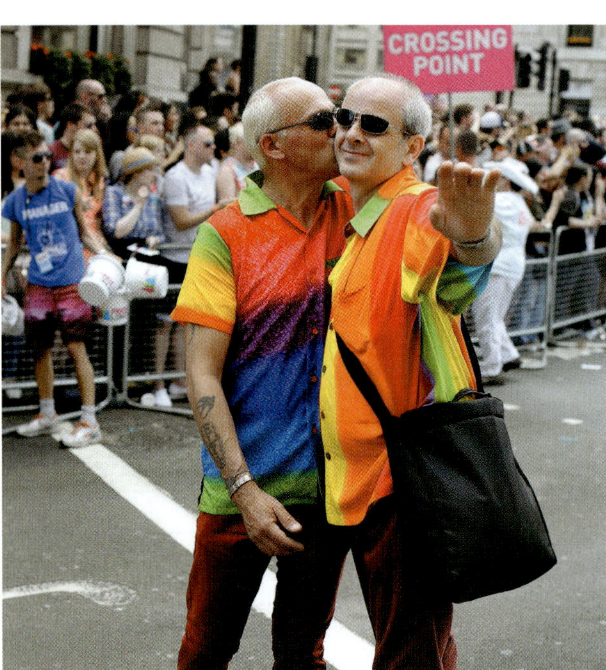

Sung Kuk Kim/Alamy Live News

Valuing and respecting diversity can be demonstrated by supporting an inclusive environment

Social and community inclusion can be considered a determinant of wellbeing, as it contributes to the capacity of individuals to:

- participate in and contribute to the life of the community
- make decisions that are relevant to themselves and their own lives
- define their own goals
- identify their own place within the community and the world.

In the workplace, inclusion translates to providing fair and equitable service for all clients regardless of difference. Further, it relates to respect for diversity and accommodation of the needs of individuals. Antidiscrimination and inclusivity are linked concepts; however, the prevention of discrimination on its own isn't sufficient. Diversity won't accrue benefits for the organisation, its employees, individuals and other stakeholders unless employees adhere to the notion of inclusivity.

A culturally safe workplace invests in developing effective employment programs and strategies that support diversity. The workplace should be an inclusive environment and celebrate the diversity that is present, implying that people won't be marginalised or disadvantaged because of differences.

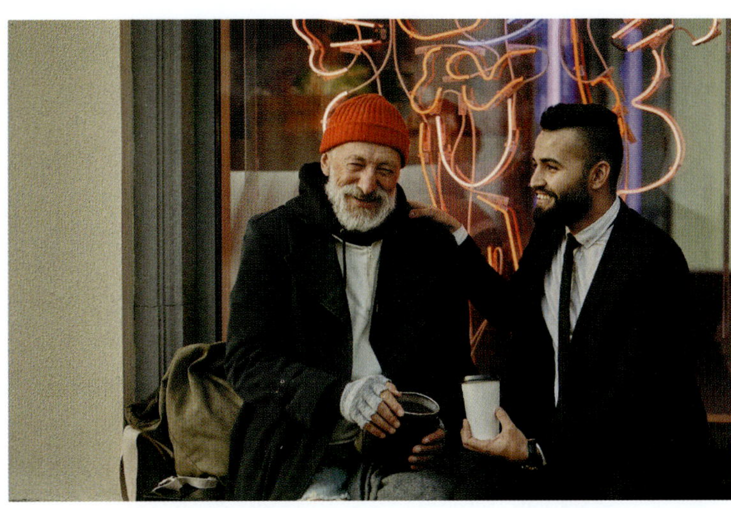
UfaBizPhoto/Shutterstock

Social and community inclusion is a determinant of wellbeing

In all areas of work, it is necessary to value and respect diversity. To build relationships with diverse people, it is necessary to appreciate their diversity and to understand the need for inclusivity. Inclusivity takes the concept of diversity and embraces it, makes it workable and useful with regard to interaction between workers in an organisation and between workers and individuals.

Care workers and other staff must contribute to the development of workplace and professional relationships based on an appreciation of diversity and inclusiveness. Most organisations understand that they require a diverse workforce–people who have, among them, a wide range of skills, attitudes and perceptions. These differences contribute to the organisation's ability to be flexible, to generate problem solutions, to relate effectively to a wide range of individuals and to provide a balanced range of services. The same principles apply to work life and interactions in the workplace.

In a socially inclusive society, people feel valued and valuable regardless of their diverse characteristics. Differences are respected and people are supported to live their lives in the way that best meets their needs in a culturally safe manner.

DIVERSITY WITHIN CULTURAL GROUPS

There is great diversity within cultural groups, such as gender identities, age, religion, beliefs, socioeconomic circumstances, ethnicity, language, sexual preferences, education, migration experiences, generational differences, history, cultural beliefs and practices. It is good to know about the characteristics of broad cultural groups, but never assume that all people from that group are the same.

As a care worker, you should treat each person as an individual and avoid stereotyping. When you learn a little about a culture, you can use this knowledge to start a conversation and learn more about that individual.

DIVERSITY WITHIN SOCIAL GROUPS

It is important to acknowledge that political, socioeconomic and cultural diversity in Australia impacts on many different areas of work and life. Diversity provides many social and economic advantages.

- It creates employment.
- It contributes to shared prosperity.
- It enables creative, innovative and artistic exchange.
- It facilitates communication across state, national and international boundaries.
- It enables identification of issues that require political action (e.g. Australia's ageing population).
- It facilitates global connections and the expansion of opportunities for global trade and investment.
- It challenges societal stereotypes of diverse and marginalised groups and can facilitate a collective change in thinking.

PRACTICE POINT

The following are some simple ways to support diversity at work.

- Ensure culturally specific foods are available.
- Follow traditional methods for handling and preparation of food.
- Support fasting and other requirements of different traditions or religions.
- Encourage staff to wear traditional garments.
- Observe cultural expectations.
- Respect that certain parts of the body may be required to be covered.
- Support and celebrate occasions and special events, remembering that not all people will want to celebrate every event.
- Organise religious visits as requested.
- Play music from a range of cultures.
- Support local cultural visits from the community.
- Display art from a variety of cultures.
- Include cultural opportunities in the activity program.

Workplaces can tap into the rich diversity of Australia that can contribute to organisational success and a strong workplace culture. Managers, supervisors and team leaders are required to work with all people in the organisation and to ensure that they actively encourage cooperation and acceptance of diversity and don't instil competitiveness or exclusion. It is essential that care workers and other staff identify and reflect on their own social and cultural perspectives and biases.

Some practical and social ideas for providing such an environment include identifying practical skills around food, music, art and clothing and using these to build cultural competence, strengthen relationships between diverse people and meet people's individual needs.

CULTURAL AND SOCIAL AWARENESS

We must all be aware of our own cultural values, beliefs and perceptions. Managers, supervisors, team leaders and care workers must demonstrate respect for diversity in a range of activities and situations, such as by:

- dealing sensitively with persons of diverse race, ethnicity, class, ability, sexual preference and age
- working and dealing equitably with people of different genders
- accommodating people's cultural and spiritual needs
- complying with duty of care requirements
- providing information that can be readily understood by people from a range of different backgrounds and with different educational abilities
- communicating effectively with workers, individuals and other stakeholders
- providing appropriate care in terms of physical, psychological and end-of-life care that meets the needs of individuals
- supporting social justice
- protecting the personal belongings of individuals and workers
- ensuring food services suit the needs and preferences of individuals, including observing taboos.

Workplace diversity can bring many benefits, including:

- greater customer satisfaction
- better market positioning
- successful decision making
- an enhanced ability to reach strategic goals
- improved organisational outcomes
- enhanced family satisfaction
- possible improved health outcomes.

Everyone in the organisation will be focused on providing high-level care and catering for individual needs regardless of diversity. Quality care will reflect respect for diversity and support for inclusiveness across all areas of work. It will contribute to the development of effective work and professional relationships.

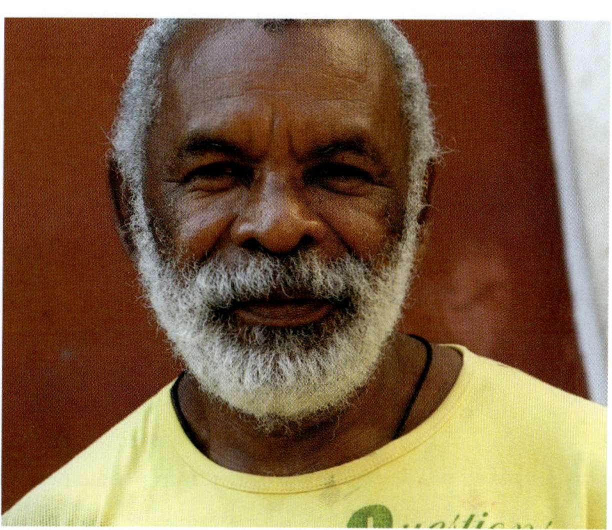

foodfolio/Alamy Stock Photo

Quality care reflects respect for diversity and support for inclusiveness across all areas of work

Acceptance of diversity and support for inclusivity will contribute to the development of:

- a workplace where exclusive clubs and cliques are unacceptable
- a focus on collaboration
- a workplace mentality that will break down any developing silos
- competitive advantage
- new or fresh outlooks on problem solving and decision making in individual teams and the whole of the organisation
- the ability to cater for and accommodate the communication, cultural and personal needs of individuals using aged care services and the diverse workforce
- a positive work environment and care environment
- decreased attrition and absenteeism of workers (increased retention of useful and valuable employees)
- the perception that this is a workplace where people want to work (improved quality of applicants for positions)
- a well-regarded public image
- a culturally safe workplace
- ultimately, sustainable business success.

A diverse and inclusive workforce enhances the quality and depth of decision making and improves collaboration and teamwork at all levels of the organisation. An inclusive and fair work environment, free of discrimination and harassment, has a positive impact on the wellbeing of employees, job satisfaction, productivity, and staff retention within the organisation.

The workplace must have suitable policies, procedures, frameworks and instruments available to encourage and support diversity. Strategies used to eliminate bias and discrimination in the workplace will be grounded by legislation.

In alignment with legislation, organisational policies and procedures will be developed. All staff must comply with these policies and procedures. Breaches of legislation or failure to carry out responsibilities can result in litigation and the loss of a job.

Aged care organisations are governed by industry and organisational codes of ethics and practice, which provide guidelines for the expected behaviour of staff. The code of conduct is not enforceable by law, but it does carry an expectation of compliance.

A shared vision will ensure a cohesive workforce, and this includes a shared set of workplace values, norms and beliefs that surround the mission of the organisation. This is a workplace culture, which is different from the personal culture and personal expectations of individual care workers.

When developing ways to improve cultural awareness and to support diversity, care workers should consider the following:

- Difference is good; it's not something to fear or to avoid.
- Communication will be effective if individual differences are respected.
- Accommodating diversity includes constantly being aware of politically correct behaviour and language.
- Care workers (including managers, supervisors and team leaders) work best when they believe they are valued.
- All stakeholders will feel most valued when they perceive their differences are being acknowledged and that strategies to support effective communication are being developed.
- The ability to learn from people perceived as different is the key to empowerment and to the building of effective, mutually interdependent relationships.

WORKPLACE SCENARIO

Understanding perspective and bias: The importance of self-awareness and reflection

Care manager Jae knows that people from culturally and linguistically diverse backgrounds require a strong relationship with all staff involved in their care and support. To build these relationships, she encourages her staff to understand their own culture and beliefs. In order to do this, she asks them to think about the following questions (to which there are no right or wrong answers). She explains that their answers to these questions will help to shape their values and attitudes:

- What is your ethnic background?
- How would you describe your religion?
- What culture do you strongly identify with and why?
- What do you particularly like about your traditions and your culture?
- What other cultures interest you? What do you know about them?
- How would you describe gender?
- How would you describe sexual preference?
- How would you describe your socioeconomic class?
- What cultures would you like to know more about?
- What cultures do you know very little about?

CHECK YOUR UNDERSTANDING

1. Are all people from one cultural background the same?
2. What is meant by diversity?
3. What benefits come from diversity in the workplace?
4. What can be considered when trying to improve cultural awareness and to support diversity?

5.2 UNDERSTANDING ETHICAL AND LEGAL FACTORS

5.2.1 Ethical principles

The *Universal Declaration of Human Rights* sets out a number of articles which people should comply with if they are to uphold the philosophies of equality and human rights for all. Human rights are inalienable, basic freedoms and protections to which all people are entitled. Aged care organisations must be aware of the need for inclusivity across all areas of work, as well as their legal obligations regarding the prevention of discrimination and the application of equal opportunity requirements.

Organisational policies, procedures and practices should contribute to workplace and professional relationships that are based on appreciation of diversity and understanding of the concept of inclusivity.

5.2.2 Ethical issues

BIAS, DISCRIMINATION AND PREJUDICE

Services and organisations must operate free from cultural biases, discrimination and prejudices. This can be achieved by:

- employing workers from different cultural and linguistic backgrounds
- working with diverse work groups in committees–for example, within the organisation
- reviewing pictures, designs and literature in the workplace to ensure they don't cause offence and accurately reflect diversity
- participating in events that honour diversity, such as Harmony Day and the Sydney Gay and Lesbian Mardi Gras
- showing interest in others by celebrating special days and festivals for the diverse members of the workplace
- planning activities for the different cultural groups in consultation with them
- openly challenging discrimination, prejudice and bias
- having vision, mission and philosophy statements that reflect and acknowledge cultural safety, cultural competence, inclusion and cultural diversity.

The word **bias** means to view a person, group or experience in a way that is considered unfair, and which often occurs because of our own values and beliefs. We all have biases and some of them are unconscious; in other words, we make a judgement about someone because we automatically think we understand their viewpoint. Another type of bias is direct bias. Examples of bias include:

- *Amy thinks that all young people know how to use technology.* (Unconscious bias)
- *Rod believes that all people who receive welfare are drug addicts.* (Direct bias)

Self-reflection and introspection can help in identifying the values we hold and contribute to our ability to accept that others are entitled to their own values and beliefs. The theory of unconscious bias holds that care workers can have biases they are not aware of that influence their decision making. Day-to-day decisions are informed by stereotypical views that people are not consciously aware of having.

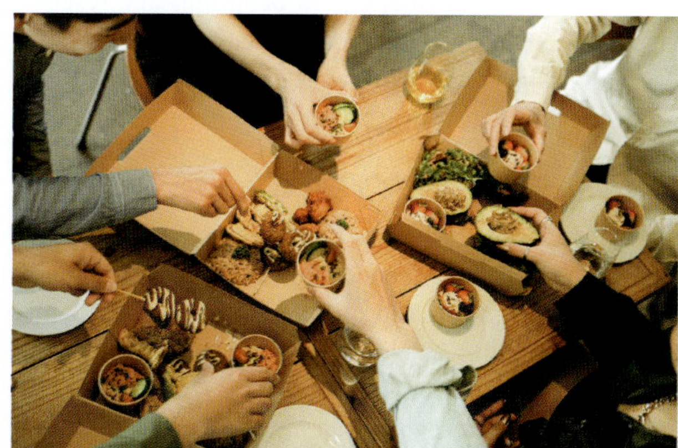

Getty Images/kyotokushige

Workplaces can show interest in others by celebrating festivals with members of the team

As a care worker, when you reflect on your own bias and associated behaviours, and the potential outcomes of removing bias, you might consider the importance of the following:

- respect and courtesy
- sharing of experiences, knowledge and skills
- fear of difference
- self-fulfilment and self-improvement
- similarities between yourself and other people from a range of cultures—looking for commonalities and meeting points, rather than differences
- questions you could ask work colleagues or older people to help them learn about different cultures
- conscious or unconscious bias
- your ability to support inclusivity
- strategies for increasing understanding of others
- ways in which you can improve yourself and your social awareness.

Care workers need to consider their own biases and increase their awareness of their own limitations with regards to diversity. The process of identifying these things and increasing their self-awareness can help a person follow strategies that enable them to understand others better, be more tolerant, improve their social awareness, and more actively and efficiently support inclusivity. The workplace must provide fair and equitable support services that don't discriminate or disadvantage any person or group. This is a requirement that is upheld by antidiscrimination and equal employment opportunity (EEO) legislation in Australia.

Aged care managers and care workers must put their own biases aside, identify their own limitations, increase their social awareness, and learn to work inclusively with colleagues, older people and their families, and other stakeholders.

Self-awareness skills include:

- recognising own strengths and areas for improvement
- identifying what is required to complete activities and tasks
- amending or addressing misunderstandings or difficulties
- being comfortable recognising and talking about your emotions
- recognising other people's feelings and needs
- acknowledging how behaviour affects others
- developing reflective practice.

In the workplace, self-reflection can facilitate skills that allow care workers to accurately judge their own performance and behaviour and respond appropriately to unfamiliar or difficult social situations. By recognising personal limitations, the care worker is better placed to seek advice and guidance from their supervisor, work colleagues, experts and other people. This will ultimately result in better outcomes for everyone involved.

STEREOTYPING

Stereotyping is the process of judging individuals on the basis of what you consider to be their cultural affiliation. Gender, sexual and racial stereotypes are often denigrating and unkind. They are also often prejudicial and untrue and don't take into account individual differences. Stereotypes can be positive or negative but are usually an exaggerated idea of group characteristics that are transferred to each of the individuals in the group.

Stereotyping can include making broad statements about people:

- *Older people are inflexible.*
- *People with disability are objects of pity and charity.*

- *Older people aren't interested in the same things as younger people.*
- *All Indigenous people are drunks and lazy.*
- *Women aren't as smart as men.*

Stereotyping can lead to **discrimination**, as it removes a person's individuality and oversimplifies their qualities. It places people into particular groups (often referred to as marginalised groups) and attributes characteristics to them that might not necessarily be attributable to them as individuals.

Stereotypes should not influence a care worker's working relationship with the people they provide aged care services to or those they work alongside. When dealing with work colleagues, people who are ageing, and their carers and families, care workers need to be sensitive to each person's sense of self-esteem. This means avoiding derogatory labelling, which can demean and dehumanise people.

MULTICULTURALISM

The original inhabitants of Australia are the Aboriginal and Torres Strait Islander peoples; however, today's Australia is home to many people from many cultures, stemming from the roots of colonisation. Contributions to Australian society from different cultures have all produced the rich variety of life that we currently enjoy. Increased access to world travel and to virtually instantaneous global communication has also added to, and expanded, our culture and cultural outlook.

Multiculturalism has provided opportunities for sharing aspects of cultures that are the fabric of the Australian experience, including arts and artistic forms, music, food and food styles, entertainment, religion and spiritual affiliations, clothing, building styles, books, crafts, interior design, education and schooling.

Multicultural Australia maximises the social, cultural and economic benefits that exist because of cultural diversity. It is based on four key principles:

- responsibilities for all
- respect for each person
- fairness for each person
- benefits for all.

As a care worker, it is important to understand that Australian diversity derives from two major social factors:

- an expansive multicultural mix
- an antidiscrimination approach, which deems illegal any attempts to prejudice the rights of individuals because of their age, gender, sexual orientation, physical qualities, ethnicity or religion.

Australia is a multicultural nation that openly enjoys the freedom and lifestyle on offer. However, there is an ongoing debate within the community and at government levels about where acceptance of cultural practices ends and a commitment to a set of national understandings starts. It is important that we all share an understanding about some basic commitments that we, as Australian citizens, accept. In Australia, individual and cultural practices must work within the framework of:

- freedom of speech
- freedom of religion
- democratic decision making through an elected parliament
- equality of men and women
- freedom from discrimination
- English as the national language.

This framework is the basis of how we conduct ourselves as a nation and culture and shapes our interactions with all other cultures.

Australia is one of the most culturally diverse countries in the world. The population is a mix of the following cultural groups and subgroups:

- Aboriginal and Torres Strait Islander cultures (First Nations people)
- Anglo-Australian (Anglo-Celtic and Anglo-Saxon) culture (the mainstream culture)
- immigrant cultures, including:
  - Chinese
  - Dutch
  - Filipino
  - German
  - Greek
  - Italian
  - Pacific Islander
  - Vietnamese.

All levels of Australian government have committed considerable resources to provide services in support of cultural difference. There is always debate about the sufficiency of such resources. Some of the concerns they seek to address in terms of culture and health and community care are:

- Indigenous health
- models of health and community care
- women's health care
- oral health care
- power roles within care provision
- disability care
- aged care
- dying and death.

5.2.3 Legislation

All employees must comply with relevant state and federal health and safety legislation. This is to ensure the physical and psychological safety and wellbeing of anyone in or associated with the workplace. Over recent times, the Commonwealth government and the state and territory governments have introduced laws to help protect people from discrimination and harassment.

The following laws operate at the federal level:

- *Age Discrimination Act 2004*
- *Australian Human Rights Commission Act 1986*
- *Disability Discrimination Act 1992*
- *Racial Discrimination Act 1975*
- *Sex Discrimination Act 1984.*

The following laws operate at the state and territory level:

- Australian Capital Territory: *Discrimination Act 1991*
- New South Wales: *Anti-Discrimination Act 1977*
- Northern Territory: *Anti-Discrimination Act 1996*
- Queensland: *Anti-Discrimination Act 1991*
- South Australia: *Equal Opportunity Act 1984*
- Tasmania: *Anti-Discrimination Act 1998*
- Victoria: *Equal Opportunity Act 2010*
- Western Australia: *Equal Opportunity Act 1984.*

Commonwealth laws and the state/territory laws generally overlap and prohibit the same type of discrimination. As both state/territory and Commonwealth laws apply, care workers must comply with both (Australian Human Rights Commission n.d.).

WORKPLACE SCENARIO

The multicultural workplace

Hannah, who has dementia, lives in residential care. She is Jewish, born in Germany in 1931. During World War II, she and her family were interned in a concentration camp. Hannah was the only family member to survive. During her time at the camp, she (like all the prisoners) stole and hid food, as food was often withheld by the guards. In the residential care facility, Hannah sometimes sneaks into the kitchen and steals food, which she tries to hide in her room.

Ng is a care worker in the facility. She was born here in 1989 to parents who escaped Vietnam on a boat to Australia. She is of the Christian faith and considers stealing a sin. One day, Ng was working in Hannah's room, tidying up and making the bed, when she found some bread hidden in the bottom drawer of Hannah's locker. Ng thought this was strange and told her supervisor. Her supervisor explained that Hannah's brain was deteriorating, due to the dementia. She thought she was back in the concentration camp, terrified of starving and doing anything to survive. The kitchen staff purposely left some food out for Hannah to "steal", the supervisor told Ng. It made Hannah feel safer to know she had food stashed away, like she did when she was a little girl in the camp.

On learning this about Hannah, Ng was filled with empathy for her. She understood that Hannah was just keeping herself safe. Ng was able to continue to be professional, but now that she knew Hannah's story and why she was behaving the way she was, Ng was even kinder to her when providing her with care.

CHECK YOUR UNDERSTANDING

1. What can organisations do to demonstrate they are free from cultural biases, discrimination and prejudices?
2. What is stereotyping?
3. List some groups that you think are marginalised in Australia.
4. What steps would you take if you found a person living with dementia in your facility stealing food from the kitchen?

5.3 RECOGNISING SOCIAL AND CULTURAL COMPETENCE AND SAFETY

5.3.1 Cultural awareness and cultural competence

Cultural awareness refers to the ability to reflect on and be aware of our own cultural values, beliefs and perceptions. As a care worker, you can demonstrate cultural awareness and competence by:

- learning about other cultures
- understanding a variety of traditions, customs, beliefs, languages, rituals and values
- appreciating how cultural backgrounds can affect the behaviour, beliefs and language skills of the people you work with.

Cultural competence refers to the ability to understand, communicate and interact effectively with a diverse range of people from different cultures and backgrounds. Cultural competence is deeper than cultural awareness. It refers to people and organisations interacting effectively in many different cultural contexts. Cultural competence enables people to feel respected, accepted and confident to express their cultural needs. Recognising and honouring differences between people is culturally competent, as is the acknowledgement of a shared humanity across diversity.

5.3.2 Cultural safety

Cultural safety can be described as an environment that is safe and supportive for people and doesn't expose them to assault, challenge or denial of their identity, needs and wants. A culturally safe environment can be created by implementing culturally safe work practices that provide care in a way that is respectful of a person's diversity and culture and is free from discrimination.

Cultural safety initiates a range of responses from a position of respect for the cultural views of another person. This means not inadvertently challenging an individual by expecting them to compromise their cultural identity. In a culturally safe environment, there is shared respect, shared meaning, shared knowledge, and the experience of learning together. Actions that recognise and respect the cultural identities of others, and safely meet their work needs, expectations and rights, are encouraged.

Cultural safety involves adopting employment strategies that support diversity and are underpinned by a strong focus on the following:

- *People:* driving the right attitudes and behaviours in the workplace to ensure that the environment is culturally and socially inclusive.
- *Linked policies:* ensuring HR (human resources) practices encourage and support the recruitment and retention of diverse candidates.
- *Engagement:* building and embracing relationships with diverse people, communities and external organisations to achieve greater outcomes and more effective and productive processes.

As a care worker, you have a responsibility to help create a safe environment by making a person feel comfortable and secure. Work practices that do this include:

- recognising and respecting the cultural identities of others
- not diminishing, demeaning or disempowering the cultural identity and wellbeing of any individual
- providing information (such as brochures or posters) in a variety of languages
- supporting a person's cultural rituals such as praying, reading religious books and meditating
- ensuring adequate nutritional intake, as cultural needs may affect nutritional requirements
- supporting a person's sexual orientation and gender
- supporting access to social activities, cultural activities and support groups
- identifying and promoting festivals, special days and events
- understanding different beliefs and behaviours about personal space and touching
- consulting with the person and their family and/or carer about decisions that will affect that person
- being aware of a person's life experiences, such as migrants who have witnessed war
- understanding there are different beliefs about physical and mental health and treatment
- following safe work practice.

Aged care services will have diversity management policies and procedures that aim to:

- meet legislative and statutory requirements
- comply with industry codes of ethics/practice
- integrate equality and diversity in policy and practice

- make the organisation a workplace of choice because it is recognised as having a culture that supports diversity
- prevent discrimination, harassment and exclusion based on personal or group characteristics
- increase employee satisfaction, health and wellbeing
- increase knowledge, capabilities and skills of employees in cross-cultural situations
- promote and recognise the value of international mobility and cross-cultural situations
- ensure that staff have appropriate training and information in equality areas to prevent and eliminate discrimination, make reasonable adjustments and promote equality of opportunity
- recruit and select staff on a fair and equitable basis
- raise awareness of stigma and discrimination around issues such as disability, mental health issues, and so on, in terms of equity
- ensure and enforce cultural safety for all.

The environment is accepted to be the surroundings that interact with a person or group of people. The work environment includes the:

- social and cultural environment
- people and institutions with which people interact
- built environment or the constructed settings that provide for human interaction
- knowledge environment, social practices, and technological and physical arrangements intended to support decision making, inference or discovery.

Everyone wants to live and work in an environment that is safe, secure and comfortable. Care workers must be able to work safely in an environment that doesn't present unreasonable dangers, including psychological harm from bullying, harassment and discrimination. A culturally safe workplace doesn't tolerate these risks of harm, and diversity policies aim to minimise risks to the mental health of consumers, their families and all staff in the same way as they aim to prevent physical harm in the workplace.

Aged care workers must use work practices that make the environment safe for individuals, their families and significant others, and for those who provide the care. This applies in all community care situations, including residential care or the provision of home care.

TRAUMA

Some people may have ongoing effects, or **trauma**, from their life experiences that have a negative impact on their wellbeing. We all have a story, and individuals from culturally diverse backgrounds may have experienced traumatic events that are linked to their culture or beliefs. They may have escaped from a war or been tortured in a takeover of their country. They may have been separated from loved ones, lived in fear, been persecuted, or not had enough to eat. These people will require extra reassurance, emotional support and understanding. They are likely to be highly anxious through any changes, or they may be triggered to remember some of the trauma they have been through. Care workers need to understand the background of the people they support, in order to develop a deeper understanding of why a person behaves in the ways they do.

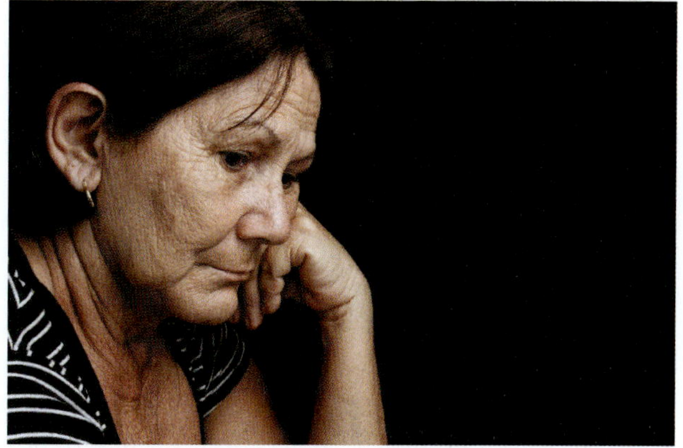

Kamira/Shutterstock

People who have experienced trauma require extra reassurance, emotional support and understanding

The person's individualised plan should detail specific strategies to guide the care worker in supporting the person to cope with the effects of past trauma. Some of your colleagues in aged care may have come from backgrounds similar to those described above, so you may find that workers from diverse backgrounds require more understanding and support from you as well. In your role as a care worker, you may also come across former child migrants, people from the Stolen Generation and others from institutionalised care.

Actions that may trigger adverse reactions include locked doors, communal showers, darkness or being cold. All of these can bring about great distress and may cause crying, withdrawal, aggression or resistance to care. A care worker will provide an environment free from potential triggers where these people feel safe and secure.

THE EFFECTS OF TRAUMA

Trauma can have a debilitating impact on the life of the individual who experiences it, and its effects can last a lifetime. The following factors have been linked to the effects of trauma:

- Increasing age correlates highly with increasing risk of trauma.
- Around 70–90 per cent of all adults over the age of 65 have experienced at least one trauma-level life event (Pietrzak et al. 2013).
- Older people are more likely to have lost very close relatives.
- Older people are more likely to have experienced life-threatening illness and medical intervention in hospital (Ganzel 2018).
- Older people are more likely to lose control over significant life choices and decisions (Van der Kolk 2014).
- Intensive care admission is associated with the development of post-traumatic stress disorder (PTSD) symptoms.
- Older people are more likely to have experienced intensive care unit admissions.
- Transition to residential care is often experienced as traumatic.

RETRAUMATISATION IN OLDER PEOPLE

Older age is often associated with reviewing life and finding meaning in past experiences. Reviewing memories may include traumatic memories and this could retraumatise the person. Illness, stress and loss of control, often associated with ageing, appear to be factors that reactivate trauma symptoms. Resurgence of the symptoms of previously experienced PTSD is significantly more common in older people.

5.3.3 Aboriginal and Torres Strait Islander peoples

Aboriginal and Torres Strait Islander peoples have very strong traditions, kinship, links to land, oral histories, languages and customs. Many languages have been lost because people were forbidden to speak their own languages after colonisation, even as recently as the 1960s. More than 200 languages existed prior to colonisation; today, only about 60 remain.

Aboriginal and Torres Strait Islander peoples have a post-colonisation history of disenfranchisement, disadvantage and discrimination. This must be acknowledged and understood when working with or for Indigenous people, because the historic and ongoing dispossession of First Nations people has resulted in significant mistrust of Western ways.

More than 500 First Nations clans exist in Australia, each having its own kinship, or social, structure. Kinship is an important social system to Indigenous people because it provides the social context of each individual's place in the world, including their relationships and responsibilities (Australians Together 2012). Service provision that is related to aged care or health matters is often developed in consultation with the person's extended family or community, whereby the Elders guide decisions. Care workers need to understand the importance of shared decision making among many First Nations communities, and how this sense of extended family affects the role of the care worker when providing care. Many Aboriginal and Torres Strait Islander people prefer to have their needs supported by their own communities rather than accessing aged or health-care systems.

First Nations people are a marginalised group in Australia, and many historic, social and stereotypical factors have created barriers to their accessing social justice. This has been compounded by racism, discrimination, socioeconomic disadvantage, lack of access to health and educational programs, high levels of poverty, poor living conditions and high levels of unemployment. Economic and social disadvantage are risk factors for poor health, disability, chronic disease, alcohol and substance abuse, suicide and high incarceration rates.

Aged care services should aim for a collaborative service approach with Indigenous communities, to enable the establishment of relationships with local Indigenous community-controlled organisations that can share valuable referral services and advice about culturally appropriate aged care services.

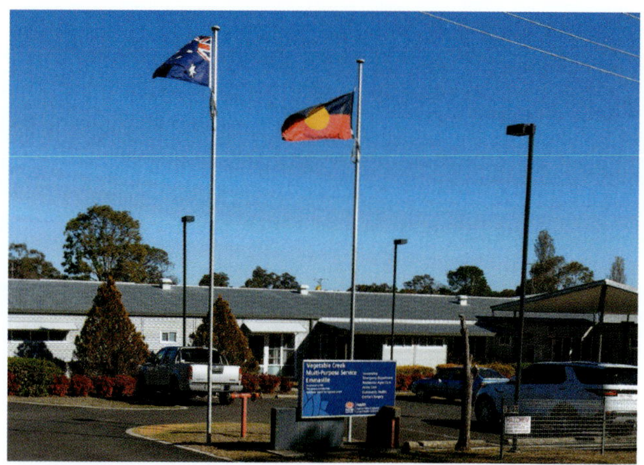

OZSHOTZ/Alamy Stock Photo

Many Aboriginal and Torres Strait Islander people prefer to have their needs supported by their own communities

Spirituality—or The Dreaming—is fundamentally essential to First Nations people. It affects all aspects of life, including sickness and ageing. Dementia, for instance, may not be recognised as a medical condition that requires care, although it might be seen as a "sickness of the soul" (Benevolent Society n.d.). Spiritual beliefs and practices will often take preference over Western health and medical interventions.

It is essential to understand that although First Nations people may share similar cultural values and beliefs, this similarity is variable among individuals. Cultural identity is much more intrinsic than what can be identified in books such as this. As a care worker, always ask the person what their preferences are and never assume that it will involve the same as other First Nations people. Although cultural identity and spirituality are fundamental to First Nations people, their interpretation of these powerful concepts will be individual.

When supporting First Nations people and working with First Nations colleagues, non-Indigenous aged care workers will require an understanding of the:

- importance of community and extended family in decision making
- diversity within the Indigenous population
- impact of living in remote areas (where relevant)
- results of restricted access to education, employment and economic stability
- historical and current impacts of colonisation
- customs, lore, laws and life expectations of the group of populations with which they work
- behaviours that signal respect for elders and culture
- procedures that should be followed to ensure suitable consultation with communities and their elders when designing and delivering services.

WORKPLACE SCENARIO

Aboriginal and Torres Strait Islander peoples

Donna is an Aboriginal woman who prefers to use health services that display the Aboriginal and Torres Strait Islander flags. The flags tell Donna that she is welcome, and that the service acknowledges her people. She doesn't feel comfortable if the workers at the service present as very official, because experience has taught her that people in some positions can use power against her.

(Continues)

When Donna needs to attend any health or aged-related service, she prefers to yarn with an Aboriginal health worker because she feels more comfortable sharing with them information about her health and wellbeing. She always takes one of her aunties with her as support during a visit to the service. Today, Donna and her Aunty Marie are enquiring about Indigenous organisations that can provide home care services for one of the Elders in their community.

CHECK YOUR UNDERSTANDING

1. What is cultural competence?
2. What is cultural safety?
3. As a care worker, you have a responsibility to help create a culturally safe environment. List three ways you can do this.
4. Some culturally and linguistically diverse people have experienced trauma in their past. How might this affect their ability to receive care, and how will you manage this in the workplace?

5.4 COMMUNICATING WITH PEOPLE FROM DIVERSE BACKGROUNDS

5.4.1 Respectful communication

Communication is the process of passing and receiving messages. These can be verbal, non-verbal or both. We communicate in order to:

- give instructions
- discuss problems
- ask for information
- entertain others
- meet our own needs
- meet the needs of other people
- create situations (to inspire or influence others) which result in action being taken
- share information or inform others.

Effective communication is the key to good service provision to individuals and to good work relationships. As a care worker, it is important to develop skills in effective communication. Despite our best efforts, communication can often get lost in translation; language barriers, in particular, can result in misunderstanding, confusion and possibly even conflict. Communication is a very important part of a care worker's role, as they will communicate with work colleagues, health professionals, people with disability, family/and or carers, and other members of the community. It is essential that a care worker is familiar with the many methods of communication available and uses the most appropriate one for the task. However, communication requires the recipient of the message to understand its meaning as it was intended. If it is not understood as intended, then effective communication hasn't occurred.

In the aged care context, all forms of communication must show respect for diversity. When working with individuals from diverse backgrounds, or with those who may have communication difficulties due to physical or cognitive issues, it is important for management and staff to take extra care with communication. Showing respect for diversity in communication with all people involves realising that people are all individuals and have different perceptions, values and expectations. Every person is unique.

Furthermore, various cultural groups have different rules or practices regarding:

- the use of humour and irony
- when to say "please", "thank you" or "excuse me"
- when the words "yes" and "no" are used
- conversational rules and conventions (e.g. who can speak to whom, and who can start the conversation)
- deference to others
- body language, gestures, personal space
- gender issues (relating to women's business and men's business)
- conventions applicable to written communications
- the use of touch.

Simply being aware that there are customs, rules and social behaviours that apply to different cultures, without knowing exactly what these customs are, can help to overcome some of the barriers associated with difference. By being culturally aware and demonstrating cultural competence, a care worker can engage in open and respectful communication.

Verbal and non-verbal communication must be used constructively to establish, develop and maintain effective relationships, mutual trust and confidence. Person-centred care is dependent on responsive relationships, trust and rapport. The workforce in aged care services will be diverse, and it is important that communication between all staff is clear and understood and is used to build effective work relationships.

The organisation in which a care worker is employed also has a responsibility to show respect for diversity in the workplace. This can occur by:

- promoting courtesy and good manners, such as saying "good morning" to others
- providing workplace information that is relevant to a person's role
- ensuring all employees feel valued in their position and role in the organisation
- having all contributions valued and respected
- ensuring all employees receive fair and equitable treatment.

Regardless of what form of communication is used, an essential skill for communicators is active listening. An active listener:

- demonstrates understanding and develops rapport with the person speaking
- stays focused on the person speaking, including attending to their body language and voice
- ensures the person can talk uninterrupted
- demonstrates an interest in and enthusiasm for what is being communicated
- provides feedback to the person to confirm understanding.

Non-verbal messages affect verbal communication. In fact, the greater percentage of effective communication is non-verbal. This means that gestures, facial expression, body language, paralanguage (tone of voice) and appearance all convey a great deal of meaning when people speak.

When accommodating diversity, it is important to understand that the gestures and verbal familiarities that one person finds acceptable might not be acceptable to individuals or co-workers from other countries or other cultures.

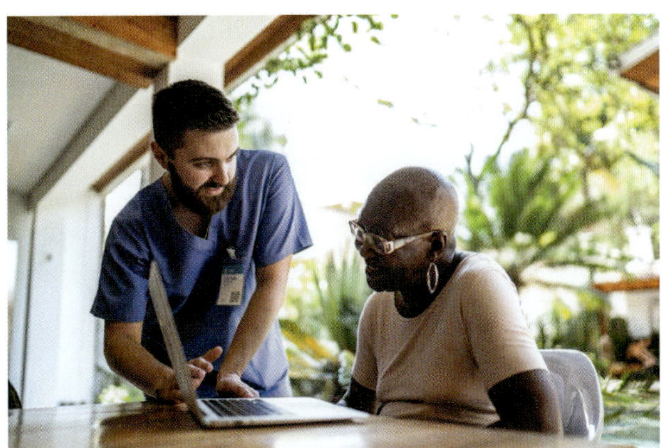
Getty Images/E+/FG Trade

By being culturally aware and demonstrating cultural competence, a care worker can engage in open and respectful communication

In many situations, people deliberately use body language to communicate. Hands, fingers and arms can be communication channels for an entire language. The most complex is the sign language of hearing-impaired people. In everyday communication, however, people tend to use facial expression and hand gestures to emphasise or explain what they are saying. In some cultures, hand gestures are used more extensively than in others–to support and to clarify what is being said. In different cultures or regions, specific hand gestures or signals can have different meanings. It is important to take care and to have some understanding of the differences that might affect the outcomes of a communication.

Most often, and in normal communication situations, people's non-verbal communication is unconscious. Yet, for communication to make sense, the verbal communication (words, sentences and projected concepts) and body language must be congruent. Nodding and shaking of the head are universally understood gestures. However, what would happen if someone was answering "yes" to a question, but was shaking their head at the same time? It would cause confusion. This is a minor and simple example of incongruent verbal and body language. Sometimes people from non-English speaking countries will nod their heads, to indicate friendliness and willingness to communicate. Unfortunately, this doesn't indicate understanding of a particular communication.

Facial expressions are part of a person's body language. For example, a smile indicates any or even all of these:

- warmth
- friendliness
- liking
- willingness to help
- amusement
- willingness to cooperate.

People convey a wide range of emotions and reactions, such as anger, pain, discomfort, happiness, love, excitement, boredom and more, through their facial expression. A simple smile, when communicating with individuals and workers, including those from other cultures, can be indicative of friendliness and willingness to help. Awareness of basic, simple communications can assist in coping with diversity. Tone of voice (paralanguage) conveys a great deal of meaning in verbal communication. Research indicates that specific voice characteristics are commonly associated with feelings/meanings (see Table 5.1).

Managers, supervisors and care workers must be aware of the way they sound and of the need to match paralanguage with verbal content. When listening to others, they also need to be aware that these are not necessarily hard-and-fast rules. Some people have particular speech habits–for example, they might speak very rapidly all the time; as this is their habitual way of speaking, it doesn't necessarily denote enthusiasm or excitement.

TABLE 5.1 Voice characteristics and feelings/meanings

Paralanguage	Probable feeling/meaning
Monotonal speech	Boredom, condescension
Slow speed, low pitch	Depression, thoughtfulness
High voice, empathetic and rapid speech	Enthusiasm, excitement
Ascending tone	Astonishment, fear
Abrupt speech	Defensiveness, impatience
Terse speech, loud tone	Anger, fear
Highly pitched, drawn-out speech	Disbelief

5.4.2 Barriers to effective communication

Care workers may be required to identify and resolve potential language and communication barriers. Solutions for overcoming such barriers can be found by using a simple problem-solving model:

1. Clearly identify barriers.
2. Collaborate to identify possible solution/s.
3. Select a solution/s that everyone agrees upon.
4. Implement the solution/s.
5. Review and evaluate the solution/s.

If managers or supervisors have difficulty understanding the spoken English of a worker or individual, they can ask the person to repeat what they said or perhaps ask them to write or draw diagrams to help clarify the message. They can encourage workers to use the same techniques when they are communicating with individuals, individuals' families and colleagues. A map or diagram could also be a valuable aid, and communication might be illustrated by gestures and hand signals.

Don't make assumptions about people and their intelligence based on their ability to read written English or to understand communications (or instructions) in a language that is not their own. There is no point in shouting at people who don't understand you; they are neither deaf nor stupid, and shouting at them is inappropriate. When communicating with individuals with a hearing, sight or other disability, treat each person as an individual and don't assume that their disability impairs their intelligence.

OVERCOMING BARRIERS

Reducing potential language and communication barriers requires us to:

- speak slowly and clearly, with careful pronunciation
- constantly check that there is mutual understanding
- avoid the use of jargon and industry terminology
- ensure understanding of common terms
- choose the correct mode of communication
- provide information through a variety of sources
- be patient, as communication across cultures takes more time
- seek assistance and support, as required.

Symbols are a visual language that can overcome many language barriers. The signage and symbols used in the workplace should be clear and universally understood. Charts, graphs and tables (of content) can also be used to overcome communication barriers. Charts and graphs provide visual representations and don't necessarily require sophisticated language skills.

Written information (instructions or information relating to client needs, menus, etc.) can be presented in different languages, taking into consideration the predominant languages of the community within which the organisation operates. If necessary, signage can also be translated into Braille, which is a distinct language for visually impaired individuals. In some cases, and in large community establishments where a particular need has been identified, bilingual or multilingual staff might need to be employed. The workplace should have a database containing information about, and contact details for, translator/interpreter services, embassies, the Office of the

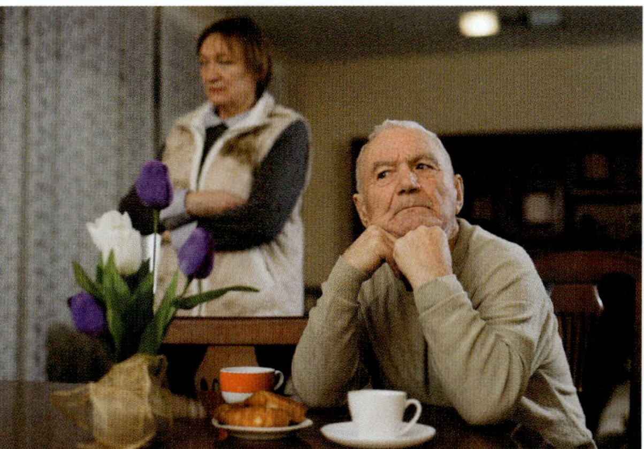

Iakov Filimonov lamy Stock Photo

People convey a wide range of emotions through their facial expression and body language

Commonwealth Ombudsman which oversees the immigration functions of the Department of Home Affairs, advocates, and legal and other advisory services. If these services are required by individuals, workers can help them contact the relevant service.

PRACTICE POINT

The goal of interpersonal and intercultural communication is to improve the communication experience. The following are some strategies for demonstrating person-centred care and culturally relevant communication.

- Learn a few words in the person's own language.
- Remember that not all people can read and write, even in their own language.
- Using picture cards could be useful.
- Check with the person how to properly pronounce their name.
- Understand the non-verbal nuances among different cultural groups, such as whether it is acceptable in a certain culture to look directly at or to touch someone.
- Use trained interpreters as appropriate.

5.4.3 Communication strategies

Communication requires active listening, attending behaviours, empathy, reflective listening, paraphrasing, summarising, questioning and non-verbal communication to support the verbal message. Cultural sensitivity and religious awareness are required. The care worker also requires awareness of Australian norms and of the cultural norm of the person they are supporting.

Generally, communication strategies include:

- *Verbal:* what you say or hear.
- *Written:* what you read or write, which can also include signs or posters.
- *Body language:* the physical actions you make when talking.
- *Signing:* using hand movements to communicate.
- *Augmentative:* expands upon existing communication methods and may be either technology-based or non-technological.

Strategies for effective communication include:

- Consider the goal of the communication.
- Consider your verbal and non-verbal body language.
- Consider your audience and adapt your communication styles accordingly.
- Be respectful, professional and considerate.
- Increase your credibility by being clear and accurate.
- Create confidence by being direct and cooperative.
- Develop trust and rapport by being honest and genuine.
- Show integrity by being consistent in your behaviours and approaches.
- Take the time to review the communication to identify if it served your goals.
- Use both verbal and non-verbal communication.

Communication strategies have been discussed in detail in Chapter 4, and the same guidelines apply when you are working with diverse peoples. The care worker needs to be able to recognise differences and to adjust their own communication to meet the needs of the person they are communicating with.

5.4.4 Using interpreters

If a care worker is in a situation where language is a barrier to communication, they will need to seek assistance. There may be times when it is appropriate to have family, friends or bilingual colleagues translate for the care worker, but the most effective source of assistance is a professional interpreter service. It is highly recommended that a trained interpreter is used wherever possible, as this will ensure that the information provided is accurate and isn't tainted by personal biases or values.

Professional interpreters are bound by codes of conduct, including confidentiality. Organisations that care for people from more than one culture will generally maintain a register of interpreters. Where possible, an interpreter of the same gender as the person is used, particularly for discussions involving questions of a personal nature.

When considering using an interpreter, take into account the following:

- Interviews and discussions take much longer.
- Professional interpreters can be costly.
- An interpreter can ensure that the person understands everything, including consent.

When using an interpreter, implement the following guidelines:

- Always face and speak to the person, not the interpreter.
- Wait until the interpreter has finished talking before you start again.
- Use words that the interpreter is likely to understand.
- Don't use complex medical jargon.

The Australian government, through the Department of Immigration and Citizenship, provides a service called the Translating and Interpreting Service (TIS National). This interpreting service is for people who don't speak English and for the English speakers who need to communicate with them.

WORKPLACE SCENARIO

Person-centred care and the importance of culturally relevant communication

Ben, a care worker, noticed that Catalina was becoming agitated as she tried to communicate with him. Catalina is a resident at the local aged care facility, and she does not speak English. Ben knows that Catalina uses a picture book to tell staff what she needs, and he uses the picture book to ascertain that Catalina wants to call her family. A smiling Catalina confirms that the picture book is an effective method of addressing the communication barrier.

CHECK YOUR UNDERSTANDING

1. Define communication and explain why we communicate.
2. What can you do to demonstrate person-centred care and culturally relevant communication?
3. What can you do to reduce potential language and communication barriers?
4. What might a smile mean? (List three different possibilities.)

5.5 PROMOTING UNDERSTANDING ACROSS DIVERSE GROUPS

5.5.1 Resolving misunderstandings and conflict

One of the most common causes of misunderstanding or difficulty in communication is language barriers. These occur when an individual has difficulty explaining to another person what they want to say or need, in a way that the other person understands. Even if people are communicating in the same language, language barriers may still exist because of differences in pronunciation and dialect, or the person may have forgotten parts of their original language. When communication misunderstandings or difficulties occur, a care worker needs to identify what caused the problem, what strategies there are to overcome it, and what is their role in resolving the problem.

Communication misunderstandings or difficulties can occur where there is conflict. Sources of conflict include:

- different verbal communication styles
- different non-verbal communication styles
- diverse attitudes towards conflict
- different ways of doing things
- challenges to decision-making abilities and roles.

Conflict can occur:

- between the care worker and the older person's family member or carer
- between the care worker and a work colleague
- within a group of people
- between the care worker and their supervisor.

The relationship between the people involved in the conflict needs to be considered, and then the most suitable strategies for managing the conflict can be determined.

5.5.2 Strategies to promote understanding

ORGANISATIONAL STRATEGIES

Aged care organisations must provide services in a culturally appropriate, client-centred manner. Staff at all levels must communicate effectively with individuals from a wide range of backgrounds, including those for whom English is a second language (ESL), those who come from culturally and linguistically diverse (CALD) backgrounds, or those who are living with a disability that affects their ability to communicate.

Care workers need to communicate effectively with each other, as some care workers will come from ESL or CALD backgrounds. Managers and supervisors need to identify issues that are likely to cause communication misunderstandings or other difficulties. If there are communication issues in the workplace, it is a good idea to consider the impact of social and cultural diversity. In the workplace, role ambiguity, lack of clarity regarding the roles and responsibilities of others, confusing work instructions, outdated or incorrect procedures, and so on, can all contribute to misunderstandings, as can cultural and social diversity.

Organisations will recruit for diversity. Skilful managers will coordinate employees' different abilities to maximise performance and production, but misunderstandings and conflict between individuals and workers or between workers and colleagues can occur for many different reasons. In workplaces where there are significant numbers of staff from different cultures, cross-cultural training is important to prevent unnecessary conflict and to provide staff with appropriate strategies, skills and knowledge to meet clients' and families' needs. Cross-cultural training and a workplace culture that actively supports inclusion will help alleviate problems with differences.

Implementing a range of activities that encourage people to learn about each other's cultures can help increase feelings of comfort and understanding. Examples include shared meals with foods from different cultural backgrounds, team bonding activities and celebrations of special occasions. Educating each other about other cultures helps people to identify similarities rather than differences.

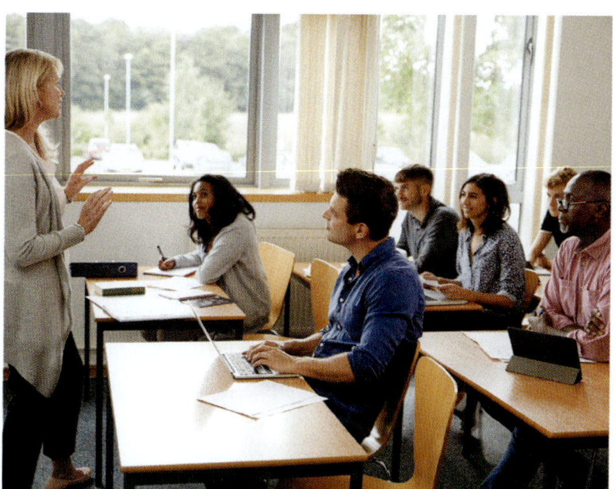

MBI/Alamy Stock Photo

Cross-cultural training is important to provide staff with appropriate strategies and knowledge to meet clients' needs

Cross-cultural training might be delivered:

- within the organisation by suitably qualified and experienced staff members
- by contracting external trainers and consultants
- online, or as a blended training program
- through attendance at workshops or training programs delivered by a range of registered training organisations
- as part of a nationally recognised qualification that relates to the community services industry (aged care sector) in which the organisation operates
- as part of a coaching or mentoring program.

It is important for an organisation to invest in developing effective employment programs and strategies which support a culturally safe and harmonious work environment that is inclusive and celebrates diversity.

Cross-cultural training can make a positive contribution towards identifying areas where misunderstandings may arise and informing the strategies adopted to prevent or address misunderstanding. Cross-cultural training should encourage employees to examine their own cultural identities and attitudes.

INDIVIDUAL STRATEGIES

It will sometimes be easy to identify the causes of misunderstandings, and issues can be readily resolved. For instance, a misunderstanding or a misinterpretation of what was said or written can be resolved if the people involved are simply given the opportunity to clarify and explain.

In some other instances, it will be necessary to determine whether there are specific diversity factors involved. Poor communication, poor listening skills, lack of patience, making judgements about the values and expectations of others without being properly informed, and holding stereotypical ideas about people can all result in misunderstandings and communication breakdowns. When communicating with individuals and workers, it is necessary to consider our own biases and attitudes and to reflect on what might need more work.

An open mind and flexible attitude will contribute to:

- better understanding of differences
- acceptance of diversity in the workplace
- clear, value-free, open and respectful communication
- development of trust-based and effective work relationships
- recognition and avoidance of stereotypical barriers
- being prepared to engage with others in a two-way dialogue where knowledge and understanding are shared.

All individuals within a workplace must accept responsibility for building a socially inclusive working environment and contributing to cultural safety. Employees in such organisations will demonstrate the attitudes and behaviours that are essential for a productive workplace and that act to support the work of others, regardless of background or difference.

WORKPLACE SCENARIO

Promoting cross-cultural understanding

Team leader Rachel noticed that new staff member Arpa always spent her breaks on her own and did not seem to interact much with the other staff. The staff had approached Rachel to say that while Arpa is often smiling, she always looks away from them when they talk to her. Rachel informed the staff that prolonged eye contact is believed to be very rude in some cultures and she made a note to herself to investigate options for including cross-cultural training in the staff education calendar.

CHECK YOUR UNDERSTANDING

1. What causes cultural misunderstandings?
2. What do you need to do when communication misunderstandings or difficulties occur?
3. What strategies can you call on to resolve cultural misunderstandings?

SUMMARY

- This chapter has discussed the requirement for care workers to develop skills and knowledge in the following areas:
  - reflecting on culture and diversity
  - complying with ethical and legal requirements
  - ensuring cultural safety and cultural competence
  - communicating with people from diverse backgrounds
  - promoting understanding across diverse groups.
- An essential skill in care and support is being able to understand how a person's culture may inform their values, beliefs and behaviours. Recognising that we are shaped by our cultural background will help us to become culturally aware. Our cultural background influences the way we see the world around us, the way we relate to others, and the way we perceive ourselves. You don't need to be an expert in each and every culture to be culturally aware; it is your cultural awareness that helps you to explore cultural issues with those to/with whom you provide care and support.
- Your cultural competence will contribute to people feeling respected, accepted and confident about expressing their cultural needs. You will go on to recognise and honour differences between people and acknowledge a shared humanity across diversity.

REVIEW QUESTIONS

5.1 What is the purpose of the Aged Care Diversity Framework?

5.2 Outline the impact of stereotyping people from diverse backgrounds.

5.3 Think about your own social group and culture.

- **(a)** What features are obvious and observable?
- **(b)** What features are invisible?

5.4 List aspects of diversity that exist within cultural groups.

5.5 List the ethical principles that underpin supporting people from diverse backgrounds.

BIBLIOGRAPHY

Aged Care Quality and Safety Commission, *Charter of Aged Care Rights*, https://www.agedcarequality.gov.au/consumers/consumer-rights, accessed 5 March 2020.

Australian Association of Gerontology, https://www.aag.asn.au/, accessed 26 April 2022.

Australian Government, Department of Health, *Aged Care Diversity Framework*, https://www.health.gov.au/resources/publications/aged-care-diversity-framework, accessed 11 April 2022.

Australian Government, Department of Health, *Aged Care Diversity Framework Initiative*, https://www.health.gov.au/initiatives-and-programs/aged-care-diversity-framework-initiative, accessed 15 March 2020.

Australian Human Rights Commission, *A Quick Guide to Australian Discrimination Laws,* https://humanrights.gov.au/our-work/employers/quick-guide-australian-discrimination-laws, accessed 21 April 2022.

Australian Institute of Health and Welfare (AIHW), *Australia's Youth: COVID-19 and the Impact on Young People*, 25 June 2021, https://www.aihw.gov.au/reports/children-youth/covid-19-and-young-people, accessed 26 April 2022.

Australian National Audit Office, *Indigenous Aged Care*, 31 May 2017.

Australians Together, *Indigenous Kinship*, 2012, https://australianstogether.org.au/discover/indigenous-culture/kinship, accessed 21 April 2022.

Benevolent Society, *Working with Older Aboriginal and Torres Strait Islander People*, Research to Practice Briefing 8, www.wimmerapcp.org.au/wp-gidbox/uploads/2014/02/Working-with-Older-ATSI-People2013.pdf, accessed 27 April 2022.

Centre for Cultural Diversity in Ageing, www.culturaldiversity.com.au, accessed 26 April 2022.

Ganzel, B.L., "Trauma-informed hospice and palliative care", *The Gerontologist* 58(3), 2018, pp. 409–19, https://doi.org/10.1093/geront/gnw146.

Hobbs, K., *Indigenous Aged Care*, 2016, Australian National Audit Office, https://www.anao.gov.au/work/performance-audit/indigenous-aged-care, accessed 26 April 2022.

Horwood, G., Adams, N., Barrett, S., Blackwell, N., Campbell, N., Chamberlain, J., Docker, K., Greene, R., Reilly, W. & Tavender, J., *Individual Support in Australia: Ageing, Disability, Home and Community Care*, TAFE NSW, Orange, NSW, 2016.

Pietrzak, R.H., Van Ness, P.H., Fried, T.R., Galea, S. & Norris, F.H., "Trajectories of posttraumatic stress symptomatology in older persons affected by a large-magnitude disaster", *Journal of Psychiatric Research* 47(4), 2013, pp. 520–6, https://doi.org/10.1016/j.jpsychires.2012.12.005.

Skatssoon, J., "Diversity plans target marginalised groups", *Australian Ageing Agenda*, 18 February 2019, https://www.australianageingagenda.com.au/clinical/social-wellbeing/diversity-plans-target-marginalised-groups/.

Van der Kolk, B., *The Body Keeps the Score: Mind, Brain and Body in the Healing of Trauma*, Penguin Books, 2014.

YouTube videos:

- *Cultural Diversity: Tips for Communicating with Cultural Awareness:* https://www.youtube.com/watch?v=ZDvLk7e2Irc
- *Cultural Competence Program:* https://www.youtube.com/watch?v=YI9J4NxQ-Zc3:29 / 7:53
- *How Body Language Differs between Cultures:* https://www.youtube.com/watch?v=EqmOAjd4Kd8/ 13:46
- *Incompetent vs. Competent Cultural Care:* https://www.youtube.com/watch?v=Dx4Ia-jatNQ
- *Non-Verbal Communication:* https://www.youtube.com/watch?v=E6NTM793zvo

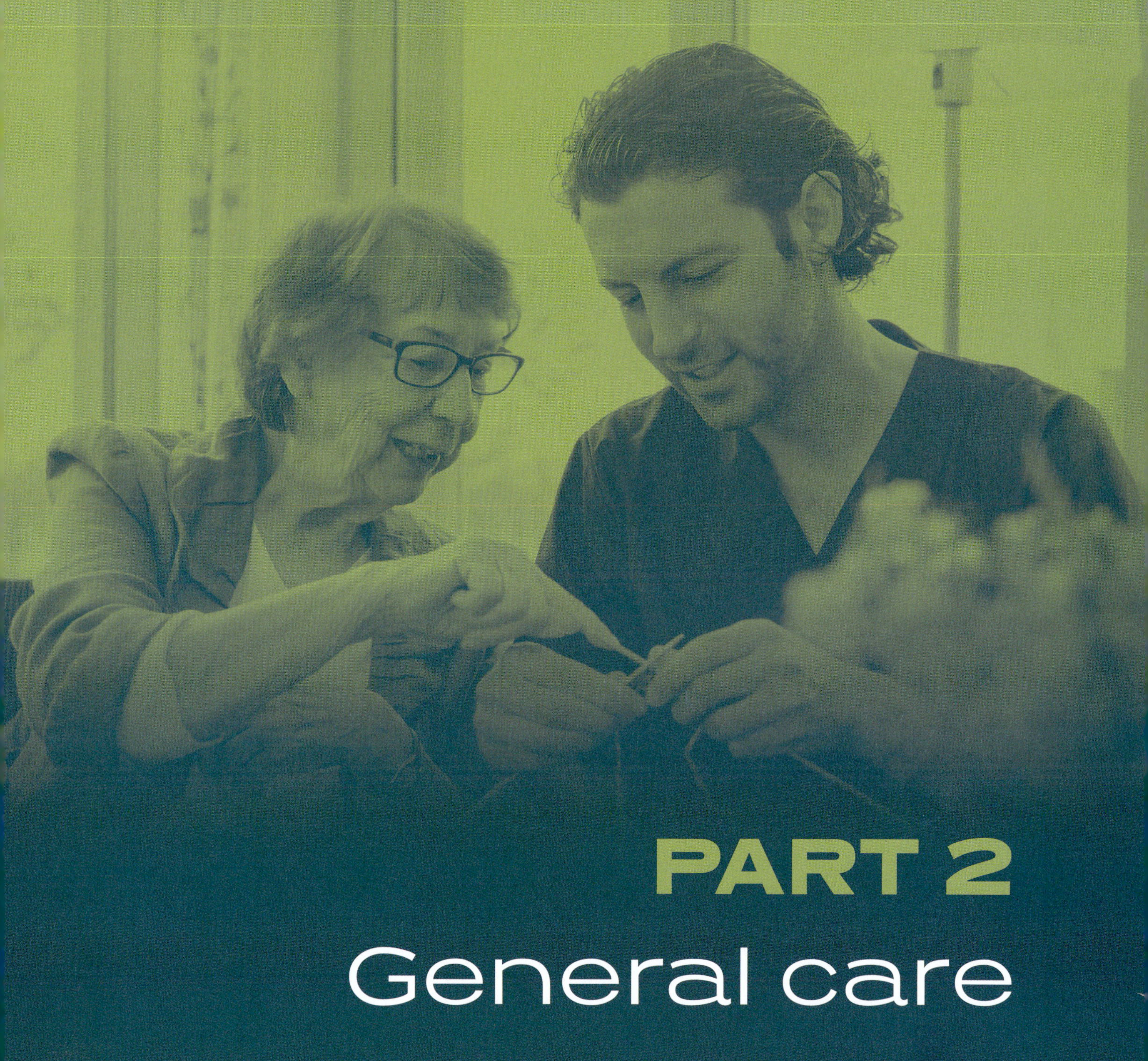

PART 2
General care

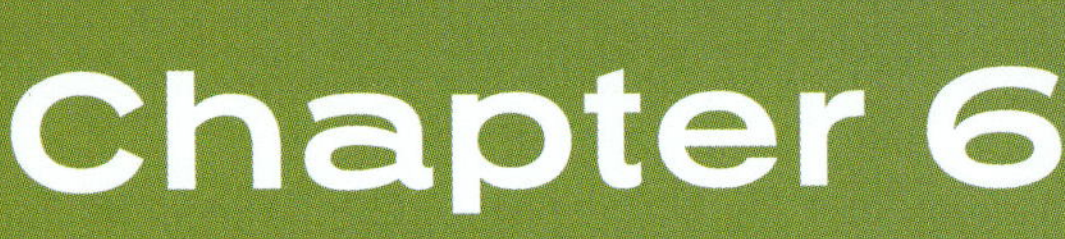

Chapter 6

Providing care and support

LEARNING OBJECTIVES

6.1 Determine support needs

6.2 Provide personal support

6.3 Monitor support

6.4 Prepare documentation

INTRODUCTION

AS OLDER PEOPLE NAVIGATE the ageing process and the social issues associated with ageing, they may require support to remain as independent as possible with their day-to-day activities. Older people who also contend with chronic disease, comorbidities or a life-limiting illness may need to access aged care services such as a residential aged care facility (RACF) so they can be provided with the intensive support they need to continue their lives in a meaningful and dignified way.

Aged care services aim to provide support to older people in a way that maintains their integrity, promotes informed decision making and focuses on their preferences. The types of support, and the way the older person wishes those supports to be offered, will differ for every person. Older people are all unique individuals with their own needs and preferences.

INDUSTRY IN FOCUS

The increasing complexity of support needs

Australia's population is ageing. Thanks to medical, scientific and technological advances, people are living longer than we ever have lived before. This is all good news; however, for aged care, it can increase pressure on an already stressed system.

Older people have complex medical and health conditions requiring support that is often clinically skill based and time consuming. As people live longer and move towards needing aged care services, they rely on services that can support their complex and chronic problems.

Older people need access to services that provide support to maintain their independence and enable them to continue to live in their own home for as long as possible. The services available may assist the person directly, such as with personal care needs, or indirectly. Aged care services can assist in the context of supporting chronic and complex health problems, for example by helping the person to continue treatments, scheduling and arranging transport for appointments, and liaising with health professionals for in-home procedures such as complex wound care and oxygen support.

Residential aged care facilities have registered nurses available for chronic and complex care support, and depending on specific state and territory legislation, many facilities are partnered with the emergency departments of hospitals to ensure timely and appropriate clinical care interventions are available for the older person.

Some organisations train care staff to perform clinical procedures such as urinalysis, recording vital signs and performing basic wound care, which address some of the complex care needs of the people receiving support. The recommendations of the Royal Commission into Aged Care Quality and Safety include further training of care staff to expand knowledge and skills, therefore offering a diversity of skill mix that can maximise the available support for the chronic and complex care needs of older people receiving aged care services.

6.1 DETERMINING SUPPORT NEEDS

It is important that every older person who requires individualised support has their needs determined through a process that is underpinned by effective communication and validated assessments. Assessment of and discussion with the person can help to identify their needs, preferences and goals, which can then be documented into their individualised plan.

6.1.1 The individualised plan

The individualised plan is a document that is developed in consultation with the older person and, if they wish, their carer or family. The person with changes to cognition may have a substitute decision maker who will be included in the consultation process.

The individualised plan is known by various other names, depending on the organisation and the service type. Those names include service delivery plan, personal profile plan, health plan and care plan. Some plans are very concise and address a specific issue. These plans might be found in in-home care, while others (such as those in RACFs) are more comprehensive and address many aspects of the older person's wellbeing.

An individualised plan may include information regarding the following:

- *Physical wellbeing:* information about the person's medical and health conditions; medications; clinical needs and technical procedures; nutrition and hydration.
- *Personal wellbeing:* information about the person's personal support needs, such as assistance with showers, continence care, and so on; needs surrounding sexuality; mobility; sleep.

- *Psychological wellbeing:* information may include behaviour support; mental health conditions such as depression; support for maintaining mental health; dementia support needs.
- *Spiritual wellbeing:* information about the person's spirituality and how this is maintained.
- *Cultural wellbeing:* information about the person's cultural wellbeing and cultural considerations.
- *Social wellbeing:* information about the person's social network, which may include friends, family and community connections.
- *Palliative wellbeing:* information about the person's choices and preferences for care that is associated with a life-limiting illness and palliation needs at end of life.

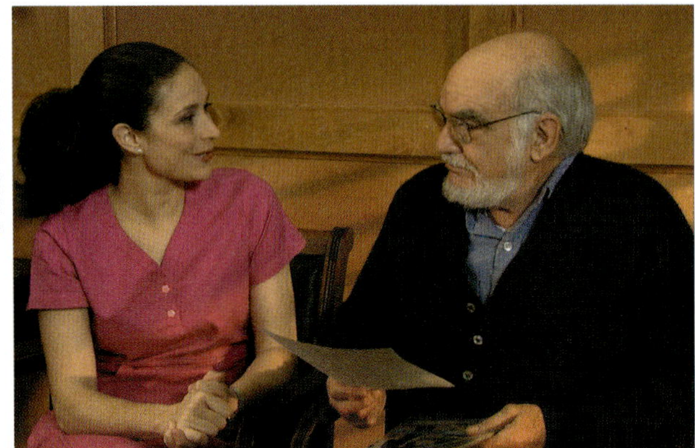

A person-centred approach embraces the uniqueness of each individual

PRINCIPLES UNDERPINNING INDIVIDUALISED PLANNING

The older person is their own expert, and their preferences are at the very core of the planning process. The following principles underpin the planning development and implementation processes.

INDIVIDUALISED PLANNING IS PERSON CENTRED

The person-centred approach to providing support is a principle that acknowledges the older person as their own expert regarding their own life. This approach focuses on involving the person and their supports, such as family and friends, as partners in service provision. The approach embraces the uniqueness of each older individual, including the person's culture, beliefs, self-identity and life experience, perspective and environment. The person-centred approach is the foundation for other principles of care, such as the strengths-based, enablement and consumer-directed care approaches.

INDIVIDUALISED PLANNING IS STRENGTHS BASED

In alignment with person-centred care, the strengths-based approach focuses on what the person can do, rather on what they cannot do. Supports are put in place to assist the person to maintain what they can do for themselves. A strengths-based approach acknowledges the older person's autonomy and ability to make informed decisions about their needs, which empowers them to remain as independent as possible rather than become a passive recipient of services.

INDIVIDUALISED PLANNING TAKES AN ENABLEMENT APPROACH

An enablement approach to services supports older people to take control of their own life by assisting them to do something, rather than doing it for them. When an individual is enabled to achieve a goal as independently as possible, they may feel empowered and in control of their needs and preferences, compared to feeling completely dependent on others for the same task, which may include feelings of helplessness. An example of enablement is assisting the person to source modified cutlery and dinnerware so they can continue to eat independently following a stroke, rather than being fed by a staff member because the person can no longer use standard cutlery or dinnerware. This type of information can be found in an individualised plan.

INDIVIDUALISED PLANNING IS CONSUMER DIRECTED

Consumer-directed care (CDC) is a flexible approach to aged care service delivery that enables the individual to influence and control how their government-funded home care package budget is used and which organisations will provide those services. Aged care facilities are required to be upfront about all the services they offer, including the associated fees, to support consumer-directed care principles.

INDIVIDUALISED PLANNING INCLUDES CULTURAL CONSIDERATIONS

Older people come from diverse cultural, spiritual and social backgrounds, and individualised plans must recognise and support all aspects of the individual's wellbeing. Our identity is shaped and influenced by our life experience, culture and social networks.

The older person's culture must be considered when developing and implementing an individualised plan for them, to ensure their psychosocial wellbeing. It is important that culture is relevant to ethnicity and religion; however, it is also relevant to any group of people with shared values and beliefs. Sporting groups can be a culture; the lesbian, gay, bisexual, transgender, questioning, intersex and asexual (LGBTQIA+) community is a culture; and other groups that a person values may be considered a culture. It is important to understand the aspects of culture that the person values and to integrate respect for these needs and preferences in their individualised plan.

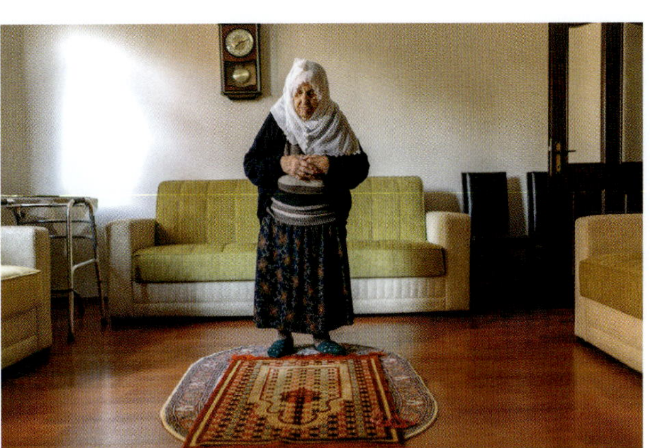

Getty Images/E+/Ergin Yalcin

It is important to understand the aspects of culture that the person values

INDIVIDUALISED PLANNING REQUIRES EFFECTIVE COMMUNICATION

Respectful, collaborative and inclusive communication is an important underpinning principle of developing and implementing an individualised plan for an older person. Effective communication that shows respect and reflects genuine empathy can build rapport and trust between the person, their carer or family and the organisation as a whole.

Discussions about the person's goals, needs and preferences should be open and honest, and be aimed at supporting them to take control and ownership of the types of support they need. It is essential to remember that older people's reactions to accepting support will differ, for several reasons. Some older people may experience disbelief and shock that they find themselves in need of aged care services–for example, after experiencing a major health event such as sudden loss of mobility after a fall, or vision loss due to a traumatic event.

Loss of independence can have a profound impact on an individual, including causing feelings of grief. Communications with the older person must be sensitive to and acknowledge their feelings about the fact that they need aged care services.

Communication that reflects the strengths-based approach is the fabric of person-centred support and should be used in all interactions with older people, including in the development of individualised plans. The way language is used can have a profound impact on the interpretation of meaning. Communication should support the older person's self-determination and be respectful of their needs and preferences regarding their support. Table 6.1 provides some examples of effective communication.

People generally accept that services do their best to accommodate their particular needs and preferences, and that the occasional need to compromise is also part of inclusive outcomes. For example, the older person may be very happy to engage the support services of an aged care organisation that they have chosen; however, the organisation may not be able to provide services on a day that suits the person. A compromise in this scenario may involve the person agreeing to receive services on a different day until their preferred day becomes available.

The older person and their substitute decision maker will have a sense of control when problem solving is shared, and informed decision making is facilitated, during any communications about service provision.

6.1.2 Organisational requirements

POLICIES AND PROCEDURES

Every organisation has policies and procedures in place to instruct and guide staff on providing personal support to older people, safely and respectfully, in the context of their job role. Policies and procedures are

TABLE 6.1 Examples of person-centred communication

Language to avoid	Try this instead
No doubt you have had UTIs before.	Have you experienced urinary tract infections in the past?
You tell me you have chronic knee pain. Don't worry. We can get our staff to rub liniment on your knees every morning before you get up.	You tell me you have chronic knee pain. What do you currently do to manage the pain?
It's easier for me to shower you so that you don't need to worry about falling.	If you are worried about falling in the shower, we can organise some grab rails to be installed on the wall so that you can steady yourself. We can also get you a handheld shower nozzle and a shower chair so you can sit while you shower. In the meantime, we can help you to shower safely. Is this something you might be interested in?
We have more staff available to visit you in the mornings, so I'll book that in. Is that okay?	Our staff can visit you in the mornings or the afternoons. What time would you prefer?

written in alignment with legislation and best practices within the industry, and they serve to document the legal and ethical obligations of the organisation in service provision.

Many policies and procedures apply to multiple areas of work practices. The following policies contain information relevant to providing support to older people.

- *Infection control policies:* Providing personal support can involve being exposed to hazards and risks, such as coming in contact with the body fluids of people receiving support, handling sharps or contaminated linens, and disposing of contaminated waste. Infection control and prevention policies and procedures serve to remind us to prevent and manage infection by implementing standard and transmission-based precautions. Many organisations will have a separate policy and procedure regarding hand hygiene, due to the importance of handwashing in the prevention of infection and infectious outbreaks.
- *Manual handling policies:* Providing support often involves manual handling tasks such as moving a person from one place to another using wheelchairs, hydraulic hoists and slide sheets. Manual handling techniques such as repositioning a person in bed, and even making a bed, are supported with procedures to keep care workers and the older person safe. Manual handling policies and procedures are indoctrinated into all aged care services.
- *Equipment, aids and assistive devices policies:* Any equipment that is used to provide support to people will require ongoing maintenance, cleaning and safe use. Policies and procedures relevant to equipment, aids and other assistive devices will be included in the organisation's suite of workplace policies.
- *Privacy and confidentiality policies:* The aged care industry is required to apply the principles of Australian privacy legislation with regard to how personal and sensitive information is used, stored and shared. All workers, including care workers, must understand their responsibilities for managing the older person's private information.

PLANNING PROCESSES

Organisations that provide in-home care and/or residential services will ensure that the people who use their services have access to care that is unified and continuous. The individualised plan (the care plan) provides real-time access to information about the person that is relevant to the support provided to them. The care plan is a living document that changes as the person changes. It ensures that all care workers are following the same plan for care and support, creating continuity and building trust.

The planning process involves the following people:

- the older person being supported
- the person's carer and family (at the wishes of the older person)
- the person's substitute decision maker or enduring guardian, or maybe a public guardian
- health professionals such as RNs, allied health practitioners and doctors
- care workers
- supervisors and managers.

The people involved in the development of the care plan will reflect the needs of the older person. For example, an older person may or may not require the services of a dietitian or physiotherapist.

Organisations use information collection techniques such as clinical and non-clinical assessments to help the person identify what needs they may have that require support. The strategies that are used to support the person's needs are discussed with the person and their family in an inclusive manner to determine how the person's preferences can be met in service delivery. Assessments are often conducted by the RN or team leader (TL) within an RACF, or by a TL or supervisor in the community aged care sector. Outcomes from these assessments provide valuable information that can help in developing the person's plan.

It is important that the person's autonomy and ownership of the plan are respected and encouraged.

EQUIPMENT AND ASSISTIVE DEVICES

The care plan will identify the types of equipment, aids and assistive devices the person uses to remain as independent as possible. Care workers will be required to use some of these items as part of their job role to ensure their own and the older person's safety. The organisation can reasonably expect workers to abide by manual handling policies and procedures as a legal and ethical obligation of the job role. This may include using hoists or other mechanical devices to lift people who are immobile. The care plan will indicate, based on a mobility assessment, what type of hoist should be used, its weight capacity and the type of sling the person should use. It will also state how many staff are required to perform the task.

The plan will identify in each section the specific type of equipment the person needs in that area. For example, the use of hoists will be documented in the plan's mobility section, incontinence aids will be documented in the elimination (or toileting) section, and hearing aids will be documented in the sensory needs section. Remember that all individualised plans will look different and contain different sections, depending on the organisation. Some plans are documented on paper and others are developed using digital software.

6.1.3 Needs and preferences

The individualised plan is constantly monitored and evaluated to ensure that the person is receiving support that is appropriate to their needs and preferences, and that all staff have a current point of reference for the support they provide in their role. Planning provides information that tells care workers and other practitioners what the person needs to happen, how and when it will happen, and why it needs to happen. Individualised plans should always align with the older person's needs; therefore, in the event the person's needs change, the plan must change to reflect this.

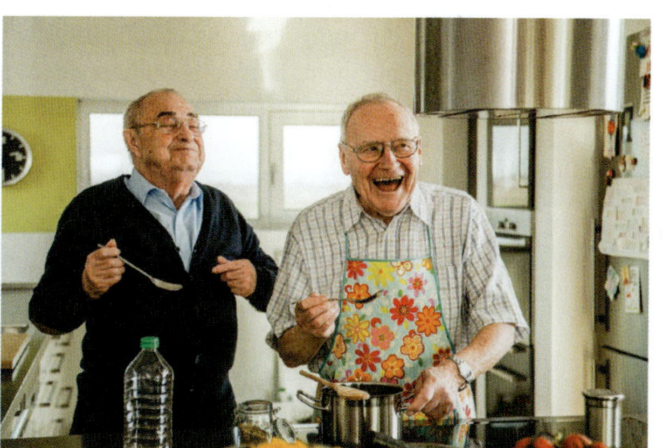

Getty Images/Westend61

The level of support a person requires will vary based on their own abilities, needs and preferences

The person-centred model of care and the underlying strengths-based approach to providing support are the focus of supporting the needs and preferences of older people. The goal in providing support is to enable older people to retain their level of independence by supporting them to do what they can do for themselves.

6.1.4 Promoting independence

We are all an expert on ourselves and have the right to live our lives the way we choose. While ageing can make us vulnerable to disease and frailty, it should not take this right away from us. Strengths-based support can help us to maintain all the independence we can individually manage on a physical and psychosocial level.

Care workers are the key people who provide personal support to older people. Remember that your goal is to support the older person to maintain their skills and abilities by following their care plan.

Having independence is a state of having some control over the ability to care for oneself; it is not defined by how much the person can or cannot do for themselves. The level of support that a person needs will vary based on their own abilities and their needs and preferences. Person A may be able to shower independently, with some help to wash and dry their legs because they cannot reach down safely. Person B may be able to wash their own face with a washer in the shower but requires help with the rest of their body because they have dementia and have forgotten what to do. The key practice here is to continue to wash and dry the legs of person A, and always to place a washer in the hand of person B when they are in the shower, to encourage their independence.

Regardless of how much or how little the person can do for themselves, they should be encouraged to continue to do so. Just as care workers can enable a person to participate in their support activities, so too can they disable a person when they constantly take over the task from the individual and do it for them. This may save a little time in the day; however, the long-term result is an increase in the person's dependence on others and a decrease in their sense of autonomy.

6.1.5 When to seek advice and assistance

Sometimes, the support that is required can be ambiguous, or the person may request the care worker to do something for them that is not in the individualised plan. Care workers should always seek clarification from an RN or TL if they are unsure about what to do. Some examples of when to seek advice or assistance include:

- The person refuses the support.
- The worker doesn't know how to use the necessary equipment, aids or assistive devices for the person.
- The person's ability to participate has changed.
- The person experiences a fall or a medical incident during the support.
- The worker is at risk of harm as a result of providing the support.
- The worker needs clarification on the support that is to be given.

Asking questions, seeking clarification and instruction, and reporting concerns are all positive aspects of risk management, and care workers should be encouraged to do this. It is better to ask than to attempt something that may have a negative outcome.

WORKPLACE SCENARIO

Incorporating cultural needs in personal care support

Mrs Ayad has dementia and can become easily upset. She was admitted to the RACF four days ago for two weeks of respite care while her husband was admitted to hospital for surgery. Mrs Ayad can speak English; however, she has reverted to her first language of Arabic as her dementia has progressed.

Care worker Cory is working on the afternoon shift at the facility when he notices that Mrs Ayed has been incontinent of **faeces** and her clothes are soiled. When Cory tries to help Mrs Ayad into a shower, she becomes distressed and begins to scream hysterically in Arabic. Staff run to her room to see what is wrong, only to find Mrs Ayad backed into a corner with her fists raised and Cory looking flustered.

The team leader calls Cory out of the room while a female care worker calms and reassures Mrs Ayad. Cory tells the TL that he had been trying to get Mrs Ayad into a shower, as she was incontinent. The TL replies: "If you had read Mrs Ayad's care plan, you would know that she will only undress and shower in the presence of female staff. As part of her culture, she won't allow a male other than her husband to see her naked. This whole incident could have been avoided. I'm sure she must feel very upset, and even more confused now, because you were trying to undress her. I know your intentions were helpful, Cory, but it's essential that you read the care plan in future. Please document this incident in Mrs Ayad's notes."

CHECK YOUR UNDERSTANDING

1. What are two principles that underpin the development of an individualised plan?
2. Why is respectful communication necessary for planning support to older people?
3. List three workplace policies that are related to providing older people with individualised support.
4. How can a care worker promote independence for the people they support?
5. Why should a care worker seek advice and assistance if they are unsure about the type of support required?

6.2 PROVIDING PERSONAL SUPPORT

The care plan can inform staff of the type of support that is required for the person; however, the care worker also needs to understand all the factors that are involved in providing safe and respectful support. The point at which support is provided is where the skills and knowledge of the care worker come together.

Providing support to older people is not task based; rather, it is an interface of legal and ethical obligations, of skills and planning abilities, and of an inherent understanding of age-related issues.

6.2.1 Factors to consider when providing support

Care workers apply a multifaceted approach to supporting older people that includes legal and ethical considerations, risk management processes, and the ability to communicate in a way that fosters the self-determination and autonomy of the older person. Table 6.2 identifies common legal and ethical considerations that all care workers are obligated to respect and abide by.

MAXIMISING PARTICIPATION

The older person, their carer and their family (if the person chooses to involve them) are the key components of the process of developing the person's individualised plan. They are an important part of identifying the needs of the older person and of helping to develop strategies to meet those needs. Goals are developed using a collaborative approach based on the person's needs and preferences.

Putting the individualised plan into action should also continue the momentum of collaboration. The older person should be encouraged to participate as much as possible in the delivery of their support. People will have varying levels of ability that will impact on the level of participation they can manage; however, the smallest effort to participate is a measure of independence and should not be ignored.

When an individual sets a goal to remain independent with an activity of daily living, the care plan will identify to care workers what support the person needs to help them reach this goal. Remember that the

TABLE 6.2 Common legal and ethical considerations for care workers

Consideration	Explanation
Duty of care	Care workers have a duty of care to do what is reasonably practicable to prevent foreseeable harm to those they support, other people and themselves when at work. This means that when providing support, the care worker must follow the care plan as well as the workplace policies and procedures. This ensures that duty of care obligations are met in the context of providing personal support.
Dignity of risk	This term is used to describe the right of older people to make decisions about their lives, even where there is an element of risk attached to that decision. Older people are supported to make informed choices that aim to minimise risk. Duty of care must be measured carefully against dignity of risk and not be used to prevent an older person from making an informed decision that may involve risk, if they have the capacity to understand the consequences of their decisions.
Privacy	Care workers are legally obligated to protect the privacy of the older person's sensitive information. An older person's health information can only be disclosed for specific purposes, according to Australian privacy laws. Workplace policies will identify what information may be disclosed and under what circumstances. Physical privacy must be maintained when the older person is being provided with support. Closing their door, knocking before entering, and covering the person when they are naked are all examples of maintaining the person's physical privacy.
Professional boundaries	All care workers have professional boundaries and a code of conduct to abide by. The code ensures that care workers apply skills and knowledge in a manner that is respectful and aligns with the behaviours that are expected within the health and community sectors. Most organisations also have their own code of conduct that sets out the expectations in the workplace of how staff will represent the organisation with their behaviour, their dress, and other aspects of employment that align with organisational visions.
Compulsory reporting	Under the Serious Incident Response Scheme (SIRS), all staff working in RACFs are legally obligated to report known or suspected abuse of older people. This system is due to become mandatory within the community aged care services later in 2022 (as of the time of writing). The SIRS is discussed in detail in Chapter 14.
Discrimination	Australia's discrimination laws prevent people being discriminated against based on their age, gender, race, disability or sexuality. Care workers must not display any form of discrimination in the workplace—for example, by refusing to provide support to a person or by favouring one person over others. We all have our own sets of beliefs, values and attitudes as individuals, and this makes us all unique. Discriminating against an older person, or trying to force them to do things differently because of our own values and beliefs, is ethically wrong. In the event a care worker feels that their own beliefs are diametrically opposed to those of the older person, the care worker should discuss their options with their RN or supervisor. At no time should an older person be made to experience shame because of their beliefs or way of life.
Scope of practice	To work within one's scope of practice means to work within the boundaries of your qualifications, workplace policies and procedures, and your job description. If an older person's care plan requires providing support for a procedure that you are not qualified to provide, you are required to report to the RN or supervisor that you are not trained to perform the task. It is always best to seek additional training, or delegation from the RN, in order to acquire new skills, thereby expanding the scope of practice, rather than to attempt something new and cause harm to the older person, to others or to yourself. Working outside of your scope of practice is breaching your duty of care.

person is in control of their supports, and that the care worker's role is to supplement the person's abilities to reach their goal. For example, it has always been Mr Allen's preference to maintain his appearance by shaving every morning using a razor. Now that his Parkinson's disease is progressing and he has tremors in his hands, he can no longer use a razor safely. Mr Allen's plan may require care workers to set up his electric shaver by the bathroom mirror to enable Mr Allen to continue to shave independently. This example demonstrates how the person's participation can be maximised to continue their autonomy and independence and reflects a risk-based approach to providing support.

When people participate in their own care, regardless of their abilities to do so, they may feel:

- empowered
- autonomous
- valued
- motivated
- determined.

When the option of participating in their own care is removed, they may feel:

- disempowered
- devalued
- as if they are a burden on others
- useless or worthless
- depressed
- sorrowful or grief-stricken
- suicidal.

As a care worker, when you provide support to an older person, encourage them to safely participate in their care. The care plan will often state how the person chooses to be involved. All older people can participate in some way, including those who are experiencing dementia. Remember: the important point isn't always *how much* the person can do; sometimes it is that they *can* do something.

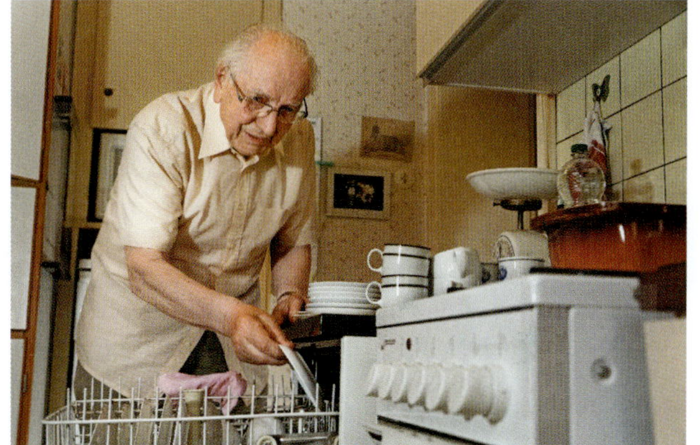

Ingo Bartussek/Shutterstock

Independence facilitates empowerment

ENVIRONMENTAL AND PERSONAL SAFETY

Maximising participation and minimising risk are two important principles of providing support to older people. It is important to be competent in the skills and processes of providing personal support; however, all support activities must be practised with a risk-based attitude.

Risk minimisation is an essential focus of working in aged care, and the prevention of harm is at the forefront of everything you do as a care worker. The workplace will have policies and procedures for addressing risk-related activities and processes, and aged care organisations are bound by compliance requirements and other regulations that ensure workplace safety is a priority.

Environmental safety relates to the place where you provide support. This may be in the older person's own home, a day respite service or an RACF. Hazards are those factors in the environment that can cause harm to the person receiving support, the care worker or others. Environmental hazards can coexist with personal safety risks. All hazards and risks are managed using the hierarchy of control, as discussed in Chapter 3.

Any risk of harm to you, as a care worker, is a threat to personal safety and must be managed with risk minimisation protocols. Table 6.3 provides examples of common environmental and personal hazards and risks.

INFECTION CONTROL

As a key component of work health and safety (WHS) requirements, infection control and prevention are a perpetual focus when working with older people, because they are both vulnerable to infection and more likely to experience profound and catastrophic outcomes as a result.

TABLE 6.3 Common environmental and personal hazards and risks

Hazard	Risk	Environmental or personal?	Control
The person's shower at home has a hub to step over. The hub is the hazard.	The person may trip over the hub and fall onto tiles. The care worker may trip over the hub and fall when assisting the person to shower.	*Environmental:* The person's bathroom is the workplace for the care worker. *Personal:* The care worker can become injured if they trip or fall, or if the older person grabs them when experiencing a fall.	The care worker can initiate discussions about bathroom modifications to remove the hub and minimise risk by arranging for the installation of grab rails and a handheld shower nozzle.
The person with dementia becomes confrontational when the care worker tries to assist with dressing. The confrontation is the hazard.	The care worker may experience a physical injury.	*Personal:* The care worker may be harmed if the older person punches, kicks or hits them, or throws items.	A behaviour support plan can assist to minimise the risk of confrontation.
Equipment, aids or assistive devices are damaged or broken.	Both the older person and the care worker can be injured.	*Environmental:* The equipment is part of the workplace and is used by others (RACF). *Personal:* There is a risk of personal harm (e.g. from falling, burning, pinching, musculoskeletal injury).	Equipment, aids and assistive devices should be cleaned and maintained as part of a maintenance program in RACFs. Items in the person's home can be repaired or replaced by the manufacturer.
Blood and other body fluids are contaminated.	The care worker can be contaminated with an infectious disease.	*Personal:* Infection can be due to direct or indirect contamination.	Infection control policies, procedures and protocols can be put into effect.
Smoke detectors in the person's home are non-functional.	Fire can cause burns, smoke inhalation or death.	*Personal:* There is a threat to safety.	Provide information that encourages the older person to replace batteries in smoke detectors.

Hand hygiene practices are embedded into daily work routines as part of standard precautions. Many older people require personal support with intimate procedures that involve body fluids. All procedures that can expose the care worker to blood and body fluids require the use of personal protective equipment (PPE) such as gloves, gowns and face protection. Personal support activities that can expose a care worker to body fluids include:

- caring for the **perineum**
- cleaning up vomit or diarrhoea
- changing incontinence aids
- emptying bedpans, urinals and catheter bags
- cleaning teeth and dentures
- assisting with toileting
- managing wounds
- handling soiled linen
- managing spills such as blood

- using sharps such as razors, insulin pens or glucometers
- handling contaminated waste
- providing support to a person who is known to scratch, bite or spit.

Infection control practices should be continuous whether or not the person is known to be infectious. The organisation's infection control and prevention policies and procedures serve to provide workers with valuable guidance on infection-related matters. It is good practice to make it your business to understand your obligations regarding infection control in the workplace by familiarising yourself with these policies and procedures. The principles of infection control and prevention are discussed in detail in Chapter 16.

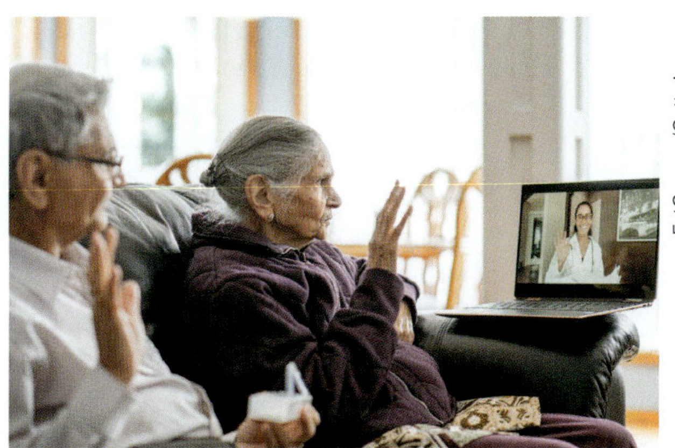

FatCamera/Getty Images

A collaborative approach to care support ensures that the person's needs and preferences are being met

INCLUSIVE COMMUNICATION

Inclusive communication gives the older person, their carer or family the opportunity to have open and transparent discussions about the needs of the person who requires support in an environment where they feel empowered to do so. When providing support to the older person, inclusive communication is essential for maintaining the person's participation and to demonstrate respect for their autonomy.

Before assisting a person with a support activity, always ask them for consent. The person (or their substitute decision maker) has participated in the development of the care plan and the support strategies in the care plan have been collaboratively agreed upon. This is a type of formal consent; however, it is good practice to ask the person if they are happy to proceed with a particular support activity at that particular time. This reflects common courtesy, as the person may not be feeling well enough to shower, or they may want to eat their meal in their own room instead of going to the dining room.

During the support activity, check in with the person with questions such as: "Is the water warm enough for you?" or "Is your pad positioned comfortably?" This type of communication reflects genuine empathy for the person's experience in that moment and can contribute to their sense of wellbeing.

Inclusive communication can also provide feedback from the older person and their carer or family about the services that are provided. The person may feel that an aspect of their plan needs to change. This collaborative approach to care support ensures that the person's needs and preferences are being met on an ongoing basis.

TIME

One of the biggest challenges for aged care workers is time management. The needs and preferences of older people are paramount, and care workers work within a routine or a work plan to ensure that all activities that are required are able to occur.

Support practices must be carried out in a timely but safe manner. Care workers in RACFs or in the community sector have a set amount of work to complete in any given shift, so an incident such as a person falling in the facility or a traffic jam producing lengthy delays in the local community can disrupt the work routine.

All support activities require care workers to apply their skills in an environment that can constantly change. Communication with team members can therefore assist when time is poor. A contingency plan may include working in pairs to get the work done safely and effectively or contacting the office to phone ahead to the older person who is waiting for you in the community. There may be a care worker who is close by who can provide support to the person if you are running late.

Even when the routine is going smoothly, time management is still important. When providing support, care workers are required to work efficiently, not hastily. Here are some ways a care worker can manage their time well:

- Follow instruction from your TL.
- Prioritise your work within your routine. Do what you can do individually and set aside time for bigger tasks if possible. Ask for help in advance—for example: "Will you have time at 11 o'clock to help me with Mrs Gibson's bed bath?"
- Sometimes you have to say "no". When you try to please everyone or try to help everyone else to get their jobs done, you may find that you have less time to complete your own work.
- Stick to your routine or work list.
- Stay focused and avoid distractions. (Care workers have no reason to have their personal mobile phone with them when at work.)
- Ensure you take your break.

Time management is a skill that takes a while to develop, and even the most seasoned care worker will have this skill challenged occasionally.

CULTURAL NEEDS

Providing support to older people requires the care worker to understand the support needs as well as other needs the person may have. People's cultural needs are outlined in their care plan and will be unique to every person, and it is important not to assume that all people of a similar culture will practise or follow their culture in the same way. For example, an older individual may state they are a Christian because they believe in God and Heaven and Hell; however, they may not follow the religious protocols of Christianity, such as going to church.

The following cultural needs are relevant to personal support.

- *Gender-specific supports:* Some cultures have specific requirements that request male or female workers to attend to personal support. For example, Islam requires women to be bathed, dressed or medically cared for by a woman wherever possible.
- *Language barriers:* Culturally and linguistically diverse (CALD) people may use English as a second language, or they may not speak English at all. The plan will state how language barriers can be overcome. Staff may learn some key words in the person's preferred language, such as "eat", "shower" or "toilet", or they may use a picture and word book, or a translation device, to assist communication.
- *Modern history:* Land dispossession and the loss of family of Indigenous people can lead to a distrust of Western processes. Older people who experienced war may also have difficulty with trusting people from other cultures.
- *Food practices:* Certain types of food are important in the diet for people from some cultures. Food is also used in a ritualistic way and within the context of worship. Cultural celebrations are a great way to share a person's culture. Eating with the hands is viewed as very disrespectful in some cultures.
- *Understanding body language:* This is an important aspect of providing support. For example, while most people see eye contact as a mark of respect, it is disrespectful to maintain eye contact with an Indigenous man. It is also considered disrespectful in some Asian cultures to use a fork instead of chopsticks.

LEVELS OF ASSISTANCE

The type of assistance the older person needs will vary according to their level of independence. It is because the person has difficulty attending to an activity of daily living that they need help. Some people need very little support and remain largely independent for activities of daily living, while others require a high level of care support because they are dependent on others to ensure that their needs are met.

People with high care support needs are often experiencing chronic disease or comorbidities. The person may have lost their ability to function independently due to stroke, trauma or a neurological condition such as Parkinson's disease, dementia or multiple sclerosis. As the level of assistance increases, the less the person is able to do for themself. This doesn't indicate that they should not be encouraged to participate in their care. This option is always offered and encouraged.

The care plan will be specific about the type of support the person needs and how it is to be provided. For example, if the person is unable to weight bear, the plan will state that the person is to be transferred from chair to bed using the lifter and two staff.

The care worker will need to read the person's personal hygiene plan to determine that they prefer to take a shower, and when. They will also need to read the person's mobility plan to determine how to assist them into the bathroom and onto the shower chair. In addition, the care worker needs to be aware of the person's cultural plan to determine if they have specific cultural requirements for showering.

The level of assistance that a person requires can fluctuate, depending on factors such as incidents and illnesses. For this reason, the individualised plan is constantly updated to reflect the changes that the person is experiencing in real time.

6.2.2 Types of support

ACTIVITIES OF DAILY LIVING

Activities of daily living (ADLs) are activities that people do every day and which are necessary for health and wellbeing. ADLs are basic self-care activities that people learn as children and continue to do throughout life. They include:

- showering/bathing
- using the toilet and performing toilet hygiene
- brushing teeth
- eating and drinking
- getting up and moving around
- grooming
- dressing and hygiene.

When an older person experiences difficulty with any ADL, this can indicate that they are experiencing a health issue. This issue may or may not be known to the person or their doctor, so any change in the person's ability to perform ADLs should be reported and documented for further investigation. Older people need help with ADLs for many reasons, including pain, joint and dexterity issues, mobility problems, cognition changes such as those seen in dementia, vision loss and, above all, frailty.

INSTRUMENTAL ACTIVITIES OF DAILY LIVING

Instrumental activities of daily living (IADLs) are those activities that people do often and which involve planning and organising. If an older person is experiencing difficulties with IADLs, they should be referred to their doctor to determine why. Difficulty with IADLs can be an indicator of dementia, particularly Alzheimer's disease. IADLs include activities such as banking, meal planning and preparation, shopping, performing domestic chores and managing medications.

6.2.3 Providing personal support

Providing personal support to older people requires specific skills and knowledge to ensure the person feels safe, respected and in control of the support they receive. Care workers must never take for granted how the person may be feeling about the support they need. Some older people will gladly and openly accept personal support, while others may be hesitant and embarrassed about receiving care. As a care worker, always try to imagine how the older person is feeling and provide support in a professional and respectful manner.

THE ROLE OF THE CARE WORKER IN RELATION TO PERSONAL CARE

The provision of personal care requires care workers to assist with ADLs for an older person. The person may be feeling many different emotions about receiving care, especially as some care procedures are very intimate and personally intrusive. The need to be reliant on others for the basic tasks of living can be humiliating, embarrassing and demoralising. However, many people who require support look forward to personal care because it provides an opportunity for social interaction. Many older people live alone, and the care worker may be the only person they interact with all day.

Care workers who are skilled in effective communication can minimise the older person's negative feelings and help them to take back control by encouraging them to participate and be autonomous wherever possible. The types of personal support you may need to provide to an older person will include assisting them to:

- bathe or shower
- use the toilet, including wiping their bottom or genitals
- dress and undress
- clean their teeth or dentures
- manage incontinence, including cleaning up faeces and urine and changing incontinence pads
- change position in bed; mobilise (walk, get in and out of bed, etc.)
- eat their meals
- shave; apply makeup; wash and comb hair.

The level of assistance required will vary depending on the person's needs and preferences; however, the care worker should always apply cultural awareness, inclusive communication and the person-centred approach when providing personal care.

ASPECTS OF PERSONAL CARE

SKIN CARE

Ageing skin is vulnerable to breakdown due to changes to the layers of skin over time. Ageing affects all three layers of the skin. For example, the dermis—the middle layer—loses valuable apparatus such as oil glands, sensory receptors and elastin. The skin becomes wrinkled and less supple, and this can affect its healing potential.

Skin care is an important part of the care plan, and most older people benefit from the application of a daily moisturiser that hydrates the skin. Care workers may assist the person to apply a topical moisturiser, wearing gloves as an infection control measure. Applying moisturiser is a good opportunity to assess the older person's skin integrity (i.e. the overall condition of the skin).

Skin tears occur when the layers of the skin become separated due to opposing forces, such as when the person removes tight clothing over elbows. The top layer of skin (epidermis) separates from the dermis, or even from the bottom layer (hypodermis), causing a wound. Skin tears are very common in older people due to their aged skin and should be reported immediately for management and dressing. The sooner a skin tear is dressed correctly, the less likely it will deteriorate and become ulcerated.

Usually, skin tear dressings are within the scope of practice of the TL or the RN. Any changes in the skin, such as a new rash or skin tear, should be reported to the RN or supervisor and be documented in the person's file. Skin tears should also be reported in the RACF incident management system and the medical officer notified regarding assessment and management.

BED BATHING

There are times when the older person is too frail or too unwell to get out of bed for a shower or bath and will be offered a bed bath—that is, they are washed while they remain in their bed. This procedure can be actioned by one care worker if the older person can assist by rolling onto their side when asked; otherwise, two care workers will be required. How much assistance the person needs will be noted in their care plan.

The equipment needed for a bed bath includes:

- a warm-water basin
- soap and other toiletries
- washers and towels; fresh clothing
- fresh continence aid, if required
- fresh bed linen, if required.

Be aware of the room temperature. You may need to close windows or turn on an air conditioner to suit very cool or very hot weather conditions. If the person is using a hydraulic bed, it is good practice to raise the bed height to the level of your hips. This can assist with minimising the risk of overstretching or bending too low, which increases the risk of a musculoskeletal injury. Sensitivity and privacy are key factors when attending to a bed bath, and you should ensure the person's door is closed.

After washing and drying your hands, put on disposable gloves. Then, using soap and water, gently wash the person's face, neck and ears. Use a towel to pat them dry. Leaving one side of the person's body covered with the bedsheet, wash and then dry the exposed side of their body, starting at the shoulder and upper body and working down to their leg and foot. Ensure the skin is fully dry. Take the opportunity to check for skin issues such as persistent redness and broken areas of skin. Cover this side of the body and repeat on the other side.

After ensuring the person is safe to leave, refresh the water basin and washer. Replace your gloves and attend to hand hygiene. The person's genitals are the last part of the body to be washed, after covering the top half of their body with a dry towel or bedsheet. Always wash female genitalia from front to back to prevent infection and irritation. When washing male genitals, ensure the testicles are washed and dried. When washing uncircumcised men, ensure the foreskin is retracted and cleaned, and the area is thoroughly dry, before replacing the foreskin over the glans penis.

Ask the person to turn onto their side to enable you to wash and dry between their buttocks. If two workers are actioning the bed bath, then the procedure for turning a person over in bed should be followed. Replace gloves and attend to hand hygiene.

Apply the person's preferred deodorant and fresh clothes and comb their hair. Support them to clean their teeth or perform oral hygiene for them. Place soiled and wet linen into a linen receptacle, or in the person's laundry if they are in their own home. Remove gloves and perform hand hygiene.

PRACTICE POINT

Perineal care is the term given to washing and drying the genitals and buttocks. It can occur as part of a bed bath or by itself as part of continence care. It is essential that the person's dignity is maintained during this procedure. Always explain to them what you are going to do, even if you have done this many times.

When cleaning male genitals, the penis may start to become erect. This is a natural physiological response and isn't always related to the man's sexual feelings. Attend to the procedure thoroughly yet swiftly, ensuring you remain professional at all times. Sensitivity is very important when attending to perineal care.

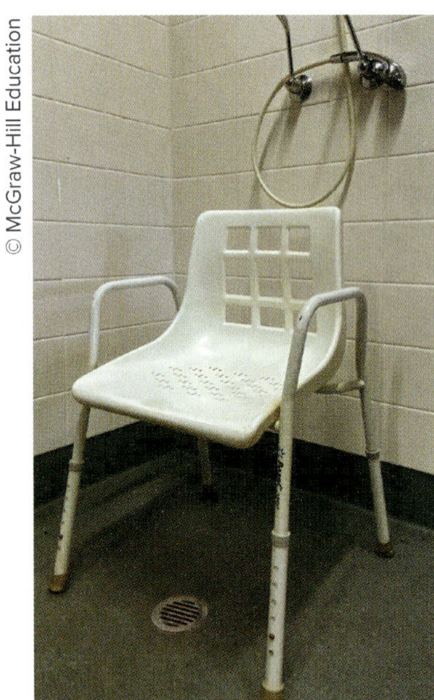

Shower chair

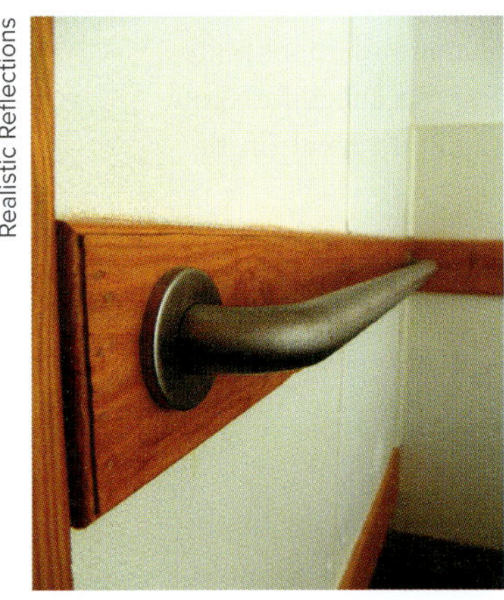

Grab rails

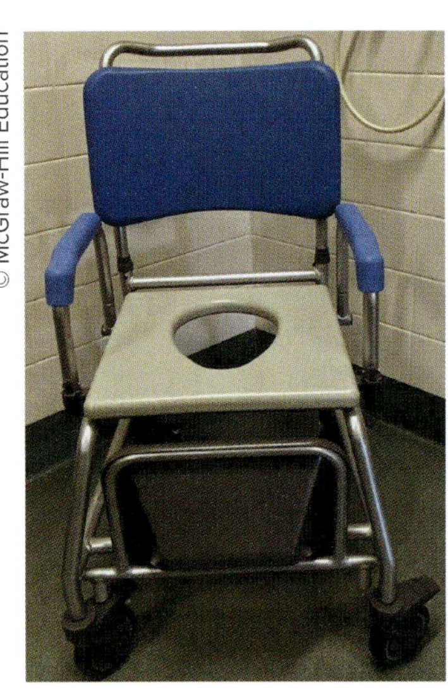

Commode/shower chair

SHOWERING

Providing support with showering can involve very minimal assistance up to full assistance. Some older people need the care worker to assist them into the shower, run the water and assist them out of the shower when they are done. Other people require semi or full assistance in the shower, which involves the care worker moving the person into the shower, washing part or all of their body, shampooing their hair, and then removing them from the shower and drying them.

When washing a person, always wash their face, ears and neck first, followed by their body and, lastly, their genitals and buttocks.

When showering a person, ensure they are safe by checking the temperature of the water, putting brakes on shower chairs that have wheels when in use, and by not leaving the person unattended if the care plan documents this.

The care worker should prepare for the shower by ensuring that everything that is required is ready for use before the person is naked and has entered the shower. This means that washers, towels, toiletries and fresh clothing are within easy reach, so the care worker doesn't have to leave the room to pick up forgotten items. In the event you have forgotten something you need and are unable to leave the person, always use the call bell for assistance.

The following equipment, aids and assistive devices are used to assist with showering.

- A shower chair—a plastic chair with holes on the seat—allows the person to sit while showering. The chairs are lightweight and height adjustable to ensure the person has their feet on the ground when showering.
- A handheld shower nozzle on an extendable hose allows the person to move the water to them instead of having to move around on the slippery floor to shower.
- Grab rails on the wall of the shower enable the person to stabilise their balance when standing.
- A commode/shower chair is used frequently in RACFs. The "over the toilet" chair on wheels has a toilet seat. The person can be placed over the toilet before their shower and then pushed into the shower recess where they can shower with assistance. The seat allows the care worker to access the person's buttocks to be washed and dried.

Sensitivity and privacy are key factors when showering a person. Ensure the door or shower curtain is closed. Cover the person's bottom half with a towel when you are drying their top half, and the reverse when drying their bottom half.

DRESSING AND UNDRESSING

Many older people require some or more assistance with dressing and undressing. These ADLs can be difficult to complete due to physical limitations such as arthritis and pain, and cognitive decline can make putting clothes on in the right order more difficult.

The level of assistance the person needs will be stated in their care plan and will vary for every individual. Some people may only need assistance with clasps and zippers, while others may require quite a lot of assistance. When assisting people to get dressed, remember to ask them what they want to wear. Choice is essential to autonomy and every older person has the right to choose their clothing, including people with dementia. However, offering limited options to someone with dementia (e.g. asking, "Do you want to wear the blue or the red top?") can minimise their confusion and maximise their wellbeing. If you are dressing the person and they are unable to or don't wish to choose their clothing, be aware of the weather. Select clothing for the person with their comfort and the climate in mind.

When dressing the person, ensure they are in the sitting position if they are able to sit up. If they are in bed, raise the bed head up to a sitting position and lower the bed. Assist the person to sit on the side of the bed so their feet are touching the ground.

Undress and dress the person's top half first, being sure to apply deodorant if they choose to use it. Ask and assist the person to stand while you take their pants, skirts or underwear down to their knees, then ask and assist them back to the sitting position. Remove the clothing from their legs. Without standing the person up, help them into their underwear, trousers or skirt, followed by socks and shoes. Ensure the shoes are fitted correctly before asking the person to stand. When standing, continue to pull up their underwear, trousers or skirt. Assist them to adjust their clothing so they are comfortable.

PRACTICE POINT

Assist a person with weakness to one side of their body (hemiparesis) as follows when undressing and dressing them:

- *Dressing:* Insert the person's affected arm into the sleeve of clothing, followed by their head, then the unaffected arm. This is helpful, as the person will have more dexterity, strength and range of movement in the unaffected arm to help with adjusting their clothing and minimising stress on the weaker side of their body.
- *Undressing:* Reverse the procedure for dressing, so that the sleeve of clothing is removed from the affected arm last.

Use terms such as "affected arm" and "unaffected arm", rather than "bad arm" and "good arm". Words can be powerful motivators when a person is struggling with their independence.

Older people can use many types of assistive devices to maintain independence with dressing and undressing, including extended shoehorns, magnetic zippers and zipper pulls, Velcro or shoelace fasteners, sock aids and dressing sticks. An occupational therapist (OT) can provide information and education about assistive devices and aids for personal support.

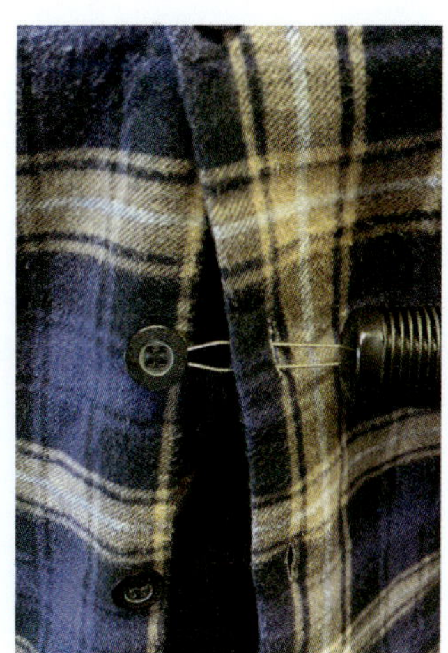

Button and zipper aid

HAIR CARE

Hair care is an important part of our hygiene and daily routine, and some older people need assistance with managing their hair. As a care worker, you may be required to shampoo, brush or style the person's hair, or assist them to access a hairdresser.

Shampooing, brushing and combing the hair are important for hair health, but they are also important for self-esteem and body image. The care plan will direct care workers when to shampoo the person's hair based on their needs and preferences. Use the person's preferred shampoo and conditioning products. Note that the scent of shampoo can be a positive sensory experience for people with dementia. Don't rush the procedure; human contact is important for the person's wellbeing. When shampooing the person's hair, be mindful of their eyes; shampoo can sting!

Many people like to have their hair styled a certain way and the care plan can assist the care worker with this. Ultimately, the older person's preference should be considered when combing or styling their hair. Some people won't have any preference, and the care worker can style their hair as they think best suits them. Brushing and combing someone's hair should not be a painful experience. It is best to comb sections of the hair gently, and to move from one section to the next, if the hair is tangled. Always use the person's own brush, comb and other hair accessories.

ORAL HYGIENE

Poor oral health can lead to gum infection and tooth decay and can make eating and drinking difficult. Dysphagia can also result from poor oral health. The teeth and gums need to be cleaned at least twice daily, and this should occur regardless of whether the older person has their own teeth or dentures. People with dementia cannot verbalise that they have a toothache or painful gums, so oral care is particularly important for preventing distress for these people. All older people can benefit from an assessment of their mouth and teeth, and dental check-ups are encouraged to be scheduled annually and whenever needed.

- *Cleaning teeth, gums and tongue:* The role of the care worker in assisting the older person with oral care may include assisting them with loading their toothbrush with toothpaste and ensuring they have access to water; or the care worker may be required to perform the entire task of brushing the person's teeth, gums and tongue. The tongue can accumulate bacteria and therefore should be brushed gently with the toothbrush when oral care occurs.

  It is important to abide by standard precautions in the realms of infection control and prevention when brushing teeth. After attending to hand hygiene, the care worker should put on disposable gloves and wear a face shield or eye protection. The person may splatter **saliva** during the oral care procedure or, potentially, blood if they are taking blood-thinning medications and the gum is brushed a little too hard. The mouth and gums are rich in blood vessels and bleeding can occur quite easily. Always brush gently, starting at one side of the mouth and working towards the other. Encourage the person to rinse and spit at intervals during the procedure.
- *Care of dentures:* Dentures are artificial teeth and usually comprise a top and bottom set of teeth. They are removed from the mouth and cleaned manually with a toothbrush and denture-specific toothpaste. Everyday-use toothpaste can be abrasive to dentures and may damage them over time. It is good practice to encourage the person to brush their own dentures; however, many older people will require the care worker to do this on their behalf. Leaving the cleaned dentures out of the mouth for a period of time (usually overnight) can give the gums a rest. Dentures are often left to soak in water and an active cleaning agent when they are not in use.

  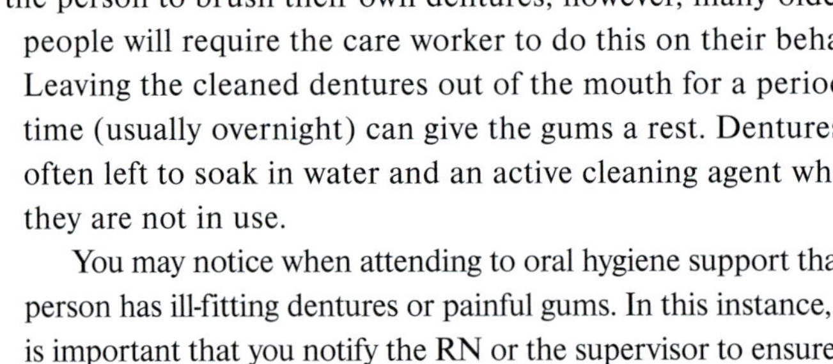

  You may notice when attending to oral hygiene support that the person has ill-fitting dentures or painful gums. In this instance, it is important that you notify the RN or the supervisor to ensure the person has a dental review. Document your observations according to policy and procedures.

  Older people may have xerostomia, a condition where the salivary glands don't produce enough saliva. Saliva is important for moistening the mouth and preventing bacteria in the oral cavity. It is also important for warming and moistening the food we place in our mouth. If the person cannot chew or swallow safely, they are at risk of aspirating food or fluid into the airways and of malnutrition.

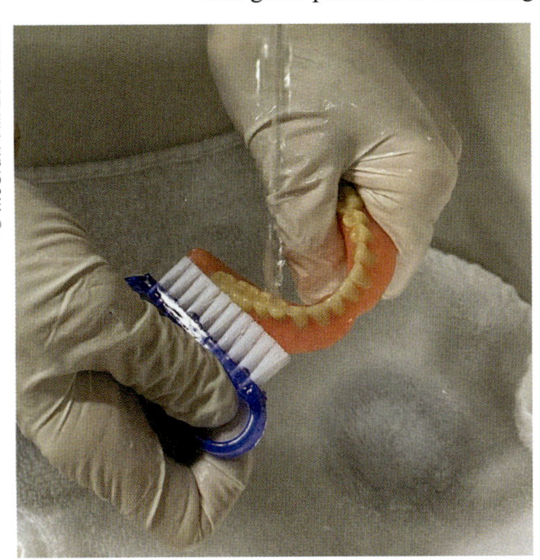

Denture cleaning

Common aids and assistive devices used for oral care include modified-handled toothbrushes that enable the person to hold the toothbrush securely, electric toothbrushes, denture brushes and artificial saliva.

SHAVING

Shaving is a component of the person's grooming routine and contributes to their wellbeing. Many older men have shaved every day for their entire adult lives, and this routine should be continued into aged care services if the person prefers. Some women also shave areas of their face, and their preference for shaving or using other hair removal techniques should be discussed during development of their individualised plan.

The care worker may be required to provide minimal assistance to the person to shave or they may have to shave the entire facial area if the person cannot do it themself. Some men prefer to have a wet shave using warm water, shaving foam and a handheld razor, while others prefer to use an electric shaver. The second option is safer, as it minimises the risk of cutting the face and exposing blood. With the first option, infection control protocols should be implemented to reduce the risk of blood exposure. The person's preference should be discussed and documented in their care plan.

PRACTICE POINT

Always be aware of the person's preferences. If the person has dementia, it can be helpful to ask their substitute decision maker what the person's hair removal preference is. An older woman with dementia who has always used tweezers to remove chin hairs may be shocked or distressed if a visiting beautician waxes her chin.

EYE CARE

Our eyes and the surrounding areas are very sensitive and can become irritated easily. The ageing process can see a decrease in eye lubrication, and the eyes can become dry, sore and scratchy. Many older people require artificial tears, or eye drops to moisten the eyes. Eye infections such as conjunctivitis are common, and infection control procedures need to be adhered to constantly when attending eye care. Not all discharges of the eyes are infectious.

- *Eye care:* Eye care involves assisting the person to clean their eyes using a saline-dampened gauze swab. Hand hygiene and the wearing of disposable gloves are essential before assisting any person with eye care. The gauze is wiped from the inner corner of the eye to the outer corner and is then discarded. It must not be rubbed back and forth over the eye, which can introduce infection or irritate the eye. A new gauze swab is used for each wipe. This clinical procedure may be referred to as an *eye toilet* or *eye bath* and is often used when the eyes are infected. Eyes can be cleaned in the shower, using the washer in the same way as the gauze, as part of everyday personal hygiene requirements.
- *Care of spectacles:* Spectacles (glasses) are prescribed by an optometrist to ensure that a person's vision is optimal. Part of the care worker's role is to ensure that the glasses of a person who requires support are clean and intact, and that the person can access them at all times. It is helpful to have the person's name engraved on their glasses if they reside in an RACF, in case they go missing or another person has a similar-looking pair. Older people should be encouraged to have an eye check-up every 12 months unless otherwise stated by their optometrist.

EAR CARE

Ear care is important for maintaining quality of life in older people. Over 75 per cent of people over age 65 have some form of hearing loss. It goes undetected in half of people living in an RACF and the proportion is even higher for people with dementia (Bellekom n.d.). Hearing loss can be linked to social isolation, even if the person lives in an RACF, because communication can be difficult and awkward. Staff tend to misinterpret what the person says, or they don't converse as much with them as they would if the person could hear them correctly. Many older people miss out on social activities and find it harder to develop relationships with others due to their hearing loss. It is within the care worker's role to report to the RN or their supervisor any concerns they may have about a person's hearing to ensure they can be referred to an audiologist to have their hearing status reviewed.

- *Care of hearing aids:* People are prescribed hearing aids by an audiologist to optimise their hearing. Many people manage their own hearing aids, but if a person needs assistance, the care worker should:
  - clean the hearing aid according to the manufacturer's instructions and ensure it is not blocked
  - ensure the hearing aid has working batteries in situ
  - ensure the hearing aid is correctly assembled
  - encourage the person to keep the hearing aid in its case when not in use, to keep it clean and safe
  - encourage the person to wear their hearing aid.

HAND AND FOOT CARE

Hand and foot care is a component of personal support and is necessary to prevent issues of the skin and nails and to minimise the impact of mobility problems. The hands can be affected by painful joint and bone issues that make movement and use of the fingers and wrists difficult. Older people may need help trimming fingernails and applying moisturiser to the skin on their hands. This is a great opportunity to sit and chat with the person.

Foot care is essential because our feet take the burden of our mobility. Painful, ulcerated and infected feet can prevent an older person from being able to walk or even to stand, causing a decline in their ability to self-function. Diabetes can cause chaos on a cellular level within the blood supply and in the skin around the feet and lower limbs of the older person. The care worker should take particular care when providing foot care to diabetics.

Feet should be washed and dried meticulously every day. This is a great opportunity to spend time chatting to the person and to check out their feet, toes and toenails, and between the toes, for any issues with skin breakdown or infection. Any observation that you make regarding changes to the feet will require prompt reporting to the RN or supervisor.

If the workplace policies and procedures support you to do so, care workers can trim the person's toenails; however, any person who is diabetic will require specialist foot and nail care from a podiatrist. To be clear, a care worker should not trim the toenails of a diabetic person.

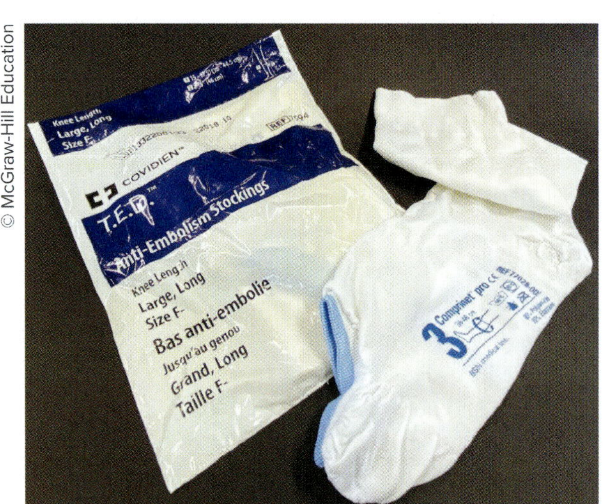

Anti-embolim stockings

- *Applying anti-embolism stockings:* Anti-embolism stockings are designed to minimise the risk of blood clots in the deep veins of the legs by increasing circulation through the application of a low-gradient pressure. This pressure helps the valves in the veins to continue to work properly. Anti-embolism stockings are applied to the lower half of the leg, below the knee to the toes; however, longer ones can extend to the thigh. Different sizes and lengths are available, and they are prescribed by a doctor for people who have recently had surgery or who are not very mobile. Anti-embolism stockings are not suitable for everyone and must be prescribed and fitted by a health professional.

  The stockings are medical grade, and the care worker will need to check that the person is not experiencing discomfort or possible skin breakdown from the pressure of ill-fitting stockings. Anti-embolic stockings can be tricky to apply, and the use of an applicator is advisable. They can also be applied by:

1. turning the stocking inside out and grasping the heel
2. positioning the foot into the sock with the heel in the correct position
3. pulling the sock up the leg
4. making sure any visible wrinkles are smoothed out.

Any noticeable skin changes in colour or temperature, swelling at the top of the stocking or broken areas of skin must be reported to the RN promptly. Anti-embolic stockings usually don't cause any problems; however, issues may occur if they are incorrectly sized.

- *Footwear:* Footwear that is well fitting and secure is advisable for older people, as good shoes can minimise the risk of falls and support people with neuropathy (nerve damage) of the feet, such as that caused by diabetes. Heeled shoes or shoes with laces can increase the risk of trips and falls among older people. Ill-fitting shoes and slippers can flop about when the person walks and may also cause a fall.

  A podiatrist is the health professional who can assist with helping the person walk safely by prescribing orthotics and other shoe modifications, based on assessment.

EATING AND DRINKING

Older people may have a slower metabolism due to the ageing process and many will eat smaller amounts of food than younger people. While the person may require smaller amounts of food, the food they consume needs to be nutrient dense to ensure the body has the energy it needs. Older people benefit from a healthy and nutritionally balanced diet that includes ample water, just like any adult.

There are many factors that can affect eating and drinking, and some older people will require varying types of assistance to ensure they access the nutrients they need. For example, the person may:

- find that eating is difficult, due to a painful mouth
- have difficulty chewing food, due to inadequate dentition
- have dysphagia (difficulty in swallowing)
- have cognition issues and forget how or when to eat
- not be able to access food or prepare meals.

The care worker can assist the person with eating and drinking by:

- helping them to prepare and heat meals
- ensuring they are positioned correctly to eat safely—upright, with their head inclined forwards
- providing them with a meal tray in their room
- arranging the meal tray in a way that enables them to reach and consume their meal
- setting the dining table to ensure the person has access to the cutlery and dinnerware they need
- serving them their meals
- encouraging them to drink water
- assisting them to eat their entire meal
- monitoring their food and fluid intake
- supporting them with tube feeding if the workplace policy enables them to do so.

Refer to the care plan to determine the required support for all eating and drinking activities. When feeding the person, sit facing then at eye level, and apply a clothing protector to the person if required. Give the person time to swallow after each mouthful and offer sips of drink frequently. Communicate with the person and determine what they would like to try from their meal. Sometimes, people will use assistive devices and aids to support eating and drinking independently. This topic is discussed further in Chapter 10.

Dysphagia is a difficulty in the swallowing response. Any change in the person's ability to swallow safely must be reported to the RN immediately. If you notice that the person is chewing or eating differently than usual, you should ensure they have swallowed the mouthful and not proceed with the meal until the person has been reviewed by the RN. People who have dysphagia will require assessment from the speech pathologist (or speech therapist) to determine the type of food consistency that is safe for them to consume. If the person requires a modified-texture diet according to their care plan, ensure they are offered each type of food from their meal. Don't blend the foods into a mixture in the bowl and expect the person to eat it or enjoy eating it. Eating should be a pleasant experience for the person, not a task to be hurried for the convenience of the care worker. Signs of dysphagia include dribbling, pouching food in the mouth, taking a long time to swallow, coughing, choking or gagging. Dysphagia is discussed in detail in Chapter 10.

TOILETING

Toileting involves the elimination of urine and faeces from the body and is an ADL that we learn to do independently when we are very young. Going to the toilet is a process that many of us take for granted because we toilet ourselves every day; however, it is one that involves a combination of planning and awareness.

We need to be able to recognise that we need to go to the toilet, then we need to locate a toilet. People with dementia have difficulty with these first steps and care workers will need to interpret the person's needs through observing their behaviour. The person may be holding themselves or pacing or may appear anxious with a sense of urgency.

Once we locate a toilet, we need the dexterity and muscle coordination to open the toilet door and close it behind us. We then need to be able to balance while we take down our clothing and bend to sit on the toilet. Once we use the toilet, we then need to use toilet paper and be able to bend and twist to wipe ourselves. Then we need to stand up, balance, and have the dexterity to adjust our clothing. More balance is needed to turn around and flush the toilet, and to wash our hands. Finally, we need to navigate our way out of the toilet and go on our way.

So, using the toilet involves planning, navigating, dexterity, muscle strength and coordination, bending, twisting and gripping. It is easy to understand that older people with chronic disease, obesity, reduced muscle mass, poor vision, limited mobility, confusion and pain may have some difficulty with using the toilet.

- *Assessing toileting needs:* The person's toileting needs can be determined using validated assessment tools and effective communication. Validated assessments are those that are known to the industry to be reliable and are viewed as best practice. They can indicate the person's usual pattern when using the toilet and can also indicate if there are particular times when toileting may be needed, such as before bed or in the afternoon. Some people may require more frequent toileting assistance due to the type of medication they take, and others may need a longer time to use the toilet if they are constipated. Bowel motions are recorded in an RACF to ensure the person receives support for constipation and other bowel-related issues such as bowel impaction and diarrhoea.
- *Providing assistance:* The care worker may be required to assist the person at any point during the toileting process, in alignment with the person's care plan. Assistance may include reminding the person to use the toilet, helping them—or using lifters and commodes to assist them—on and off the toilet, attending to their toilet hygiene and encouraging them to wash their hands.

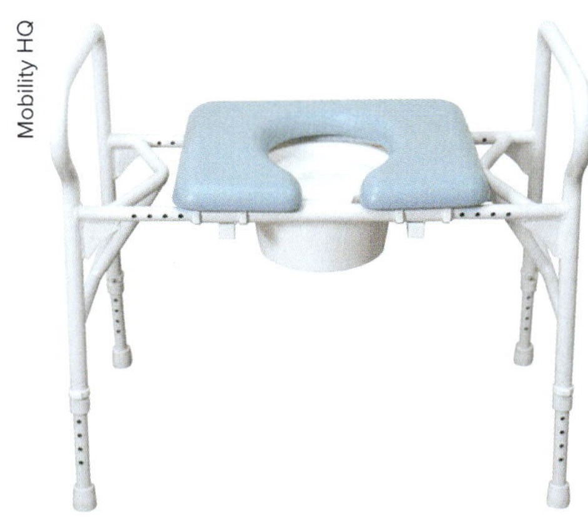
Mobility HQ
Over-toilet frame (raised toilet frame)

Toileting assistance also includes applying and emptying the bedpan and urinal for people who are in bed or unable to get to the toilet in time. Some older people prefer to use a bedside commode during the night, and care workers are required to empty the contents of the commode for the person.

Another key aspect of the care worker's role is to promote a regular toileting routine that can help to minimise episodes of incontinence. During toileting, it is important to report any observations that the person may be experiencing discomfort or possible urine infection. You may notice that their urine is very dark in colour, and it may smell offensive. The person may tell you that they feel a burning or stinging sensation when they pass urine.

You may also notice that the person appears to be having problems with their bowels. Excessive and painful straining can indicate constipation or other bowel-related issues and should be reported. Likewise, very loose and fluid bowel motions also indicate health issues. Bleeding from the anus can be caused by haemorrhoids but can also occur for many other reasons. Always report your observations to the RN or supervisor and document them in the appropriate notes or assessment charts.

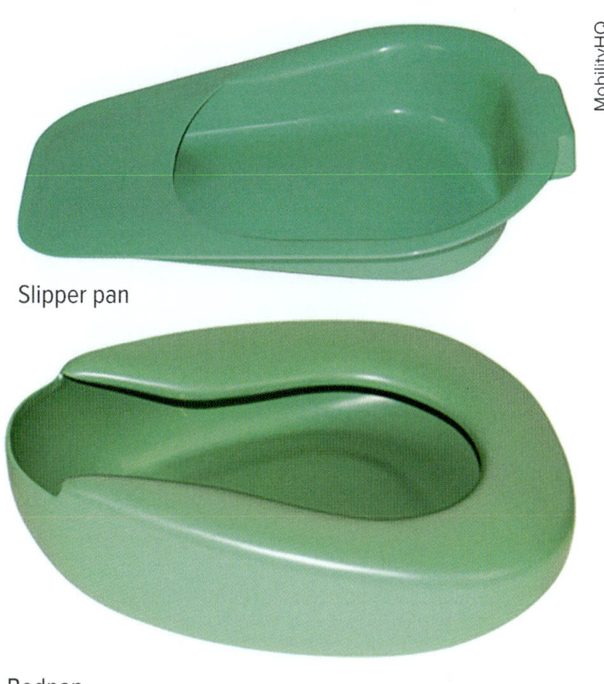

Slipper pan

Bedpan

MobilityHQ

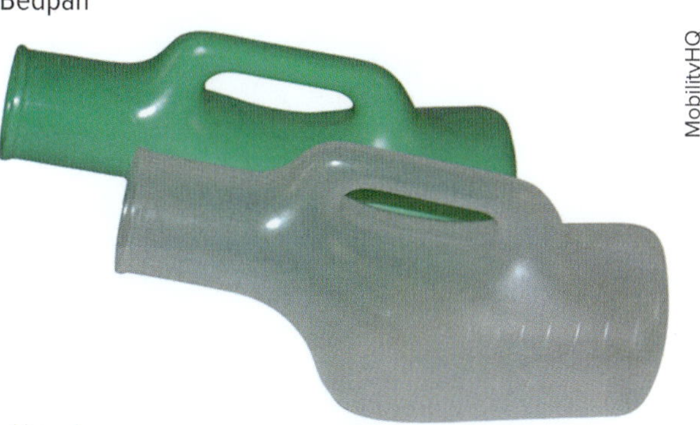

Urinals

MobilityHQ

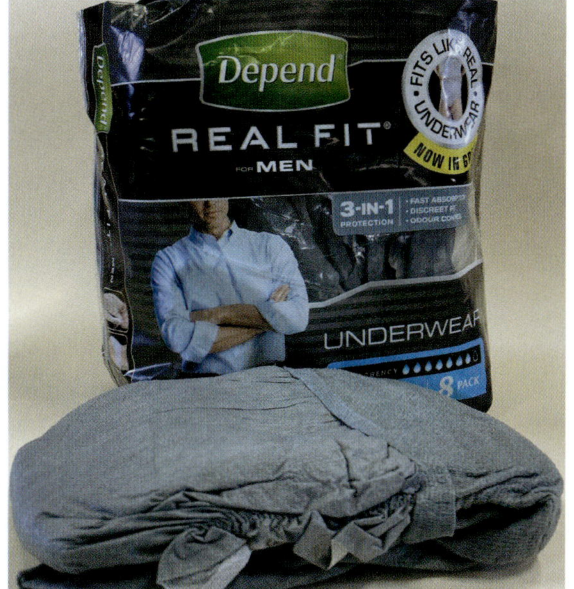

Incontinence pads

Incontinence

Incontinence occurs when the person has limited or no control over the elimination of urine or faeces from the body. People may experience urinary incontinence, faecal incontinence or both. Incontinence isn't a normal part of ageing; however, because of dementia and progressive neurological conditions, many older people who are incontinent are unable to participate in a continence program that aims to retrain the bladder.

Incontinence can cause social isolation of the older person as they retreat from social and enjoyable activities due to feelings of embarrassment and shame. Incontinence can create an unpleasant odour and, because of this, many older people feel unable to participate in social activities such as outings. The role of the care worker is to use effective and inclusive communication to ensure the person's feelings are acknowledged and to encourage them to participate in their continence management. The person may benefit from a referral to a continence nurse specialist who can offer information and strategies for managing or even reversing some types of incontinence. Supporting all older people who are incontinent to be clean and dry will minimise odour and prevent skin excoriation and infection.

There are several types of incontinence, and many require specific management strategies. Table 6.4 identifies types of incontinence and their causes.

The way an older person's incontinence is managed should be according to their needs and preferences. Everyone will have different needs due to their varying medical conditions, medications and lifestyles. Ultimately, continence management must fundamentally support the dignity and autonomy of the person. Some people may require support with accessing continence aids such as pads, sheaths and

TABLE 6.4 Types of incontinence and their causes

Incontinence type	Cause
Stress incontinence	Small amounts of urine are passed involuntarily when abdominal pressure increases, such as when a person laughs, sneezes, lifts something heavy or coughs. Pregnancy and menopause can cause stress incontinence in women, and men can experience it after prostate surgery. It can be managed or cured with support from a health professional.
Urge incontinence	There is a strong urge to urinate when the bladder isn't full, and the person may pass the urine before getting to the toilet. Conditions that affect the message system of the brain that tells us the bladder is full can contribute to urge incontinence. Some medications in unison with a bladder training program can be helpful in managing this type of incontinence.
Functional incontinence	The person has a cognitive or physical disability that prevents them from accessing the toilet, resulting in incontinence. The person may have problems recognising and accessing a toilet or managing their clothing. Environmental issues can also cause functional incontinence. People who experience this type of incontinence may have dementia, intellectual disability, or physical disability that affects mobility and dexterity.
Nocturia	This type of incontinence involves waking during the night to urinate. It may be caused by caffeine in the diet, fluid medications or drinking large amounts of fluids before bed. Nocturia increases the risk of falls as people are not fully awake when they get up to use the toilet or commode.
Post-micturition incontinence	Men who have an enlarged prostate or problems with the muscles that cause the urethra to contract may have difficulty emptying the bladder. Referred to as "after-dribble", this type of incontinence results in urine leaking involuntary from the penis after the man has urinated.
Faecal incontinence	The involuntary passing of faeces (involuntary bowel movements) is caused by some medications, heavy lifting throughout life, some surgeries, and neurological disorders that interrupt messaging systems of the brain related to defecation.

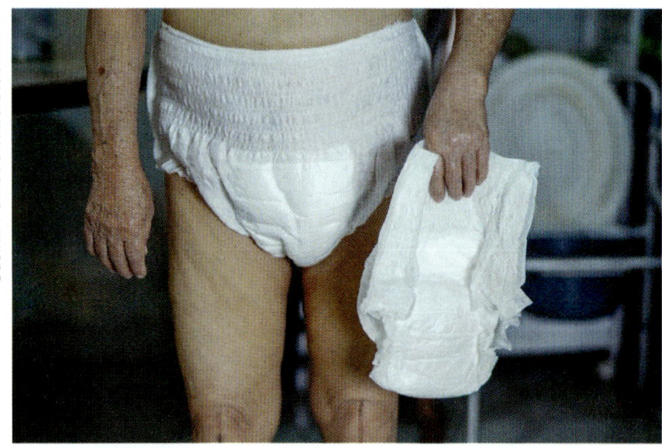

Sasirin Pamai/Shutterstock.com

Pull-up incontinence pants

bed protection, and others may require full support that includes perineal care and the application of aids. The person's care plan will indicate how they manage their incontinence.

Continence aids are items that assist the person to manage incontinence. If incontinence is related to disability, the person may be able to access continence aids through the National Disability Insurance Scheme (NDIS) as part of their funding allocation, and older people who have permanent or severe incontinence can apply for the federal government's Continence Aids Payment Scheme (CAPS) which provides a payment to the person to assist with the cost of continence aids.

Continence aids include pads of various types, pants, sheath drainage and bed protection. Care workers may be required to assist with any or all of these continence aids. Remember: always be aware of the person's dignity and use empathy in all your interactions.

PRESSURE INJURIES

A pressure injury is damage to the skin that occurs when the skin is exposed to pressure for extended periods of time or from shearing and friction forces. All cells need oxygen, nutrients and water for survival, which are contained in the blood supply. Blood supply is prevented from accessing the cells in the skin when the skin is compressed, much like a kinked garden hose that doesn't let water through. Cells can become compromised and cause tissue death, resulting in a wound.

Shearing is a mechanical force that occurs when the person's skin and their underlying bony structure move in opposite directions. For example, a person who remains sitting up in bed will slide downwards, causing the skin of their buttocks to move downwards while the bone of their pelvis stays put. The resulting opposing force causes tissue damage at the deep levels of the skin where it is attached to the muscle fascia.

Friction is another mechanical force that can cause pressure injuries. When skin is dragged across a surface such as bed linen, the top layer (epidermis) can become damaged, leaving the skin susceptible to further deterioration. When pressure, shear and friction coexist, the risk of pressure injury is extremely high.

Pressure injuries often occur on bony prominences such as the hip, shoulder, **sacrum**, heel and spine when a person is immobile. Ageing skin is already very thin, so damage can occur very quickly and healing can take much longer.

PREVENTING PRESSURE INJURIES

Pressure injuries are largely preventable; however, they continue to be an ongoing issue in aged care. Pressure injury risk assessment tools, such as the Braden Scale, the Norton Scale and the Waterlow Scale, are helpful for predicting the level of risk an older person has of developing a pressure injury. These tools can be used as a baseline and should be used again when the person's condition changes. Factors that increase a person's risk of pressure injury include immobility, incontinence, anti-inflammatory and steroidal medications, malnutrition, age and comorbidities, and inadequate nursing care.

Prevention methods include:

- using a pressure injury risk assessment tool
- thorough skin assessment on a daily basis
- reporting any reddened areas or skin changes to the RN immediately
- requesting a dietitian to review the person's nutritional status
- encouraging the person to consume a nutritional diet or referring them to a doctor for multivitamins or nutritional supplements
- implementing dedicated repositioning regimes to prevent prolonged exposure to pressure
- using positioning techniques to minimise pressure on pressure points
- following excellent continence care to ensure the skin isn't compromised to breakdown from urine or faeces
- requesting a pharmacist to review the person's medications
- employing equipment, aids and assistive devices to prevent pressure injury, such as using air mattresses and other supportive surfaces, air cushions for wheelchairs and recliners, skin protectors, and padding for pressure created by callipers and other prosthetics.

TYPES OF PRESSURE INJURIES

Pressure injuries are classified into stages in an attempt to unify management strategies globally. A stage I pressure injury can develop into a stage II wound within hours, so any reddened area that is observed must be reported to the RN promptly. The deeper the tissue injury, the higher the risk is for prolonged healing, pain, increased costs and infection. Chronic wounds can have a negative impact on the quality of life of older people, and prevention is always better than cure.

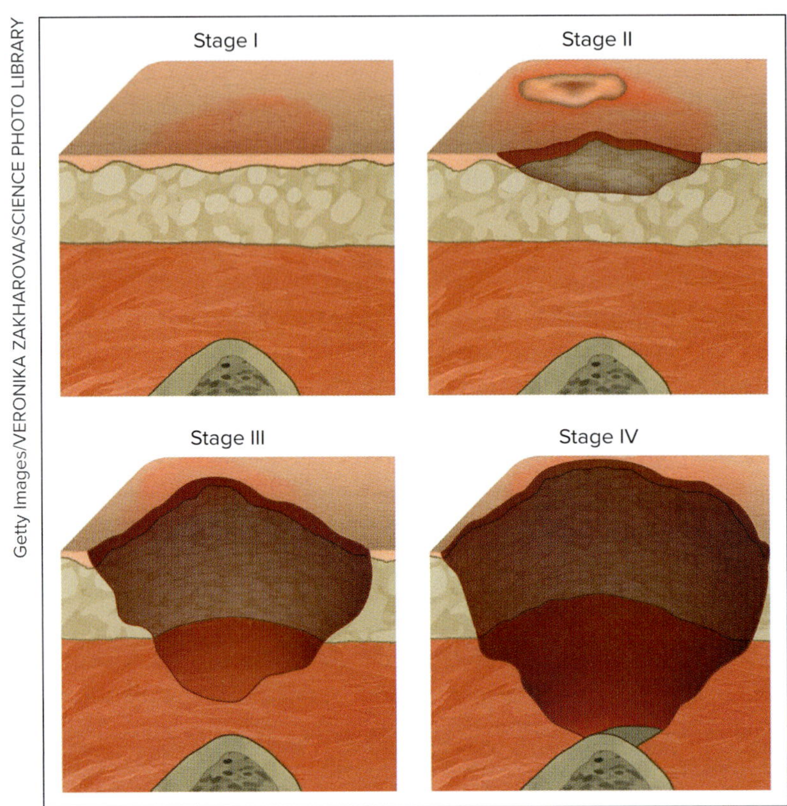

Pressure injuries are staged from I to IV, depending on the extent of tissue damage. Stage I pressure injuries do not break the skin, but damage occurs on a cellular level in the skin. Stage II pressure injuries involve wounds that have extended into the dermis but not into the hypodermis. Stage III pressure injuries involve tissue damage at a depth not further than the hypodermis. Stage IV pressure injuries involve tissue damage that may or may not extend to underlying structures such as muscle, tendons and bone.

MANAGING PRESSURE INJURIES

Management of pressure injuries is complex and multifaceted and differs between individuals. Healing can be affected by many factors and any open wound can create an environment for infection. Infection can overwhelm the immune system of the older person, leading to long-term complications. Death can sometimes occur due to multi-organ failure as a result of sepsis.

Pressure injuries are managed according to the person's wound management plan, which includes the wound dressing plan and regimen, a photographic timeline of the wound, and other strategies to address the cause of the wound such as the use of assessment tools, the implementation of a repositioning regimen, and the incorporation of assistive devices such as surface protectors. Wounds require specific vitamins and minerals to assist the healing process and nutritional supplements are often prescribed by the person's doctor or a dietitian.

The ideal way to manage a pressure injury is to implement prevention strategies based on risk assessment.

COMFORT, REST AND SLEEP

Ageing affects people differently; however, research suggests that it often has an impact on sleep. Sleep is important for healthy bodies and overall wellbeing, and as we age the rhythm of sleep can change. Older people may wake earlier and become tired earlier. Older adults may also sleep less deeply as they experience changes in the stages of sleep. Sleeping periodically during the day isn't uncommon for older people; however, excessive daytime naps can affect the night-time quality of sleep. Older people should be aiming for around seven to eight hours of sleep a night (Hirshkowitz 2015).

Care workers can support the person to sleep and rest by following their care plan. People have their own bedtime routine, and this is part of the preparation phase of sleeping. When routines are disrupted by an incident or even an upset, it can be difficult for the person to fall asleep and stay asleep. Lack of quality sleep can increase their risk of falls and accidents.

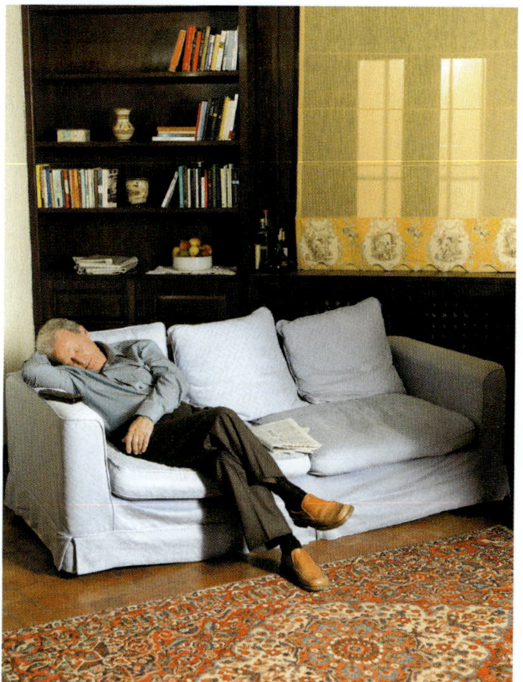

Cultura/Image Source

Excessive daytime napping can affect the quality of night-time sleep

People with dementia may have issues with sleeping, as their sleeping rhythm is disrupted by the effects of dementia on the brain. Redirecting people back to their room if they have left their bed can be helpful, as well as ensuring that the environment is conducive to rest and sleep. This may involve minimising harsh lighting (but ensuring safety), minimising noise, and incorporating other relaxation techniques such as aromatherapy or music.

The care worker should consider the person's level of comfort in all the support they provide, not just when the person is sleeping or napping. Ensuring comfort includes asking the person if they are comfortable or if they would like any changes to the support. Such changes may not necessarily be complex and may include just checking in with the person to ask about their comfort. For example:

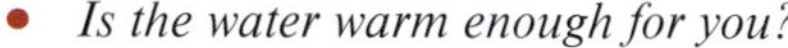

- *Is the water warm enough for you?*
- *Do you feel dry enough?*
- *Would you like a snack?*
- *Do you want another blanket?*
- *Can I adjust that strap for you? It looks a little tight.*

Communication is key to effective and person-centred support that puts the person at the centre of their care according to their needs and preferences.

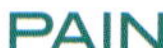

PAIN

Pain is an issue for many older people, for many reasons, and it affects each person differently. Because it is subjective, it is impossible to fully understand how another person is feeling pain. The way people interpret pain can be influenced by factors such as their culture, life experience, medications and available social supports.

TYPES OF PHYSICAL PAIN

Physical pain can have a direct impact on the person's quality of life, functional abilities and relationships. When a person is in physical pain, they may struggle to manage ADLs and require support.

There are different types of pain.

- *Nociceptive pain:* pain that is common to almost everyone. Nociceptors send messages to the brain that something hurts, and we have nociceptors throughout our body, especially the skin. An example of nociceptive pain is a burn from hot water or a cut from a sharp object.
- *Visceral pain:* occurs from within the body and affects organs. This type of pain is described as a pressure or cramping type of pain. Appendicitis pain is an example of visceral pain.

- *Acute pain:* occurs suddenly and lasts for a short time. Acute pain occurs usually for a specific reason, such as childbirth or a bone fracture.
- *Chronic pain:* lasts over a period of time (more than six months) and requires ongoing management and planning. Chronic pain can increase in intensity at any time and can impact quality of life. Energy and motivation can be affected by chronic pain, and the person's mental health can also be impacted in a negative way. Examples of chronic pain include back pain, arthritis and neck pain.
- *Neuropathic pain:* also known as nerve pain. Damaged nerves can produce sensations such as tingling, burning and stabbing pains. An example of nerve pain is shingles.
- *Somatic pain:* occurs when deep tissue pain receptors are activated to send a message to the brain that something hurts. Somatic pain affects bones, ligaments, joints and muscles. An example of somatic pain is tissue damage from a sprained ankle.
- *Total pain:* when a person is experiencing a combination of physical, emotional, social and even spiritual pain.

EFFECTS OF PAIN

Pain can affect mobility, movement, dexterity and flexibility, making it difficult for the person to brush their teeth or get dressed. Pain can affect the person's quality of life by:

- challenging their mobility
- decreasing their ability to perform ADLs or IADLs
- causing feelings of anger, resentment and frustration
- socially isolating the person from participating in relationships and social activities
- creating emotional pain by predisposing the person to feelings of worthlessness and uselessness, resulting in depression, anxiety or suicidal thoughts.

SIGNS AND SYMPTOMS OF PAIN

The way a person expresses pain is influenced by their culture, social norms and life experience. People with dementia cannot always verbalise that they are in pain, and the care staff need to be aware of changes to the person's behaviour that may indicate they are feeling pain.

Common signs and symptoms of pain include grimacing, guarding the part of the body that hurts, voicing and expressing pain, not eating or drinking, changes in behaviour, restlessness and irritability.

ASSESSING PAIN

Validated pain assessment tools are used in aged care services to assist in identification of pain and appropriate pain management strategies. Pain assessments are indicated when a person is admitted into an RACF to obtain a baseline of information about their pain, if they have a change in their condition, or when pain is suspected. According to the Pain Management Guide (PMG) Toolkit for Aged Care, a pain assessment should occur every three months (Savvas et al. 2021).

MANAGING PAIN

Pain management is unique to the individual because everyone experiences pain differently. The type of pain a person experiences is also relevant to the appropriate pain management strategies that can be implemented. End-of-life pain management is unique and is discussed in Chapter 12.

Medications that reduce or relieve pain are one component of pain management, and they are prescribed cautiously by the person's doctor because many side effects of strong pain medications can cause falls and delirium, and place pressure on the ageing respiratory system. The doctor will often prescribe pain medications that have lower risks before stronger painkillers are introduced to the person's pain management plan. Non-pharmaceutical strategies for pain management include:

- eating a nutritional diet and drinking adequate water
- staying as active as possible

- aromatherapy
- massage
- music therapy
- breathing exercises and mindfulness activities
- meditation
- counselling and support groups
- spending time in nature
- incorporating strategies indicated by allied health professionals, such as physiotherapy.

Remember that pain is unique to the person, and so pain management strategies and supports need to be tailored to the individual and their needs and preferences. The care worker has a valuable role in monitoring the effectiveness of the person's pain management plan and reporting any observations that indicate it is not effective.

6.2.4 Mobility

Mobility is important for independence and autonomy. It includes the ability to walk and to transfer one's position from one place to another. When a person's ability to mobilise changes, they may require support from others to participate in ADLs and IADLs. Limited mobility and immobility can affect a person's quality of life.

Mobility can be affected by many factors, including injury, falls, the fear-of-falling phenomenon, illness, diseases that affect movement such as Parkinson's disease and Huntington's disease, dementia and other progressive neurological diseases, some medications such as anti-psychotics, obesity, pain and depression.

Older people should be encouraged to remain as active as possible and to participate in programs that support the maintenance of their mobility. There are many community- and RACF-based exercise programs that provide support to older people in maintaining their muscle and joint strength and dexterity. These types of programs also offer social interaction which can boost the wellbeing of older people.

Individual strategies to improve or maintain mobility are located in the care plan. Strategies may include the use of mobility aids, pain management and exercise programs. Individual physiotherapy plans may also be included in the mobility plan and are developed collaboratively between the person and the physiotherapist. Care workers may be required to learn how to assist with the physiotherapy plan—for example, learning how to perform range-of-movement exercises (ROMs) for the person. ROMs are helpful in preventing a person's limbs from becoming stiff and painful and involve the care worker physically moving part of the person's body in repetitions. When the person performs ROMs independently, this is referred to as *active* exercise; however, care workers may be required to perform ROMs when a person has limited mobility. This is an example of *passive* exercise.

ASSESSING MOBILITY

Mobility assessment is necessary to determine information about the person's ability to move freely and safely. Assessments are validated tools that identify aspects of the person's mobility status and include identifying the factors that may affect their mobility, such as their history of falls, the types of medication they take, and what health conditions they have that may contribute to their abilities or disabilities in regard to movement.

There are different types of mobility assessments, and they may be utilised by doctors, hospitals, physiotherapists, and other allied health practitioners and aged care services. In the context of aged care services, a mobility assessment should occur at the point of service entry, whenever the person experiences significant changes in their condition or if they are experiencing falls and near misses, and every three months as part of a monitoring and evaluation process.

MOBILITY AIDS

Mobility aids enable the person to maintain independence and to mobilise safely, and each type of aid will provide a specific type of support. The person's need for a mobility aid should be based on assessment and involve a physiotherapist or an RN. Mobility aids need to be of the correct height, weight and overall purpose for the person. **Bariatric** equipment is required for people who are morbidly obese to minimise the risk of injury to themselves and to staff. A body weight of 125 kg and more requires equipment that is larger and designed to bear a heavier weight.

WHEELCHAIRS

Wheelchairs provide an opportunity for the person to travel distances that would otherwise be difficult if they walked independently. They can be pushed manually by a care worker or be self-propelled by the person, or they can be electric. An electric wheelchair is fitted for the person's body shape and weight and is usually charged overnight to ensure plenty of battery life so the person can use it the following day. Electric chairs are often used for people with limited or no ability to mobilise independently.

PRACTICE POINT

- When pushing a person in a wheelchair, ensure they have their elbows safely tucked inside. Many older elbows have sustained nasty skin tears from being bumped on doorframes.
- Never pull a person backwards in a wheelchair, especially if they have dementia or are confused. Remember that a wheelchair has wheels. When the chair is not in motion, the brakes must be on. (Be aware of your service's policy on using wheelchairs at the dining table; it may be a restrictive practice.)
- When assisting a person into a wheelchair, ensure the brakes are on and the foot pedals are upright and turned away from the person. Replace them into position when the person is sitting in the wheelchair and carefully assist the person to place their feet on the foot pedals. This prevents skin tears to the lower legs if the person should bump them.

FRAMES

Older people use frames to provide support and stability while they walk independently. Distinctive styles of frames provide varying levels of support and are selected based on a mobility assessment. A risk of injury arises when the person forgets to use their frame and tries to walk without it, or if the person becomes aggressive and throws the frame at or towards others.

Care workers should ensure that the person has their mobility frame within reach at all times. Some people may require standby support when using their frame. This means the care worker walks alongside the person who is using their frame to offer encouragement and guidance with mobility.

Figure 6.1 illustrates common types of frames used by older people to maintain independence with mobility.

CRUTCHES

Crutches are only helpful for mobility of older people if the person has the upper body strength, coordination and capacity to use them safely and properly. Crutches may be preferred by some people to use as stabilisation when walking; however, they can increase the falls risk of an older person. If crutches are required, forearm support and hand grips are preferred over underarm crutches.

FIGURE 6.1 Mobility frames

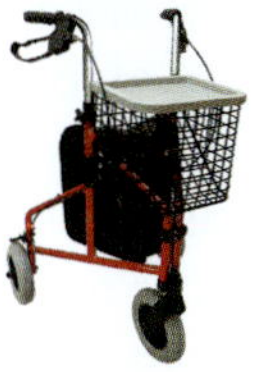

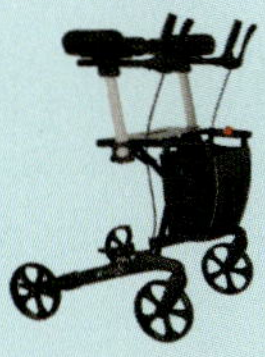

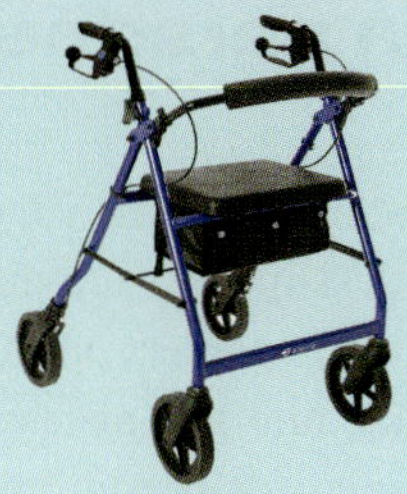	Four-wheeled walker: • is foldable • has automatic brakes and handbrakes • includes seat • assists stability.
	Three-wheeled walker: • is foldable • is lightweight • has handbrakes • assists stability.
	Forearm support frame (FASF): • provides forearm support • offers more stabilisation • is often rigid • is adjustable in height.
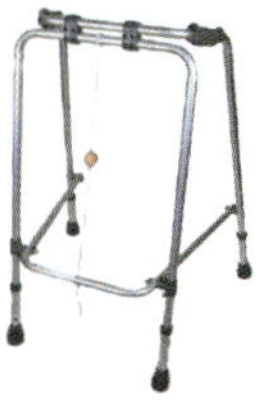	Zimmer frame: • is lightweight • guides mobility • is adjustable in height • is often rigid.
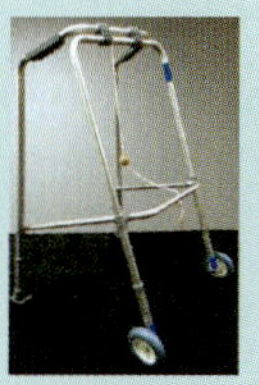	Glider frame: • can be detachable • aids mobility on carpeted areas • is helpful for people who use a walker indoors and who push, rather than lift, the walker.

Images: MobilityHQ; (bottom image) © McGraw-Hill Education

WALKING STICKS

Walking sticks–also referred to as canes–are used when a person needs minimal mobility support or only for a short period of time, such as following an injury. Walking sticks come in a variety of styles that have different purposes in the context of safe mobility and should be used on the side opposite the weakness or injury.

Some common walking sticks used in aged care include the standard walking stick, which is a handled support rod to help the person balance as they walk; and the quad stick, which is a walking stick with a four-pronged base to offer more stability. Quad sticks are helpful for people who have a weakness on one side of their body (hemiparesis).

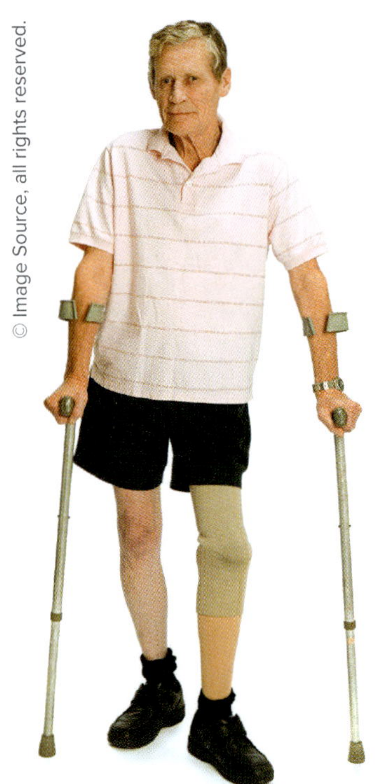

Forearm support crutches

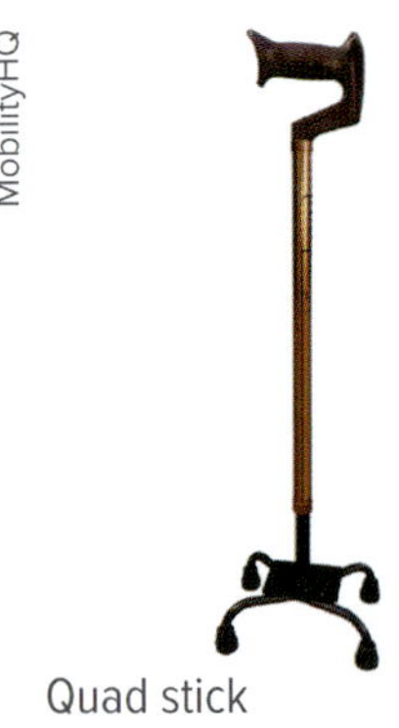

Quad stick

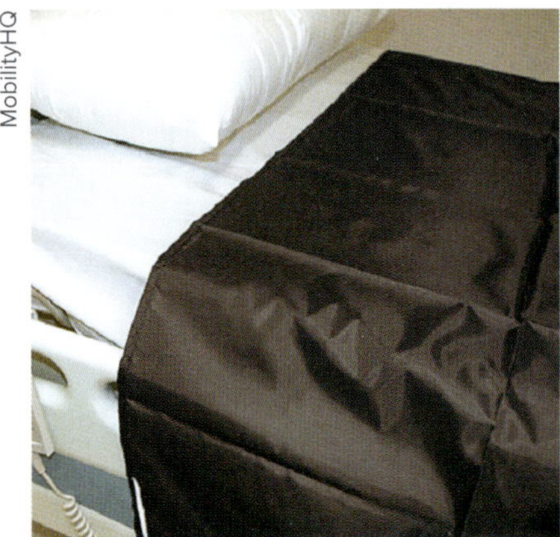

Slide sheets

Walking sticks must be height adjusted and have a comfortable hand grip. Many styles will collapse down for transport purposes.

6.2.5 Manual handling in personal care support

The amount of support older people need with ADLs will vary, based on many factors. When assisting people with support activities that require manual handling, it is essential that care workers always refer to the person's care plan to determine the risks, and the necessary risk management strategies, that have been determined for preventing injury. The organisational policies and procedures also support safe work practices in the context of manual handling and all care staff need to have a sound understanding of their content.

Providing personal care support involves manual handling when the care worker has to move the person in any way or has to use their own musculoskeletal system to carry out hazardous manual handling tasks. This may involve:

- repositioning a person in their bed for pressure injury prevention
- moving a person from bed to chair when they are immobile
- assisting a person to transfer from a chair to standing position
- making a bed with a person in it
- pushing a person in a wheelchair
- assisting a person from bed to chair.

Any activity that involves pushing, pulling or repetitive movements has the capacity to cause a musculoskeletal injury to the care worker; therefore, risk minimisation procedures must always be followed. Take the time to use equipment correctly and according to the care plan.

MANUAL HANDLING EQUIPMENT

Manual handling equipment used in activities that are associated with personal support include slide sheets, hoists, slings and lifters.

SLIDE SHEETS

Slide sheets are used to move a person in bed, including repositioning them from one side to the other, and up or down the bed. The sheet is made of polyester fabric with a fine coating that provides a slippery surface. It is designed to be used to manoeuvre someone in a bed or a chair, not to lift them. Slide sheets reduce risk of injury to the person and the staff as they minimise the need for heavy manual handling of the person. Infection prevention and control protocols require that each person has their own slide sheet, and they are not used communally. Two care workers use the slide sheet together to reposition a person, taking care to have full control over the manoeuvre so as to move the person safely. Slide sheets are a slip hazard and an infection control hazard if left on the floor.

LIFTERS, HOISTS AND SLINGS

Older people who are immobile will be fully dependent on others for all their mobility needs. Mechanical lifting equipment minimises risk of injury to the care staff and the person when used correctly. The terms "lifters" and "hoists" are used interchangeably in the workplace. Common types of mechanical lifting equipment are lifting hoists, standing hoists and slings.

- *Lifting hoist:* This hoist is used to lift a non-weight-bearing person up from the bed or chair by means of a sling. It is mobile and allows movement with the person, such as moving them from bed to chair, and enables the care worker to attend to the person's personal hygiene needs; however, it is not recommended the person remain suspended in the hoist for extended periods of time. Some aged care organisations use ceiling hoists, which (as the name suggests) are attached to the ceiling over the person's bed.
- *Standing hoist:* This hoist is used for people who have some ability to stand up or weight bear, but who need some support to do so. The hoist will assist the person to stand, allowing the care worker time to adjust their clothing or assist them onto the toilet. A sling is used to support the person's back during the motion of standing up. The standing hoist is mobile, which enables it to be used in bathrooms, dining areas and other areas away from the person's room.
- *Slings:* The slings that are used for lifting and standing hoists are designed for a specific purpose. Different-coloured loops, or handles, are hooked into place on the mechanical lifter according to the size of the person. This specific information can be located in the person's care plan. The *general-purpose sling* is a hammock-like sling used for people who cannot physically participate in the moving procedure. It cocoons the person safely when it is applied correctly. A toileting sling can be used for non-weight-bearing people who can assist with the lifting procedure. It is important before using this type of sling to assess whether the person has the upper body strength to participate in the lift. The *standing hoist sling* is used by people who can take some of their weight and are able to actively participate in the lift. The sling supports the person's mid-back area, coming up under the armpits where it attaches to the standing hoist. The person is supported to place their feet on a footplate to ensure they are secure when they are assisted to stand.

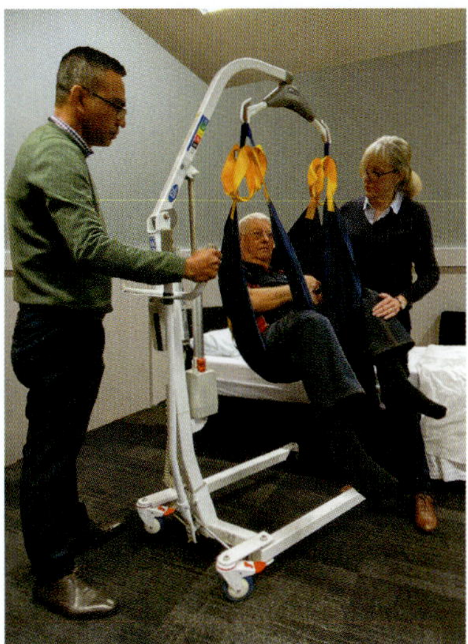

Hoist lifter with sling

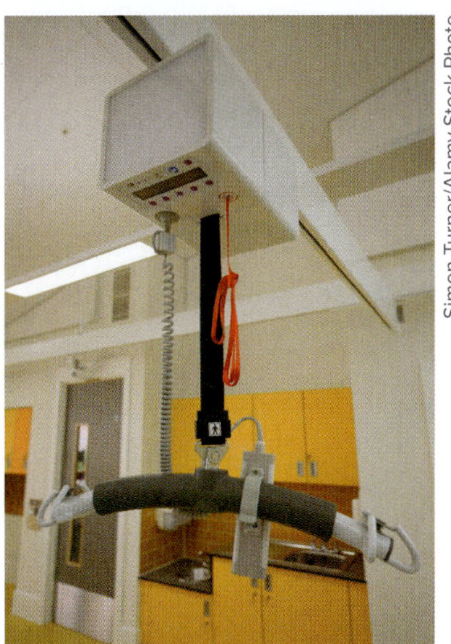

Ceiling hoist

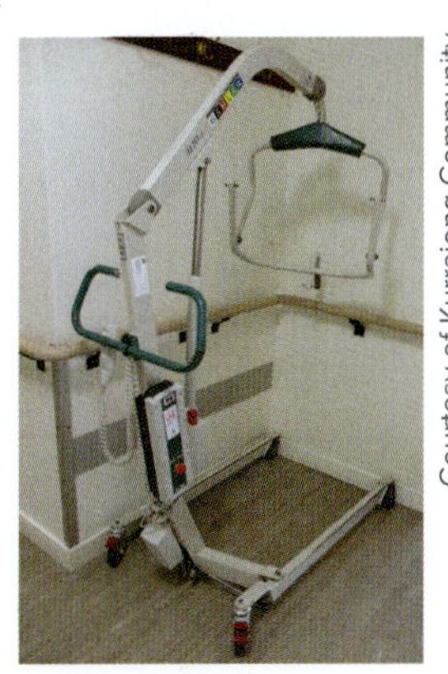

Stand-up hoist

Older people have their own dedicated sling if they require the use of a hoist, as slings are not shared communally.

Lifting hoists have a specified weight limit and care workers must check they are using the appropriate hoist for the person, in accordance with their care plan. Severe injury and death of older people has occurred as a result of inappropriate use of hoists and weight loading. Check the person's care plan, or the manufacturer's information, and clarify with the RN or supervisor if you are in doubt about which hoist to use.

All care staff are required to participate in yearly education that includes manual handling to ensure that equipment is used safely.

TRANSFERRING A PERSON

Some people have limited mobility and can walk unassisted, or assisted with a mobility aid, for short distances, while others cannot mobilise but can weight bear for a short period. Care workers will learn transfer techniques during their qualification and within the workplace. Common techniques for transferring people include:

- transferral between bed and chair, or commode or wheelchair
- transferral from a seated to a standing position
- transferral into and out of a car
- falls recovery.

Each technique has a specific process to ensure the safety of both the older person and the assisting care worker. Key principles of transferring a person include performing a risk assessment of the area before and after the transfer, ensuring the person's dignity is maintained, and being mindful that the person may feel anxious about falling. Providing clear instructions during the transfer, along with reassurance and encouragement, is helpful.

6.2.6 Restrictive practices

Restrictive practices are interventions that effectively restrict the rights or freedom of movement of a person receiving aged care services. These practices include chemical or environmental restraint, mechanical restraint, physical restraint and seclusion.

Restrictive practices must only be used as a last resort after all behaviour supports and strategies have been tried. The reason for using these practices is to prevent serious harm to the person or others as a result of their behaviour and associated actions.

LEGISLATIVE AND REGULATORY REQUIREMENTS

The use of restrictive practices must be compliant with the *Aged Care Act 1997* and the *Quality of Care Principles 2014* which were updated in July 2021 to reflect the new legal and regulatory expectations surrounding the use of restrictive practices. The Aged Care Safety and Quality Commission is the regulatory body for all compliance matters, including the use of restrictive practices.

An approved health practitioner who knows the person must assess the need for the restrictive practice, which must then be documented in the person's individualised plan. Informed consent for the use of restrictive practices must be obtained from the person or their decision maker in the event the person doesn't have capacity to make informed decisions. If the restrictive practice is used, the person's decision maker must be informed.

POLICIES AND PROCEDURES

The policies and procedures of aged care organisations are aligned with regulations and legislation, and in the context of restrictive practices, the policies cover factors such as consent for the use of such practices, and the requirement that the least restrictive practice is used and that the person to whom the practice is applied is monitored to ensure their safety.

ETHICAL CONSIDERATIONS

The use of restrictive practices in aged care has ethical considerations. These practices must be used as an absolute last resort and only in the context of protecting the person or others from harm, due to their behaviour. It may be considered abuse when restrictive practices are used as a first line of intervention, rather than as the last.

The care worker must always work in alignment with the person's care plan, the Quality Care Standards, the Charter of Resident Rights, and the policies and procedures of the organisation to ensure they are meeting the legal and ethical requirements of their role (see Chapter 2).

ALTERNATIVE STRATEGIES

As a legislative requirement, all other strategies identified in the person's behaviour support plan must be implemented before a restrictive practice is applied. These strategies may include using diversion, talking to the person, removing known triggers for the person's behaviour, massage, or other activities that are known to de-escalate or avert a behaviour of concern.

DOCUMENTATION

Documentation of the use of restrictive practices is a legal requirement and may include completing an incident report, documentation of the incident in the person's notes, further behaviour assessments and care plan updates.

If any use of a restrictive practice is inappropriate, the incident may be reportable under the Serious Incident Response Scheme (SIRS).

WORKPLACE SCENARIO

Providing personal care for a person with dementia

Alice, who has dementia, has been living at the residential aged care facility for three months. She prefers a morning shower and usually requires some assistance from care workers to run the water and provide her with soap, a washer and towels. The care staff also lay out Alice's clothes on her bed in the order in which she will put them on. After her shower, Alice usually gets dressed independently; however, she needs help with fastening her bra.

This morning, Ze, one of the care workers, notes that Alice is just standing under the shower and appears not to know what to do. Ze provides assistance and helps her to shower. She notices that Alice passes urine in the shower that is dark in colour and smells offensive.

After her shower, Alice becomes distressed. She begins to shake and picks up her clothes and throws them across the room. Ze wonders if Alice has a urinary tract infection that has changed the usual way she does things and is affecting her behaviour. Ze picks up the clothes, and gently reassures Alice while she helps her to put on one item of clothing at a time. Alice appears to feel calmer and sits in her recliner to nap. Ze reports her concerns to the RN and Alice is referred to the doctor for review. Ze makes sure to document her observations in Alice's notes.

CHECK YOUR UNDERSTANDING

1. How might an older person feel when they participate in their own care, regardless of their ability?
2. Why is inclusive communication important?
3. List four examples of activities of daily living.
4. What type of equipment or assistive devices might be used to assist a person with their shower?
5. What are "restrictive practices"? Give one example.

6.3 MONITORING SUPPORT

The older person requires support that is based on their needs and preferences. Once their care plan has been developed, it will continue to change according to the person's needs. As time passes, the person may experience significant changes to their health and wellbeing, requiring modifications and changes to their support needs.

The care plan needs to be monitored to ensure the person is having their support needs met and that any transient changes in their condition are addressed. Monitoring the support that is provided to the person is an ongoing process and should occur formally on a regular basis as well as incidentally.

6.3.1 Maintaining high standards

As a care worker, you should aim to work in a legal and ethical manner at all times. Working in accordance with your duty of care and your code of conduct will support you to work professionally within your role.

Older people are reliant on care workers to support them with their personal needs and preferences in a way that upholds their rights, dignity and autonomy. Delivering high standards of care support provides the older person with confidence and promotes trust, facilitating a good rapport between the care worker and the older person.

Self-reflection is an effective way to ensure that you are maintaining high standards within your role as a care worker. Seeking feedback from others is also helpful for professional development. It is good practice to ask yourself what your strengths are as a care worker, as well as what areas of your role you can improve on.

6.3.2 Responding to situations of risk

When providing support to older people, the care worker may identify situations of risk to themself, the older person or others. All workplace policies and procedures must be followed in regard to risk assessment and managing situations of risk; however, not all risk is foreseeable. It is good practice to always have the mindset to expect the unexpected.

Situations of risk may include the following:

- The person becomes abusive towards you.
- A family member becomes angry towards you.
- Aggressive dogs aren't restrained when you visit the person's home.
- Equipment isn't appropriate to the task.
- The environment is poorly lit.
- You are exposed to infection or possible infection.

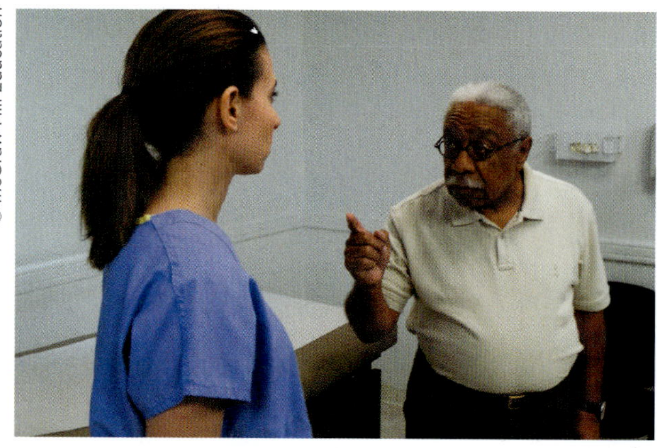

Confrontation is a situation of risk

Policies and procedures exist to ensure that legislation is followed and, ultimately, to minimise risk. The care worker will develop a risk-based mindset that supports the constant process of risk assessment in practice.

Always ensure your own safety when working and seek help in the event a situation becomes dangerous or threatens your safety or that of the older person or others.

6.3.3 Responding to unmet needs

During the process of providing support, the care worker is in the ideal position to recognise and report when a person's needs are not being met. Observations that indicate a change in the person's behaviour or functional abilities generally identify an unmet need. The person may tell the care worker when their needs are not being met; for example, they may state that they are having difficulty chewing their food because their dentures are loose. It is important to report these types of conversations to the RN or supervisor so the unmet need can be assessed and addressed in the person's care plan.

You may be involved in planned review meetings with the RN, the person, and their carer or family to discuss the person's care plan and to determine what is working well and what is not. The person should be encouraged to discuss openly any needs they feel are not being met and be supported to identify actions or strategies that could meet them.

The following observations may indicate unmet needs.

- A person who has dementia may appear to be visibly distressed, panicked or agitated. This may indicate an unmet need such as pain, hunger, thirst, discomfort (e.g. feeling hot or cold), wanting to use the toilet, or anxiety that requires reassurance.
- A person may continually spill food from their plate while eating, indicating they may need an assistive device, such as a lip plate, to maintain their independence.
- When a person is unwell or injured, they may choose to remain in bed for longer periods of time. When reddened areas are observed on the person's heels, hips or other bony prominences, they have the unmet need for pressure injury prevention.

Many unmet needs can go unidentified, and it is most often the care worker who will make an observation about the person's support that requires interventions such as assessment and management. As a care worker, always report and document your concerns according to your workplace's policies and procedures.

6.3.4 Managing contingencies when providing personal care

Planning for the unexpected is also an important aspect of your role as a care worker. While the person's care plan contains valuable information to inform care workers how to support the person, it may not include information about what to do when things don't go to plan. In this case, you will need a contingency.

Workflow is important, due to the demands on the time of care workers and other health practitioners. A care worker who works within community in-home care will have multiple people to support during the day, so it is essential that they adhere to allocated time frames if they are to arrive at the next person's home on time. Staff who work in an RACF are also generally time poor, even though they work as teams to ensure that people who require support are provided quality support whenever they need it. When the workflow is disrupted, planning processes need to be revisited and prioritised.

Having a contingency plan means identifying alternative options when the original plan is disrupted. A contingency plan for providing support may be required when:

- there is a staff shortage
- temporary staff are not familiar with the work routine or the needs of the older person, requiring other staff to work differently to compensate
- the older person has a fall or a medical incident requiring changes to the workflow
- the person refuses support
- the person may be experiencing distressed behaviours that puts the care worker at risk of harm
- there is an outbreak of an infectious disease
- staff are injured while providing support
- equipment and assistive devices are broken or missing.

Contingency planning often needs to be done spontaneously. However, the RN or TL will provide care workers with help in planning and prioritising their workflow, in a way that supports inclusive communication with the people who use the service.

Depending on the incident, contingency planning may include:

- accessing extra staff, such as casual or agency staff
- postponing staff meetings to free up time
- rescheduling activities that are not urgent, such as scheduled staff education sessions
- postponing outings or in-house activities for the day.

As a care worker, you may find that the contingency you need is relevant to the individual support that you are providing to an older person. The person may refuse the support, and they have the right to do so; however, it is helpful if you can determine why as you may have a solution to their reason for refusing. In any case, you must document and report the person's refusal of services. If the person becomes aggressive or uncooperative, it is safer not to attempt the support and to report the incident to the RN or supervisor. People who have experienced behaviours of concern such as aggression will have a behaviour support plan as a component of their overall individualised plan. When people display these types of behaviours for the first time, it is important that the RN is informed. Sudden changes of behaviour may indicate a clinical issue such as infection, or the person may be feeling frustrated, angry or depressed.

PRACTICE POINT

A key indicator of depression in older people is their frequent refusal to participate in care activities such as showering, eating and being mobile. If you notice that an older person is refusing activities, report your observations to the RN or supervisor promptly. Depression often goes undiagnosed in older people.

6.3.5 Promoting self-determination and respecting privacy

An individual's self-motivation to be actively in control of the support services they receive can facilitate quality-of-life outcomes. Care workers can promote the self-determination of older people in many ways, and ultimately support their autonomy and individuality in all support activities.

The person is their own expert on their own needs and preferences. The care worker's job is to support people in meeting their needs in the least intrusive way and to ensure the care they receive is person centred and strengths based. Encouraging the person to participate in their support is important for maintaining their independence and for respecting their rights to autonomy and to privacy.

Privacy is a basic right that we can take for granted until we don't have access to it. Always be mindful of the person's right to privacy when supporting them with personal care. Examples of respecting privacy include:

- closing the door when assisting the person to bathe, shower, dress and undress
- ensuring the door is closed, or the room curtain is pulled closed, when attending perineal and incontinence care
- arranging for the person to eat their meal in the privacy of their own room if that is their preference
- ensuring the person isn't left sitting on the toilet with the door open
- not calling or yelling out when talking to the person about their care—for example, not calling out something like "Harry, have you done a wee yet?"
- not sharing information about the person without their consent and in alignment with policies and procedures surrounding privacy and confidentiality.

Remember that the person is using their money, or their funding, to be provided with a service that supports their needs and preferences. Care workers and other staff don't have the right to tell people how to live their lives or what they should do. Our job is to provide support in a way that is respectful to and empowering for the person.

WORKPLACE SCENARIO

Monitoring and reflecting on your own work

Liza is a care worker who works for a community organisation that provides personal care to older people in their own homes. Last week, she was helping Mrs Lantry with her shower when she heard her work mobile phone ringing from her workbag in another room. Liza thought it must be important, so she asked Mrs Lantry to quickly sit on the shower chair while she answered the phone.

While Liza was walking back to the bathroom after answering her phone, she saw Mrs Lantry stand up and slip over, hitting her shoulder on the tiled floor.

Liza is thankful that Mrs Lantry wasn't seriously hurt, and she feels bad about putting her at risk. She realises now that she should have let the phone go to voicemail, where she could have checked it later when Mrs Lantry was safely showered, dressed and sitting in her armchair. She also appreciates better now how something that is potentially very dangerous can happen so quickly. Liza has decided that she will never again put at risk any of the people she supports.

CHECK YOUR UNDERSTANDING

1. Why is self-reflection good for professional development?
2. What are two examples of a situation of risk that a care worker may be exposed to?
3. What are three ways to respect the person's privacy when providing support?

6.4 PREPARING DOCUMENTATION

Documentation is a legal requirement for aged care organisations that provide services that are subsidised by the government. Documentation provides information that can be applied to a continuum of care and support regarding the needs and preferences of the person receiving services and can be used in many formats and contexts.

6.4.1 Ongoing assessment and observation

Documentation can be used in ongoing assessments and observations when the person has needs and preferences that require monitoring. Ongoing assessment can provide valuable information about the person's needs and help to identify if support strategies are adequate or if new strategies need to be developed. The person, their carer and their family are all part of the consultation that surrounds the ongoing assessment processes. An example of ongoing assessment and observation that requires documentation is behaviour. When a person experiences behaviours of concern, the care worker may be required to observe and monitor the behaviour and document their observations on behaviour charts. The chart can provide information that suggests a pattern of behaviour that may also identify possible triggers for it.

Documentation relating to ongoing assessment and observation may include:

- developing the person's care plan using documentation on validated assessment tools
- monitoring the person's care plan that requires ongoing assessment or reassessment
- using documentation for assessment purposes that are related to funding
- documenting referral letters and medical reports that are relevant to ongoing assessment processes.

It is good practice to document with integrity and to ensure that the content of any documentation is objective–meaning it is factual.

6.4.2 Personal care support: recording and reporting

During the provision of personal care support, the care worker may be required to record and report information that is relevant to the person's needs. The types of record-keeping and reporting processes that occur often are those that are relevant to the ongoing care of the person. They can serve as part of a monitoring process or they can identify an unmet need that requires further investigation and assessment.

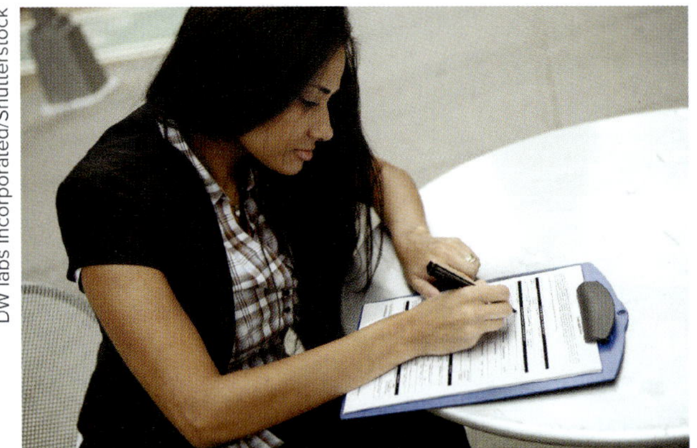
DW labs Incorporated/Shutterstock

Always ensure that your documentation is clear, current and factual

As a care worker, you will be required to use documentation every time you go to work. It may include recording information such as charting bowel activity on a bowel chart, documenting food and fluid intake on a fluid balance chart, completing incident reports and writing progress notes.

All forms of documentation that are relevant to service provision for older people are considered legal documents and can be used in a court of law. Always be sure that your documentation is clear, current and factual.

6.4.3 Confidentiality

As has been mentioned in other chapters, all care workers are bound by legal and ethical requirements to maintain the privacy and confidentiality of the person's information. Written information must be managed according to the privacy laws of Australia and the workplace.

Care workers are in a position of trust and privilege in the context of knowing the person's private and personal information. They must never breach the duty of care requirements of their position by failing to maintain the confidentiality of that information.

6.4.4 Organisational policies

In the context of documentation, organisational policies and procedures are the workplace documents that provide workers with legal and ethical information that enables them to:

- safely store documentation by using a digital passcode when documenting electronically or by ensuring that paper-based documentation is locked away
- determine which documentation is used for particular purposes, such as tasks, assessments or incidents

- adhere to specific documentation processes and requirements for reporting under the SIRS
- follow guidelines for documenting in-progress notes
- disclose requirements around documentation.

Always refer to the policies and procedures of the workplace for clarification of the documentation requirements for the specific issue at hand. Specific documents may be required for particular procedures. For example, the procedure for supporting a person after a fall may instruct the worker to complete an incident report to document the circumstances surrounding the fall and what observations may need to be recorded if the person hit their head during the fall. Policies provide valuable information to all staff relevant to both their day-to-day work expectations and to those things that are unexpected.

WORKPLACE SCENARIO

Observing and assessing the person in your care

Noah and Emma are working as a pair in the residential aged care facility. They have 12 people to provide personal support to during their morning shift. They also have responsibilities to document in the progress notes for the people in their care who require support.

Mid-morning, Noah looks at Emma's earlier observation about Mrs Koll's behaviour in her behaviour chart.

"You have documented that Mrs Koll was disruptive and pacing the hallway during the first part of our shift, but I know she was still napping in her chair at that time," he says.

Emma responds that she wasn't sure what she had to write. "I just wrote what other staff have been writing. I didn't want to write something that would make me look stupid."

Noah explains to Emma the importance of accurate and factual documentation. "Falsifying notes can have serious legal consequences", he says. "Not to mention consequences for Mrs Koll!"

He suggests that they talk to their TL about Emma having some training to ensure she understands the purpose of behaviour charts and how to document her observations in them correctly.

CHECK YOUR UNDERSTANDING

1. What are three types of documentation that may be relevant to ongoing assessment and observation?
2. Why are reporting and recording important in personal care support?
3. Why is it important to maintain confidentiality of the person's information?
4. Which workplace documents provide workers with legal and ethical information?
5. Give three examples of workplace policies and procedures that are relevant to documentation.

SUMMARY

- The older person is their own expert and is actively involved in developing their individualised plan to identify their needs and preferences. The person may choose to involve their carer or family in the development of their plan.
- Key concepts of providing support include empowering the older person to participate in their care and promoting dignity of choice and autonomy. Care workers aim to enable, not disable.
- Providing support to older people involves supporting them to remain as independent as possible while assisting them with identified activities of daily living, including personal hygiene. The care plan provides information for care workers regarding how to provide the support the person needs according to their preferences.
- Legal and ethical considerations must always be applied in practice when providing support. A risk-based approach to working will ensure that the risk of harm to the person, to staff and to others is minimised.
- It is important for care workers to observe, report and document any concerns they have about the person's support, as this may identify any of their needs that are not being met. This, in turn, will enable the person to have access to the assessment and communication processes that are required to ensure their needs are met.

REVIEW QUESTIONS

6.1 List three principles that underpin individualised planning.

6.2 Outline the role of the care worker when providing care.

6.3 List four factors to consider when providing support.

6.4 **(a)** Outline the importance of maximising a person's participation in personal care.

(b) Identify ways in which you can maximise a person's participation in personal care.

BIBLIOGRAPHY

Bellekom, S., *Submission to the Royal Commission into Aged Care Quality and Safety*, Ear Science Institute Australia, https://agedcare.royalcommission.gov.au/system/files/2021-01/AWF.001.05519.01.pdf, accessed 22 January 2022.

Hirshkowitz, M. et al., *National Sleep Foundation's Sleep Time Duration Recommendations: Methodology and Results Summary*, 2015, https://pubmed.ncbi.nlm.nih.gov/29073412/, accessed 15 January 2022.

Savvas, S., Dang, C., Peck, A., Vaughan, M. & Scherer, S., *Pain Management Guide (PMG) Toolkit for Aged Care,* 2nd edition, 2021, Melbourne: National Ageing Research Institute, and Sydney: Australian Pain Society.

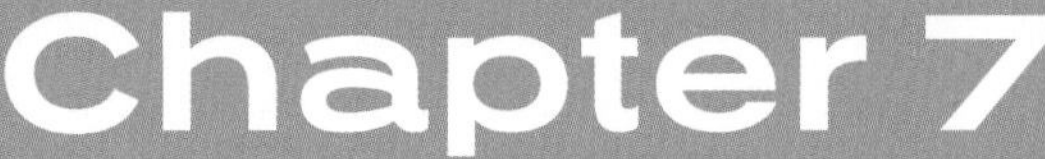

Chapter 7

Promoting choice and self-determination

LEARNING OBJECTIVES

7.1 Empower people who require support

7.2 Promote human rights

7.3 Facilitate choice and self-determination

INTRODUCTION

OLDER PEOPLE WHO USE AGED CARE SERVICES are unique individuals with their own life story. As individuals, older people have the same human rights as everyone else and all interactions with older people, within the role of care worker, should reflect the **rights-based approach** to service delivery. We are our own expert on ourselves, and age doesn't change this. The person-centred philosophy of providing aged care services always places the older person at the centre of decision making and the development of care strategies that promote the rights of the person. The empowerment of older people supports the principles of autonomy and self-determination, and care workers can facilitate the empowerment of older people by following the person's individualised plan and by employing person-centred communication skills.

INDUSTRY IN FOCUS

Consumer-directed care

Consumer-directed care (CDC) is a model of care that was introduced to community aged care services around 2015. The model focuses on the principle of autonomy and empowerment by facilitating choice for the service user.

Under CDC, the person who is eligible for a government-subsidised home care package can select what organisation will provide their services and how they will be provided. This ensures that aged care services are transparent in their approach to offering home care package management for older people. It also ensures the older person is making the decisions about how their allocated funding is used.

The principles of CDC are:

1. The person has the right to exercise choice in the services they receive.
2. The person's rights are respected.
3. The person works with the service provider in a way that is respectful and balanced.
4. The person has the right to participate in the development and implementation of services as much or as little as they choose.
5. Wellness and reablement are a focus of service provision.
6. The person has full knowledge of how their funding is used, in alignment with full transparency from the provider.

The legislative framework that supports CDC includes the User Rights Principles 2014 and the Charter of Care Recipient's Rights and Responsibilities—Homecare (the Charter). As part of CDC, providers help the person to determine how their funding is spent by providing a budget for the person that will assist them to make their choices. Each person who is funded for a home care package will also receive a monthly statement of how their funding is being used.

All providers of home care packages provide support to the person in deciding on and setting goals that can be achieved using the allocated funding. The goal is for providers to work with the person to determine how the person's needs and preferences can be met from the sum they are allocated.

CDC is a model of care that is predominantly used in community aged care services or in-home care. The philosophy of this model is incorporated into residential aged care facilities in the way some services are offered. This may include offering the individual flexible dining times rather than set times, flexible activities, and individualised plans that are directed by the older person or their family. CDC will take time to evolve in the residential aged care system as it will require a move away from traditional approaches to care that are driven by routines and tasks, and the needs of the organisation, towards support for the dignity, autonomy and independence of people in care and their individual preferences.

The aged care sector in Australia is undergoing major changes that are based on the expectations of older people and society in general. Aged care services today are embracing the rights-based approach to delivering services that are reflective of the person's autonomy and individuality. The person-centred philosophy is essential in order to meet the rich diversity of our ageing population.

7.1 EMPOWERING PEOPLE WHO REQUIRE SUPPORT

To be able to respond to the needs, goals and aspirations of older people, it is essential to provide the individual with the "process of taking control and responsibility for actions that have the intent and potential to lead to fulfilment of capacity" (WHO 2010). This is also known as **empowerment** and plays a key role in **holistic** person-centred care.

Empowerment can be achieved by expanding the knowledge and skill base of those supporting the person in care. Care workers and health-care professionals have a legal and ethical role and responsibility to provide information and to ensure that a person receiving care isn't denied their rights.

When practising person-centred and consumer-directed care, **autonomy** becomes a key principle. It is through autonomy that rights, risks and responsibilities become balanced, and a person becomes enabled to act on their own values, interests and choices. Autonomy allows for individualism and uniqueness, and for a person to optimise their power and decision making. Autonomy also allows for an individual to practise independence and for individual strengths and abilities to be maximised. An older person's independence can be promoted and encouraged through day-to-day care, and this supports the individual to be in control of how their needs and preferences are met, rather than be influenced by the decisions of others.

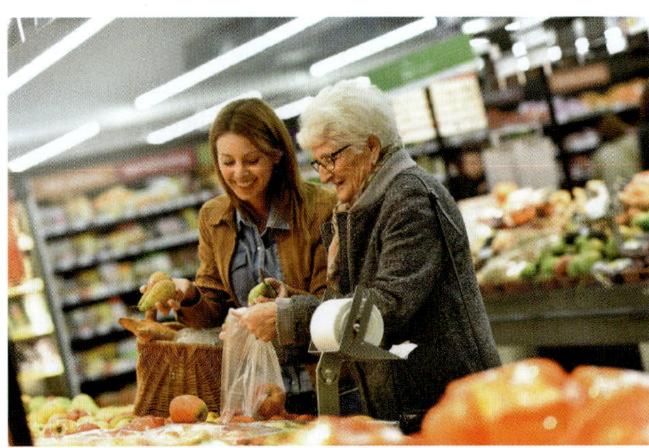

goodluz/Shutterstock

Older people should feel empowered to make choices and decisions that meet their own needs and desires

The concept of **self-determination**, whereby an individual determines their own choices and behaviours without direct influence of others, aligns with the concept of autonomy. These concepts ultimately empower the person to exercise their rights and capacity to make choices and decisions that meet their own individual needs and desires. The capacity of an older person to make decisions and to understand the potential consequences of those decisions can be affected by cognitive decline caused by illness, disease or injury to the brain. A health professional such as a doctor or a psychiatrist can assess an individual's capacity for making safe decisions. Capacity also means having the ability to understand and interpret information and to make decisions based on that information without influence or coercion from another. People with changes to cognition will have another person such as a carer or family member to assist with decision making, and some people will have an appointed public guardian to make decisions on their behalf.

7.1.1 The impact of personal values and attitudes on providing support

Our own values and attitudes will be different from those of the older people we are providing care and support to. It is extremely important that we don't impose our beliefs on them or use our beliefs to coerce the person into thinking or behaving in a certain way.

If conflict arises between the care worker and the older person receiving services, the care worker should examine their own values and attitudes to determine if they are having an impact on the relationship. Values are subjective and vary between people and cultures; in many ways, they are aligned with beliefs and belief systems. Personal values develop very early in life and are often derived from groups or systems such as cultural and religious groups and political party associations. A person's family, nation, and general and historical environments all help to influence their personal values. Each one of us has values that influence our thoughts, feelings and actions.

Our life experiences also influence how we view the world, and the views of others can clash with our own. As a care worker, it is important that you keep your personal views, values and beliefs to yourself, and it is essential to seek advice from your manager in the event you are unable to work in a situation that challenges your wellbeing.

7.1.2 Concepts relating to empowerment

SOCIAL JUSTICE

Social justice is closely linked to human rights and is the opposite of discrimination. It can be described as fairness within society and includes the concept that all individuals have access to social justice based on the principles of rights, access, equity, participation and inclusion. Examples of social justice include access to housing, employment and health care. Older people have the same right to social justice as any other age group and should not be discriminated against based on age alone.

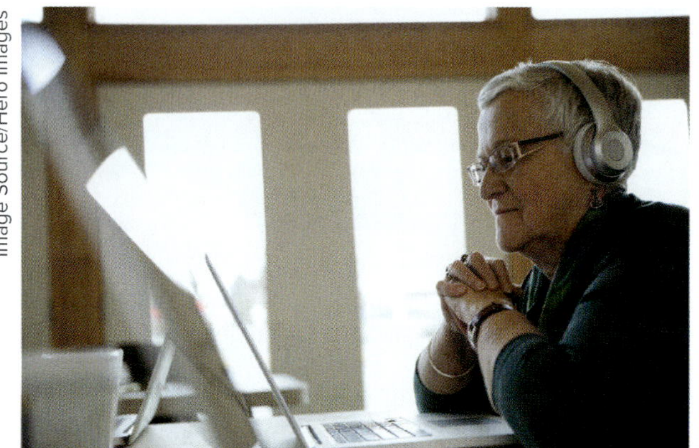

Image Source/Hero Images

Older people should always be supported to live their best life

AUTONOMY

In the context of aged care services, the word "autonomy" means to self-govern or to have control over one's care services. Autonomy is the foundation of independence and individuality. Care workers can support the person's autonomy by promoting the concepts of self-determination, empowerment and the strengths-based approach during interactions with the person and their family.

SELF-DETERMINATION

Self-determination is a concept that supports a person's autonomy and individuality. Older people should always be supported to live their best life by making their own decisions about how their needs and preferences can be met, and by setting goals that support their wellbeing. As a care worker, you can support self-determination by putting the strengths-based philosophy into action. You can do this by supporting the person to do what they can without taking over, and by supporting them with aspects of care services they cannot do independently. Self-determination is a concept that is important in all aspects of aged care service delivery; however, it is also regarded as a positive practice when working with people who have dementia.

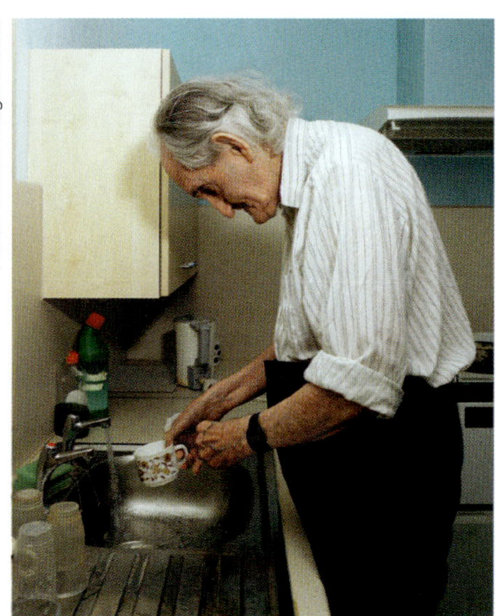

Haris Artemis/Image Source

Independent older adults can complete activities with little or no assistance from others

INDEPENDENCE

Being independent is about being able to initiate, perform and complete activities with little or no assistance from another. The level of independence someone has is influenced by factors such as their physical, cognitive, environmental, social and financial abilities. In the context of aged care, physical independence refers to the ability of someone to physically perform activities of daily living (ADLs) such as moving, eating, drinking, showering, dressing and grooming. This includes being able to plan, choose and coordinate appropriate clothing and grooming for any given situation. Choosing and coordinating forms part of the cognitive ability to be independent, along with decision making and risk taking.

CAPACITY

In the context of supporting older people, capacity can be described as physical capacity and cognitive capacity. The term "physical capacity" refers to the physical capabilities of an individual to attend to their physical needs and ADLs. The ageing process, chronic disease and pain are examples of factors that can affect physical capacity. "Cognitive capacity" refers to the ability of a person to process information and to make an informed decision based on their understanding of that information. The person has capacity when they are able to understand the possible consequences of the decision-making process. People with dementia and other conditions that affect cognition will have reduced capacity and may require a substitute decision maker. Changes to physical and cognitive capacity can be temporary, transient or permanent.

QUALITY OF LIFE

As we are all individuals, the definition of quality of life is difficult to determine. People decide what quality of life means to them based on their values, beliefs and personal expectations. Beliefs that have been influenced by culture, family and life experiences can define what each of us believes is a good life.

Care workers can support the quality of life of older people by ensuring they have an understanding of the person and of what is important to them. Sometimes, a person has their wishes documented to ensure their quality of life is recognised in the event they don't have a voice, such as in dementia or stroke and at end of life. The person's wishes must be respected, even if they don't align with the care worker's beliefs about what quality of life means to them.

ENABLEMENT AND REABLEMENT

Enablement and reablement are approaches that are specific to encouraging independence by focusing on the ability or capacity of an older person to improve, gain or regain abilities by focusing on what they want to be able to do and what they can do.

Enablement focuses on providing a person with adequate authority, means, opportunity and resources to make decisions and choices, and to take actions, that will enhance their life. Enabling is an ongoing and ever-changing process when caring for the older person and encouraging their independence. For example, if the person has a weakened grip due to a stroke and cannot hold a spoon, providing them with modified cutlery so they can continue to eat independently rather than be fed by a care worker is enabling independence.

Reablement focuses on returning one's capabilities to the usual state after a period of illness, disability or change in lifestyle. Reablement, just like enablement, focuses on all areas of physical, cognitive, social, cultural and financial ability. For example, if the person returns home from an extended stay at their son's house and finds they now have difficulty preparing their own meals, which they didn't have to do while staying with family, the care worker can support them with meal planning and preparation, gradually withdrawing that support as the person feels more confident to do this independently.

Working with an older person to identify physical, cognitive, social, cultural and financial enablers and disablers that are impacting on their health outcomes and quality of life is key to the success of encouraging independence and holistic person-centred and consumer-directed care.

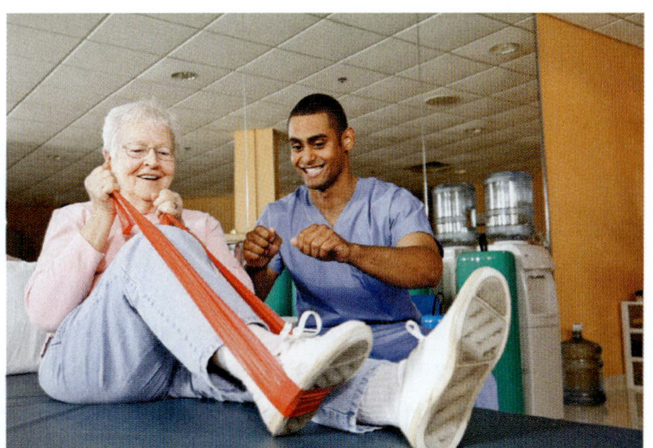

Getty Images/E+/kali9

Reablement encourages independence by helping the older person to gradually regain their capabilities

PRACTICE POINT

At all times, it is essential to minimise risk of harm to the older person, your colleagues and yourself. When providing support that is designed to enable or reable an older person to increase their independence, be sure to work in alignment with the person's individualised plan.

Sometimes changes to the plan aren't documented in a timely manner, such as when the person returns from a hospital admission. Their level of independence may have decreased during their time away, and they may need more support with some activities. You may be the first person to recognise these changes.

This is the opportunity for reablement. Always refer your observations to the registered nurse (RN) or your supervisor and be confident in your observations about the person. The RN or other qualified personnel will determine if reablement is appropriate based on the person's individual needs.

7.1.3 Obstacles to empowerment

The environment in which a person lives as they age also influences the level and type of independence they have. If they reside in an environment such as an extended family home, their carers sometimes take over; even though they feel like they are helping the older person, unknowingly, they are limiting their independence. Likewise, if the older person is receiving care in a residential aged care facility (RACF), nurses, carers and visitors may unknowingly limit their independence by rushing activities and by making decisions before consulting the person. For example, they may lay out clothing for the person to wear for the day without asking them what they would like to wear.

Social and financial abilities overlap somewhat, as it is often a person's financial status that influences their ability to be social or to socialise. Social independence in aged care is often limited for the older person, as the activities in an aged care facility or service are organised into groups and schedules. However, with increased consumer-directed care we are seeing changes in this area, with persons in care being enabled to choose their own activities and set their own schedules.

Physical disability and chronic disease can also be a barrier to independence; however, the care worker should adopt a strengths-based and person-centred approach to service delivery to optimise the independence of the person. Another barrier to empowerment is language. Communication is essential for interacting with people, and strategies that support effective communication in the context of language barriers should be adopted according to the organisation's policy.

STEREOTYPING

Older people are often perceived by society as frail, useless and as no longer participating in the world but merely being onlookers. This stereotyping can be a barrier to the empowerment of older people, both individuals and collectively. Attitudes that misrepresent the individuality of older people can have a direct and negative impact on their self-esteem, sense of value and inclusivity, and overall mental health and wellbeing.

As a care worker, you can counteract this stereotype with attitudes that empower older people by infusing the principles of autonomy, dignity, respect and human rights into every interaction you have with the person.

7.1.4 Facilitating empowerment

It is the care worker's role to promote and encourage an older person to maintain their independence for as long as possible, as the benefits to the older person are many. They include promoting confidence, self-esteem and self-worth; increasing autonomy and accountability; promoting and maintaining physical abilities; and encouraging **inclusivity** within the community. An older person can experience feelings of fear, anxiety, frustration and worthlessness when their opportunities for independence are limited. Encouraging and promoting independence can contribute to building trust, rapport and a therapeutic relationship between the care worker and the older person.

This role of the care worker is pivotal. Their day-to-day recognition of an individual's uniqueness and particular abilities helps in designing and redesigning approaches to promoting that person's independence. Individuality is an important concept to consider when empowering the person. We are all different, with different needs and preferences that require specific care and support interventions. Support practices will vary among people, due to many factors; for instance, people may have conditions that are genetic or linked to a disability, they may have experienced physical or psychological trauma, or they may live with a chronic disease or have experienced a brain injury. Needs are unique, and the strategies that care workers implement when providing support must be in alignment with the person's individualised plan.

People with cognitive decline have the same rights as those who do not. The principles of person-centred care, autonomy, dignity and self-determination are still relevant and appropriate to the person's care. Changes to cognition can occur due to injury, genetics, illness and disease, but cognitive changes do not mean that the person cannot be empowered.

Choices should always be offered in a way that doesn't overwhelm the person, and information is always provided in a simplified and understandable manner. Communication and dementia is discussed in Chapter 11. Duty of care and dignity of risk applies to supporting people with cognitive changes, and it is important to remember that people with cognitive changes may not have the capacity to understand the consequences of decisions they make. The person should be supported as an individual to meet their goals in a way that doesn't take from their sense of self and autonomy but doesn't put them in harm's way. The person's carer or family are often involved in decision-making processes where risk is evident.

Methods of encouraging independence are listed in Table 7.1.

TABLE 7.1 Encouraging independence

Method	Implementation
Introduce aids and assistive devices	Check the individualised plan for needs that require adaptive aids and equipment
Support the person to have and make choices	Consult the person when selecting clothing for the day, activities for the day, and food choices
Modify or adapt their physical environment	Provide the person with information about home modification processes and adapting their living space in a way that promotes independence, such as repositioning of furniture
Encourage their participation in service support	Verbally prompt the person's support and assist them but don't take over
Provide ample time for them to complete activities	The older person may require time to be independent with support activities
Focus on their abilities	Abilities facilitate independence
Communicate with the person	Communicate with the person and relevant people in a way that promotes the person's independence and autonomy
Recognise and acknowledge their independence	Verbal recognition or a compliment encourages self-satisfaction and a sense of achievement

WORKPLACE SCENARIO

Empowerment and cognitive decline

Omar is a care worker who provides home care services to 69-year-old Verity, who has early stages of dementia. Verity has lived alone since her wife died three years ago and she has no family. Verity has recently surrendered her driving licence, and Omar has noticed that she appears withdrawn and that her memory loss seems to have increased. Omar sits with her and asks how she is feeling. By the end of the conversation, he realises that Verity is feeling sad because she cannot visit her beloved wife's gravesite, as she had always done on Tuesdays, because she can no longer drive.

Omar discusses Verity's options for using other means of transport that would maintain her independence. Community transport is organised to collect Verity from her home every Tuesday at 9.30 am, drop her at the cemetery and return an hour later to take her back home.

Omar marks this on Verity's calendar and sets reminders for her every Monday when he visits. Soon, he notices that Verity appears to be happier and more talkative since being empowered to maintain her routine.

CHECK YOUR UNDERSTANDING

1. Why is autonomy important for older people receiving aged care services?
2. What should a care worker do if their own values and beliefs clash with those of the person they are supporting?
3. Explain the terms "physical capacity" and "cognitive capacity" in the context of aged care services.
4. Explain the terms "enablement" and "reablement".
5. List three barriers, or obstacles, to empowerment.

7.2 PROMOTING HUMAN RIGHTS

The rights of older people, and how to support these rights, are core to the *Aged Care Act 1997* (Cth) and its principles. The aged care sector works continuously to uphold, respect and protect the older person's rights by undergoing processes such as accreditation, audits and inspections and by participating in reforms. The regulatory framework that exists in the aged care sector is rigorous, and compliance with regulation is heavily focused on the rights of the older person using the services.

7.2.1 Human rights

Under Australian law, every individual has basic universal human rights regardless of their age, gender, race, sexual orientation, religion, ethnicity or financial status. These rights include and are aligned with those declared by the United Nations in 1948 and shown in Table 7.2.

7.2.2 The rights of an older person

The Aged Care Quality and Safety Commission (the Commission) is part of the Australian Department of Health and Aged Care's portfolio. The Commission functions to protect, enhance and improve the safety,

TABLE 7.2 Basic universal human rights

Human right	Explanation
Dignity	The right to be treated with dignity, without being subjected to humiliating, devaluing or derogatory behaviour
Equality	The right to be treated fairly and equally regardless of age, gender, ethnicity, religion, sexual orientation, cultural background, or past experiences and behaviours
Respect	The right to be treated with respect in all areas regardless of ability in physical, cognitive, social, psychological, cultural, spiritual, sexuality and financial arenas
Safety and security	The right to be and to feel safe and secure in one's own environment; the right to security afforded by policing and legislative mechanisms
Shelter and clothing	The right to access shelter and clothing at a satisfactory or minimum level
Food and water	The right to access food and water at a satisfactory or minimum level required for survival
Democracy	All people over 18 have the right to vote, and to vote according to their beliefs and values without undue pressure and influence
Freedom	The right to physical freedom (free of unnecessary confinement) and to freedom of speech
Privacy and confidentiality	The right to privacy and confidentiality (e.g. physical, financial, social, cultural, medical)

Source: Extracted from United Nations, *Universal Declaration of Human Rights* (1948).

health, wellbeing and quality of life of people receiving aged care. The functions of the Commission are aimed at ensuring that all aged care providers who receive government subsidies are legally and ethically compliant. The Commission currently independently accredits, assesses and monitors aged care services and the sector, conducts home care audits, and determines compliance requirements to be imposed on providers when breaches of compliance are evident (e.g. sanctions). The Commission also has the responsibility for approving providers to operate, for monitoring reportable incidents and for managing complaints. The Aged Care Quality Standards (the Quality Standards) developed by the Commission have the purpose of ensuring safe and quality aged care services that place the older person at the centre of decision making.

A right is an entitlement, and a responsibility is something a person has a duty to do. Older people have both rights and responsibilities. Older people who know about their rights will be more likely to recognise situations where their rights are at risk and to take action to ensure they are upheld. A number of legal and ethical frameworks outline the rights of people receiving aged care services. It is important that care workers are familiar with the policies and procedures of their organisation that support the rights of older people, so they can put them into practice in their workplace and recognise when the rights of the person are not being upheld.

Information about the older person's rights during care and receipt of aged care services can be found in:

- legislation relevant to aged care services, such as the Aged Care Act
- the Charter of Aged Care Rights
- industry and organisation service standards
- industry and organisation codes of practice and ethics
- the Aged Care Quality Standards
- codes of conduct
- international and national charters
- organisational policies and procedures.

The rights of people receiving aged care services include the right:

- to safety and not to be abused or neglected
- to receive care that promotes optimal physical, cognitive, social, psychological, cultural, spiritual and financial wellbeing
- not to be discriminated against on the basis of age, gender, race, colour, religion or cultural beliefs
- to freedom of speech, movement and association
- to equity and access to services that are afforded to all people
- to make decisions about and participate in all aspects of their life
- to access information about their care
- to make a complaint or raise an issue and to use the services of an advocate
- to privacy and confidentiality.

Another document that supports the rights of older people is the Charter of Aged Care Rights (the Charter), which replaced all other charters of aged care rights in July 2019. The Charter focuses on 14 core rights for all older persons receiving care or support regardless of subsidy or type of subsidised care. The aim of the Charter is to provide a clear, comprehensive, concise guide to expectations and standards of care.

There are specific situations where a right can legally be denied–for example, when a person is at risk to themselves or others. People living in an RACF with dementia may have restrictions placed on their freedom of movement to prevent wandering and entering other people's rooms. This denial of right in this situation aims to protect privacy and safety, not only of the individual but also of others.

7.2.3 Human rights and sociocultural identity

Everyone receiving care and support is an individual with their own background, history, life experiences, culture, religion and family. Every person will have a different medical history and care needs. No two people are the same. However, all persons have certain rights in common: the right to privacy, confidentiality, dignity, respect and quality care.

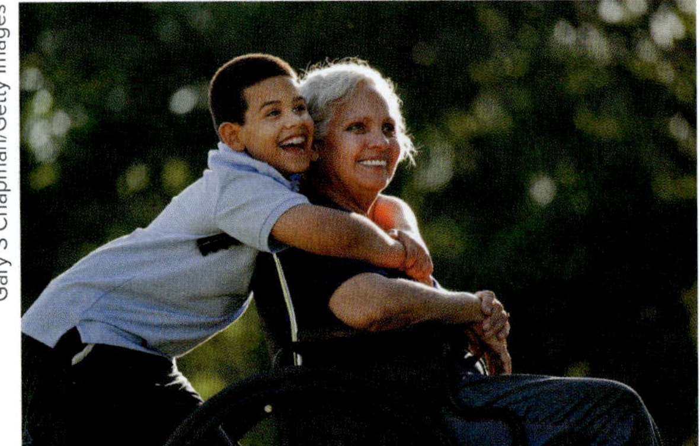

Gary S Chapman/Getty Images

Everyone has the right to receive quality care

At all times, it is the role of the care worker to uphold the rights of the older person, including the rights that are ingrained in a person's sociocultural identity. Sociocultural identity refers to shared beliefs and values such as religion, sexual identity, ethnicity and language. The uniqueness of individuals is the fabric of diversity and should be respected and acknowledged for the wellbeing of the person and of society in general. Diversity provides many benefits, including learning opportunities and personal connection and empowerment.

7.2.4 Abuse, neglect and empowerment

The alleged or actual abuse of an older person is an absolute violation of their rights and must be reported in line with organisational policies and procedures. Under the Serious Incident Response Scheme (SIRS), all aged care workers are mandatory reporters of suspected, alleged or actual incidents of abuse of older people. The SIRS is discussed in detail in Chapter 14.

The older person and their family can be empowered throughout the reporting process of the incident when they are provided with support and empathy, and when effective communication is used to provide appropriate information about the available options for the person regarding extra services that may be required or the processes that are involved in a criminal investigation.

7.2.5 Structural support for a person's rights

The Aged Care Quality and Safety Commission is the regulatory body that manages complaints from older people, and their advocates, who are receiving government-funded aged care services. Of the eight Quality Standards, Standard 6, "Feedback and Complaints", specifically focuses on the expectation that an organisation has a structured process in place that supports the person to make a complaint without fear of reprisal.

The Commission also focuses on open disclosure and continuous improvement as positive components of complaint resolution processes. Open disclosure is a process whereby the organisation manages complaints and incidents in a transparent manner and takes accountability. Working with the person, their carer and family, the organisation then makes genuine attempts to resolve the issue and learn from the outcomes. This will then develop into a continuous improvement process whereby new lessons are learnt, and even new practices emerge, from the original incident that was the basis of the complaint.

7.2.6 Advocacy services and complaints mechanisms

The care worker provides assistance to the older person to uphold their rights, within their scope of practice and in alignment with the workplace policies and procedures. This may include supporting a person, or their family, to make a complaint by providing information about the organisation's grievance process. It may also include providing information to the person about their rights or explaining that external services are available to provide advocacy services when necessary.

If the rights of older people are not upheld, a grievance policy and procedure should be followed. While procedures can vary slightly between providers, most grievance procedures include the following steps:

1. Speak directly to the person involved.
2. If the matter isn't resolved, report it to the RN or supervisor.
3. If the matter still isn't resolved, report it to a senior manager.

It is essential to ensure that the older person (or their advocate) is aware of the channels and mechanisms by which they can lodge a complaint, raise a concern or voice a potential conflict.

Older people, their carer and family may be required to access support for complaints that doesn't come from within the aged care service itself. External agencies and services include legal entities and advocacy organisations, such as the National Aged Care Advocacy Program (NACAP), which is provided by the Older Persons Advocacy Network (OPAN) across Australia.

TRAINING AND SKILLS DEVELOPMENT

Aged care organisations are aware of their legal and ethical obligations that surround the rights of older people who use their services. Part of the framework that organisations have in place to protect the rights of older people includes staff education and training. This ongoing education provides staff with knowledge of how they can uphold the rights of older people. This education and training includes, but is not limited to:

- specific policy and procedure focus sessions
- recognising and responding to abuse (compulsory reporting)
- the use of restrictive practices
- the Aged Care Quality Standards
- open disclosure
- incident management
- managing complaints.

Some education and training occurs every year, while other learning occurs according to the service's training schedule; or it may be opportunistic, such as when new legislation is introduced into the sector.

7.2.7 Breaches of human rights

When a person's rights are breached, the person may experience physical and psychological injury. All incidents that involve the breaching of the person's rights must be reported according to the organisation's policies and procedures, and in a timely manner. Examples of breaching an older person's rights within an aged care service may include:

- all incidents that are reportable under the SIRS
- inappropriate use of physical restraint, such as not following protocols regarding the use of physical restraint or using it as a convenience
- inappropriate use of chemical restraint, such as administering PRN antipsychotic medication without adequate clinical assessment to determine the need for such use
- withholding information from the person that is relevant to their wellbeing
- inappropriate disclosure of information about the person
- not reporting complaints that the person or their family may have
- not reporting health-related issues about the person to the appropriate person in a timely manner, such as failing to report that the person has had a fall.

All care workers have duty of care and mandatory reporting obligations that require breaches of the person's rights to be reported to the RN or supervisor, or other personnel or entity, according to policy.

WORKPLACE SCENARIO

A person's rights

Wilhelm and Martina are moving into residential aged care after their daughter, Johanna, moves interstate for work. They have lived with Johanna for some years and have decided that a move is necessary due to their increasing frailty and declining health.

When Wilhelm and Martina meet with Maria, the care manager, she provides them with information about their rights and responsibilities as "consumers" of the services provided by the facility. They discuss the various rights listed in the Charter of Aged Care Rights, and Wilhelm and Martina explain that they are particularly concerned about being treated with respect and maintaining their independence to the extent they are able. Maria reassures them that being treated with respect and promoting independence are fundamental to providing support. She also explains that the Charter works with their legal rights, as well as the Aged Care Quality Standards, and that they both have the right to live as they choose, even if their choices involve a degree of risk.

They discuss Wilhelm and Martina's responsibilities, which include:

- treating others with respect
- being aware of the care staff's safety
- sharing any information relevant to their care
- paying the agreed fees on time.

Maria gives them each a copy of the Charter, which she has signed. She explains that they have the option to sign it too and that this is in addition to their aged care agreement. She clarifies that they are not obligated to do so, but that by signing it they acknowledge they have each received it and understand their rights. Wilhelm and Martina sign the Charter and are given a copy. They tell Maria they will share this information with Johanna.

CHECK YOUR UNDERSTANDING

1. List four places, or resources, where information about the rights of older people can be found.
2. Which of the eight Aged Care Quality Standards supports the rights of older people to make a complaint about the services they receive?
3. What is the care worker's role in upholding the older person's rights in the context of making a complaint?
4. What are five examples of how an older person's rights may be breached while receiving aged care services?
5. In the event that a care worker observes that the older person's rights are breached, what action should they take?

7.3 FACILITATING CHOICE AND SELF-DETERMINATION

7.3.1 PROMOTING HEALTH

The aged care industry follows a philosophy of positive ageing. Ageing well involves the consideration of physical, cognitive, social, psychological, cultural, religious, spiritual and financial factors of each individual. An important component of positive ageing is supporting individuals to have healthy lifestyle practices. Care workers have a role to play in assisting and supporting the older person to adopt healthy lifestyle practices that are within the scope of their needs and preferences. All forms of encouragement must come from a space of genuine support for the older person, not from the values or beliefs of staff.

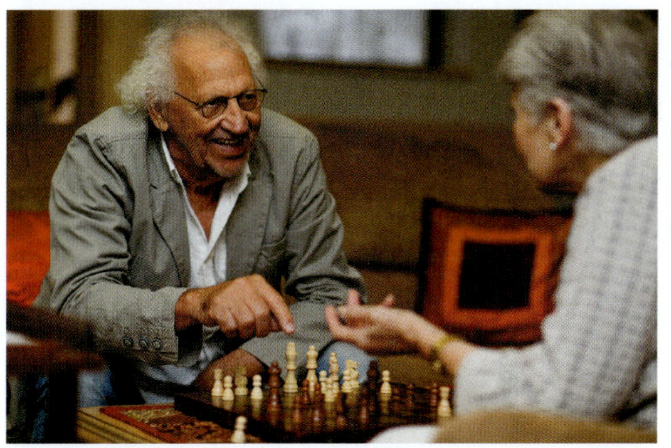

Westend61/Image Source

Care workers can support positive ageing by ensuring older people can attend activities in which they are interested

It is appropriate to follow a care plan that contains details of what the older person's interests are and how they will be supported. Care workers can support an older person's interests by:

- encouraging them to talk about their interests
- keeping them connected with other people who share similar interests
- ensuring they can attend relevant activities to pursue their interests.

A healthy and positive lifestyle that is characterised by choice and community inclusion can be facilitated by providing guidance in the form of current and accurate information that endorses healthy ageing. Older people can be supported to adopt strategies for healthy lifestyle practices, and this increases the likelihood of the person having not only good physical health but also a happier, more fulfilling lifestyle.

7.3.2 Duty of care and dignity of risk

Although the older person has the right to make choices and to take risks for themselves, the duty of care a care worker has is to ensure that the older person is fully informed and empowered to make such choices and to have dignity of risk assured. *Duty of care* refers to the care worker's legal obligation to do everything practicable to prevent foreseeable harm to those they provide aged care services to, and to their colleagues. *Dignity of risk* refers to the legal right of every person, including those with a disability, to make choices and take risks to learn, grow and have increased quality of life despite another person, such as a carer, support worker or family member, considering it harmful or detrimental in some way.

Care workers must balance duty of care obligations and the dignity of risk rights of the older person. Duty of care and dignity of risk are discussed further in Chapter 2.

7.3.3 Assistive technologies that promote autonomy and independence

Assistive technology supports autonomy and facilitates independence for older people. When technology is integrated into service provision, it can support self-determination. Assessing, planning, consulting, collaborating and implementing are all key to promoting and supporting independence. The digital world can support independence by providing information to an older person that empowers them as individuals. Access to the internet opens many learning and creative opportunities for the person to improve their physical and mental wellbeing, and their overall quality of life, according to the individual's viewpoint.

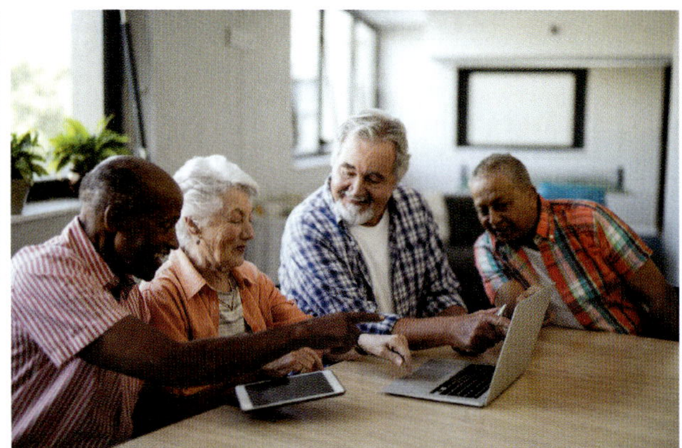

wavebreakmedia/Shutterstock

The digital world can support independence

Any consideration of introducing assistive technology into the person's life should be made after consulting with the person and the care team regarding the individual's needs and preferences. Factors that must be considered include appropriateness, safety, cost, policies and procedures, and the wellbeing of the person on a physical, cognitive, social and cultural level.

Assistive technologies that assist with autonomy and independence are also covered in Chapter 6.

WORKPLACE SCENARIO

When facilitating individual choice conflicts with the needs of the group

It is movie night at the aged care facility and several residents gather with their snacks to watch the movie together. This group of people have joined each other for movie night every Friday night for the past several weeks. Tonight's movie is a love story and Harold isn't impressed. He complains loudly that he is sick of watching gushy movies and wants to watch an action movie instead. Some of the women look around in dismay and roll their eyes. Robina states that she hates action movies and wants to watch a thriller.

Liu is the care worker on shift. Sensing that it is going to be difficult to select a movie that will please everyone, she has an idea. She approaches the group and asks if anyone has ideas that could help the movie night be enjoyable for everyone. She explains that while everyone has the right to watch a movie of their choice, some compromise is necessary as the group genuinely enjoys each other's company.

The group begin chatting together and start laughing as they discuss the options. Finally, they decide they want to form a movie committee that will organise a fortnightly movie night that will be themed. They might even produce a monthly program, they say, so that people know what films are coming up.

Liu is impressed by the group's problem-solving abilities and congratulates them on their great idea.

CHECK YOUR UNDERSTANDING

1. List three factors of holistic health and wellbeing that are important for healthy ageing.
2. How can a care worker support an older person's interests?
3. What two important legal obligations must a care worker balance when providing support for the older person?
4. What are the benefits of using assistive technologies in service?
5. What factors should be considered when introducing assistive technologies into a person's life?

SUMMARY

- Care workers can promote the autonomy and self-determination of the older person by implementing the person-centred approach to care. The older person's individualised plan will guide the care worker on how they can empower the person.
- Human rights are entitlements that are extended to everyone, regardless of age. The rights of older people who receive aged care services are protected by legislation and regulations as governed by the Aged Care Quality and Safety Commission.
- Enablement and reablement are essential components of empowering older people to increase, maintain or regain their independence.
- The care worker has an important role in ensuring that any breach of the older person's rights is reported according to policy and procedures, and that the person is supported to make a complaint without fear of reprisal.

REVIEW QUESTIONS

7.1 **(a)** What concepts relate to empowerment?

(b) Choose three empowerment concepts and provide an example of each in a residential aged care context.

7.2 Why is empowerment important in aged care?

7.3 You observe a colleague using a sheet to tie a person in a chair. When you question your colleague, they respond: "It's so they don't get up and have a fall."

(a) What personal right is being breached by your colleague?

(b) What is tying a person in a chair an example of?

(c) After your colleague answers your question, what do you do?

BIBLIOGRAPHY

Australian Government, Department of Health, *Charter of Aged Care Rights* (information for providers), 2019, https://www.agedcarequality.gov.au/providers/provider-information, accessed 10 June 2020.

Australian Government, Department of Health, *Quality Standards*, 2019, https://www.agedcarequality.gov.au/providers/standards, accessed 10 June 2020.

Australian Government, Department of Health, *Aged Care Reforms and Reviews*, 28 February 2020, https://www.health.gov.au/health-topics/aged-care/aged-care-reforms-and-reviews, accessed 10 June 2020.

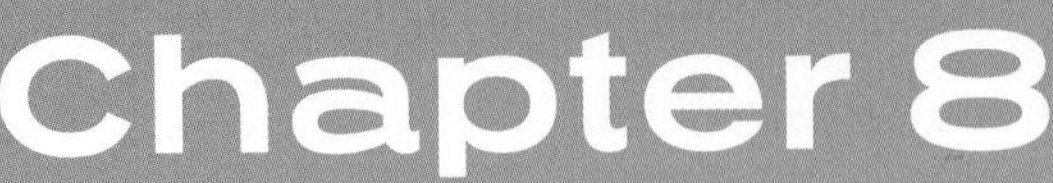

Chapter 8

Promoting independence and wellbeing

LEARNING OBJECTIVES

8.1 Understand ageing

8.2 Respect individual differences

8.3 Encourage independence

8.4 Promote physical wellbeing

8.5 Promote social, emotional and psychological wellbeing

INTRODUCTION

PEOPLE SEE THE WORLD from their own perspective, which is influenced by their society and culture, including life experiences and social connections. We are all individuals with our own unique needs, preferences, attitudes and beliefs, and all people—including older people—are the experts of their own life. Individuality develops and morphs throughout the life span, and older people continue to develop individuality as they age.

Every older person has the right to be respected as an individual and to be supported to maintain their autonomy over decisions that affect their lives. Care workers can support older people to live their lives the way they prefer by using approaches to service delivery that place the person at the centre of care decisions and facilitate philosophies of care that are person centred and strengths based. Providing services in a way that encourages self-participation can have a positive impact on the older person's sense of self and promote their optimal physical and emotional wellbeing.

INDUSTRY IN FOCUS

Support for expressions of identity and sexuality

Sexuality is an important component of wellbeing and remains so into old age. Society holds the view that older people are not sexy, and that they don't need sex and intimacy. These views culminate over time among generations and are influenced by media exposure such as advertising and film.

Older people are not asexual; in fact, intimacy and companionship are important factors in a healthy and positive ageing experience. However, it is difficult for older people who live in residential aged care facilities (RACFs) to express their identity and sexuality. Reasons for this may include a lack of privacy, judgemental attitudes of staff, inadequate knowledge of the needs of lesbian, gay, bisexual, transgender, questioning, intersex and asexual (**LGBTQIA+**) people and misunderstood intimacy needs of people with dementia.

The aged care industry and the government have developed and built upon various strategies and initiatives to support identity and sexuality for older people in aged care, including the LGBTI Ageing and Aged Care Strategy 2012–2017. This strategy was developed through a consultative process to determine the issues that older LGBTQIA+ older people experienced when navigating and using aged care services and later became part of the Aged Care Diversity Framework. Older people who identify as LGBTQIA+ now have a more inclusive experience as an aged care services consumer than before the strategy; however, cultural awareness and cultural competence are still evolving within the industry.

Sexuality among older residents of facilities can be acknowledged and supported with staff education and cultural training. Some organisations use a sexuality assessment to identify how the person can be supported to express their identity and meet their sexual needs. Many facilities now provide rooms for cohabitation or have procedures to support the person to have an overnight visitor. Many older people engage the services of a sex worker, either within their own home or within the facility they reside in.

Sexuality in aged care has become a topic of open discussion and recognition compared to even a decade ago. Older people are sexual beings, even if they have a life-limiting illness. Sexuality is a human trait that expresses identity, the need for intimacy and companionship, and contributes to wellbeing; however, sexuality and the elderly is a concept that needs to be normalised in society.

8.1 UNDERSTANDING AGEING

8.1.1 What is ageing?

Ageing is a natural process that occurs from the moment we are conceived and involves complex physiological processes within our bodies that are influenced by our genetics and our environments. Ageing affects people differently and there are many factors that contribute to how well a person will age. Many individuals remain independent and physically fit well into their later years; however, many people experience ageing in a way that can have a direct effect on their ability to live and function independently.

LIFE EXPECTANCY

"Life expectancy" is the term that refers to the period of years that an individual is expected to live. This can be different among different population groups and cultures. According to the Australian Bureau of Statistics (ABS), in Australia, as of 2021, the life expectancy for females is 85.3 years and for males is 81.2 years (ABS 2021). In 2017, life expectancy for Aboriginal and Torres Strait Islander people was 75.6 years for females and 71.6 years for males (AIHW 2020).

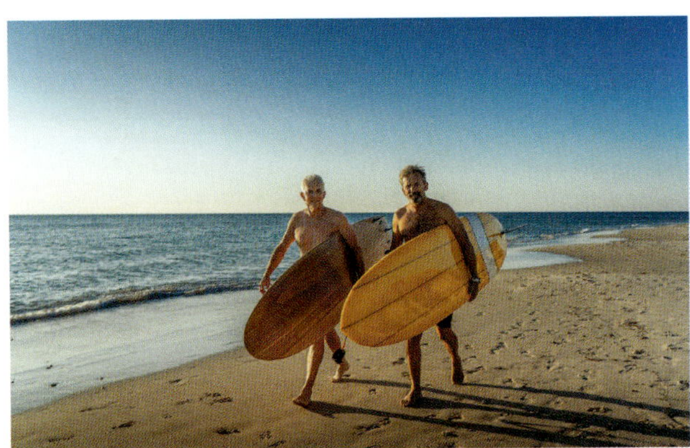

Sam Wordley/Shutterstock

Ageing affects people differently and many factors influence how well a person will age

CHRONOLOGICAL AGE AND HEALTH AGE

Age can be viewed in different contexts and a person's chronological age and health age can be two different experiences. "Chronological age" refers to an individual's age that is measured in years; for example, a person may be 58 years old according to their date of birth. "Health age" refers to an individual's state of health and wellbeing, and to their ability to participate in their life. Health age is impacted by lifestyle, illness, disability and chronic disease. For example, a person may be 58 years old but may be considered frail, like an 85-year-old, based on their physiological health and wellbeing.

Health domains include the physical, psychological, cultural, social, spiritual and sexual aspects of being human. Each domain has specific needs, and each domain is affected by ageing. Common issues of ageing can manifest across multiple domains; for example, a person with a psychological issue such as depression may experience physical issues as a result, such as consuming too much alcohol or overeating to feel better. The care worker may make observations about one or more issues about the person that fall into the health domains, and these observations should be reported to the registered nurse (RN) or supervisor. Changes and issues associated with ageing may be common, but they will be experienced by all people differently as individuals.

8.1.2 The ageing process

THEORIES OF AGEING

BIOLOGICAL THEORIES

Biological theories of ageing focus primarily on ageing processes that are based on physiological phenomena. While genetics is known to contribute to ageing, many scientists are researching different theories, or ideas, that may explain the ageing process in people. Some of these ideas include programmed theories that state humans have a biological timeline causing cellular and hormone changes within the body or that the immune system is programmed to deteriorate as we age, making us susceptible to infections and illnesses. There are many biological theories on ageing from around the world and many researchers are making interesting discoveries about our bodies.

PSYCHOSOCIAL THEORIES

Psychosocial theories of ageing are those that look at other areas of life that may contribute to the ageing process. These areas may include factors that relate to a person's mental health and social wellbeing, such as stress, social connection, determination and motivation. Some examples of psychosocial theories on ageing include the disengagement theory, activity theory and continuity theory.

STEREOTYPING AND AGEISM

A **stereotype** is a view of a group based on assumptions. These groups are perceived to have specific traits and behaviours and are deemed to be different from the majority of society. Examples of stereotypes include thinking that people with a physical disability have below average intelligence, that all Aboriginal peoples have issues with alcohol, and that people who are homeless brought it upon themselves by not working hard enough to rent or own a house.

In Australia, older people are also stereotyped by society, and ageism is a common component of this stereotype. Ageism is a form of discrimination based on the chronological, or perceived health, age of an individual. All older people are grouped together under this umbrella of discrimination, and ageism can

TABLE 8.1 Common myths and facts about older people

Myth	Fact
Depression is normal in old age.	Depression isn't a normal part of ageing. Ageism can contribute to an older person developing depression.
Older people are **asexual**.	Older people are human, with a need for intimacy, comfort and sex. Ageing doesn't remove the libido.
Older people cannot learn new things.	Older people are absolutely capable of learning new things and of making new memories.
All older people are heterosexual.	Many older people identify as part of the LBGTQIA+ community.
Older people should not be allowed to drive.	The majority of older people drive well and without incident. Factors of ageing that may affect driving include reduced dexterity, vision and hearing issues, and slower reflexes. These changes are individual, and the need to give up driving is essentially based on individual needs.
Older people have nothing to offer to society.	A big myth! Older people have a wealth of knowledge and experience that supports their skills and abilities. Older people can provide incomparable mentorship to other workers.

occur anywhere in society, including in the workplace, in social gatherings or communities, in cultures and even in families. Stereotypes largely develop from the bias that is portrayed to people within society, and the media have played a huge role in creating ageist attitudes. Older people are often portrayed as frail and useless, and as not contributing to society, instead of as experienced and valued assets of the community. Table 8.1 describes some myths and facts about older people that are commonly believed in Australia.

Australia has legislation that exists to protect people from discrimination. It includes:

- *Age Discrimination Act 2004* (Cth) (people cannot be discriminated against on the basis of age)
- *Disability Discrimination Act 1992* (Cth) (supports the rights of people with disability)
- *Sex Discrimination Act 1984* (Cth) (people cannot be discriminated against based on gender or sexuality)
- *Racial Discrimination Act 1975* (Cth) (people cannot be discriminated against based on skin colour, race, ethnicity or culture).

Ageism continues to condone the stereotype of old age in society. Until we can all appreciate the value and integrity that older people bring to the community, older people will continue to be devalued and patronised in the final years of their story.

WORKPLACE SCENARIO

The problem with stereotyping

Les is a 78-year-old man who is supported to live independently at home with home care services. Before retirement, Les worked as a computer technician for a big corporation. Since then, he has continued to repair computers for people in his local community.

When care worker Lisa arrives to hang out the washing for Les, she finds him to be quiet and sad. When she asks him if he feels okay, he responds that he is past his "use by" date and should just sell up

(Continues)

and move into a residential facility. On further discussion, Lisa learns that Les tried to enrol in a course in computing technologies so that he could keep up with the latest changes. However, the person processing enrolments told him that numbers in the course were limited and that he should leave his place for a younger person who needed to find a job. Lisa is upset to hear this, and to see the effect the comment has had on Les, who loves repairing computers for the community and making social connections by helping others.

Lisa explains to Les that the person was completely out of line and that he has every right to enrol in the course. She explains his rights to Les, saying there are laws in place to prevent this sort of discrimination against older people.

Les agrees to take the matter further with the advocacy of the home care service and is soon happily studying the computer course and looking forward to putting his new skills to use.

CHECK YOUR UNDERSTANDING

1. List three of the health domains that can be affected by ageing.
2. What is a stereotype?
3. What is ageism?
4. Many people feel that older people have nothing to offer to society. Why is this belief incorrect?
5. Which antidiscrimination legislation prevents discrimination against individuals based on age?

8.2 RESPECTING INDIVIDUAL DIFFERENCES

8.2.1 Philosophies of aged care

The key philosophy that guides aged care services is the person-centred approach. Put simply, this approach places the older person and their carer and family at the centre of decision making about their services. The person is consulted in a way that respects that they are their own experts, and that they know best what their needs and preferences are. The multidisciplinary team will work with the person and their carer or family to develop appropriate planning of services that ensure their needs are met. The person is continually consulted throughout the planning and delivery of services and is the driving force of managing their own care services.

The person-centred approach is manifested in other principles and philosophies of aged care service delivery, including consumer-directed care, the strengths-based approach to care service delivery and the rights-based approach to service delivery.

The entire philosophy of providing aged care services is aimed at promoting the dignity and autonomy of the person receiving the services. It is not intended to disable the person by taking away their abilities and independence, but rather to enable and re-able them to remain as independent as possible for as long as possible by utilising their strengths and abilities.

MODELS OF AGED CARE

Models of aged care relate to the way aged care services are delivered, and models will be different depending on the needs of the older people who use them. The traditional settings and models for aged care service delivery in Australia are evolving and the future of aged care is focused on the individual needs and preferences of the person. For example, dementia care has traditionally been provided within an RACF with communal living areas and corridors lined with bedrooms. Some models are now reflecting the specific needs of people with dementia and focus on environments that are more personal and intimate, such as shared cottage residences. The more the world learns about the specific needs of aged care service recipients, the more the industry will transform to be user friendly and specific. Some models of care include:

- residential aged care facilities
- Commonwealth Home Support Programme
- small-scale domestic living
- dementia villages
- community-based shared living arrangements
- Montessori approach
- teaching nursing homes
- intergenerational communities.

8.2.2 Social trends

The aged care sector has changed significantly over the past several decades, driven by a combination of demographics, changing care needs, increased funding for community care and restructuring by service providers. The most important trends have been an increasing number of older Australians requiring care and an increasing emphasis on home care packages. Within aged care facilities, there is a greater proportion of residents in high-level care.

The philosophy of "ageing in place" is a key component of aged care services in Australia. Many aged care services are focused on providing services and support that optimise the independence and autonomy of older people as they get older. In-home care and support models strive to provide the necessary support that will enable the person to maintain the skills and abilities they have regarding activities of daily living (ADLs) and instrumental activities of daily living (IADLs), while ensuring the person is supported in areas of living that require assistance. This type of service delivery model provides opportunity for the older person to age at home, rather than gradually lose their functional abilities and become increasingly dependent on others, requiring admission to an RACF.

Access to financial assistance for aged care support depends on the type of help a person requires, the provider they choose, their financial situation and the services they currently receive. A person is expected to contribute to the cost of their care if they can afford to. The types of fees and costs payable depend on what type of care the person has been assessed as eligible for. People who use home care services are expected to contribute a small amount to the costs of the care package. Others who reside in RACFs are also required to contribute to services; however, these payment procedures are more complex, and contributions are variable based on multiple factors.

8.2.3 Individual differences

"Identity" is the term used to encompass all aspects of an individual that make them unique. Identity includes the person's likes and dislikes, their values and belief systems, their self-concept and self-esteem, their life experiences, and their influences. Identity is important because it validates our belief of who we are on a very personal level and explains how we see the world. Identity doesn't fade away as we age; in fact, identity evolves continually. Older people have had a long time to develop their identity, and part of a care worker's role is to preserve and respect the older person's preferences, including when those preferences change. Care of the older person involves more than the personal care routines of the ADLs. There needs to be a significant focus on supporting the older person to maintain a quality lifestyle.

Our values are principles or beliefs that serve as guidelines to help us make decisions about actions, behaviours and life choices. They reflect what we value and how we feel about the rightness or wrongness of things. Care workers must avoid imposing their own values and attitudes on older people, as this is both unethical and unsafe. Everyone has a right to their own values and attitudes. By imposing our own values on a person, we may make them feel judged or condemned. This could negatively impact on their self-esteem, and/or cause conflict or anger towards the staff member.

Individuality is expressed in many areas of the person's life:

- *Socially:* Many older people enjoy socialising with other people, while some older people prefer their own company or limited exposure to social events. People prefer to socialise with others who have similar values and beliefs, such as community groups. Social health includes interacting with others both informally and formally, and individual preferences must be respected. If an older person is forced to participate in a social event against their wishes, they may be exposed to anxiety and other negative emotions. Always ask the person what their preferences are with regards to events and interactions with others on any level.
- *Spiritually:* Religion and religious rituals are important for wellbeing; however, spirituality encompasses more than religion. Spirituality involves those aspects of a person's belief system that reflect how they identify with the concept of the human soul or spirit. This may be expressed with organised religious beliefs and practices such as baptism and prayer, or by individual beliefs and practices such as meditation and energy healing. Spirituality is deeply personal and should not be criticised, as it contributes to our identity.
- *Physically:* Our identity is expressed physically in many ways. Individuals express their uniqueness by:
    - the type of clothing and accessories they wear
    - tattoos and piercings
    - hair styles and colours
    - makeup and nails
    - beard and moustache styles.

  Older people may embrace the effects of ageing on their physical appearance, or they may struggle with the concept of the loss of their youthful appearance. Remember that our physical perception of ourselves plays a huge role in our emotional wellbeing, and this doesn't exclude older people. Always ensure the person is supported to meet their preferences and needs that support their physical identity.
- *Psychologically:* Individual differences occur on a psychological level because we are all exposed to different experiences and opportunities as we navigate life. Risk and protective factors of mental health play a role in shaping the way we think, and while some older people will have a strong sense of self, others may experience poor self-esteem and lack confidence due to a past **traumatic** experience that has left them with unique psychological needs and preferences. It is important to understand how you can encourage self-esteem for those you support. The first step in this is to understand the person's needs.
- *Sexually and through gender identity:* Sexual desires and needs don't disappear because we age. Sexual expression in older people carries with it a wide range of social prejudices, such as:
    - Older people are sexually unattractive. Sex is only for young people.
    - Women past menopause are not interested in sex.
    - Sex between older people is immoral.
    - Older men wishing to enjoy sex are just "dirty old men".

EyeEm/Alamy Stock Photo

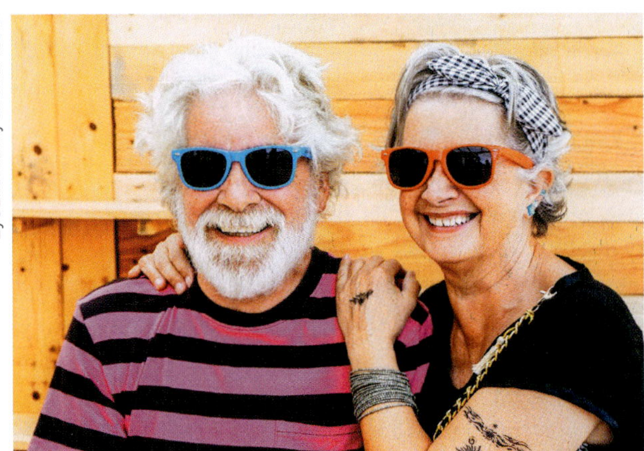

People's perception of themselves plays a huge role in their emotional wellbeing

Sexual relationships should be reciprocal, be based on respect, and should never be coercive or exploitative. All persons have the right and obligation to make responsible sexual choices.

Regardless of the care worker's attitudes towards sexuality, they must respect different expressions of sexuality, which can be diverse. A care worker must remember that older people need to have the opportunity for private conversations, emotional expression, sexual companionship and intimacy. Sexual needs are not just about sexual intercourse; they include warmth, love, touching and sharing between people.

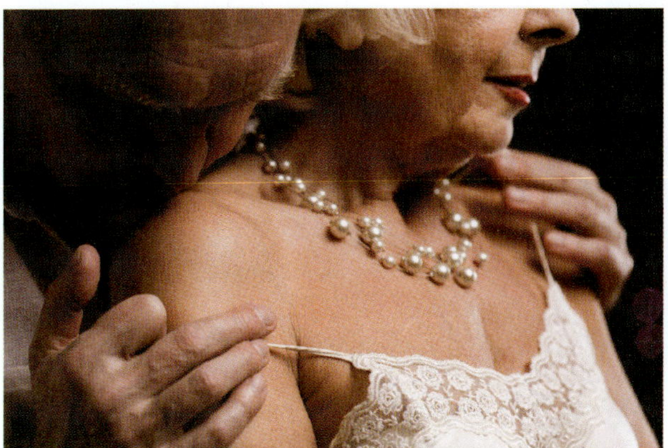
KatarzynaBialasiewicz/iStock/Getty Images Plus

Sexual desires and needs don't disappear as people age

Older people are increasingly being supported to express themselves sexually by acknowledging their right to such relationships and by providing encouragement and privacy for sexual expression. As a worker, to ensure privacy and dignity for a person, there is an expectation to knock and wait for an invitation to enter a person's room.

Historically, individual gender was biologically based as female, male or **intersex**; however, in today's society a range of gender identities exist that are not traditionally male or female. All gender identities of older people must be respected, regardless of the values and attitudes of care workers. Care workers who cannot support a person based on their own values and attitudes should seek a discussion with the organisation they work for to collaboratively look for a solution. The older person's wellbeing must not be compromised due to the opinions of service providers and employees.

- *Culturally:* Cultural sensitivity in aged care is particularly important. Within society, groups of people come together to interact because of shared interests, beliefs and values. We align culture to family groups, religious or spiritual affiliations, peer groups, race, gender, sexual orientation, age, nationality, etc. Within these groups, people learn behaviours and gain information that endorses their beliefs and ways to express their feelings. For many cultures, there is a predominant religion that is a principal element in the lives of those people.

All people should always be treated with respect, which includes an acceptance of their cultural and spiritual preferences. A care worker must also not assume that beliefs or values are the same for everyone. Many people tend to interpret the words and actions of others in terms of their own beliefs and cultural norms, and with the understanding that they are shared. As a care worker, find out what is important to the person, what values they hold and how they interact with their environment. Find out the needs of the person and work to address those needs.

8.2.4 Supporting individual differences

PERSONAL DEVELOPMENT

All people have needs that result from the layers of their individuality. Personal needs identify an area of the person's life that needs to be addressed for a goal to be achieved. For example, the person may have social needs that involve participating in the community to achieve the goal of having purpose and inclusion in their life. Having purpose and inclusivity can have a positive effect on wellbeing and be a protective factor for mental health.

When we discuss the needs of individuals, we can refer to Maslow's hierarchy of needs as a guide to identifying different types of needs (see Figure 8.1). The hierarchy defines the categories or levels of needs an individual has as they age and aspire to reach a point in their life where they have "self-actualised"—in other words, the person has become the best version of themselves. The basic level of needs is those that a person

FIGURE 8.1 Maslow's hierarchy of needs

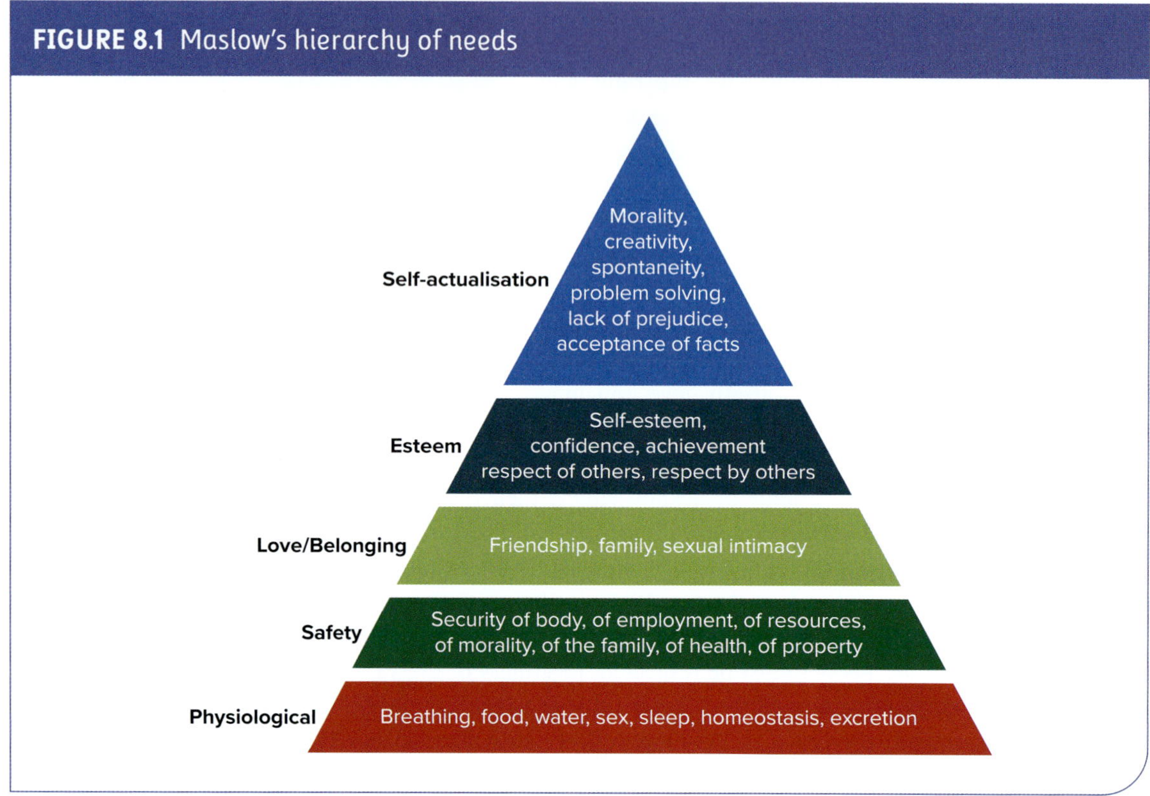

needs to maintain life, such as food and shelter, while other levels of the hierarchy define those needs that are seen as important for wellbeing.

We continue to have needs into old age. Although some older people require support to have needs met, the focus on providing support should be grounded in the empowerment and self-determination of the older person to meet their goals as independently as possible.

To deliver an appropriate service, a care worker needs to be able to assist the person to identify their own personal needs and has an ongoing duty of care to monitor if those needs are being met. If the person's needs have changed, the care worker should inform the RN or supervisor.

NEEDS AND PREFERENCES

Part of planning services into a care plan is to identify the needs and preferences of the older person. The person, and their carer or family, is pivotal in determining their needs and setting goals for care service delivery. The person's self-determination and sense of autonomy must be promoted at every opportunity when developing a care plan. It is essential that interventions and care strategies don't detract from the person's abilities and strengths; however, their needs must be met in a way that can empower them to remain as independent as possible for as long as possible.

When identifying the needs of the older person, it is important for a care worker to consider the diversity of people in late adulthood and to go beyond chronological age and examine whether a person is experiencing optimal ageing, normal ageing (in which the changes are similar to most of those of the same age), or impaired ageing (referring to someone who has more physical challenge and disease than others of the same age).

While a person's key capabilities may diminish as they age, it is important for the care worker to acknowledge that the person is generally still capable of making decisions and choices. These can be about simple day-to-day matters and/or more complex life decisions. Taking responsibility for making one's own decisions is a major area of risk that we face in our lives; so, when we discuss people who are ageing taking risks, we also mean the risk of choice and decision making. All decisions, simple or complex, are important. The right to make decisions and choices can affect an individual's quality of life. For example, what would it mean to a person's wellbeing if a care worker always decided on how the person spent their time, the places they went and with whom they socialised?

The degree and nature of a person's capabilities could mean that they are not able to make minor or major decisions completely on their own. Every effort, however, must be made to ensure they can participate in steps of the decision-making process. Knowing the person's strengths, interests and personal preferences is important when involving them in the decisions that affect their life. Decision making will only be empowering when the person is a part of it and feels a part of it.

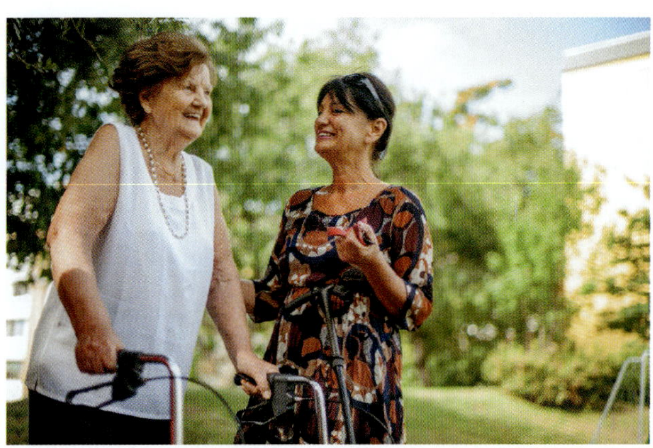

CasarsaGuru/E+/Getty Images

An advocate will speak out for the person so that their interests are represented

Involving someone who knows the person well and who will act as an advocate further increases the person's participation in decision making. Essentially, the advocate's role is to support the person and to speak out with them or for them so that their interests are represented. In the case where the person is unable to make decisions, their authorised person (their carer, guardian or person having power of attorney) will be responsible for their welfare. They should, therefore, be consulted and be actively involved in decision making on behalf of the person.

Care workers can use the following to help promote a person's increased participation in decision making:

- provide time to decide
- identify the relevant information needed
- explore the options
- limit their choices when necessary
- identify the results or consequences of a decision
- break enormous amounts of information into manageable chunks
- avoid suggesting answers
- check for understanding
- support decisions
- provide assistance without undue influence
- seek support from others when necessary.

When supporting decision making, a care worker will be guided by their organisation's policies and procedures, which are endorsed by legislation and regulatory requirements, including the Aged Care Quality Standards (the Quality Standards). The purpose of these standards is to ensure that care provided is of an excellent quality, and that consumers are encouraged to live as they wish and to participate in a range of social experiences. The Charter of Aged Care Rights also supports dignity of risk in decision making. Resources to assist an older person in making decisions are available from the Older Person's Advocacy Network (https://opan.org.au).

8.2.5 Participating in activities

Activities that reflect the person's individual physical, social, cultural and spiritual needs can provide benefits to their wellbeing. Individuals participate in activities that are important and relatable to them, and which offer values of autonomy and self-determination. Activities may include ADLs such as attending to personal hygiene needs or meal preparation, or IADLs that include shopping and managing finances. Other activities include physical, social, cultural and spiritual-based activities such as ceremonial and ritualistic activities, social gatherings with friends and family, and self-improvement activities.

Examples of activities that are not related to ADLs or IDLs include:

- self-improvement activities such as short courses of interest
- spiritual activities such as beach meditation or prayer groups
- social activities such as craft sessions, group outings or picnics, and group cooking activities
- physical activities such as walking groups, gym memberships and water activities.

When people participate in activities, they may experience feelings of inclusivity and purpose. As we are social beings, the social connection of many activities can boost a person's sense of self and overall emotional wellbeing.

When organising activities for the older person, it is essential that they are consulted and included in the planning process. The care worker should have an understanding of the individual's needs and preferences before attempting to develop an activity for them or to include them in an activity that doesn't suit their needs. For example, an 82-year-old man with dementia may be embarrassed to sit with others and use colouring pencils to make Christmas cards; however, he may be happy to sit with others and work on puzzles or small tinkering jobs with tools. It is difficult to establish a sense of empowerment and positive self-esteem in an individual by providing activities for them that they dislike. Activities are designed to promote a person's strengths and sense of achievement, not to disable these or to devalue their integrity and individuality.

WORKPLACE SCENARIO

Finding the balance between focusing on tasks and focusing on the individual

It is a busy morning shift at the RACF and Zac is already behind with his routine because his colleague has called in sick and a replacement care worker hasn't arrived yet. Zac needs to help Myrtle, a resident, to get out of bed and to shower before breakfast. Myrtle is quite independent but needs some minimal help and supervision because she is at risk of falling due to her frailty. Zac realises he doesn't have time to give to Myrtle before breakfast unless he takes over the tasks that she can do by herself. He decides to explain the situation to Myrtle and to give her the option of having breakfast in bed and a shower after breakfast, when he has more time. Myrtle is quite thrilled to have breakfast in bed. Zac assists her to use the toilet and to get back into bed, ready for breakfast. He is able to give Myrtle the time she needs after breakfast, by which time the staff replacement has arrived.

CHECK YOUR UNDERSTANDING

1. Why should care workers not impose their values and beliefs on the older people they support?
2. List three ways in which an older person might express their physical identity.
3. How does Maslow's hierarchy of needs group human needs?
4. List four ways in which a care worker can promote increased participation of the person in decision making.
5. Why is participation in self-care and activities beneficial for older people?

8.3 ENCOURAGING INDEPENDENCE

Older people are the experts on themselves. The fundamental philosophy of providing aged care services is that of supporting the person to maintain independence, to enable them to use their strengths and abilities, and to promote the values of self-determination, autonomy and dignity. When these values are stripped from the older person, intentionally or not, the person is vulnerable to feelings of being devalued, loss of self-esteem and self-worth, and depression. As a member of the multidisciplinary team, the care worker is a key element in supporting the person's autonomy and right to oversee their own life.

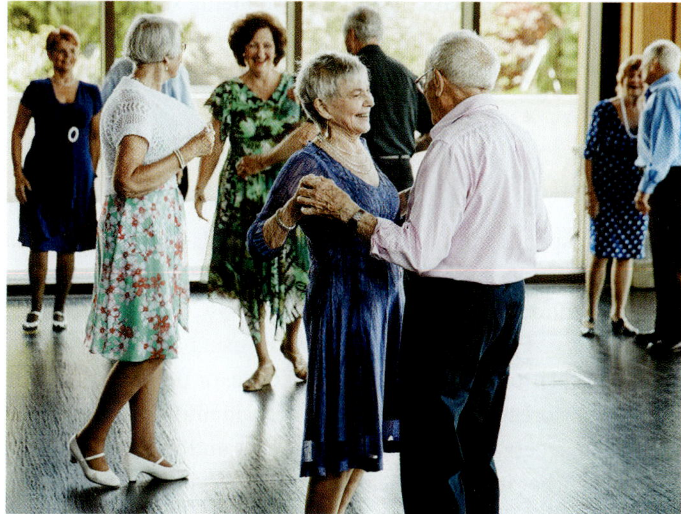
Thomas Barwick/Getty Images

Supporting older people to maintain their independence is a fundamental philosophy of aged care services

8.3.1 Supporting self-care

An older person has the same rights as all other members of our community. Both the person and their care worker should know what those rights are, so that the person is provided the optimum standard of care. The older person's rights are evident in the Charter of Aged Care Rights and in the Quality Standards (Standard 1 Consumer dignity and choice), which underpin the compliance requirements of government-funded aged care services. People have the right to:

- maintain their personal independence and personal choice wherever possible
- be supported in taking personal responsibility for their own actions
- have their personal dignity respected by others in every way possible and to be treated as individuals, whatever their frailties or disabilities
- participate in decisions about daily living requirements, within the scope of capacity
- have privacy, for themselves, their belongings and their affairs
- be consulted about any changes that might be proposed and to have a genuine say in services policies
- have their cultural, religious, sexual and emotional needs accepted and respected, as well as the whole range of their commonly accepted needs
- expect management and staff to accept that a degree of personal risk is involved in these principles, and that their personal independence should not be unnecessarily or unreasonably restricted for fear of such risk.

Aged care legislation enforces a framework that ensures quality of care. A care worker and the organisation for which they work must function within these legal structures and be familiar with this legislation. Formal advocacy services are also available for older people when they need support to complain or make a grievance when their rights are withheld. These organisations function independently of aged care services.

8.3.2 Support services

The aged care services that the person is engaged with may not offer specific types of support that the person requires. The aged care service can provide information about services that are external to them and, in many instances, they can offer a referral to the external services on behalf of the older person.

TYPES OF SUPPORT

The types of support that services offer will be many and varied. However, they often include:

- physiotherapy and other allied health support
- legal advice
- advocacy
- specific health and wellbeing services such as psychology
- specialist medical services such as cardiologists and neurologists
- sex services
- hydrotherapy
- community programs.

Services are designed to support the older person to meet their needs and preferences that are specific to their physical, cultural, social, emotional and spiritual domains of wellbeing. Other support services are those that are subsidised by the government and include respite care, residential aged care and home care.

People can access services using a referral system from a health professional or organisation, via digital platforms such as My Aged Care, or they can self-refer with information provided to them by a carer or a care worker. Where the person can identify positive lifestyle practices, the care worker should ensure they have access to the necessary support and resources. In some cases, the person might need assistance to identify what is likely to help them sustain a positive lifestyle prior to providing support and you can assist by working with the person to identify requirements.

BARRIERS TO ACCESSING SERVICES AND SUPPORT

The person has a right to decline any offer of information or referral to a service; however, they may be hesitant for many reasons. Barriers to accepting other services may inhibit the person's opportunities for a positive experience. Barriers may include:

- disbelief about the benefit of the support and/or resource
- belief that the costs are too high
- belief that the benefits of the support mechanism will be outweighed by its disadvantages
- belief that the initiative will take up too much of their time
- belief that the suggested support will require too much effort on their behalf
- feelings that the initiatives conflict with their values
- feelings that initiatives are not in their best interest
- fear that utilising the support mechanism will lead to a reduction of benefits
- fear of being given inaccurate advice
- fear of conflict or confrontation.

Barriers can be eliminated or reduced with valid and reliable information. A care worker may provide information about the services such as location, fees and general information that can be found on websites or in brochures, but they cannot give advice. Advice must be provided by an RN or health professional when the service is relevant to the person's general wellbeing. Barriers to accepting services may be removed by demonstrating to the person that the service will meet their needs, and by explaining that the benefits of initiatives outweigh any negative effects.

A care worker should ensure the information they provide considers the person's privacy, preferences and aspirations by asking them whether they have or will inevitably find the information useful and easy to utilise.

The person should be consulted and asked to contribute to the decision-making process. They may become more likely to utilise the service when they have a greater sense of ownership. Their right to refuse to use a service should be respected at all times.

WORKPLACE SCENARIO

Self-management of services

Harold lives in the family home with his wife of 50 years, Lucy. Both Harold and Lucy receive home care services. Harold is a double amputee, and he needs help with showering. When care worker Riley is visiting to help Harold in the shower, Harold tells Riley that he has been diagnosed with post-traumatic stress disorder (PTSD) as a result of serving in the Vietnam War. He tells Riley that he has been referred to see a psychologist, but that he feels unmanly if he goes to see "the shrink".

Riley takes the time to talk to Harold about mental health and stigma. In today's society, he tells Harold, psychology is a common aspect of self-care. Riley shows Harold how to find accurate information about mental health online, referring him to organisations such as Beyond Blue and The Black Dog Institute.

As Harold learns more about mental health and PTSD among defence force personnel, both past and present, he agrees to see a psychologist occasionally, though he doesn't always keep his appointments. He prefers to continue to manage his PTSD on his own terms. However, he finds a PTSD support group for veterans that he attends and participates in to be very helpful for his wellbeing.

CHECK YOUR UNDERSTANDING

1. Aged care services strive to support the person to maintain independence, to enable them to use their strengths and abilities, and to promote the values of self-determination, autonomy and dignity. What is the impact on the person when this doesn't occur?
2. What are some rights of the older person who is receiving aged care services?
3. List four types of services that an older person may be referred to use outside of the aged care service.
4. List four barriers to using supports and services.

8.4 PROMOTING PHYSICAL WELLBEING

8.4.1 Wellbeing

The term "wellbeing" refers to a state of feeling content, happy or comfortable. Wellbeing involves a balance of the domains that make us human, such as our physical, emotional and social health. Older people are prone to physical decline if they don't eat a well-balanced diet or have a sedentary lifestyle or one or more chronic diseases. People have different perceptions of wellbeing, and this is because we are all individuals. An older person who doesn't exercise and sits watching television all day may feel their wellbeing is just fine. However, a person who is forced to rest after being injured won't experience their sedentary state as one of wellbeing, because they can't get around or move as they usually do.

Care workers can promote physical wellbeing in many ways, such as by:

- supporting the person with a physical improvement program
- encouraging a healthy diet

- encouraging the person to cut down or stop smoking
- providing opportunities for the person to participate in physical activities suitable to their overall health condition (with approval from the person's doctor or the RN)
- supporting the person to have their medications reviewed annually
- supporting the person to have regular health check-ups
- promoting good sleep by making the sleep environment conducive to rest
- supporting the person to maintain oral care
- supporting the person to maintain skin integrity.

To support a person to make lifestyle decisions in the context of physical health and wellbeing, a care worker should first gain an understanding of their physical health and emotional wellbeing, as this could relate to a change in their health status. Basic requirements for good health include:

- healthy diet
- regular exercise
- a healthy, active lifestyle
- good hygiene
- oral health
- sleep
- pleasure and happiness
- maintaining health.

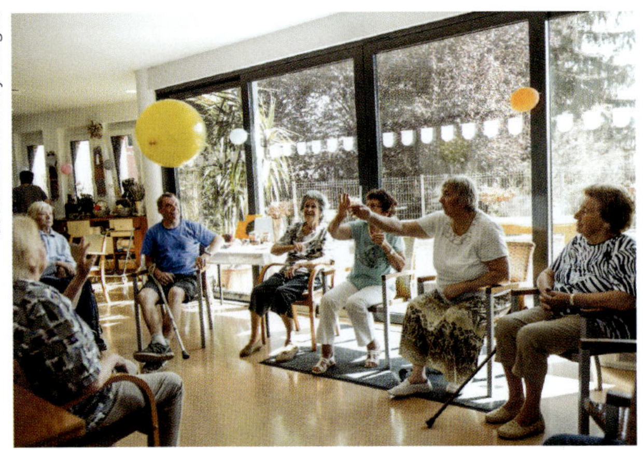

CasarsaGuru/Getty Images

Care workers can promote physical wellbeing through an exercise program

A healthy diet includes fibre, protein, carbohydrates, vitamins and minerals, fats and oils, and plenty of water. An active lifestyle is also recommended for people who can exercise, as it increases bone and muscle strength, increases circulation, and increases energy and general wellbeing.

A person can be assisted to make decisions about their physical health and wellbeing by ensuring they are provided with adequate information. Information about what constitutes a change in physical health status could be helpful, along with any other information relating to physical health and wellbeing. For example, the person may be advised by the physiotherapist that tai chi is helpful to improve balance and minimise risk of falling. The care worker can assist by providing brochures and other validated information about tai chi to assist the person to make their decision.

Regular consultation with the person can ensure the care worker facilitates decision making that is relevant. A care worker could consider consulting with other stakeholders who have an interest in the decision-making process. Liaison with the person's medical practitioner might be appropriate with the permission of the person, or the care worker could consider discussing the person with their supervisor.

FACTORS THAT IMPACT ON PHYSICAL WELLBEING

Physical wellbeing can be impacted by multiple factors, such as chronic illness, poor mental health and pain. It can be challenging to improve physical wellbeing when motivation is influenced by an inability to move without distress or discomfort, and loneliness can compound inabilities to achieve physical wellbeing as social isolation affects mental health.

INDICATORS OF A CHANGE IN WELLBEING

It is important for care workers to identify any variation in a person's condition and to report this to their supervisor, as it could potentially be lifesaving for the older person. Variations in a person's physical condition might include:

- reporting feeling unwell
- weight loss or weight gain
- changes in skin tone and colour
- aches or pain
- oral health anomalies
- tiredness
- swelling of feet or ankles
- frequent colds
- gastrointestinal problems
- seizures
- skin conditions
- vision or hearing problems
- urinary issues.

A person feeling unwell could indicate they have a medical problem, and prompt reporting to the RN or supervisor will ensure the person is referred to their doctor.

8.4.2 Ageing and health

The ageing process has an effect on all body systems (see Table 8.2) and we all age differently. The decisions people make throughout their lives can influence how ageing will affect them in the future. For example, smoking can lead to lung cancer and emphysema, and an ageing respiratory system and immune system may struggle with the biophysical demands of such chronic diseases and illnesses. A healthy lifestyle is a key aspect of healthy ageing and is also beneficial in old age.

The following practices contribute to a healthy lifestyle:

- A healthy diet ensures adequate nutrition. Older people need to eat less, but food needs to be nutrient dense.
- Exercise/fitness improve circulation and, therefore, oxygen transport to vital organs. Exercise should be approved by the person's doctor to ensure the person is physically safe to participate.
- Hygiene helps to prevent infection, skin breakdown and dental issues.
- Oral health is essential for safe swallowing, and the prevention of infection and dental issues such as decay.
- Sleep provides nourishment and rest for the body.
- Activity that includes social group activity can assist with physical strength and muscle dexterity.

Maintaining health is important to prevent a loss of independence. Health can be maintained with regular check-ups, vaccinations against diseases, preventative health screening and by implementing healthy lifestyle activities.

Managing illness and disease is important for maintaining health. It is important that chronic disease and illness are kept in check and that the person is supported to manage these conditions appropriately. Care workers can support the person to manage chronic illness by assisting with assessments and observations such as taking their blood glucose levels (BGL) when required for monitoring diabetes, by using assessment tools to monitor pain, and by assisting with physiotherapy for people with chronic airway limitation.

TABLE 8.2 Physical changes associated with ageing

Body system	Age-related changes	Common illnesses and other health problems	Signs and symptoms	Treatment/management
Cardiovascular	• Changes in size and walls of the blood vessels • Decreased blood flow to vital organs • Effectiveness of pumping action of the heart compromised	• Hypertension • Heart disease • Anaemia • Arteriosclerosis • Cerebrovascular accident (stroke) • Oedema • Hypotension	• Dizziness • Fainting • Falls • Swollen ankles • Leg ulcers • Delayed wound healing	• Encourage the person to do regular, gentle exercise • Ensure good fluid intake • Maintain regular body temperature • Monitor nutrition/diet (not too high in cholesterol/fat) • Administer medication as prescribed • Avoid sudden movements • Be aware of symptoms
Musculoskeletal	• Changes in muscle mass and bone structure alter posture, gait, height and weight	• Fractures • Arthritis (osteo and rheumatoid) • Gout • Kyphosis • Scoliosis • Osteopenia (low bone mineral density) • Osteoporosis (porosity and fragility of the bones) • Muscle wasting	• Pain • Changes to mobility and dexterity • Falls • Enlarged joints • Decrease in height	• Ensure the person retains mobility • Ensure ongoing review of the person's mobility by a physiotherapist • Assist the person in undertaking appropriate exercise (where necessary, passive exercise is still beneficial) • Provide sufficient time for activities • Use hip protectors • Maintain a safe environment
Integumentary (skin)	• Skin becomes dry and less elastic • Loss of circulation impairs healing abilities	• Pressure injuries • Loss of skin integrity • Skin tears • Ulcers • Skin cancers • Scarring • Excoriations	• Redness • Tenderness • Discomfort • Feeling of burning • Pressure injuries • Dry and itchy skin	• Consult a pressure injury prediction scale • Relieve pressure • Moisturise and care for the skin • Regularly move and reposition the person • Ensure good nutrition • Maintain the person's fluid intake • Maintain a clean, dry bed • Use a special air mattress • Use sheepskins under the bedlinen • Monitor the person constantly

Body system	Age-related changes	Common illnesses and other health problems	Signs and symptoms	Treatment/management
Respiratory	• Reduced mobility in the rib cage • Loss of elasticity • Decreased blood flow to the lungs • Alveolar deficiency • Changes in the lungs and chest • Lungs become more rigid • Amount of air that can be expelled after full expiration is reduced	• Chest infections • Respiratory complications • Shortness of breath • Flu and pneumonia complications • Lung cancer • Chronic airways limitation (emphysema, asthma, bronchitis)	• Reduced cough reflex • Shortness of breath at rest • Frequent cough • Rattly chest • Frequent chest infections • Changes in pallor • Cyanosis (bluish tinge around the lips and fingertips) • Lower oxygen saturation rate • Increased respiratory rate • Anxiety	• Encourage the person not to smoke • Maintain the person's posture • Encourage the person to participate in active and passive exercises • Assist the person in wearing adequate clothing • Ensure the person has regular vaccinations (e.g. flu shot) • Have oxygen available (if required) • Transfer a bedridden person to a recliner several times a week • Regularly turn the person in bed • Always follow the physiotherapist/ other specialist's directions as recorded in the individual care plan
Gastrointestinal	• Ingestion less efficient • Slower peristaltic action of the intestines due to decreased muscle tone • Fat absorption and absorption of fat-soluble vitamins decreases • Decreased and thicker saliva • Stomach functions less efficiently • Decrease in gastric juices and digestive enzymes • Reduced blood flow to the intestines	• Chronic constipation • Bowel obstruction • Tooth decay due to decreased saliva • Stomach ulcers • Falls due to medication malabsorption • Malnutrition • If the person has chronic conditions, swallowing difficulties may be experienced • Dry mouth syndrome	• Constipation • Reduced absorption of nutrients • Poorer tolerance to certain foods • Poor digestion • Reduced appetite • Oral problems • Bloating and gas • Nausea • Dysphagia • Faecal incontinence • Bowel cancer • Gastroenteritis	• Serve an adequate and varied diet • Provide appetising food with adequate fibre • Encourage the person to follow good oral hygiene • Ensure the person takes medication for indigestion and constipation (if necessary) • Administer vitamins and minerals • Raise the bed head for sleeping if gastric reflux is a problem • If the person is bedridden, ensure they sit upright during meals and after meals for a period of time (designated in the individual care plan) • Consult a speech pathologist, if required • Consider vitamising food and using food or fluid thickeners

(Continues)

TABLE 8.2 Physical changes associated with ageing (continued)

Body system	Age-related changes	Common illnesses and other health problems	Signs and symptoms	Treatment/management
Nervous	• Decreased reaction times as cerebral processing is slower • Decreased blood flow to the brain • Neurons are lost • Organs degenerate • Synthesis of information is slower (but intelligence does not decrease)	• Memory affected (short term) • Less sensitive to pain • Slower reflexes • Decreased sensory perception • Dementia • Stroke • Transient ischaemic attack • Parkinson's disease and other neurological disorders	• Headache • Neuralgia (nerve pain) • Tremors • Changes in behaviour • Changes in balance • Speech changes • Swallowing changes • Changes in consciousness	• Remind the person of tasks and outings (e.g. appointments, taking medication) • Encourage the person to reminisce • Encourage mental exercise
Special senses	• Sensory perception decreases • Sensitivity to touch and temperature reduced	• Pain threshold increases • More illumination is required to stimulate the sensory receptors in the eyes • Number of taste buds reduces • Smell receptors work less efficiently • Less enthusiastic about eating as taste and smell diminish • Hearing receptors work less efficiently, affecting communication and socialisation • Alteration in perceptions of space and depth	• Overstepping objects • Using more salt or other condiments when eating • Not responding appropriately when in conversation • Falls • Squinting or holding objects with arms outstretched to see them • Changes to sensory functions	• Ensure the person has appropriate eyewear (glasses) • Ensure their eyewear is clean • Provide comfortable seating • Ensure the person wears and maintains a hearing aid, if required to wear one • Ensure communication is clear • Provide sufficient time for the person to process what is being said • Check that withdrawn behaviour is not due to hearing difficulties • Provide an appropriate diet with food that is well prepared and tasty • Take care of the person's nails and hands/feet
Reproductive	• Females: decreasing oestrogen levels, drying and shrinking of the organs and tissues • Males: decreased testicular function, decreasing testosterone levels	• Females: breast cancer, fibroids, uterine/cervical cancer • Males: benign prostatic hyperplasia; prostate cancer	• Females: thickening or a mass in the breast, loss of bone density, lower libido • Males: changes to urination, erectile dysfunction	• Females: HRT, regular breast screening, regular Pap smears, report any abnormal discharge from nipple or vagina • Males: regular prostate assessment, report changes to urination and sexual function • Medication

Body system	Age-related changes	Common illnesses and other health problems	Signs and symptoms	Treatment/management
Endocrine	• Decreased glucose tolerance • Thyroid: basal metabolic rate tends to go down • Thymus: immune response less effective • Body increasingly destroys its own healthy cells • Pancreas: production of insulin and glucose decreases • Blood sugar levels increase • Females: decrease in oestrogen (causing the vaginal walls to thin and secretions to diminish) • Males: blood levels of testosterone decrease	• Diabetes • Low blood pressure • Feeling tired • Difficulty regulating temperature • Less active or alert • Males: stimulation of the penis is slower; ejaculation may be restrained • Autoimmune reaction • Hyper- or hypothyroidism • Females: vaginal inflammations	• Signs of hypoglycaemia (e.g. tiredness, irritability or even unconsciousness) • Excessive thirst • Frequent urination of large volumes • Feeling excessively hot or cold • Feeling lethargic or hyperactive	• Provide the person with assistance in the regulation of diabetes • Provide the person with assistance in temperature regulation • Measure the person's blood pressure (regularly)
Urinary	• Kidneys decrease in size; scars replace renal cells and renal concentration is poorer • Kidney function and efficiency reduced • Reduced bladder capacity • Medication cumulation in the blood	• Loss of urinary bladder muscle tone • Bladder wall becomes increasingly irritable • Bladder emptying becomes less efficient • Filtration ability reduced • Urinary infections • Males: enlarging of the prostrate and bladder dysfunction • Declining bladder capacity • Incontinence • Stress incontinence (leakage of urine) • Prostate cancer • Benign prostatic hypertrophy • Kidney/urinary tract infections • Kidney failure	• Frequent need to urinate during the night • Incontinence • Pain • Frequent urinary tract infections • Abnormal urinalysis • Difficulty passing urine, especially males • Retention of urine • Minimal urinary output • Change in behaviour (delirium)	• Establish toileting schedules • Help the person to control their fluid intake (increase fluid intake) • Provide appropriate aids for incontinence • Encourage the person to exercise as appropriate • Empty urine bags in line with the organisation's infection control procedures • Take care of catheter lines and bags when transferring or turning the person
Lymphatic/ Immune	• Lymphatic vessels suffer problems arising from loss of control over permeability (what can pass through the vessel walls) • Muscle cell atrophy, aged lymphatic vessels • Decreased ability to produce new, mature T-cells in the thymus	• Lymphoedema • Infections • Autoimmune diseases (Crohn's, rheumatoid arthritis, lupus) • Lymph nodes degenerate and become fibrotic, making it harder for immune cells to mount an acceptable defence against pathogens and cancers • Decrease in the normal capacity to react against foreign organisms	• Fever • Delayed healing • Recurrent infections • Lethargy • Delirium	• Provide the person with plenty of fluids and nutrients • Encourage the person to exercise • Encourage the person to have regular massages • Encourage the person to take medication (as prescribed) • Encourage vaccinations

8.4.3 Reporting changes to a person's physical condition

Care workers can identify and report changes to a person's physical condition to the RN or the supervisor. When a care worker becomes aware that something is different about the person's wellbeing, it is essential that the person is provided assessment, and medical intervention if required, as soon as possible. Regardless of how insignificant the change may be, it could have catastrophic outcomes for the older person. All variations of a person's physical condition must be diagnosed by a qualified health-care practitioner, especially since serious disease might not always be accompanied by overt symptoms.

ASSESSING PHYSICAL CHANGES

Physical changes that the care worker may notice may include the following.

- *Weight loss:* This refers to a decrease in body fluid, muscle mass or fat. A decrease in body fluid can come from medications, fluid loss, lack of fluid intake, or illnesses such as diabetes. A decrease in body fat can be intentionally caused by exercise and dieting, such as for obesity. Unexplained, unintentional weight loss is often a result of illness and should be evaluated by a health-care professional. Weight loss might mean that a person isn't eating well because of dental pain or painful swallowing.
- *Dysphagia:* Refers to changes in the way the person swallows food or fluids. Dysphagia places the person at risk of choking, aspirating food or fluids into the lungs, and malnutrition. Signs that need to be reported include trouble chewing or swallowing, coughing during or after a meal, becoming tired during a meal and being unwilling to finish it, avoiding certain foods or textures or temperatures, and having a runny nose or sneezing during the meal. The health-care provider needs to know if these symptoms are occurring.
- *Weight gain:* This can be caused by eating too much of the wrong foods or not exercising enough, or by health conditions such as hypothyroidism, food sensitivity, Cushing's syndrome, organ disease, prescription drug use, anxiety, blood sugar imbalance, and essential fatty acid deficiency. Thyroid hormone deficiency can decrease metabolism of food, causing appetite loss with modest weight gain.
- *Skin changes:* Changes to skin tone or colouration should be reported promptly, as they can indicate various medical conditions and need a medical investigation. New wounds or abrasions should also be reported immediately, as the smallest injury can deteriorate quickly.
- *Poor sleep patterns:* Sleep is important for staying healthy. Lack of sleep can cause tiredness during the day and daytime napping. It is helpful for the health-care provider to know when there is a change in a person's sleep pattern, whether it is an increase or a decrease in the amount of time spent sleeping. Having trouble falling asleep might be a symptom of depression. Having trouble getting comfortable without adding extra pillows might mean a person has a new health problem. Many trips to the bathroom during the night could indicate a prostate problem or a urinary tract infection. Waking up several times during the night and then going back to sleep might mean a person has sleep apnoea, which means they stop breathing for short periods of time while sleeping, which causes them to wake up briefly.
- *Heart conditions:* Swelling of the feet and ankles, or being cold to the touch, might be a sign of a change in a person's circulation. A grey or blue colour to the lips or nails might mean poor circulation as the result of heart problems. This is referred to as cyanosis. When a person has this symptom while exercising, or if they develop chest, jaw or left arm pain, it is a more urgent situation that the health-care provider needs to know about. Continuation of these symptoms can be a life-threatening emergency.
- *Symptoms of colds, coughs, sneezes or trouble breathing:* It is not normal to have frequent colds, coughs, sneezes or trouble breathing, but some chronic conditions might increase the

frequency of these symptoms. These conditions include asthma, cardiac disease, allergies and aspiration. It is important to report such symptoms to the supervisor. Tests or medications might be prescribed by the medical practitioner to reduce the frequency or severity of the symptoms.

- *Gastrointestinal or bowel complaints:* Sudden abdominal problems are often the cause of a person being admitted to hospital. Significant abdominal pain isn't normal and should be considered an urgent problem. Frequent vomiting, burping and heartburn can indicate a developing problem with the stomach or oesophagus. Increased constipation might result in a life-threatening bowel obstruction. Frequent loose stools (or diarrhoea) might be caused by infectious bacteria. Prolonged diarrhoea can result in dehydration. Blood in the bowel movement could be a sign of hemorrhoidal bleeding or of cancer.
- *Poor oral health:* This can result in sensitive teeth, gum and tooth infections, and tooth loss. Tooth loss might mean a person cannot eat a balanced diet. Good dental health is vital to overall good nutrition and good health. Bad breath might be a sign of oral infection. Certain medications can cause a person to have bleeding gums, which can cause mouth pain and infections. Poor oral hygiene can lead to multiple tooth decay and removal, affecting the person's ability to chew and to swallow safely.

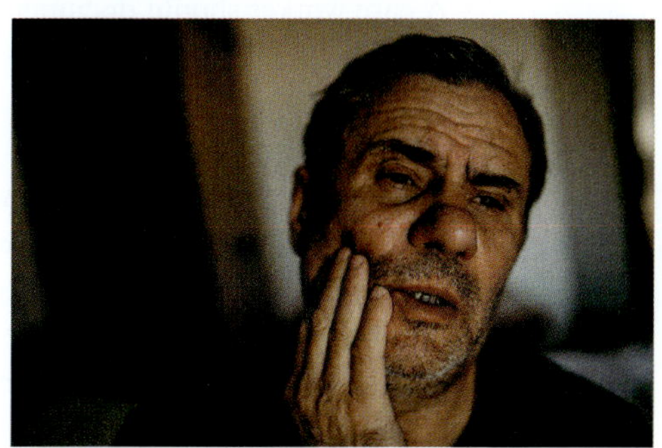
Getty Images/E+/Nes

Good dental health is vital

- *Vision and hearing problems:* Vision and hearing are very important to a person's ability to be involved in and benefit from their daily activities. Many individuals have conditions that affect their vision and hearing. Usually this happens gradually, so care workers need to be very observant to notice changes. Any sudden change is an urgent situation. Redness of, or drainage from, the eye might be a sign of an infection. Redness and pain might be a sign of glaucoma, which is a serious problem with pressure in the eye. These are urgent situations that require a visit to a doctor or eye specialist. Squinting, or needing to move into better light or to sit closer to the television, might indicate a change in eyesight. It might be time for new glasses.

  Drainage from the ear is always a problem that must be referred to a doctor. Many people have problems with wax build-up in their ear canals, and ear wax can affect hearing or decrease the ability of a hearing aid to work. Loss of hearing can cause a person to have unusual behaviour, including depression, and can impact their quality of life.
- *Urinary changes:* It is important to note a person's normal pattern of urination. A change from their normal pattern needs to be reported to the RN or supervisor. Urinary tract infections (UTIs) are a common problem, especially if the person is incontinent and wears protective underwear. A strong, foul odour, frequent visits to the bathroom and burning on urination are all signs of a UTI. Increased accidents might also indicate a UTI.
- *Pain:* Aches can indicate muscle strain, which might require some physiotherapy. Pain can indicate that something is wrong internally, which could be quite serious. Pain should always be followed up by an examination by a medical practitioner unless it is caused by something obvious and is dealt with easily, such as when the elastic in clothing is too tight or an object in the person's shoe is rubbing on their foot.

Care workers have a duty of care to report variations in a person's condition to ensure they have the opportunity to receive assistance. Reporting should occur according to the organisation's policies and procedures, and in a timely manner. Verbal reports of variations in the person's condition should be documented accordingly.

OTHER CHANGES

In the process of delivering services, it is likely that a person will have multiple needs, including those that are not directly catered for by their individual care plan and yet will impact on its likely outcomes. These needs may be related to housing, finances, legal issues, or personal and family relationships. The possibility of comorbidity must also be considered in terms of a person's needs and referrals to other services.

Although the main focus will be on delivering services to address primary needs, a care worker should always be receptive to any additional needs or issues, particularly when they are likely to have an impact on the person's engagement, commitment and motivation, or on the outcomes of a planned service.

A care worker should document the person's needs and contact the appropriate professionals or service, following their organisation's accepted practices. They might need to contact a service on behalf of the person, make an appointment for them, provide referral information to them, or attend initial appointments or interviews with them.

Much of the communication with the person will be verbal. However, staff can also provide written information, including brochures and fact sheets that will assist them in making decisions about their future directions and service options. If staff provide the person with written information, they must be prepared to assist with explanations so that the person fully understands what they have been given.

Staff must ascertain the support that is needed, not only by the person, but also by family members and significant others who are involved in the person's care, and then identify the support services available to them. The support needed by families will depend on the issues the person is facing, and on the impact such support will have on the family unit or significant others. There are numerous support services available; however, they differ from state to state.

WORKPLACE SCENARIO

Encouraging practices that contribute to health

Ziva, who resides in a residential aged care facility, has type 2 diabetes and requires insulin. Even though she can walk using a frame, she chooses to mobilise around the facility in a self-propelled wheelchair, as she currently requires intensive wound care for diabetic ulcers on her left foot that won't heal.

Ziva loves to eat and has a sweet tooth. Staff often find her at the vending machine buying her favourite chocolate bars, even though Ziva knows that, as a diabetic, she shouldn't eat them.

Zeva's wounds have become **gangrenous**, and the doctor requests a meeting with her and her family. The doctor informs them that Ziva's choice of diet is contributing to her problems with diabetes. If she doesn't make changes, she may well end up with a limb amputation, the doctor says. Ziva is given information about diabetes and circulation and is offered referrals to a dietitian to review her diet, and to a physiotherapist to review her ability to participate in an exercise program.

Ziva decides to make some health changes that can improve her diabetes management and accepts the referrals.

One week later, a care worker, Lia, is tasked with escorting Ziva to her appointment with the dietitian. She notices that Ziva has two chocolate bars on her bedside table. Lia reminds Ziva of the doctor's advice about diet and diabetes. Ziva tells Lia she completely understands, and that she will try to adhere to the doctor's and the dietitian's advice. However, just as they are preparing to leave, Ziva turns to Lia, smiles and says, "I'll just nick downstairs and have one last Mars Bar before I see the dietitian!"

CHECK YOUR UNDERSTANDING

1. List five ways a care worker can promote physical wellbeing for an older person.
2. What are the basic requirements for good health?
3. List three practices that contribute to a healthy lifestyle.
4. Why do care workers need to report observations about variations in the person's condition?
5. Following the organisation's protocols, how might a care worker support an older person with needs other than those in a care plan?

8.5 PROMOTING SOCIAL, EMOTIONAL AND PSYCHOLOGICAL WELLBEING

8.5.1 Self-esteem, confidence and security

We all have emotional and psychological needs that, if not met, can negatively impact on our wellbeing. Circumstances that can impact on personal wellbeing include the person's standard of living, health, achievements, relationships, security, community involvement, financial situation, and spirituality.

Emotional needs might include the need to be supported when coping with loss and grief, for understanding and support for managing the anxieties of life, and for freedom from loneliness. A sense of security, contentment and belonging is important for emotional wellbeing, and so is freedom from feelings of shame, regret and guilt.

Psychological needs of older people might include the need to have a sense of control over their own life and have an opportunity to be useful and to contribute to society. Self-determination and autonomy are key factors of psychological wellbeing, as they contribute to a positive self-esteem and personal identity. Empowering a person helps them to take control of aspects of their life that they may have given up on, due to feeling hopeless or overwhelmed by circumstances such as grief.

If a person's standard of living is low due to their poor financial situation, this can cause them to fear falling into homelessness or into a state where they are unable to afford the necessities of life. This can lead to feelings of hopelessness, anger, anxiety and depression, and may result in more significant mental health issues and concerns.

Stress can also impact the lives of older people who are ill or struggling financially, especially if they don't have a support network. For example, war veterans might be suffering from post-traumatic stress disorder (PTSD) and depression. War widows and widowers might suffer from depression because of caring for a partner with PTSD or from having lost a partner in the war.

In the event the care worker observes that the person is being negatively impacted by their circumstances, they should report their concerns to the RN or supervisor to ensure that processes, actions and circumstances can be identified and implemented to assist the person.

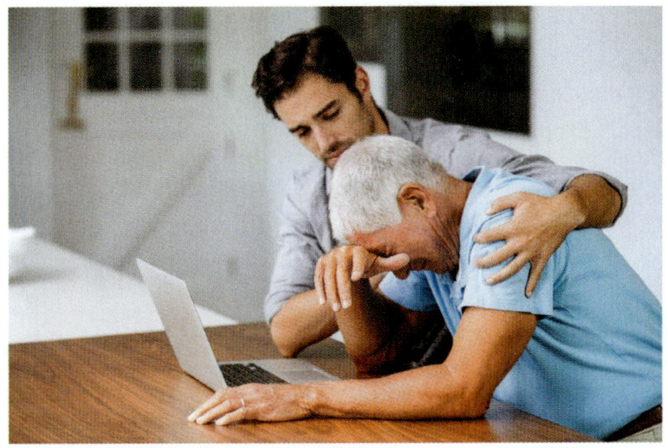

Wavebreak Media ltd/Alamy Stock Photo

Older people should be supported with kindness, compassion and a listening ear

An ageing person might experience grief over the loss of their ability to do something they could do before, or over the loss of their independence or of their home if they go into care. Grief is a normal response to loss, but it is a very individual process and can involve periods of crying, depression, anger and isolation. People can be supported through grief with grief counselling and support groups, and with kindness, compassion and a listening ear.

When providing support to a person, it should be given in a manner that promotes the person's self-esteem. People should be treated with respect, understanding and compassion at all times.

8.5.2 Reporting changes to a person's social and emotional wellbeing

Care workers must work within their job specifications in order to be in line with their organisation's policies and procedures, and to be responsible in terms of their duty of care to the people they care for. If supporting a person's emotional wellbeing falls outside the scope of the care worker's job role, the worker must seek support from an appropriate staff member, such as the RN, the person's case manager or the worker's supervisor. Even if a task or situation falls within the scope of the care worker's job role, they must still seek clarification and guidance from an appropriate person if the task or situation is outside their own knowledge or skills. Staff training might be required in such circumstances.

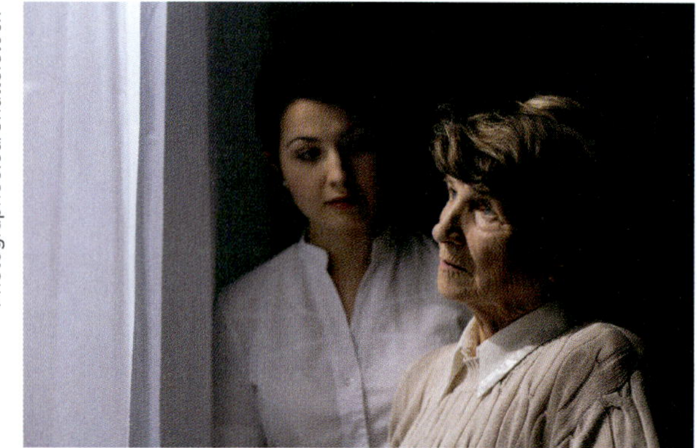
Photographee.eu/Shutterstock

A care worker may be required to seek guidance when supporting the emotional wellbeing of older people

Situations where a worker should seek support might include those where the person's emotional wellbeing has varied, because in such situations the person is likely to need the possible intervention of professional counsellors or medical practitioners.

8.5.3 Risk factors and protective factors for mental health

A risk factor is something that increases the likelihood of harm being caused to a person, while a protective factor is something that decreases the probability of harm. Protective factors act as a defence or buffer against the effects of risk factors. When working with a person, it is necessary for the care worker to reduce the likelihood of future harm by interacting with them to increase their protective factors by supporting, enhancing or developing their capacity, motivation and competence.

It is important for a care worker to understand the factors that place a person at an increased risk of mental health issues and those that can be utilised to protect them from mental illness. Table 8.3 provides some examples of risk and protective factors in the context of mental health conditions.

8.5.4 Cognitive changes

People don't become confused and disoriented due to ageing. Cognition doesn't change dramatically due to the ageing process; however, mild cognitive impairment (MCI) can be common. This means that older people may experience difficulty with multitasking or it may take them longer to recollect some memories; however, MCI doesn't usually have an impact on the person's ability to function.

8.5.5 Psychological changes associated with ageing

Older people do experience psychological challenges that are founded in illness, disease, mental health conditions and disorders. Table 8.4 describes some psychological and mental health issues that older people may experience.

TABLE 8.3 Risk and protective factors in the context of mental health conditions

Risk factors	Protective factors
A biological relative with mental illness	Feeling part of a family (or group)
Exposure to violence or conflict	Feeling connected with others
Unresolved loss or grief	Access to support services, resources and networks
Effects of trauma	Having a strong cultural identity
Substance abuse	Having economic security
Financial difficulty	Experiencing family stability
Poor family functioning/environment	Participating in community activities
Isolation	Having positive coping skills
Discrimination	Having strong spiritual beliefs
Physical or sexual abuse	A healthy lifestyle
Lack of access to support services or a support network	Financial stability

There are many types of mental health conditions that older people may experience, just as younger adults do. Dementia affects cognition, which is the way we think and organise our behaviour. Dementia affects the ability to plan, organise and understand contexts and consequences; however, it can also have psychotic features, where the person loses touch with *their* reality.

Regardless of the type of psychological issue the person is experiencing, the care worker should be observant for changes to their behaviour. These changes may include changes to the way the person interacts with others, eats and sleeps, dresses or behaves. Any observation the care worker makes about the older person that is different from usual can be regarded as a sign that something isn't as it should be.

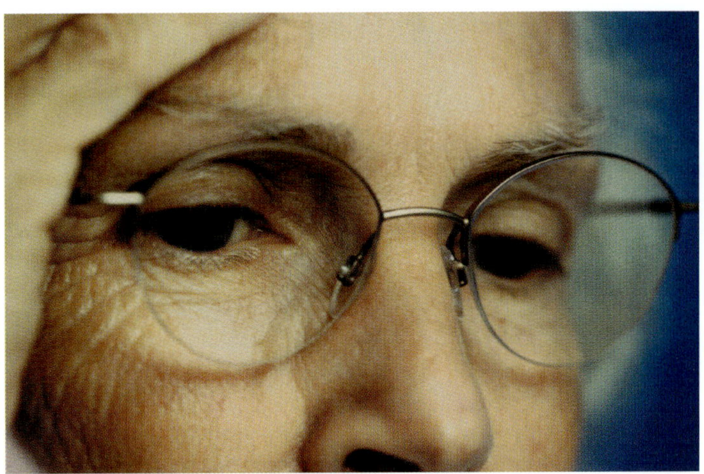

Depression is under-diagnosed in the older population

PRACTICE POINT

The person may make death statements, such as "I won't need that anymore" or "I wish I was dead". These statements are not attention-seeking behaviour; they are expressions of emotional pain and are to be taken seriously. Always trust your judgement regarding the mental wellbeing of the older person. You don't have to be a mental health expert; just report your concerns about the person to the RN or supervisor.

TABLE 8.4 Psychotic and non-psychotic conditions and illnesses experienced by older people

Condition	Description
Adjustment disorder	Adjustment disorders are mental health conditions whereby people cannot cope well with significant changes in life, such as the death of a loved one or a move into a long-term facility. Like most mental health conditions, these disorders also involve depression and anxiety.
Anxiety disorders	Most people experience anxiety; however, many experience it on a level that interferes with their lives. Different anxiety disorders are defined by the impact they have on the person, and each disorder has its own defining characteristics. Examples of anxiety disorders are generalised anxiety disorder, obsessive compulsive disorder and post-traumatic stress disorder.
Bipolar disorder	This psychotic disorder is characterised by extreme mood swings, from profound depression to mania and feelings of euphoria. Bipolar disorder is managed by a psychiatrist, and episodes of depression and mania can be managed with medication and psychological treatments. Some people have very few episodes in life, and others may have more.
Delirium	Delirium is a sudden onset of confusion that is often associated with an infection or other organic cause, resulting in changed behaviour, potential hallucinations and lack of awareness. It can be experienced with or without dementia. Any new behaviour a person experiences should alert staff to consider delirium and begin the process of assessment to ascertain why the delirium is occurring.
Depression	With this mental health condition, a person experiences feelings of profound sadness, futility and apathy. Depression is often linked to other mental health issues, and is under-diagnosed in the older population, especially in residential aged care facilities. Symptoms of depression include: • feelings of sadness or of being down, or crying more than usual • reduction or loss of interest or pleasure in things and people • significant weight or appetite gain or loss • agitation and anxiety or sluggishness • fatigue and loss of energy • feelings of worthlessness or excessive guilt • irritability and anger • recurrent thoughts of death or suicidal thoughts. Depression and anxiety often coexist.
Psychotic illnesses	Psychotic illnesses are those that require intense treatment such as inpatient mental health care, medications and psychiatric intervention. Many psychotic illnesses can involve psychosis, an intense mental state whereby the person loses touch with reality. Examples of psychotic illnesses include bipolar disorder and schizophrenia.
Schizophrenia	Schizophrenia is a complex psychotic illness that is characterised by feelings of paranoia and psychosis. This illness has nothing to do with a split personality as it is portrayed by Hollywood. Schizophrenia requires specific psychiatric treatment and medications, and hospitalisation is necessary when the illness is exacerbated. People with schizophrenia are supported to live under the guidance of the psychiatric team.
Substance abuse and addiction	It is important to understand that many people experience alcohol and other drug dependence. People may become addicted to substances they use over time to manage emotional pain and trauma. The more a person "self-medicates" with alcohol and other drugs, the higher the risk of addiction and dependence. Specialist rehabilitation that includes administration of withdrawal medications may be required for the person in the event they request help.
Suicide	According to data from the Australian Bureau of Statistics, interpreted by the Australian Institute of Health and Welfare, men over age 85 have the highest rate of suicide, and both sexes in the over-65 age group have one of the highest age-specific rates of suicide in comparison to other age groups.

WORKPLACE SCENARIO

Depression in aged care

Cora is 82 years old and lives in a residential aged care facility—initially with her husband, Edgar, up until his death nine months ago, and now alone. Cora's five daughters visit her regularly.

The family has requested a meeting with Cora's doctor and the care team, as they have been worried about Cora's recent lack of interest in joining in conversations and activities. They have also noticed that she is refusing most of her meals and has lost a noticeable amount of weight. Cora attends the meeting at her daughters' request.

During the meeting, care worker Debbie says that Cora has been reluctant to shower lately, and that the staff feel she only showers to keep them happy. For the last week, Debbie says, it has also been difficult to convince Cora to go to Bingo, which is an activity she enjoyed in the past.

The daughters learn that Cora has complained to each of them separately that she is in pain, and that she asked each of them to bring her paracetamol when they visit, so that she doesn't have to "bother the busy staff". It is determined that each daughter brought Cora a packet of paracetamol in the last two weeks. The RN is unaware that Cora is experiencing pain and asks her why she has accumulated so much paracetamol. Cora suddenly bursts into tears and says she has had enough of being lonely and useless. Everyone would be better off without her, she says.

Cora's doctor explains gently to her that she feels Cora has depression, which can be treated with medications and psychotherapy. Cora's daughters and the care team all rally around Cora and support her with her recovery.

Six months later, Cora still has her "bad days". However, she has been able to resume her social activities such as Bingo and to enjoy visits from her daughters. Staff are aware of Cora's diagnosis and know to report any variations in her wellbeing to the RN for follow-up.

CHECK YOUR UNDERSTANDING

1. What are emotional needs?
2. List four risk factors for developing poor mental health.
3. List four protective factors for preventing the development of poor mental health.
4. What is delirium?
5. What are some key observations a care worker may make about an older person that might indicate a problem with their wellbeing?

SUMMARY

- Ageism is a form of discrimination that treats a person unfairly based on chronological or perceived age. It is a contributing factor to the stereotype that portrays older people as asexual beings who have nothing to contribute to society in general. Far from reality, ageism and the myths that accompany stereotypical attitudes of older people can have a negative and destructive impact on the wellbeing and self-esteem of an older person, leading to depression and other forms of mental ill-health.
- All people have the right to autonomy and positive self-esteem. The care worker can empower older people to feel secure and confident by respecting their identity and empowering their self-motivation and strengths for self-care.
- The care worker can support healthy ageing in many ways, but especially by identifying and reporting variations in the older person's physical, emotional and psychological wellbeing.

REVIEW QUESTIONS

8.1 What is the difference between chronological age and health age?

8.2 Name three models of aged care in Australia.

8.3 List practices that contribute to a healthy lifestyle.

8.4 List factors that contribute to social, emotional and physical wellbeing.

BIBLIOGRAPHY

Australian Bureau of Statistics (ABS), "Life expectancy hits a new high", media release, 4 November 2021, https://www.abs.gov.au/media-centre/media-releases/life-expectancy-hits-new-high#:~:text=Life%20expectancy%20in%20Australia%20continues,Bureau%20of%20Statistics%20(ABS), accessed 7 March 2022.

Australian Institute of Health and Welfare (AIHW), "Indigenous life expectancy and deaths", 23 July 2020, https://www.aihw.gov.au/reports/australias-health/indigenous-life-expectancy-and-deaths, accessed 7 March 2022.

Australian Institute of Health and Welfare (AIHW), "Suicide & self-harm monitoring: Deaths by suicide in Australia", https://www.aihw.gov.au/suicide-self-harm-monitoring/data/deaths-by-suicide-in-australia, accessed 22 April 2022.

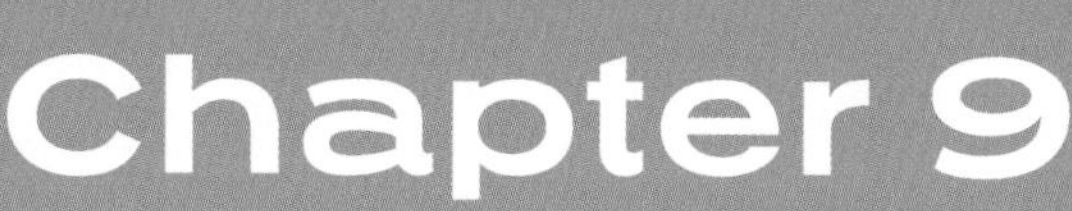

Supporting carers and families

LEARNING OBJECTIVES

9.1 Include carers and family members as part of the support team

9.2 Assess and respond to changes in the care relationship

9.3 Monitor and promote the rights, health and wellbeing of carers

INTRODUCTION

THE AGEING PROCESS AND THE PRESENCE OF CHRONIC DISEASE can create difficulties for many older people, affecting their ability to maintain complete independence with activities of daily living and instrumental activities of daily living. As Australia's population ages, the availability of aged care services may be limited due to the sheer volume of older people who require them. The demand for services may not reflect the supply of services available. Carers of older people often fill this gap in service availability when they care for their loved one at home. This may take pressure off an already pressured aged care system; however, carers can be vulnerable to stress, depression and lifestyle changes when they are not supported. This caring work is crucial to the wellbeing of those who are cared for, as well as to the Australian community and economy. Caring relationships and roles are diverse. Each care situation is unique and may emerge and change across the life course.

The role of the carer in Australia's aged care environment is crucial for quality service delivery.

INDUSTRY IN FOCUS

Supporting carers during the COVID-19 pandemic

Carers play a vital role in the health-care system. The 2.65 million people caring for a family member face pressures on their work, incomes, health and wellbeing as they strive to care for their loved ones. The COVID-19 situation intensified these pressures and poses a significant threat to all members of the Australian community. Vulnerable persons, such as people who are ageing or frail and those living with chronic illness or disability, are at a heightened risk from COVID-related complications. Many people also rely on the support of family members and friends to manage their condition and enable them to participate effectively in the community.

Assisting a vulnerable family member or friend may expose that carer to an increased risk of contracting the virus, especially where access to personal protective equipment (PPE) and clear information about how to manage COVID safely at home are limited. In many cases, physical contact with the care recipient—and other people such as paid workers—is unavoidable in order to meet a person's needs. Many health-care workers, including care workers, continue to be infected with COVID, requiring them to take time off work to isolate. Isolating protects others; however, the sheer numbers of health workers isolating at any one time is placing a burden on the ability of aged care services to provide adequate staffing numbers on any given day. Carers and family members are having to fill the staffing gaps.

Carers are often the safety net for a person when formal services are reduced or no longer available. Therefore, in the current environment, many carers have taken on additional caring responsibilities to replace formal services and to assist the person they care for to self-isolate.

A range of carer services are available nationally through the Carer Gateway; however, not all carers are aware of the support available to them or how to access it. Many carers are also too busy attending to the needs of others to reach out for support for themselves.

Carers NSW has published information for carers on how to manage COVID in a booklet titled *Caring through Crisis: COVID-19 Handbook* (available online for free download). Carers NSW has been advocating for flexible, responsive carer support, inclusive and affordable telehealth options, practical assistance with online engagements, and carer-aware policymaking and service delivery to address these issues.

Coordinated messaging regarding older people and people with disability has vastly improved since the start of this crisis; however, in many cases, information and resources applying recommendations and announcements to carers and the people they care for have been lacking. In order to support carers during the COVID-19 pandemic, Carers NSW has been advocating for:

- more balanced visitor policies
- improved testing and protection for care workers
- improved access to PPE to address these issues
- financial support for carers—in particular, to assist with access to digital technology.

COVID continues to challenge carers' ability to keep themselves and their loved ones safe; however, support resources are growing as our awareness of the issue develops.

9.1 INCLUDING CARERS AND FAMILY MEMBERS AS PART OF THE SUPPORT TEAM

It is essential that carers and families are considered as part of the support team to facilitate a continuum of support and to maintain the integrity of the relationships within the care and family environments. Carers and families can provide valuable information about how best to serve the older person based on their needs and preferences, and when included as part of the team, carers can feel empowered, respected and acknowledged with regard to their role in the older person's life.

9.1.1 The importance of carers, family and friends

CARERS

A **carer** is a spouse, family member, friend or neighbour who provides unpaid care and support to a person they know who cannot care for themselves independently due to frailty and age-related issues, disability, chronic illness or geographical isolation. According to Carers Australia, there are over 2.65 million carers in our country, making up 11 per cent of the population. A primary carer is the person who takes responsibility for most of the care and support that is needed by the older person, and the majority of primary carers provide between 20 and 40 hours of unpaid care to their loved one every week (Carers Australia 2022a).

A carer can be of any age. A "young carer" is someone under 25 years of age, but the majority of carers are middle-aged women (Carers Australia 2022b). Most people don't choose to be a carer; the role evolves due to changing circumstances. They might be the family member who lives closest to the ageing parent, they may have a nursing background and so are delegated by the rest of the family, or they might find suddenly or even gradually that their relationship with the person has become one of carer and care recipient.

Many carers report that caring is a role they find rewarding and satisfying, but many also face challenges they didn't expect to face. Each caring relationship will be different, and the impact of the caring role will differ from one situation to another and may alter over time. Carers are sometimes socially isolated or experience a feeling of being trapped. They often experience health issues (which may or may not be treated), including stress, exhaustion, chronic grief, anger and/or frustration, and are more likely to ignore their own health needs while attending to the needs of others.

When service providers (or care workers) initially become involved in providing care and support for a person who has a carer, the care worker should ensure they treat the carer with respect, by validating and valuing them and by recognising them as a crucial member of the support team. From the onset, carers should be involved in the development of the individualised care plan, and their knowledge of the person and their particular skills should be recognised and utilised in supporting the person. If the carer feels acknowledged, respected, valued and included in the care of their spouse, family member or friend, there is less likelihood that conflict will arise between the carer and the care worker and become an issue. If the carer is given the support and encouragement they require to have their own needs and preferences met, there is also less likelihood of conflict arising between the carer and the person they are supporting; and if it does arise, they are more likely to be able to resolve it, especially if counselling and mediation services are made available.

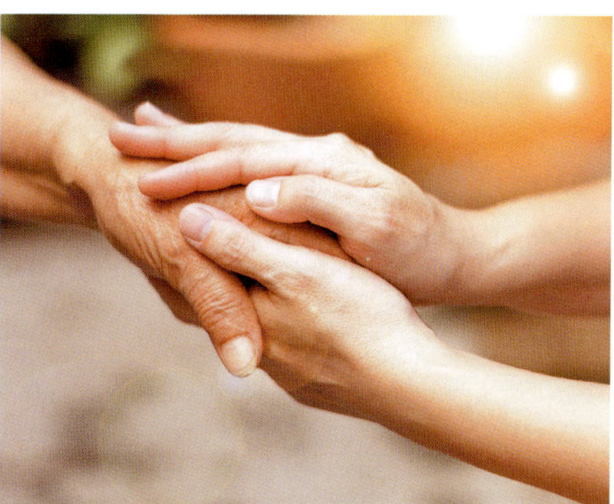
BlurryMe/Shutterstock

Many people find the caring role to be rewarding and satisfying

FAMILY ROLES AND RELATIONSHIPS

The family unit in today's society has many definitions and interpretations, and multiple people living as part of a household may refer to themselves as family regardless of

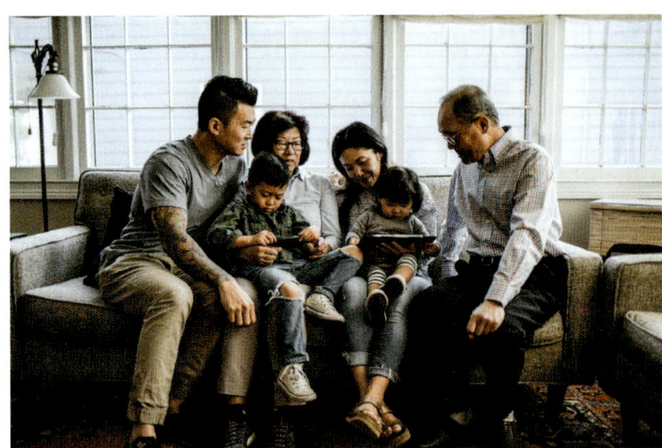
MoMo Productions/Getty Images

A person with support needs will continue to have a role to play in their family unit

bloodlines. Different family members have different family roles, and these roles are determined by lifestyle, culture, religion and generational influences. Relationships between family roles are important for the functioning of the family itself, and these relationships direct the family's rules, behaviours and way of being.

It is important to note that all families are different, and behaviours that represent normality in one family might be regarded as dysfunctional by another family. Family roles and relationships can be very important in the life of the older person, and care workers can support an older person to maintain these roles and relationships. It is important to recognise that a person with support needs might continue to have roles to play in their family unit and have relationship roles both within and outside of their family. Ageing, disability and illness can challenge the person's ability to maintain their usual roles and relationships with family members, especially with their carer. For example, the progressive changes seen with dementia can rob an individual of their personality and change the way they would normally act and behave in a family relationship. These changes can have a huge impact on the older person's roles and relationships with the carer or other family members.

An older person who requires support from a carer at home still has needs, like everyone else, and maintaining relationships within their normal roles is important for the emotional wellbeing of both the person and their carer. A person with family roles, regardless of their health needs, still wants to feel desirable to their partner and to participate in household decisions and activities, and they still want to engage in friendships where they are valued and accepted for their personality and character. These are needs common to humanity.

9.1.2 Recognising and supporting the care relationship

PERSON-CENTRED CARE AND SIGNIFICANT RELATIONSHIPS

Person-centred care is a way of thinking that promotes the autonomy and inclusion of the person during the planning and development of their required support. It is practised throughout the implementation of the person's support plan. Person-centred care regards the older person, their carer and family as equal partners in the provision of care support. This means putting the person, carer and their family at the centre of decision making and regarding them as experts, working alongside professionals to get the best outcome. Person-centred care is not just about giving people whatever they want or providing them with information. It is about considering the person's desires, values, family situations, social circumstances and lifestyles; it is about treating them as an individual and working together to develop appropriate solutions. The underlying philosophy of person-centred care is the same: it is about doing things *with* the person, rather than *to* them.

The person-centred philosophy can also be applied to the older person's carer and family members. Significant relationships between the person and others must be acknowledged and preserved where possible. Key person-centred strategies to support significant relationships include:

- using open and honest communication with the significant other
- determining what the person's needs and preferences are
- encouraging communication and inclusivity by discussing issues in a way that facilitates shared decision making between the person, their carer or other significant person
- showing empathy when the person, their carer or family member is struggling with the changes to routine, roles and relationships

- working within their scope of practice and referring to the registered nurse (RN) or supervisor if the carer or family member asks for advice or information
- giving the carer your time when they want to talk about how they are feeling, within the context of the workplace policies and procedures, and listening actively to them.

The care worker's role should meet the needs of the older person according to the care plan, and it will often extend to complementing the role of the carer. For example, the carer might provide care for the person during the evening and overnight, which might include preparing a meal for the person, administering their medication and assisting them to bed. The role of the care worker, in this case, might be to assist the person out of bed in the morning, assist them with showering and dressing, preparing their breakfast, and taking them on outings or to appointments.

PRACTICE POINT

When you involve the carer in the work you do, you are sending a message that says I have respect for the care you provide and I acknowledge how important your role is in this person's life.

In order to provide unpaid care to a loved one, a carer often has to sacrifice many of the things they need or love, such as social connections with others, their job or a career they like, or plans for an extended trip away with their partner or friends. As a care worker, the key to working positively with carers, families and friends of the older person is to acknowledge their role and their relationship, and to use effective communication to reflect respect, non-judgement and inclusivity.

ORGANISATIONAL POLICIES

Government-funded aged care services must meet legislative and regulatory compliance requirements. Policies and procedures are one component of this compliance framework.

As a care worker, it is good practice for you to know where the policies and procedures are located in your workplace so that you can access them when you need clarification regarding your work practices. Some examples of policies and procedures that are relevant to supporting carers, families and friends of the older person are described in Table 9.1.

TABLE 9.1 Policies and procedures relevant to carers, families and friends

Policy or procedure	Purpose
Grievance	States the procedure for supporting carers, families and friends to lodge a formal complaint to the organisation
Open disclosure	Discusses the requirements and processes required for the organisation to admit error, and to apologise, if an incident could have or did cause harm to the older person
Compulsory reporting	Explains the process for reporting alleged or suspected abuse of the older person by staff, residents or family
Communication	Clarifies various policies and procedures that set out how the carer is included in processes such as care plan development and review, decision making, etc.
Privacy, confidentiality and disclosure	Explains the legal and ethical requirements of all workers that surround information sharing processes
Consent	Explains what consent is and when it is to be obtained from the carer if they are the substitute decision maker for the older person

WORKPLACE SCENARIO

Including the carer in the design, planning and implementation of support

Joe has been caring for his mother, Eva, for three years. She has multiple sclerosis and needs assistance with showering and walking. Joe works from home and is an active member of the local fishing club. Since Eva's condition has intensified, Joe has been struggling to manage his work while also caring for his mum, and lately he doesn't have the energy to go fishing. Eva has been assessed as eligible for in-home support; however, Joe has been reluctant to ask for help because he doesn't want strangers telling his mother what to do. Eva knows that Joe is starting to have difficulty in supporting her and convinces him to contact an in-home care service.

A representative from the service arrives to discuss Eva's needs and to perform a safety check. Joe and Eva explain their situation and are asked about preferences for the service delivery for showering and some domestic support that would take some of the pressure off Joe. Eva is happy that her preferences are acknowledged, and Joe is happy that his mother is respected and offered choices, specifically around what time she would like a shower and what housework the service could assist with. Eva says she wants to continue to do some cleaning; however, she would like help with cleaning the floors and the bathroom and with hanging out the laundry.

CHECK YOUR UNDERSTANDING

1. Why is it important to include carers as part of the care team?
2. Why is person-centred support important when working with older people, their carers and family?
3. Why are family roles and relationships important?
4. List two person-centred strategies that can support significant relationships.
5. List three policy subjects that involve carers, families and friends of the older person.

9.2 ASSESSING AND RESPONDING TO CHANGES IN THE CARE RELATIONSHIP

9.2.1 The impact of caring

Providing care to a loved one or a friend can be life changing, and the impact on the carer's physical and mental health can have negative outcomes. Many carers don't wish to place their loved one into a residential aged care facility (RACF) and will care for them in their own home for as long as possible. There are many reasons for this, including love and commitment, religion and culture, family expectations and fear of the unknown.

Caring for a loved one or friend may start out slowly because the older person's support needs are not intensive; however, older people who need support may have one or more complex health conditions that progress over time and require intensive support and attention. Some of these conditions include dementia, emphysema, diabetes, multiple sclerosis and cancer. As time progresses, carers will be required to provide support that may include:

- showering
- dressing/undressing
- oral care
- skin care
- wound care
- medication administration
- toileting and continence care
- meal preparation and feeding the person.

Akhararat Wathanasing/Alamy Stock Photo

Carers may assist with a variety of activities

Carers not only need to assist with these activities, but may also be required to pay bills, do the grocery shopping, collect scripts from the pharmacy, organise times and transport for the older person to keep medical appointments, and attend to domestic work. It can be difficult for a carer to maintain their own employment, social networks and life as they knew it before the person needed care, and their relationships with other family members, such as their spouse or partner, and their children and grandchildren, can be impacted. Carers are more likely than non-carers to experience poor physical and mental health and disability, and rates of depression among carers are high.

PRACTICE POINT

It may be you, the care worker, who notices that the carer is struggling within their role as a carer. You may observe that they look tired, that the household isn't as tidy as usual, that the carer isn't taking care of their own physical appearance, or that they are losing weight. Report all your observations about the carer so they can be provided with information to support them. Carers have a high rate of clinical depression as a population group.

CARER'S RIGHTS

No matter what level of care they provide and the type of care relationship they are in, carers have rights. Respect, consideration, recognition and support are some of the principles that guide how government departments, local councils and government-funded services work with carers and the people they care for. Rights relating to carers include:

- being respected and recognised as an individual with their own needs, as a carer and as someone with special knowledge of the person in their care
- being supported as an individual and as a carer, including during changes to the care relationship
- being recognised for their efforts and dedication as a carer and for the social and economic contribution to the community that comes from their role as a carer
- having the carer's views and cultural identity taken into account, together with the views, cultural identity, needs and best interests of the person they care for, in matters relating to the care relationship, including when decisions are made that impact on the carer and the care relationship
- having their social wellbeing and health recognised in matters relating to the care relationship
- consideration of the effects that the caring role has on their participation in employment and education (if they are deciding on becoming a carer).

9.2.2 Strategies to minimise the stresses of changes in relationships

The relationship between the carer and the older person can change due to the transformation of roles within the relationship brought about by the support needs associated with ageing, chronic disease and life-limiting illnesses. Relationships often have boundaries, which can be blurred by caring for a person with support needs. Carers can experience depression and anxiety, and many carers can feel frustrated and resentful about being a carer, which in turn makes them feel guilty.

Care workers are in the ideal position to recognise changes to the relationship between the older person and their carer and signs this is happening may include:

- The carer states they are unhappy.
- The older person's needs aren't being met.
- The carer's demeanour has changed from their usual one to being angry, distant, agitated or despondent.
- The older person isn't happy with the carer.

If the caring relationship breaks down, the impact on the person and the carer can negatively affect their emotional wellbeing. The breakdown of a care relationship can also warrant a significant change to the person's individualised plan, especially if the carer has been providing substantial support to the person. It is important both that the older person still has their needs and preferences met if the carer can no longer help, and that the carer's needs are supported.

Other key changes that could cause the relationship to break down include:

- worsening carer health
- worsening health or behaviour of the person with support needs
- loss of formal or informal supports
- high level of carer stress
- carer providing high-intensity care (where the person has multiple complex needs)
- multiple competing role demands
- conflict in relationships with family and/or service providers
- caring for a person with dementia.

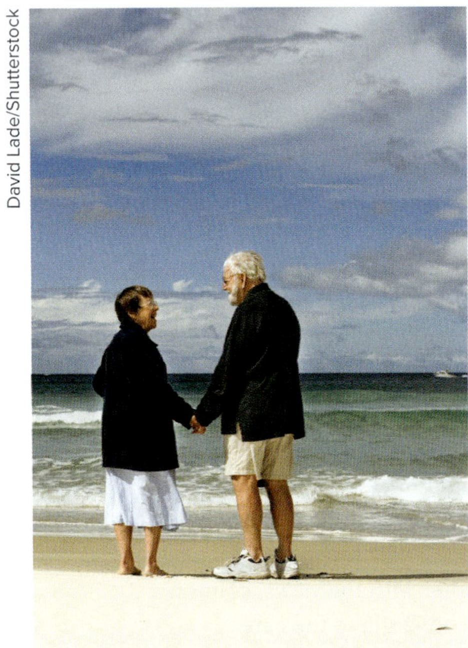

David Lade/Shutterstock

Care workers can help with strategies to minimise changes in the carer relationship

Early identification of potential relationship stressors is essential to minimise relationship breakdowns between the older person and their carer. The sooner supportive measures are put into place, the better the outcome for both the carer and the older person.

Where there are changes in relationships, the carer and care worker may need to discuss a range of strategies and options available to minimise the stress involved. Support services may need to be increased so the carer can take a break from care, or it might mean that the carer ceases to be a carer and resumes the role of a family member or friend of the person. In such a case, the person who was the carer needs to be supported and encouraged not to take on aspects of their carer role out of habit, convenience or pressure from the person. Carers might need counselling through the process due to possible feelings of guilt developing, and both the carer and the person might require counselling to process the grief of the changed relationship and resulting circumstances.

Where there is a loss of formal or informal supports, this may be compensated by increased services. For example, if a support group the person or carer was attending is dissolved, the person or carer could be referred to another group. If a family member (not the carer) who usually provided transport for the person and the carer moves interstate, a taxi service might be able to be provided, or a care worker may be assigned to cover the person's transport needs.

If a carer is suffering from high stress that is impacting negatively on the carer relationship, respite may be the answer. Respite services provide opportunities for carers to have a break from their caring role and/or support the caring role. They might be offered for a week or more to overcome the crisis level of stress, or on a regular basis (perhaps on one or two days per week). Increasing daily support services might also alleviate the stress of the carer.

For different carers, respite will mean different things. Some carers don't want to be separated from the person they care for; instead, they are just seeking a short break from their caring role, or assistance with some of their caring duties. It might be for a few hours, a day, a night or longer. Respite ideally should be individualised based on the expressed needs of the carer.

9.2.3 Indications that someone needs to move into residential care

The older person's needs may intensify to the point that the carer is no longer able to support the person at home. This can be a difficult time for the older person and the carer, as moving into an RACF is a life transition that can create stress, worry, guilt and, of course, grief. Sometimes, the older person may need to move into residential care because the carer cannot cope or is unable to safely care for the person. The carer may experience their own health issues that render them unable to provide care.

When an older person is required to transition into full-time residential care, it is important for the service provider to develop strategies that will encourage the carer, family and friends to view the transition as a challenging event with an opportunity for positive change. The following are some possible strategies.

- Encourage the carer and person to become involved in the planning and development of the care plan.
- Encourage questions and open and honest communication.
- Acknowledge anxiety, loss and grief issues and provide reassurance.
- Ensure that carers, families and/or friends have adequate information about the positive impacts of the transition, including information about the benefits of self-care.
- Provide cognitive training opportunities so that carers, families and friends can learn to process the transition event differently.
- Make referrals to specialist providers such as psychologists, social workers or counsellors so that carers, families and/or friends can talk about how the transition event has impacted all involved.

Other key strategies can be identified by brainstorming with the carer, family and friends or with colleagues and other specialist providers. These other strategies could help carers, families and friends to:

- build and utilise support networks
- look at how they can restructure their way of thinking by providing information
- solve problems
- manage stress.

Two main goals can be considered:

- Assist carers, families and friends to see the transition as a predictable and understandable process.
- Ensure that carers, families and friends are equipped with the necessary assistance during the transition, and provide support for feelings of hopelessness, grief, loss and guilt.

9.2.4 Encouraging the carer and family to be involved in the life of the older person

Older people who reside in an RACF are not exiled from the world outside; indeed, the facility will encourage the person to participate in the many social activities and outings they organise. Carers, families and friends should be encouraged to be involved in the life of the older person, just as they were prior to the person moving into residential care. Carer and family participation is important for the wellbeing of the older person and can support both the person and the carer and family to adjust to the new living arrangements.

Carers, families and friends of the older person can be encouraged to:

- visit as often as they would like
- take the older person out for day trips if able to do so
- celebrate relevant events and days with the older person in the facility
- join the person for meals
- help the person to decorate their room, where appropriate
- participate in the planning and development of the older person's care plan
- actively participate in the hands-on care of the older person, if appropriate.

Staff should be aware of opportunities to include the carer and family in monitoring and evaluating the types of support the older person receives. The carer and family are a vast source of information that can contribute to effective service delivery for the older person, ensuring their needs and preferences are met. Likewise, carers and families should be informed of incidents and issues that involve their loved one. Ongoing and transparent communication is essential to develop trust and rapport between the organisation and the carer.

9.2.5 Responding to conflict

CONFLICT BETWEEN CARERS, FAMILIES, FRIENDS AND SUPPORT STAFF

Conflict occurs when a misunderstanding arises, usually from ineffective communication or a lack of communication. Conflict can occur between carers, families and friends, and support staff for various reasons, and these incidents must be handled professionally and respectfully. Effective communication is essential to prevent conflict from escalating, and most of the time a resolution can be achieved. When a person is upset or agitated, generally they have a need to have their issue acknowledged and heard in a way that shows understanding. It is important to speak assertively without appearing rude and to make a genuine attempt to work with the person to solve the problem.

Care workers should follow their organisation's policies and procedures regarding conflict and seek the support of the RN or supervisor if necessary. When carers and family members take issue with staff, always attempt to understand what the issue is and why the carer or family member may be feeling angry or frustrated. Try to work with the person to come up with a solution to the issue. Remember that the carer may be feeling intense emotions of guilt, loss and grief because they can no longer care for their loved one at home or they are struggling with their caring responsibilities. If the issue cannot be resolved, seek support from the RN or supervisor, who may assist the person to lodge a complaint.

PRACTICE POINT

In the event you are faced with conflict from the carer or family members, remember not to take it personally. Don't raise your voice or have a screaming argument. This is futile and will make any situation of conflict worse. If you feel out of your depth, seek assistance from the RN or supervisor, and consult your workplace policies and procedures.

CONFLICT BETWEEN THE PERSON AND THEIR CARERS, FAMILIES AND FRIENDS

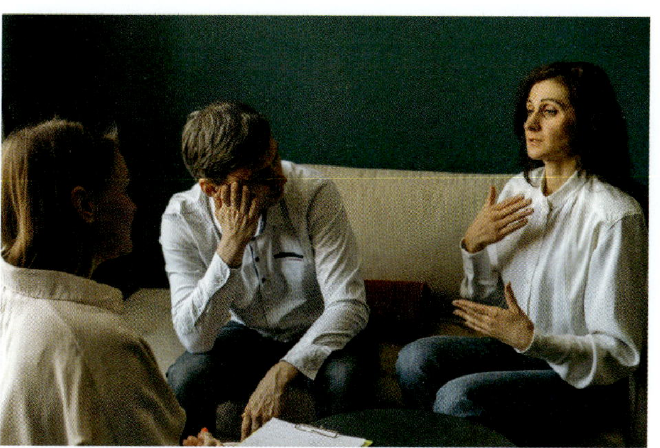

Getty Images/Fiordaliso

Frequent conflict in a family may impact the wellbeing of both the older person receiving care services and the care worker who provides the services

Generally, conflict between the older person and their carer is a personal matter; however, care staff should endeavour to report the conflict to the RN or supervisor and document their observations. If the carer or the older person directly involves the care worker, careful communication should occur that doesn't indicate the care worker is attributing blame or taking one person's side in the conflict. As a care worker, you can provide support and information; however, you cannot provide advice. Remember to work within your scope of practice and to seek support from the supervisor. The carer and the older person may benefit from counselling support; however, conflict may be indicative of the strain and pressure that the carer may be experiencing. If the older person is at risk of abuse or exploitation, the care worker should follow the procedures set out under the Serious Incident Response Scheme (SIRS) and report the matter to the RN or supervisor.

CONFLICT WITHIN THE FAMILY

Conflict occurs occasionally in most families, but some families experience a lot of conflict. Domestic violence, the effects of addiction, crime and discrimination can all have a direct impact on the way each family member functions and how they see the world around them. Frequent conflict may be "normal" in some families; however, this may impact the wellbeing of both the older person receiving care services and the care worker who provides the services. Ultimately, the care worker and the aged care service are not responsible for family conflict, though they are responsible for the safety and wellbeing of staff. If the older person is at risk of harm, abuse or exploitation, the care worker should initiate a report under the SIRS.

WORKPLACE SCENARIO

Responding to family conflict

Jill is working in the community RACF when she is approached by Mrs Rosa's daughter, Olive. Mrs Rosa was admitted to the facility a week ago for permanent residential care. Prior to her admission, Olive was her mother's primary carer.

Jill notices that Olive looks unhappy, and that her face is red. She is almost marching. She throws her arms in the air and speaks tersely to Jill. "Where is my mother's crocheted rug? It's been missing since she came to this awful place. And by the way, stop putting milk in her tea! She drinks black tea and has done so all her adult life! Twice I've had to remake her tea! My mother pays a lot of money to be here, and the services just aren't good enough!"

Jill remains calm, maintains eye contact with Olive and speaks in an assertive tone. "Yes, your mum's rug still isn't back from being labelled, and I can see how frustrating that must be. I'll contact the linen department and see what's going on, if you like. And you're right to be angry about your mum's tea. It's well documented that she has black tea, so I'll bring this up with the catering department. I'm sorry this has happened, Olive. You have a right to be upset. Do you want to make a time to talk to the RN?"

Olive feels a little better because Jill has recognised and acknowledged her issues. However, she takes her up on the offer to have a discussion with the RN about her mother's transition into care.

CHECK YOUR UNDERSTANDING

1. Care workers are in the ideal position to recognise changes to the relationship between the older person and their carer. List two ways in which this might be signalled.
2. What are three reasons that may contribute to the breakdown of a relationship between the older person and their carer?
3. Moving into an RACF is a huge transition for the older person and their carer, family and friends. What are three strategies that provide support during this transition?
4. It is important to encourage carers, families and friends to be involved in the older person's life. What are four ways you can do this?
5. What might the care worker do when faced with conflict from the older person's carer, family member or friend?

9.3 MONITORING AND PROMOTING THE RIGHTS, HEALTH AND WELLBEING OF CARERS

9.3.1 The impact of caring

For many years, there has been widespread concern about the levels of unmet needs in relation to carers. The many potential problem areas that this group might face include:

- stress
- exhaustion
- physical health and wellbeing
- unattended medical conditions
- grief and loss
- emotional wellbeing
- depression
- strained family relationships
- lack of social participation
- inability to participate in the workforce
- financial difficulties.

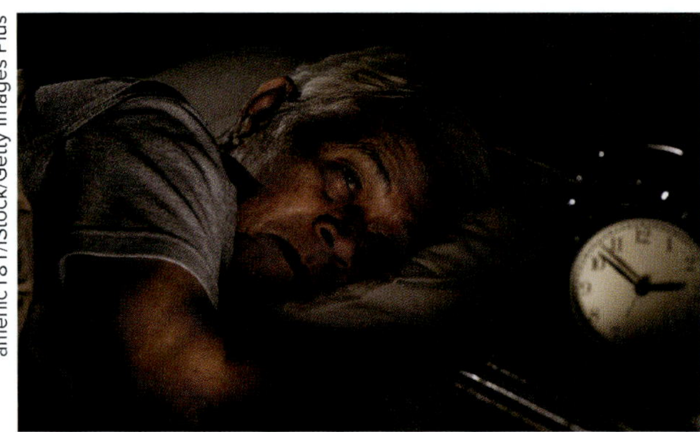
amenic181/iStock/Getty Images Plus

Carers may face stress and exhaustion

When working with a person who is ageing, the care worker needs to identify the knowledge and skills of the carer so that the care worker and carer can work in partnership to meet the needs of the older person. The care worker's role should be identified and confirmed with the supervisor so that job role boundaries are established that indicate respect for the carer's role.

The carer will be knowledgeable relating to the person's daily routines, likes and dislikes, strengths and weaknesses, behaviour management, etc. This knowledge can be invaluable to the care worker, who, by seeking this information from the carer, can make them feel valued in the caring process. The carer might also have skills that can assist the care worker in their support role. For example, the carer might be skilled at providing physical therapy for the person after performing the procedure for many years. They might also follow a procedure when administering medication that makes the process smooth and problem free.

It is important for the care worker also to identify the needs of the carer. For example, the carer might need:

- affirmation
- recognition
- education
- information
- referral assistance
- inclusion
- choice about involvement in specific aspects of care
- peer support
- respite
- workplace participation.

Care workers can support the needs of carers by providing:

- information that is clear and accurate
- information that is free of jargon
- time for the carer to consider any proposed treatment or diagnosis
- support in listening to the carer's fears and worries
- acknowledgement of the carer's expert understanding of the day-to-day needs of the person needing support and of their knowledge of the person's history
- answers to the carer's questions
- a range of options and alternatives for service provision for the carer.

Carers might also need to be included in the community and in the development of the older person's care plan and be given choices about their involvement in specific aspects of the person's care. Many carers would benefit from peer support, which may be available through carer associations and support groups.

If the carer's needs are not addressed or met, the carer might become stressed or depressed, or may resent their role, which could then have a negative impact on the person they are supporting. Inclusion of the carer in the person's support/care plan, and validating and valuing the carer, along with providing them with support and respite services, can have a positive impact in meeting the carer's needs, and thus may also benefit the person they are supporting.

9.3.2 Respecting privacy and confidentiality

Legislation protects the privacy of health information in Australia and governs its handling in both the public and private sectors, including by hospitals (whether public or private), medical practitioners and other health-care organisations. It also includes other organisations that have access to any type of health information. Health **privacy principles** are the legal obligations describing what organisations must do when they collect, hold, use and disclose health information.

Confidentiality is an ethical expectation; often a person (and sometimes their family members and friends) will, in conversation with care workers, talk about their private lives, their aspirations and their past experiences. It will generally be assumed that these conversations are confidential. That is, they are not for sharing with others–such as work colleagues or with people outside the work organisation. People have a right to expect that confidentiality regarding their disclosures will be respected unless mandatory reporting is an issue.

Other confidentiality considerations include the following:

- *Disclosure with consent:* A care worker might need to consult with another care worker to assist with improving care and treatment of a person, and the person would reasonably expect the organisation to use the information for that secondary purpose. Where possible, this should be done in a non-identifying manner. When collecting information, it is advisable for the care worker to discuss with the person how a team-based approach might affect the handling of personal information. A person's information is to be regarded as sensitive, and therefore if there is a requirement to disclose information, permission should be obtained either in writing or verbally in accordance with the Client Record Policy.
- *Disclosure without consent:* In limited circumstances, there might be a need to use or disclose personal information to lessen or prevent a serious and imminent threat to a person's life, health or safety, or a serious threat to public health or public safety. This exception allows for such uses and disclosures and generally relates to emergencies; for example, it can allow disclosures to the police or other government authorities, such as other health departments or mental health crisis teams. The exception also allows for disclosure to an individual whose life, health or safety is threatened, but only after consultation with the supervisor.

  Other examples of where an aged care provider is legally obliged to use or disclose a person's personal information include mandatory reporting of elder abuse, or the notification of diagnoses of certain communicable diseases (under public health laws). However, the health provider does have discretion. Other permitted uses and disclosures could relate to suspected unlawful activity, criminal offences or other breaches of law, or suspected improper conduct.

In any circumstances where a decision needs to be made to breach confidentiality, the care worker must, where possible, consult with the supervisor. Decisions regarding disclosure should be made on a case-by-case basis. If there is a need to disclose any information to conform with any laws or legal processes, the organisation must inform the individual of what information has been disclosed and to whom (unless informing is precluded by legislation) so that any necessary action can be taken.

9.3.3 Carer's health and wellbeing

Supporting another person who is in need may seem all-encompassing. It can also be rewarding and provide a sense of satisfaction. The impacts of caring can vary, depending on the length of time the carer has been supporting the person and the stage of the person's condition, other current events in the family's or carer's life, the carer's past experiences, and their own physical health and wellbeing. If carers, families and/or friends provide care to someone, they may experience impacts upon their own:

- emotional wellbeing
- physical health
- relationships
- employment
- education
- social life
- lifestyle
- finances.

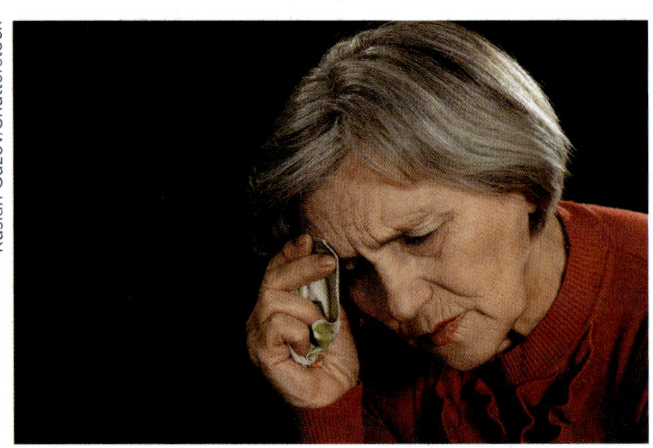

Ruslan Guzov/Shutterstock

Carers need to find a balance between caring for the older person and attending to their own self-care

Therefore, common issues for carers, families and/or friends can include looking after their own health and wellbeing, finding a balance between caring for the older person and attending to self-care, financial security, accessing suitable services and support, taking regular breaks (respite), accessing suitable accommodation, having their role recognised by health professionals, and accessing education and training. A care worker can identify these issues by communicating with the carer, family or friend. While listening to them, acknowledge their issues and consider how each one might be affecting the carer's health and wellbeing. Possibilities could relate to whether they have become depressed, financially insecure, and unable to socialise and/or have changed their lifestyle.

Impacts upon emotional wellbeing, physical health, relationships, employment, education, social life and finances can all have a negative impact on the health and wellbeing of the carer. While each impact might manifest differently for each carer, reports of changes that are negative are likely to have an adverse effect universally.

- *Focus your attention:* When communicating with carers, families and/or friends to engage them or to identify specific issues, a care worker should focus their attention by ceasing all other actions and listening actively to what the person has to say. Sometimes this can be difficult due to distractions. Minimise distractions by moving the conversation to a quiet area.
- *Position yourself appropriately:* Consider the height of the person and, if possible, sit near them and face-to-face. This will make it easier to hear the person, and they can see indicators that the care worker is interested.
- *Don't judge:* When engaging with carers, families and/or friends to identify specific issues, a care worker's intention should not be to make a personal assessment. Follow organisational policies and procedures, regardless of whether the care worker believes the issue is justifiable.
- *Listen actively:* Think about what is being said and consider the tone and speed of the person's voice as well as the content of the message. Look at their facial expression and make an assessment about what they are trying to convey verbally and non-verbally.
- *Demonstrate interest:* The care worker's body language and the way they communicate (speak) can reflect mood. Be mindful that people often gauge interest by sight and acknowledge the care worker's understanding by nodding, leaning slightly forward and speaking calmly. Don't assume it is appropriate to demonstrate interest by making physical contact. Guidelines in relation to keeping a safe and healthy distance between the person and the care worker apply.
- *Consider barriers:* Barriers to communication include those that relate to language and physical impairment. If the person is from a non-English-speaking background or is hearing impaired, ensure appropriate translation services and/or appropriate communication aids are provided.

Other strategies a care worker can use to engage with a person (and/or carer) include using open-ended questions that cannot be answered with a simple "yes" or "no" response. Begin questions by asking what, where, when, why or how, or ask the person to talk about their experiences. Paraphrasing can also be engaging. Listen to the person and repeat their message back to them using similar words to reassure the person that they have been heard and understood.

Indicators which suggest that people are engaged can include increased willingness to communicate, an interested expression, positive body language, positive verbal feedback and an increase in the accurate determination of specific issues. Where carers, families and/or friends don't engage despite the efforts of the care worker, discuss your concerns with a supervisor while being mindful of the person's right to confidentiality and to give their consent.

9.3.4 Identifying when a carer needs support

Carers have needs and preferences like everyone else, but because of the intensive role many of them perform as carers, some of their needs might not be met. It is important for a care worker to identify aspects of a carer's role that have a negative impact on their own needs and preferences so that they can inform an RN or supervisor for follow-up. If a carer's needs and preferences are not met, their emotional, mental and physical wellbeing can be negatively impacted, resulting in feelings such as frustration and depression, and even physical illness. It is important for all stakeholders to work together to find solutions that will assist the

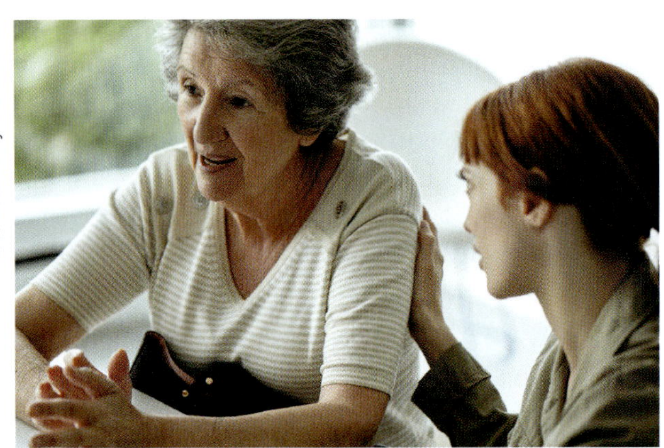
PhotoAlto/Alamy Stock Photo

If a carer's needs are not met, this can result in feelings of frustration and depression

carer to achieve and maintain positive lifestyle outcomes that reflect their needs and preferences. For example, if a physiological need for a carer is identified, it should be reported for immediate follow-up because these are the most basic needs for survival. A carer, and the person they are caring for, might be living on a very low income and doing without adequate nutrition because of limited funds. Financial assistance might be offered in such instances, or financial counselling may help the carer to better manage their funds.

9.3.5 Services for carers

When planning support of a person, a care worker or coordinator of an aged care organisation generally arranges an assessment of the person (with the carer) in their own home. They discuss how their service can best assist them with any concerns they are experiencing. After the assessment, an individualised care plan is either developed (if a person doesn't already have one developed) or reviewed using the information gathered from the person and the carer (as part of the assessment). The care plan is based on what the person and the carer report as their needs, and what support services are available. A care worker might support the person with:

- housekeeping
- personal care
- shopping
- minor household tasks, such as washing and drying dishes or hanging out and bringing in washing
- assisting the person with medication
- taking the person shopping (locally)
- taking the person out to social activities
- accompanying the person on short walks
- talking with the person
- accompanying the person to medical and other appointments.

If the carer is having difficulty showering the person or dislikes accompanying the person on social activities, the care plan should reflect this by providing support in those two areas, while acknowledging the carer's agreement to continue support in other areas such as medication assistance, shopping and housework. If the carer is happy to give full care to the person during the week but needs some time to themselves on the weekend, respite services might be planned as part of the care plan. The person might be the one to ask for support from a care worker in areas that they feel the carer is not covering adequately, or if they are concerned that the burden placed on the carer is adversely affecting their health and wellbeing.

Support services should be based around the needs of both the person and the carer. If the person is reluctant to have a care worker take over some of their care, the service provider should work with the person and the carer to facilitate a guilt-free release of the carer in such circumstances.

Other ways to support carers in their role may include introducing them to the various carer support networks and organisations that exist in the community. For example:

- **Carers Australia** represents carers of people with a disability, mental illness or chronic condition, or those who are frail or aged. It provides information, support, education, training, counselling, advice and referral to services that can assist carers in their caring role. Information is available on a wide range of topics, including home help, carers support groups, financial entitlements, support services, respite and general assistance.

- **Carer Gateway** service providers offer carers supports such as in-person counselling, peer support and emergency respite.
- **My Aged Care** is the Australian government's starting point on a person and their carer's aged care journey. The government-funded services available range from help at home or short-term care, to access to aged care homes.
- Anglicare–Dementia Care Services (Sydney) supports people living with dementia and their carers across Blacktown, Nepean, the Cumberland region and The Hills District, and offers support groups.
- National Respite for Carers Program (NRCP) contributes to the support and maintenance of caring relationships between carers and care recipients by facilitating access to information, respite care and other support appropriate to the carer's individual needs and circumstances, and those of the care recipient. The intent of the NRCP is to complement existing services and support already provided to the community under the Commonwealth Home Support Programme and other programs or information networks.
- The stated objectives of the **Commonwealth Home Support Programme (CHSP)** are to deliver timely, high-quality, entry-level support services, taking into account individual goals, preferences and choices, to help frail older people stay in their homes as long as they can and wish to do so.

The benefits of being in a support group include:

- being with people who understand the pressure of caring
- expressing emotions such as sadness, depression, guilt, exhaustion, frustration, anger and irritability, and being understood, accepted and supported
- making new friends
- expanding one's social network and helping to improve one's overall sense of wellbeing
- getting up-to-date information on developments in policies, entitlements and special events for carers.

Most support groups meet once a month for a couple of hours, usually at the same location. However, some support groups may vary the day, time and, in rural areas, the location. The groups are free, although some ask for a small contribution for refreshments. Carer support groups must respect confidentiality, and discussions of personal situations must not be disclosed to others outside the group.

A range of community-based and residential respite options are available and include:

- day (care) centres that provide respite for a half day or full day
- in-home respite services, including overnight, home care and personal care services providing respite and support
- respite in an RACF or overnight respite in a community setting
- respite for carers of people with dementia and challenging behaviours
- activity programs
- a break away from home, perhaps with a care worker visiting the home.

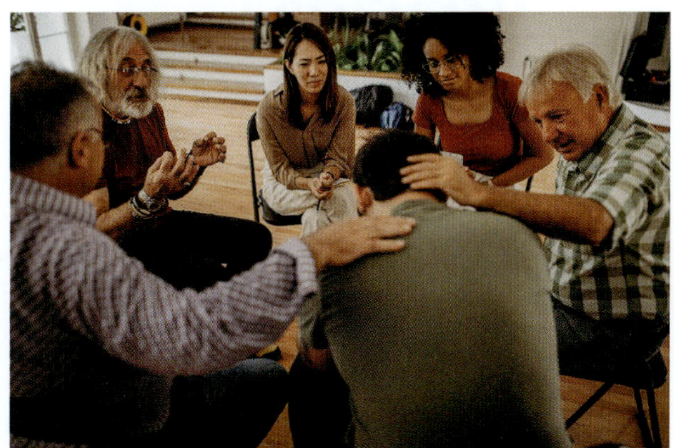

Getty Images/E+/South_agency

Being in a support group helps carers to expand their social network and improve their overall sense of wellbeing

WORKPLACE SCENARIO

The health and emotional wellbeing of carers

Damien arrives at Mrs Grey's home to assist her with her shower. When Mr Grey opens the door, Damien notices how tired he looks. He also notices that Mr Grey hasn't shaved for a few days and the house is untidy, which is unusual. After assisting Mrs Grey with her shower, Damien says to her husband: "You look very tired, Mr Grey. Are you coping okay?"

Mr Grey tells Damien that he just needs a break and a good night's sleep. His wife needs more care as her dementia progresses and it is becoming harder for him to take breaks. Damien and Mr Grey chat about the available options for respite and Mr Grey accepts Damien's offer to talk with his supervisor about working towards a respite placement in an aged care facility for two weeks. Damien acknowledges Mr Grey's feelings of guilt and reassures him that he is a wonderful husband who just needs a break. Mr Grey feels relieved that his wife will be in good care while he takes a short rest.

CHECK YOUR UNDERSTANDING

1. List four possible feelings or issues a carer may experience as a result of caring for another person.
2. What can a care worker provide to support the needs of a carer?
3. What is disclosure without consent?
4. What aspects of the carer's life might be affected by the caring role?
5. What are the benefits of a support group for carers?

SUMMARY

- Carers are people who provide unpaid support for another person who has a disability, are aged or frail, have a chronic illness or are geographically isolated. Carers are usually a family member or friend. Carers are of any age, and young carers are those under 25 years of age. Carers provide care on average of 20–40 hours per week, and they provide care on a holistic level.
- Caring for a loved one can have a negative impact on the carer, especially if the person they support has dementia or a life-limiting condition. The carer will be affected by disturbed sleep, changes to routine, changes to social support and, possibly, financial changes as a result of caring for their loved one. Carers are at risk of depression and anxiety.
- Carers should be viewed as an important component of the care team, as they can offer valuable information about the older person that can assist in ensuring that the person's needs and preferences are met. The care worker should acknowledge and identify the role of the carer as being complementary to their own role. Carers and families should be supported to be involved in the design and delivery of the person's support services.

- Carers and families may need support during times of change and transition, and the care worker can identify and respond to the needs of services required by the carer to support the care relationship with the person. The care worker may also recognise issues that may impact on the physical and emotional health and wellbeing of the carer and ensure that support is available for them. Providing carers and families with information about carer support services is helpful.

REVIEW QUESTIONS

9.1 List some of the signs and symptoms of carer stress.

9.2 Access the Carer Gateway website at www.carergateway.gov.au. What support do they provide?

9.3 What are the benefits of involving carers and families in the development of a care plan?

9.4 List three services for carers in your local area.

BIBLIOGRAPHY

Better Health Channel, *Carer Rights and Recognition*, 2015, https://www.betterhealth.vic.gov.au/health/servicesandsupport/carer-rights-and-recognition, accessed 5 January 2021.

Carers Australia, *Who is a Carer?*, 2022a, https://www.carersaustralia.com.au/about-carers/who-is-a-carer/, accessed 21 April 2022.

Carers Australia, *Young Carers*, 2022b, https://www.carersaustralia.com.au/about-carers/young-carers/, accessed 21 April 2022.

Carers NSW, *NSW Carers Strategy: Caring in NSW 2020–2030*, https://www.facs.nsw.gov.au/inclusion/carers/nsw-carers-strategy, accessed 21 April 2022.

Health Innovation Network (South London), *What is Person-Centred Care and Why is it Important?*, http://healthinnovationnetwork.com/system/ckeditor_assets/attachments/41/what_is_person-centred_care_and_why_is_it_important.pdf, accessed 12 January 2021.

My Aged Care, *Caring for Someone in an Aged Care Home*, https://www.myagedcare.gov.au/carers/caring-someone-aged-care-home, accessed 7 November 2020.

NSW Carers Advisory Council, https://www.facs.nsw.gov.au/inclusion/advisory-councils/carers, accessed 12 November 2020.

NSW Health, *COVID-19 (Coronavirus): Information for Families and Friends of Residential Aged Care Facility Residents–Fact Sheets*, https://www.health.nsw.gov.au/Infectious/factsheets/Pages/covid-19-racf-family.aspx, accessed 1 September 2020.

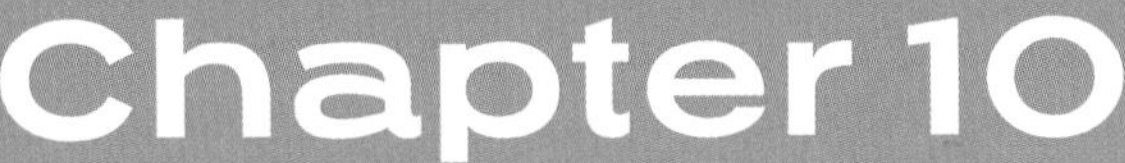

Chapter 10

Assisting with meals

LEARNING OBJECTIVES

10.1 Prepare meals
10.2 Serve meals
10.3 Understand special considerations

INTRODUCTION

EATING AND DRINKING ARE important aspects of living, and while meals are necessary to sustain life, they are also important for social and cultural engagement. Providing support for older people to access and enjoy healthy and nutritious foods is an important aspect of quality care.

Food safety is a critical component of food services within aged care organisations, and food handlers must follow policies and procedures to ensure that any hazards associated with foods are minimised.

Older people require less food than younger people; however, the food they consume must be nutritionally dense to ensure their bodily systems can function well. Unfortunately, many older people who receive aged care services suffer malnutrition because of the quality or quantity of food they have access to. The prevention of malnutrition is therefore an ongoing concern within the industry. This chapter will explore the many ways a care worker can support an older person with meal planning, preparation and consumption while also promoting the person's self-determination, dignity and self-respect.

INDUSTRY IN FOCUS

Managing dysphagia

Any problem with the swallowing process is referred to as **dysphagia.** Swallowing requires a collaboration of physiological processes to occur in a timely manner to ensure the person does not choke or aspirate. When food enters the mouth, the teeth and jaw movements tear and grind the food to a soft lump called a bolus. Saliva warms and moistens the food to help form the bolus, which is then pushed to the back of the throat (pharynx) by the tongue.

The next phase of swallowing is reflexive and involuntary, when the bolus enters the throat, causing the nasal cavity to become blocked by the soft palate to prevent food and fluids entering the nose. The voice box lifts upwards and the epiglottis (a small cartilage structure in the throat) covers the airway temporarily to prevent food or fluids from entering the lungs. The throat pushes the bolus down through the oesophagus where it is passed into the stomach.

The brain and muscles control the swallowing reflex. Dysphagia occurs when a problem, or an interruption, occurs at any point in this process. Dysphagia can result from many conditions, including illness, stroke, dementia and other neurological conditions, and cancer. Dysphagia can be temporary or permanent.

Treatment of dysphagia depends largely on assessment outcomes and the individual. Dysphagia is assessed by a speech pathologist, also known as a speech therapist, who may perform a fluorescent swallow study of the person's swallow reflex to ascertain the risk of aspiration and choking. **Aspiration** occurs when food and fluids are aspirated (inhaled) into the airways, potentially increasing the person's risk of developing aspiration pneumonia.

People who have been diagnosed with dysphagia require great care with eating and drinking due to the elevated risk of choking and aspiration. The person's care plan will state the specific requirements that are needed to keep them safe. These requirements may include:

- ensuring the person is positioned upright for meals
- providing food and fluids that are texture modified to assist with swallowing
- ensuring the person has ample time to swallow each mouthful before they are offered another (if they require feeding)
- observing and reporting for signs of aspiration, such as coughing, a wet voice or recurrent chest infections
- monitoring food and fluid intake
- tube-feeding regimens, as prescribed by the dietitian.

Managing dysphagia often starts with the observation that a person is having difficulty swallowing, and this observation is commonly made by the care worker. Always report your concerns to the registered nurse (RN) or person in charge if you notice something different about the person's swallow process.

10.1 PREPARING MEALS

10.1.1 Planning

Meal planning for older people receiving aged care services involves a multifaceted approach. Older people have specific factors that must be considered to ensure not only that they receive the nutrients they need but also that their meals address the dietary requirements of any chronic diseases they may have, such as diabetes or dysphagia. Meal planning should also support cultural diversity.

Meal planning should focus on a risk-based approach to minimise food-related incidents of harm, such as food poisoning, choking and aspiration. Minimising risk in food planning requires input from a multidisciplinary team that may include a physiotherapist, an occupational therapist, a dietitian, and nursing and care staff. Some people may have allergies or intolerances to certain foods, and this needs to be considered when planning meals for people who require food preparation services. Table 10.1 identifies some of the roles and responsibilities that may be involved in meal planning for older people receiving aged care services.

All aspects of safe consumption of food and fluids must be considered in a manner that encompasses the skills and knowledge of health workers and professionals to ensure that the older person isn't placed in harm's way. Dignity of risk should be balanced with duty of care, and ultimately at the core of safe food planning are the needs and preferences of the older person.

TABLE 10.1 Roles and responsibilities in safe meal planning

Role	Responsibilities
Older person or carer	• Guides the planning process wherever possible • Provides the team with necessary information about needs and preferences
Care worker	• Follows the care plan • Reports concerns to the RN or supervisor • Documents incidents related to eating and drinking according to their organisation's policies and procedures
Dietitian	• Prescribes food types based on nutrition need and context • Prepares appropriate menus for residential aged care services and older people in the community • Provides nutritional guidance for chronic health conditions such as diabetes, high cholesterol and heart issues • Provides strategies to manage constipation, gastric reflux and malnutrition
Kitchen staff	• Play a vital role in safe meal planning and delivery in residential aged care facilities (RACFs) • Follow the food safety plan of the organisation • Follow all food-related policies and procedures
Occupational therapist	• Provides assessment of the environment to assist with health and safe eating • May prescribe the use of adaptive equipment to support independence and a safe meal experience
Physiotherapist	• Assesses the swallow process for dysphagia • Provides information for safe swallowing • Prescribes modified food textures according to dysphagia needs
Registered nurse	• If trained, can perform a bedside swallow assessment following a medical incident • Liaises with other allied health and medical professionals regarding safe eating and drinking • Develops and amends the older person's care plan as required • Ensures a cohesive approach to meal planning

10.1.2 Needs and preferences

Today's models of care in aged care service delivery are rights based and person centred, unlike in the past when a medical model of care was employed. This means that aged care services are now founded on the rights of the older people who use them, and on meeting their individual needs and preferences wherever possible. Food planning is no exception, and the individual (with their family, if appropriate) is involved throughout the process.

The Aged Care Quality Standards (the Quality Standards), along with the Quality of Care Principles 2014, set out the compliance requirements of all government-subsidised aged care services. Of the eight Quality Standards, Standards 1 and 4 are most relevant to food planning and mealtime support. Standard 1, "Consumer Dignity and Choice", emphasises the older person's right to be treated with respect and dignity and to make their own choices about how they live their life. With regards to food planning and mealtime support, consumers have the right to be part of the planning process and to make their own decisions about what their nutritional needs are and how they can be supported. Information provided by the health-care team can assist the person to make informed decisions.

Standard 4, "Services and Supports for Daily Living", encompasses what the organisation must do to ensure the older person receives safe and effective services that focus on their optimal health, wellbeing and independence. This includes the expectation that organisations have evidence of outbreak plans for food-borne illnesses such as gastroenteritis, effective infection control systems, risk management processes that can be applied to all aspects of services provisions, and evidence which demonstrates that services are provided to older people in a way that supports their needs, goals and preferences.

The nutritional support needs of the older person are based on assessment processes, and the individual is an active part of this process. Assessment processes can identify important safety considerations that affect what the person eats, how they eat it and when they eat it. Considerations for safe and individualised meal planning include:

- oral health
- chronic disease
- food allergies
- food intolerances
- food likes and dislikes
- food restrictions
- changes in cognition.

Needs and preferences related to meal planning and preparation must consider the safety of the individual. All food-related needs and preferences are documented in the person's individualised plan (care plan) to ensure that all relevant staff are aware of the person's nutritional requirements and considerations.

Eating is often associated with pleasure, and the presentation of food is another factor to be considered when planning or preparing meals. Including the person in decision making such as menu planning or encouraging them to actively participate in meal preparation can support their individual needs and preferences. This option may not be supported in an RACF when preparing meals for the entire facility; however, cooking and food preparation activities for individuals or small groups can provide an opportunity for participation. Providing meal support in the community sector affords workers with an opportunity to support the participation of the older person.

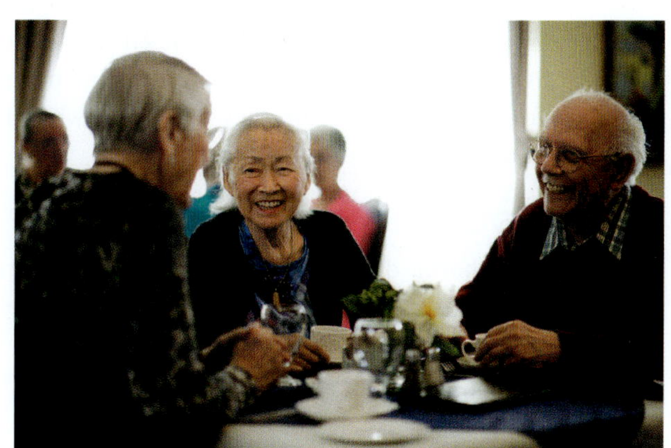

Fat Camera/Getty Images

Eating should be a pleasurable experience

10.1.3 Food preparation in aged care

Preparing food for consumption in aged care services requires processes that support choice and dignity but also minimise contamination of food. All food handlers need to be aware of the risk minimisation procedures, and some food-handling roles are required to be supported with specific knowledge and skills obtained from food safety courses. According to Food Standards Australia and New Zealand (FSANZ), a "food handler is anyone who works in a food business and who either handles food or surfaces that are likely to be in contact with food such as cutlery, plates and bowls" (FSANZ 2008).

In the context of aged care services in an RACF, food handlers may include the supplier of the food, and the kitchen staff who receive, store, thaw, cook and prepare it. Staff who serve the food to older people in RACFs are also food handlers. Care workers who are required to serve meals and to assist some people with eating their meals are food handlers, too.

Care workers who work within in-home aged care services are also food handlers if they prepare meals and serve them to the person they support. Community organisations don't require a food safety plan as meal preparation and support occur on an individual basis in the person's own home; however, staff participate in training programs related to food safety. Community aged care services are required to demonstrate safe and hygienic food practices according to the Quality Standards.

Food preparation in aged care aligns with the legislation around food safety. Part of this legislation is the Food Standards Code (the Code), which is a suite of Food Standards developed by FSANZ. The Food Standards contain information about many aspects of food safety and food handling.

10.1.4 Food safety

HAZARDS AND RISKS

A hazard is something that has a risk of harm attached to it. Hazards exist in many work activities, including food preparation. Like other diseases, food-borne diseases can make people very sick and may even result in death among some older people. Microorganisms such as bacteria, viruses and fungi can cause illness and infection. Microorganisms that are harmful are called pathogens. Pathogens are discussed in detail in Chapter 16.

Pathogens are hazards and the associated risks include sickness, disease and death. Hazard control and risk minimisation are essential to prevent food-borne illness. Pathogens are transmitted between people in various ways, the most common of which are air-borne, droplet and contact transmission. People can breathe in, absorb and swallow infectious agents.

AIR-BORNE DISEASES

Air-borne diseases are those that are transmitted to other people through coughing, sneezing or even laughing. The pathogens are carried in the air where breathing space is shared. Air-borne pathogens can travel a reasonable distance if the environment permits, such as air circulating in air-conditioning systems. A sneeze from an uncovered mouth may travel up to eight metres, suspending droplet particles in the air for a short time before they evaporate, while heavier droplets fall to the ground to contaminate surfaces, equipment and sometimes food.

FOOD-BORNE DISEASES

Food-borne diseases (also known as food-borne illnesses or food poisoning) occur when an individual consumes contaminated food or fluids. Signs and symptoms of food-borne disease will depend on the type of pathogen, but may include:

- nausea
- vomiting
- diarrhoea

- headache and body aches
- changes in kidney function
- changes in liver function
- fatigue and confusion.

Food can become contaminated by microorganisms such as bacteria, viruses, toxins, fungi and parasites at any point between the origin of the food and its consumption. Food products go through different processes before they are ready for consumption, including harvesting and collecting, cleaning, sorting, packaging, storing, delivery, preparation and serving. The food supply chain is regulated by legislation in Australia; however, contamination can occur at any point in the chain.

Common food-borne diseases that may be found in aged care facilities and in the community are described in Table 10.2.

TABLE 10.2 Common food-borne diseases

Pathogen/disease	Transmission	Symptoms
Campylobacter (bacteria)	• Consuming contaminated food • Poor hygiene techniques when handling raw chicken • Drinking untreated water • Poor hygiene after touching pets/farm animals (in pet therapy) • Person-to-person spread • Drinking unpasteurised milk	Gastroenteritis symptoms: • nausea/vomiting • diarrhoea (may contain blood or mucus) • abdominal cramping • fever
Cryptosporidiosis (caused by Cryptosporidium parasites)	• Contaminated water • Person-to-person spread (from poor hygiene, including hand hygiene) • Contained in faeces of infected people and animals • Touching pets/animals and not washing hands	Gastroenteritis symptoms: • watery and profuse diarrhoea • nausea/vomiting • abdominal cramping
Listeriosis (bacteria)	• Eating contaminated chilled ready-to-eat foods such as processed meats, unpasteurised milk and other dairy products, prepared salads, cooked diced chicken and soft cheeses	• Mostly mild gastrointestinal symptoms • Can lead to meningitis (infection of the lining of the brain) and septicaemia (blood poisoning)
Noroviruses (group of viruses)	• Eating contaminated food • Swallowing microscopic air-borne particles of vomit • Touching contaminated surfaces, then touching the mouth • Poor hand hygiene	Gastroenteritis symptoms: • nausea/vomiting • diarrhoea • abdominal cramping • fever
Salmonellosis (Salmonella infection) (bacteria)	• Eating contaminated food • Eating undercooked food • Person-to-person spread (from poor toilet hygiene and poor hand hygiene)	Gastroenteritis symptoms: • nausea/vomiting • diarrhoea • abdominal cramping • fever
Shigellosis (Shigella infection) (bacteria)	• Poor personal hygiene • Carried by flies • Eating contaminated food • Direct (touch) and indirect (e.g. chopping board) • Poor hand hygiene	Gastroenteritis symptoms: • nausea/vomiting • diarrhoea (may contain blood or mucus) • abdominal cramping • fever

Food contamination can also occur when chemicals are present in food from equipment and surfaces that have cleaning and other chemicals on them. Most agricultural pesticides are used under strict regulatory guidelines in Australia; however, fruits and vegetables should be washed before use to prevent ingestion of some pesticides.

Within the context of aged care services, most food-borne illness arises from workers' practices that may involve poor hygiene, not using appropriate equipment and personal protective equipment (PPE), inadequate food heating and other food preparation processes, the use of contaminated food utensils and food sourced from unsafe suppliers. RACFs have strict rules and recommendations about food that is brought into the facility by carers and families for loved ones. They can provide information about what types of food are safe to bring into the facility and how to keep the food at the appropriate temperature in transit between home and the facility.

In the community aged care sector, the risk of food contamination in the person's home can increase if the older person doesn't understand the principles of food safety. Care workers can provide valuable information about food safety in the community, such as recommending how to use designated food equipment to minimise contamination of foods and explaining the risks associated with using out-of-date foods. It is important to note that the care worker can also contaminate the older person's food and food preparation environment if they have poor hand and personal hygiene.

Many infectious diseases are transmitted via direct transmission, so touching objects and items in the environment that are contaminated can cause cross-contamination of the infectious agent. If you are infectious, you can contaminate the environment, and if the environment is infectious, it can contaminate you.

INFECTIOUS DISEASES

Many food-borne illnesses will only affect the person who ingested the contaminated food or water; however, some food-borne diseases are contagious. Noroviruses are a group of viruses that cause gastroenteritis (gastro). They present a high risk of transmission among older people. People living in a communal environment such as an RACF or a respite cottage are at higher risk of being infected by a norovirus. The close proximity and shared spaces create infection control and prevention challenges for nursing and care staff. Noroviruses are transmitted via direct contact with contaminated surfaces, such as equipment and objects in the person's immediate environment, and can also be transmitted if a person swallows microscopic particles of vomit or diarrhoea when caring for a person with the virus.

The ongoing practices of standard precautions are increased to include transmission-based precautions when gastroenteritis is present in RACFs. This involves the use of increased hand hygiene practices and the use of PPE. An outbreak plan for gastro is a compliance component of all government-funded RACFs and is aimed at preventing and managing an outbreak of gastroenteritis among consumers (residents).

There are other infectious diseases that contaminate food and water and can ultimately make people very unwell. For example, hepatitis A, a food-borne illness, causes an acute infection of the liver. This virus is present in the blood and faeces of the infected person and can be transmitted via direct contact. Handwashing is essential to prevent the spread of infection of hepatitis A. Some parasites that cause infection from ingesting contaminated food or water can also be contagious. These parasites live in the faeces of infected people and can be passed on with contact from contaminated hands.

DIRT, WASTE, GREASE AND PESTS

Dirt can contaminate food and water, as it may come in contact with food such as fruits and vegetables. When washing fruits and vegetables, it is important to ensure that any microscopic dirt particles are removed. Unwashed produce grown in soil may pose a risk of food contamination if the soil is contaminated with heavy metals or toxic substances.

Waste needs to be disposed of correctly, according to an organisation's policies and procedures, as contamination can occur if waste matter comes in contact with food. Waste receptacles need to be cleaned according to cleaning protocols to minimise the risk of contamination.

Greases and lubricants used in ovens, dishwashers and other food preparation equipment are also a potential hazard for food contamination. As such, all lubricants and greases use in a food-processing or preparation environment must be food-grade lubricants.

Insects such as flies and cockroaches, and rodents such as mice and rats, can contaminate food and food-related equipment and surfaces. Flies and cockroaches can spread bacteria to food, and the droppings of rodents can contaminate food and water with pathogens that cause serious disease in people. Rodents also carry infection indirectly when they shed ticks and lice that exist on their bodies.

Foreign bodies can contaminate food and are often discovered by chance. Inanimate objects such as band-aid dressings and fingernails can also find their way inadvertently into food. These events are highly avoidable when the food safety legislation is complied with.

FOOD SAFETY LEGISLATION AND GUIDELINES

Legislation and guidelines provide a framework for safe work practices to ensure the risk of food contamination and food-borne disease is minimal. They enable organisations to develop safe food-handling policies and procedures that can be incorporated into safe food practices in the workplace.

Food Standards Australia and New Zealand is the peak body for food safety legislation and guidance in Australia. The organisation developed the Food Standards Code, which contains the Food Standards. The states and territories are responsible for enforcing the Food Standards through various institutions such as health departments, food authorities and councils. The Food Safety Standards include:

- Standard 3.2.1, "Food Safety Programs"
- Standard 3.2.2, "Food Safety Practices and General Requirements"
- Standard 3.2.3, "Food Premises and Equipment"
- Standard 3.3.1, "Food Safety Programs for Food Service to Vulnerable Persons".

Standards 3.2.1, "Food Safety Programs", and 3.3.1, "Food Safety Programs for Food Service to Vulnerable Persons", require RACFs and aged care day services that prepare meals to have a food safety plan in place. The food safety plan must show how the organisation manages risk around food handling, including hazard identification, risk control and monitoring of risk controls. The organisation must be able to demonstrate, on being audited, the records associated with the program. The food safety program addresses aspects of food safety that include:

- receipt of food and the temperature of received food from suppliers
- storage of food
- transport of food
- further processing of food
- thawing of food
- prevention of cross-contamination, including equipment and utensil use, personal hygiene and waste disposal
- support programs that include maintenance, cleaning and sanitation, and pest control programs. Other support programs include staff training, internal audits and food recall programs.

Organisations in New South Wales that provide food services to vulnerable people are required to have a licence under the Vulnerable Persons Food Safety Scheme of the NSW Food Regulation 2015. An overarching legislation related to food safety, the Regulation sits under the *Food Act 2003* (NSW). This legislation states the requirements for all things related to food safety, such as licensing requirements of food services, the training and assessing criteria for food safety certificates and qualifications, and expectations of how nutritional content is displayed on food packaging.

Another risk management tool is the Hazard Analysis and Critical Control Points (HACCP) assessment plan. The HACCP identifies seven important principles in food safety that focus on hazard identification, risk control and monitoring of the implemented control measures that minimise risk. Record keeping is also an important aspect of the HACCP. The Australian Institute of Food Safety offers a HACCP Food Safety Plan kit to provide support to organisations to introduce the HACCP risk management system into their business.

STORAGE

Food needs to be stored in a way that prevents contamination and is suitable for the product. Different storage areas will be required for various food types. Some foods require refrigeration and others require dry storage. Standard 3.2.2, "Food Safety Practices and General Requirements", provides guidance on correct storage procedures, recommending compliance with ensuring that food is stored in the correct environment and under temperature control.

TEMPERATURE CHECKS AND RECORDS

Some foods are potentially hazardous, such as those that are required to be kept at specific temperatures to prevent the growth of pathogens and toxins in the food. Potentially hazardous food includes:

- raw meats, cooked meats and food containing meat
- dairy products and foods containing dairy products
- seafood and food containing seafood
- processed fruits and vegetables
- cooked rice and pasta (FSANZ 2021).

RACFs are required to demonstrate that their food safety plan includes temperature control checks and to produce records of the various temperature checks they perform. Temperature checks (or logs) may occur for refrigerators and heating devices, to ensure that foods are stored, prepared and cooked according to safe food practices.

Cold food must stay cold, and hot food must stay hot, to minimise food contamination. Cold hazardous food should be kept at 5°C or colder, and hot hazardous food kept at 60°C or hotter, within a four-hour time frame. A two-hour/four-hour guide can be applied to food that is ready to be consumed (see Figure 10.1). Bacteria can develop quickly between 5°C and 60°C, and food that is left within this zone can become unsafe after four hours. Any ready-to-eat food must be consumed within two hours in the danger zone or be returned to the safe zone (5°C for cold food and 60°C for hot food). The food must be consumed within two to four hours, otherwise it must be discarded.

All food that is cooked to serve must be cooked at the required temperatures according to the type of food, with a required internal temperature that can be measured using a thermometer. The two-hour/four-hour guide applies to food that has been cooked and is ready to be plated and served.

FIGURE 10.1 The two-hour/four-hour guide for safe food consumption

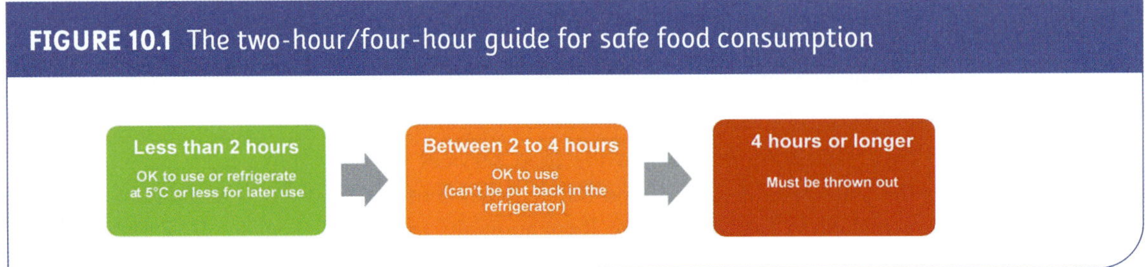

Source: The 2-hour/4-hour rule, NSW Food Authority, Newington, accessed 16 February 2022 © State of New South Wales through the NSW Food Authority, www.foodauthority.nsw.gov.au

GUIDELINES FOR REHEATING

Food that is to be reheated can only be done so once. According to the Food Standards, any food that is to be reheated must be reheated to a temperature of 60°C and kept at this temperature until served. Food that is reheated must be used within 48 hours and any leftover foods that have been reheated must be discarded.

CLEANING AND SANITISING EQUIPMENT AND SURFACES

The organisation's food safety plan will address how food-related equipment and surfaces are cleaned and sanitised. It is a requirement under Food Standard 3.2.2 that items that may come in contact with food must be cleaned and sanitised. Equipment and surfaces should be cleaned of grease, dirt and food remnants and then sanitised to destroy microorganisms. Cleaning involves washing the equipment or surfaces with warm water and detergent, followed by a rinse of warm water. Sanitising can be achieved by using a commercial-grade sanitiser or a dishwasher with a sanitising setting. Each organisation will have its own protocol for cleaning and sanitising equipment.

HAND HYGIENE AND PPE

Hand hygiene is important for reducing the risk of contamination of food. Workers such as kitchen staff and care workers who are in contact with the food that older people consume can minimise the risk of food contamination by frequent and effective handwashing. Many pathogenic microorganisms are transmitted by contact and are present on the many surfaces and objects within the organisation. The poor hand hygiene of workers will often result in severe illness for older people if they consume contaminated food.

Personal protective equipment is essential to prevent food contamination by workers. Those who are in the direct role of food preparation are required to wear PPE such as:

- hairnets to prevent hair from contaminating food
- gloves to prevent food contamination
- eye protection to prevent cleaning chemicals from splashing the eyes
- aprons to cover the torso
- beard snoods to cover beards.

PPE is an important component of personal hygiene measures required by food handlers, and the organisation's food safety plan will provide information about mandatory PPE and personal hygiene protocols to minimise risk of food contamination.

ORGANISATIONAL POLICIES AND PROCEDURES

Policies and procedures are written in alignment with legislation and regulations, and they provide workers with the tools to do their job ethically and legally. Policies and procedures support the food safety plan within the workplace and provide guidance on all aspects of food handling.

Care workers who work in any aged care setting can access the policies and procedures to seek clarification about particular food safety-related tasks, or they can ask for clarification from the RN or their supervisor.

10.1.5 Nutrition

Every cell in the human body requires air, food and water to survive and to function. The food we consume needs to address the nutritional needs of the body, and illness can ensue when insufficient or excessive nutrients are consumed. Not all food and drinks contain nutrients; eating these types of foods can affect our health and wellbeing by increasing the risk of obesity, cardiovascular disease and diabetes.

Our eating patterns are influenced by factors such as culture, socioeconomic circumstances, geographical residence and convenience. **Food security** is a daily challenge for some Australians due to geographical isolation, homelessness and social isolation.

FOOD GROUPS

To obtain optimal nutrition, we need to eat food from all nutritional food groups. These are:

- vegetables
- grains (cereals) that are high in fibre and preferably wholemeal/wholegrain
- lean meats and poultry, fish, eggs, tofu, nuts and seeds, and legumes/beans
- fruit
- milk, yoghurt and cheese (preferably reduced fat).

Nutrition Australia's Healthy Eating Pyramid is a well-known visual representation of the food groups that have nutritional value. It also illustrates the proportion of each food group that we should eat daily. The base layer of the pyramid contains the foods that should make up most of our daily diet—that is, plant foods. See https://nutritionaustralia.org/fact-sheets/healthy-eating-pyramid.

The Australian Dietary Guidelines were developed by the National Health and Medical Research Council with Commonwealth government funding. The guidelines provide information and advice about healthy eating that supports individuals and health professionals to make informed decisions about the food types they consume. The guidelines don't include specialty nutritional requirements that may be needed for specific medical conditions and illnesses. The *Australian Guide to Healthy Eating* is illustrated in Figure 10.2.

NUTRITIONAL NEEDS IN THE OLDER PERSON

We should continue to eat from the healthy food groups as we age in order to meet the specific nutritional needs of growing old. Older people need around 70 per cent more calcium than they did when they were younger (Klemm 2020) to ensure bone health and to prevent or manage osteoporosis. Vitamin D is also essential for bone health. While all older people need extra calcium and vitamin D, older women need more than men. A diet that is high in fibre and includes adequate water intake can prevent constipation in older people. Wholemeal bread, wholegrains, fruit and dried fruit can help prevent constipation.

Weight management is important for older people to support ongoing mobility and dexterity. Obesity can affect musculoskeletal conditions such as arthritis by increasing the impact of weight on inflamed joints. The risk of cardiovascular conditions and chronic diseases such as diabetes can be reduced with a healthy diet and weight that is within the healthy range.

Older people have a lower metabolism and require smaller meals than younger people; however, their meals need to be nutritionally dense.

THE IMPACT OF NUTRITION ON WELLBEING

Eating a healthy and nutritious diet not only supports good physical health, it also supports our psychosocial wellbeing. Good mental health is important for enjoyment of life and enables us to live our best life, achieve our goals and feel valued by others.

Eating patterns can be directly related to mood, and this can have a positive or negative impact on physical health. Depression and other mental health conditions can result in making poor food choices, or not eating at all. It is important to recognise when the older person shows signs that indicate their mental health is changing, so they can be provided with the support they need.

Eating well can have a positive impact on our wellbeing. Nutritionally balanced diets can improve sleep patterns and energy levels. The effects of food on mental wellbeing are an ongoing research topic globally. What is known is that some food types improve wellbeing and others can lead to worsening mental health. For example, a deficiency in many of the B group vitamins can result in poor concentration, irritability and even depression (Mental Health Foundation, UK 2017) while a deficiency in vitamin D may contribute to the signs and symptoms of dementia as well as poor sleep.

Eating has historically been, and remains, an activity that is associated with socialising. Sharing a meal or a drink with friends can improve the wellbeing of individuals and offer a sense of belonging and connection to others.

FIGURE 10.2 Australian Guide to Healthy Eating

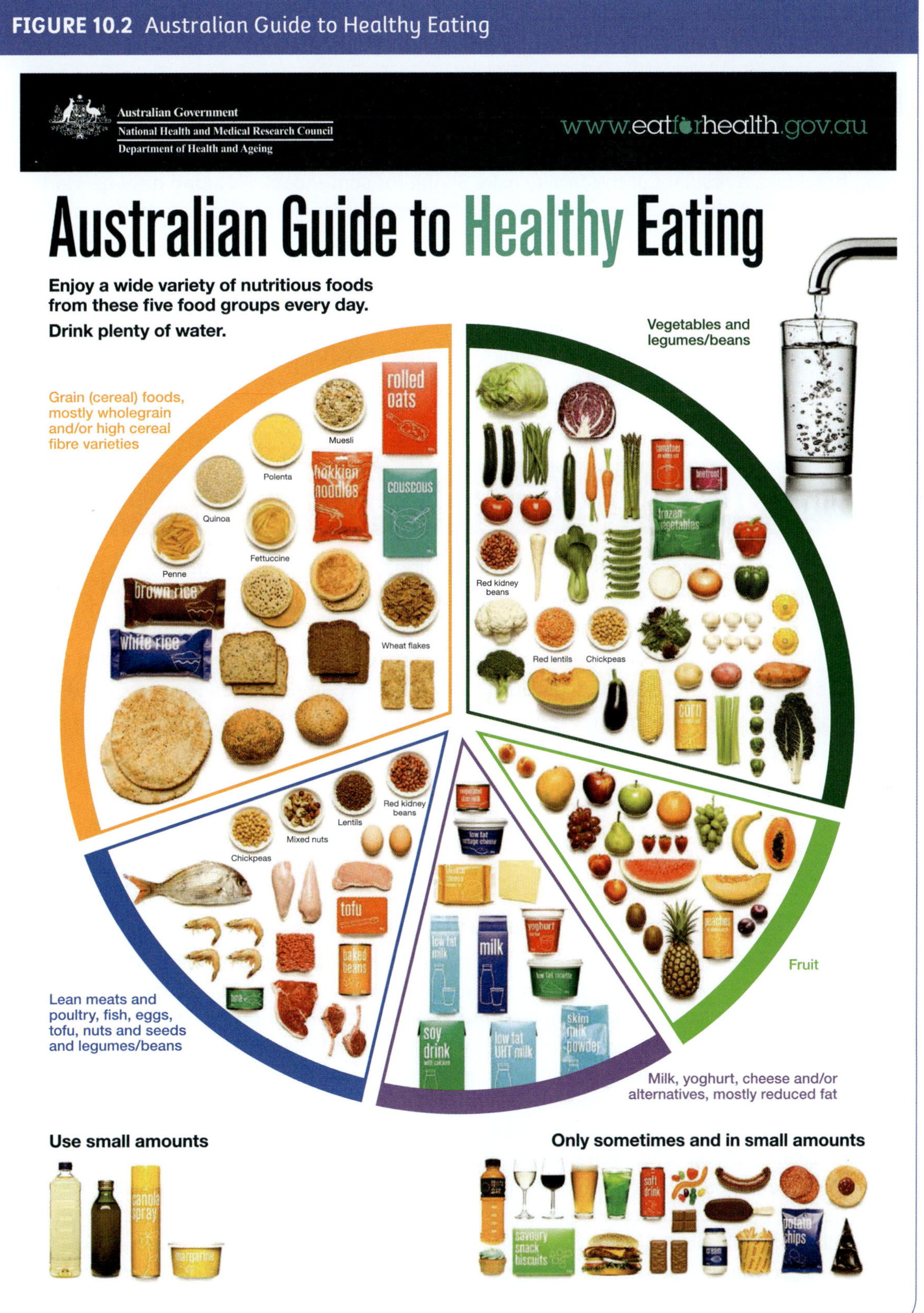

Source: National Health and Medical Research Council CC BY 4.0, https://creativecommons.org/licenses/by/4.0/

WORKPLACE SCENARIO

The importance of understanding individual needs and preferences

Sharni, a care worker who works for an aged care staffing agency, has accepted a day shift at an RACF. During breakfast, a resident at the facility asks Sharni for some toast. Not long after he starts eating, he starts gagging and choking. One of the care staff provides first aid and succeeds in removing the toast from his airway.

Sharni is required to have a meeting with the RN, who informs her that the resident has severe dysphagia due to Huntington's disease and that his care plan specifically states he cannot eat toast safely. Sharni, while shaken from the event, realises how important it is to ask for clarification about food requests, or to check the person's care plan, in order to keep them safe.

CHECK YOUR UNDERSTANDING

1. What are some considerations for safe and individualised meal planning?
2. List three signs or symptoms of food-borne illness.
3. Some foods, such as raw and cooked meats and seafoods, are potentially hazardous when consumed at the wrong temperatures. Why is temperature control important for food safety?
4. What are the five nutritional food groups that, together, comprise a healthy eating pattern?
5. Why do older people need to consume a nutrient-dense diet?

10.2 SERVING MEALS

10.2.1 Roles and responsibilities

The responsibilities of care workers who support older people with food planning and preparation in community aged care services are very different from those who work in RACFs. Community-based care workers are responsible for ensuring they follow the person's care plan and the organisational policies and procedures in the context of food services. In-home meal planning and preparation services that care workers may be responsible for include assisting the person to purchase, store and prepare healthy meals. Following safe work practices to minimise food contamination in the home is essential, along with diligent hand hygiene and personal hygiene. Organisations that provide these services may have information, such as brochures and pamphlets, about safe food handling available to offer service users.

The roles and responsibilities around food preparation in an RACF involve many people; however, the kitchen staff are the ones who are responsible for cooking and preparing the food the residents eat. These staff are also responsible for following the organisation's food plan and policies and procedures to minimise risk with food handling and preparation. Kitchen workers will plate the meal when prepared for serving. Not all older people who reside in an RACF will choose to eat meals in a communal dining area. Some older people may require a meal tray that is prepared and delivered to their room by kitchen staff.

The responsibilities of the care worker in an RACF in the context of meal service include:

- following all policies and procedures relevant to food safety
- assisting the person with opening packets if they cannot do this on their own
- serving meals to the dining table
- assisting the person into a comfortable position to enjoy their meal from their meal tray
- organising the meal tray for the person if they are unable to put milk on their cereal, butter their toast, etc.
- observing the person during meals for any difficulties, such as chewing or swallowing problems
- reporting concerns about the person to the RN or the supervisor and following their instructions
- attending to documentation relevant to food service, such as writing progress/case notes, filling out incident forms and fluid balance charts, and completing other assessment forms
- providing assistance to the person with eating while maintaining their dignity
- knowing the first-aid procedure for choking.

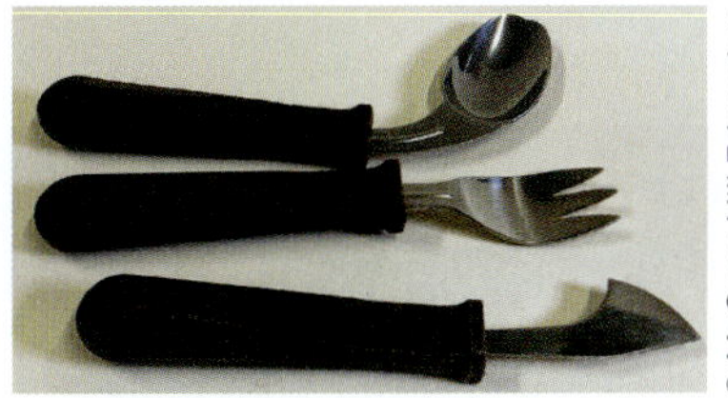

Modified cutlery

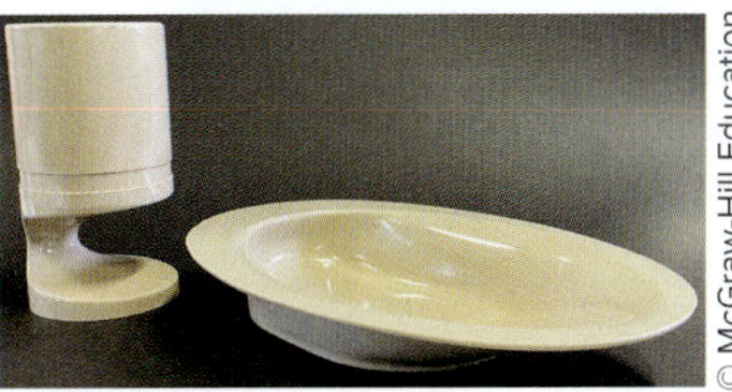

Modified plates and bowls

10.2.2 Equipment

There are many reasons why an older person may require assistance with eating and drinking, including visual impairment, certain chronic diseases and some other medical conditions. For example, the person may have difficulty using cutlery or drinking from a wide-mouthed cup due to weakness or facial paralysis.

Adaptive or modified equipment can assist the older person to maintain independence with eating and drinking and support their dignity. This type of equipment includes the following assistive devices:

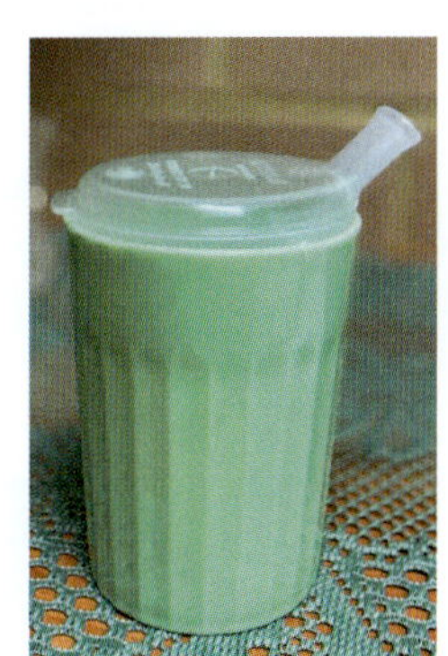

Cup with spout

- Modified cutlery is designed to enable the person to grip the handles more easily, as they are thicker or specifically shaped and require less dexterity to use. Some modified cutlery is curved to support people with getting food to their mouth when they have limited mobility in their arm or wrist.
- Modified plates and bowls are shaped to enable the person to scoop the food without it spilling over. These plates and bowls may have a detachable “lip” that provides a buffer for cutlery, enabling the person to load the cutlery with food. Other types of plates and bowls are an all-in-one-design and are moulded to achieve the same effect. This equipment is helpful for people who have limited movement and dexterity due to stroke or another neurological condition.
- Cups with spouts are helpful for people whose mouth is unable to form a seal correctly, due to facial paralysis or another structural change. Spouts may also benefit those with dementia who have forgotten how to use a cup or how to suck from a straw. The care worker can assist the person to drink safely and in a controlled manner using a spout.
- Clothing protectors protect the person’s clothing from food and drink spillage at mealtimes. Spillage may occur due to poor coordination, tremors

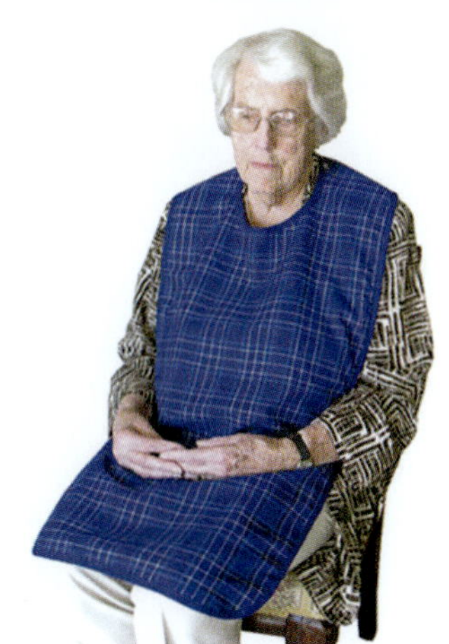

Clothing protector

and other health-related reasons. Clothing protectors may also be used when the person requires a care worker to provide full assistance (feeding) with their meals. Clothing protectors are usually made of towelling cloth and are washed after use, although some people prefer to use disposable ones.

PRACTICE POINT

Clothing protectors must not be referred to as "bibs", as this term can be interpreted as condescending. Older people do not wear bibs; they use clothing protectors.

10.2.3 Distributing meals

In an RACF, meal distribution is scheduled for specific times. The catering and kitchen staff work to a strict routine and a set schedule to ensure that all residents receive regular and healthy meals each day. People who reside in an RACF receive breakfast, morning tea, lunch, afternoon tea, dinner and supper, and each meal is prepared according to their individual needs.

A menu is planned in advance and residents can select from it daily. Meal sizes in aged care vary according to the person's care plan and are overall more than enough to meet their nutritional needs. Breakfasts often include a hot meal option or a continental breakfast of cereal, toast and fruit, and a hot meal is served at lunchtime and includes desert. The evening meal often includes sandwiches, soup and desert, or light meals such as salads and pasta.

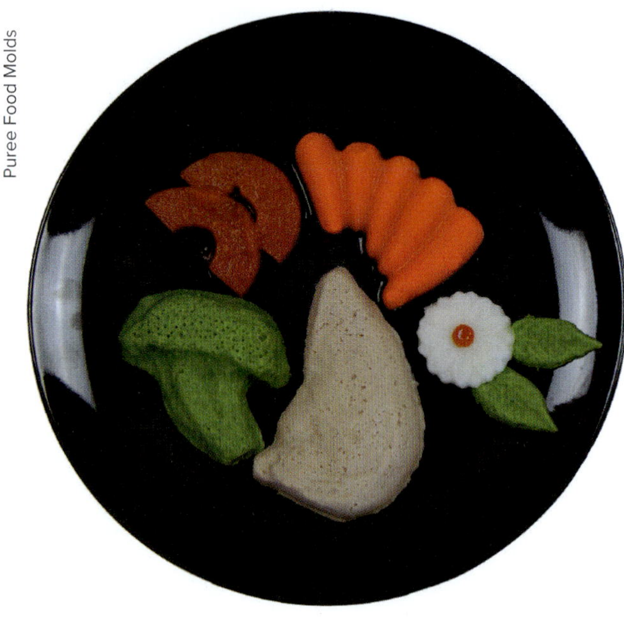

Puree Food Molds

Some facilities use moulds to enhance the look of pureed food

10.2.4 Meal presentation

Eating is a sensory experience, and the way food looks and smells can have a direct impact on meal enjoyment. Our sense of smell and taste declines as we age, so food served in aged care services needs to appeal to the older person. It may often include the use of herbs, spices and tasty sauces.

The texture of the meal is important not only for enjoyment but also for safety. **Pureed** or blended food will be presented in scoops or separate servings. For example, potato, carrots, greens and meat will be pureed separately and plated separately into the bowl or onto a plate. Each component has a different colour, smell and taste and offers a positive sensory aspect to eating. It is good practice to ask the person what they would like to try from their meal. It is unacceptable to mix the contents of the bowl into a brown pulpy mess. Mixing pureed meals together is a practice that doesn't promote dignity or choice. Because it is difficult to make pureed food look appetising, some facilities use moulds to change the way the food is viewed.

10.2.5 The importance of culture and social connection

Food has been a strong factor in cultural and social connections for millennia and continues to bring people together for many reasons. It is part of cultural and ethnic identity. Some foods are used ceremonially and ritually in different cultures and religions to initiate, celebrate, worship and mourn. Older people may use food to stay connected to their heritage and the memories that are associated with it, and it is important that aged care services recognise and encourage cultural eating habits and celebrations. Many cultural celebrations occur in aged care services such as RACFs and aged care day programs, including Christmas, Ramadan, Chinese New Year and St Patrick's Day. However, food diversity is not only for specific occasions; individual cultural and religious food preferences must be accommodated in aged care services as required.

10.2.6 The environment

Another aspect of social connection is the environment where meals are eaten. In an RACF, many older people choose to eat meals in a communal dining room. Generally, people join a table with others who they get on with; however, not everyone gets on all the time with other residents in aged care services. Conflict is to be expected when many personalities live in a shared environment. Care workers can make observations about the relationships among residents, especially in the dining room, and should report concerns about any altercations to the RN.

An environment conducive to eating will support the social wellbeing of diners. The following strategies may help to achieve such an environment.

- Reduce noise levels by turning off televisions and radios during mealtimes (or reducing their volume).
- Offer choices that promote diners' agency and dignity.
- Staff should speak in low voices.
- Display a menu board or daily specials board for ambiance.
- Offer table settings that reflect the age group of diners.
- Ensure that meals are unhurried.

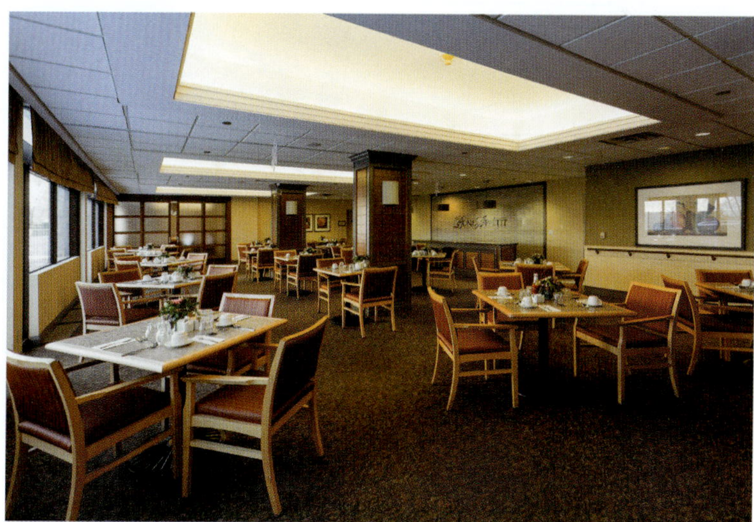

Derek Trask/Alamy Stock Photo

Many older people prefer to eat their meals in the communal dining room

Eating is a social and enjoyable experience and meals are often something that older people look forward to during the day.

10.2.7 Providing assistance during mealtimes

The type of assistance required during mealtimes will differ among individuals based on their specific needs and preferences. The person's care plan will provide care workers with the information they need to be able to provide appropriate mealtime assistance. Care workers also need to provide a safe and comfortable environment for meals. The person may require assistance with physical positioning to minimise risk of choking, or they may need to be positioned at the dining table in their wheelchair. Figure 10.3 illustrates correct positioning at the dining table.

Many older people receiving aged care services will not require any assistance with meals, while others will require full assistance such as feeding. When feeding a person their meal, always be respectful. Offer them a clothing protector, sit opposite them, and allow them enough time between mouthfuls to swallow

FIGURE 10.3 Correct positioning at the dining table when eating

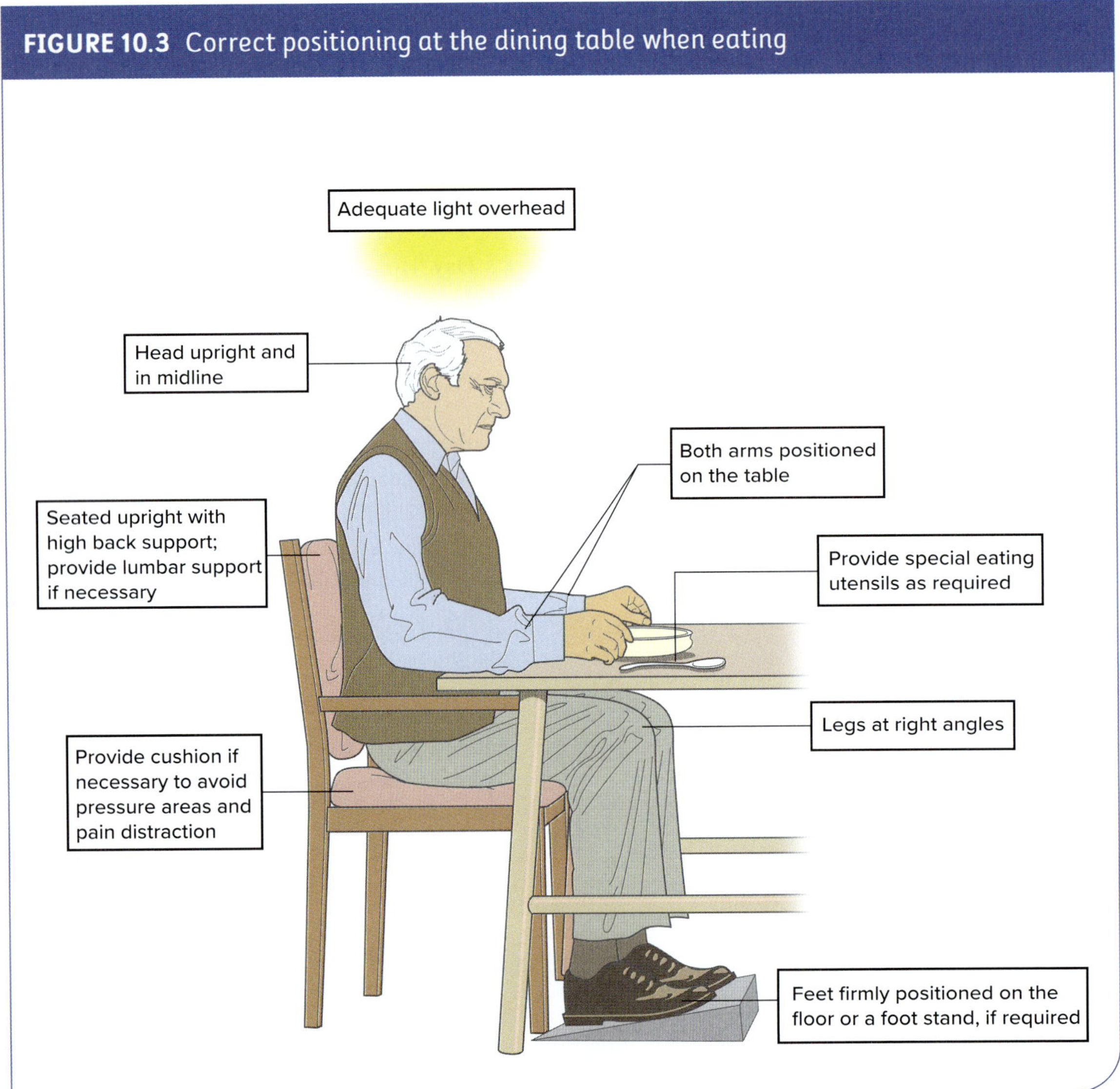

Note: Not all older people are comfortable or physically capable of sitting in this position. Always refer to the person's care plan for information that meets the person's needs and preferences for positioning at mealtimes.

safely. Always ask the person what they would like to eat next from their meal, even if they have dementia or another cognitive condition. Always ensure to remove clothing protectors after meals and ensure the person is clean and tidy. (They may require assistance to wipe their face or wash their hands.)

Maintaining the older person's dignity and independence is at the core of providing them with support. Some older people who eat independently may take a long time to complete their meal, or they may spill their meal onto themselves or onto the table or floor. The more often a worker intervenes for the sake of tidiness and timeliness, the more dependent the person will become. It is important to note that these actions can also contribute to the older person feeling embarrassed and devalued. Regardless of the type of assistance required, it is essential always to ensure the person has choice and that their dignity is preserved.

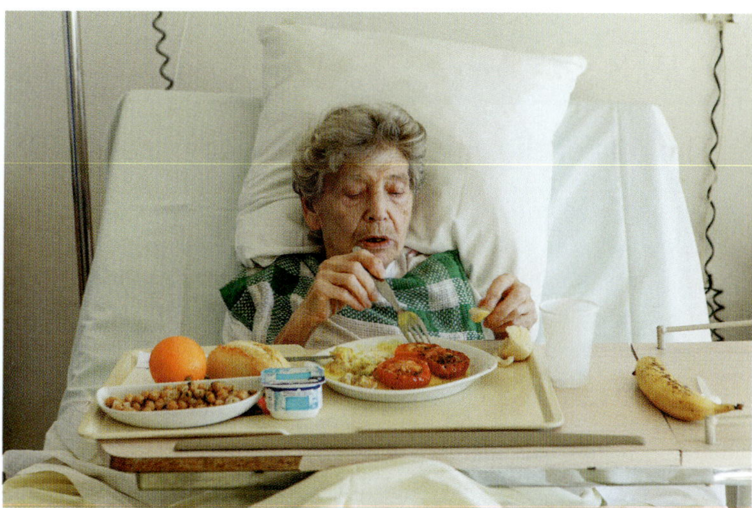

The type of assistance required during mealtimes depends on the individual

10.2.8 Collection and cleaning procedures

When assisting residents in the dining room, care workers can serve them meals, top up their drinks, and observe them for any possible eating issues. When the person has finished their meal, the care worker can collect their plate and cutlery and scrape leftovers into a waste container. Often, a trolley is set aside to collect dirty plates and cutlery for the kitchen staff to collect after completion of meals. The organisation's policies and procedures will direct how this process occurs in a safe manner, according to the food safety plan.

Meal trays are usually collected by kitchen staff and placed onto a trolley to be wheeled to the kitchen for cleaning. Sometimes, care workers will be required to collect cups and cutlery after hours when there are no kitchen staff on shift. The workplace has protocols for how this occurs, including how leftover foods and waste are managed and the cleaning procedure that should be followed.

10.2.9 Organisational policies for reporting changes to food and fluid preferences and intake

Sometimes, an older person's nutritional needs may change, along with the type of assistance they require at mealtimes. These changes may be a direct result of medical conditions and incidents and include:

- a diagnosis of diabetes that requires a diabetic diet
- a diagnosis of coeliac disease that requires elimination of gluten from the diet
- a deterioration of heart function that requires strict fluid restriction and salt reduction
- a neurological incident that affects the swallowing process, such as a stroke.

Many of these changes occur progressively, while some are spontaneous occurrences. Care workers are often the first people to notice that something is different about the older person in many contexts, including if the person is having difficulty chewing or swallowing, or if they are showing other signs of dysphagia, such as coughing when they eat. In the first instance, the care worker must stop the person from eating and report their observations to the RN. Reporting your observations is the first step in the person accessing an assessment for changing needs.

Policies and procedures will direct care workers and other staff on the requirements for reporting changes related to food and fluid intake. When an older person has had a dietary change based on assessment procedures, the care plan is updated by the RN, or the supervisor if working in in-home care. This information is also documented in the person's progress or case notes and is shared among relevant staff during handover procedures and via other communication platforms. Kitchen staff are also informed of the changes to ensure a continuum of awareness about the person's needs, to minimise risk.

WORKPLACE SCENARIO

The role of the care worker at mealtimes

Jeremy, a community care worker, is scheduled to assist Mr Duncan with preparing his evening meals. Mr Duncan lives independently, with in-home support three days a week. Today, Jeremy is assisting Mr Duncan to make spaghetti bolognaise. Jeremy is careful to follow safe food-handling practices, such as hand hygiene and surface preparation protocols.

After the meal is cooked, Mr Duncan wants to leave it on the stovetop until the morning because he feels very tired. He says he will portion it into containers in the morning for freezing. Jeremey knows that the bolognaise is a potentially hazardous food if left out. He explains to Mr Duncan that the meal should be portioned and placed in the freezer immediately, because of the risk of bacterial contamination. Before he leaves, Jeremy assists Mr Duncan to complete his meal preparation, cleans the kitchen according to safe food practices and documents the incident in Mr Duncan's case notes.

CHECK YOUR UNDERSTANDING

1. List five responsibilities of the care worker in the context of the provision of meal services in an RACF.
2. Identify and describe one type of assistive device that is used for eating or drinking.
3. List three ways the environment can support a happy, social and enjoyable eating experience.
4. Where can the care worker obtain documented clarification about the older person's mealtime needs?
5. What should a care worker do if they notice an older person is having difficulty eating?

10.3 UNDERSTANDING SPECIAL CONSIDERATIONS

10.3.1 Dysphagia

Many older people have dysphagia and are at risk of choking or aspiration. Dysphagia means the person has difficulty swallowing food normally due to medical conditions such as a stroke, cancer or a progressive neurological condition like dementia. Food can be prepared in various textures to minimise the risk of choking or aspiration, and the care plan will reflect the specific food textures an individual requires. A speech pathologist assesses for dysphagia and prescribes modified food and fluid textures.

The degree of food and fluid modification will vary among individuals based on their risk factors for choking and aspiration. The International Dysphagia Diet Standardisation Initiative (IDDSI) provides a universal framework for describing the different textures of food and drinks that are used for dysphagia. The IDDSI provides terminology and descriptions of modified foods and thickened fluids that can be used internationally, therefore minimising risk to people with dysphagia. For more information on the IDDSI framework, see https://iddsi.org/framework.

10.3.2 Allergies, food intolerances and specific nutritional needs

Individual needs regarding food and fluid types can be influenced by allergies, food intolerances and other nutritional needs.

FOOD ALLERGIES

Allergens are substances in foods, such as some proteins and food additives, that are harmless to the majority of people, but which can trigger an allergic response in others. An allergic reaction occurs when an allergen triggers the immune response in the body, causing anything from a mild allergic reaction (such as hives) to a life-threatening allergic reaction called **anaphylaxis**, which requires an adrenalin injection from an EpiPen to prevent death. Food labelling must list ingredients that can be allergens.

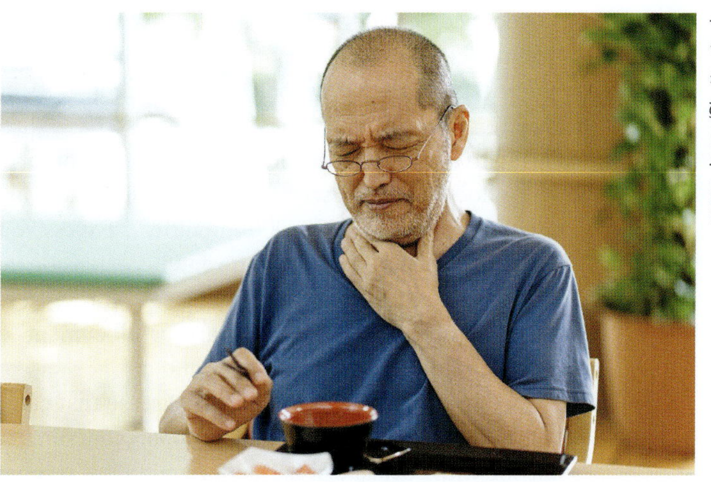

mapo_japan/Shutterstock

While some people with dysphagia may show signs that they are experiencing difficulties swallowing, others may not show any signs at all

FOOD INTOLERANCE

Food intolerance occurs when the body cannot manage components of the food normally. Different from allergy, a food intolerance may occur when a bodily process is altered in some way. For example, lactose intolerance may occur in people who have diminished amounts of the enzyme needed to break down lactose in the small intestine. (Lactose is a sugar that is found in milk and other dairy products.)

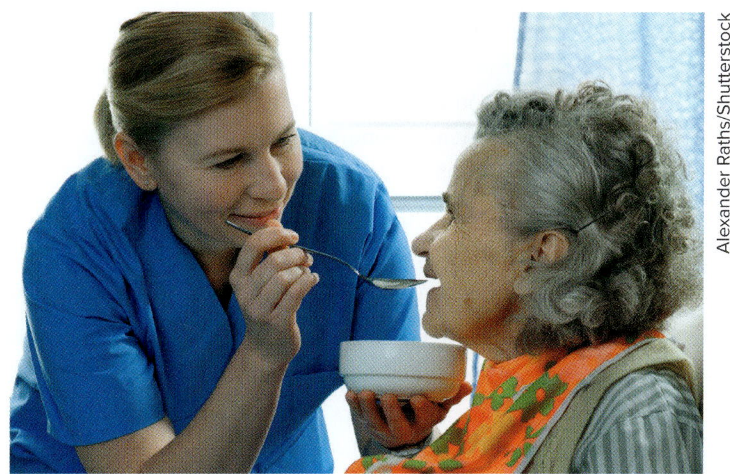

Alexander Raths/Shutterstock

It is important to position the person for safe eating when they are in bed to minimise the risk of choking

SPECIFIC NUTRITIONAL NEEDS

Some people have specific needs that are directly related to nutrition. Some foods or their vitamins and minerals are needed in specific amounts for healthy bodily functioning. For example, iron deficiency can lead to **anaemia**, which in turn can lead to fatigue and falls in older people. Excessively high amounts of some electrolytes, vitamins and minerals can have a critical effect on the body's ability to function properly. Extremely high blood levels of potassium, for instance, can affect the ability of the cells in the heart to function properly.

10.3.3 Health conditions

Chronic health conditions such as diabetes, heart disease, **hypertension** and coeliac disease require careful nutritional and hydration management. Older people with diabetes will most likely require medication or insulin to manage blood sugar levels; however, their diet is key to good diabetes management. Diabetics need a diet that is tailored to their needs by a health professional who understands the nutritional requirements of diabetes. Diabetic diets are generally low in sugars and saturated fats, and high in glycaemic index (GI) carbohydrates.

Carbohydrates are essential for energy, and they break down to become glucose in the blood. The GI describes how quickly this occurs. Carbohydrates that break down quickly are not helpful for managing blood glucose levels and maintaining energy in the body. Low GI carbohydrates such as bread, oats, fresh fruit and pasta convert to glucose at a slower rate, and this has a better impact on blood sugar levels. A person with diabetes should have a personalised nutritional plan that has been developed by a health professional specifically for them based on their particular needs and preferences.

Older people with heart disease and hypertension may have restricted diets and fluid intake on the advice of their doctor. The diet may include a reduction in salt, as salt has a direct effect on storing water in the body, and this can cause problems in the circulatory system when the heart and kidneys may be struggling to function correctly due to disease. Salt also has a direct impact on the cells of the heart, and too much salt can lead to a change in the heart's normal rhythm (arrythmia).

The doctor may prescribe a fluid-restricted diet and specify the maximum volume of fluids the person can consume in a day (e.g. 900 millilitres). Excessive fluid can cause oedema (swelling in the body tissue, including the lungs), kidney failure and hypertension, and fluid restrictions can help the heart to work better by reducing some of the load. Any person who is on a fluid-restricted diet will need to have all their fluids monitored using a fluid balance chart that documents every amount of fluid the person puts into their body, and sometimes every amount they put out.

Coeliac disease is an autoimmune disease that causes the body to have an immune reaction against itself when gluten is ingested. Gluten is a protein contained in wheat, oats, barley and rye. When gluten is eaten by someone with coeliac disease, an inflammatory response in the small intestines occurs, preventing the body absorbing and effectively using nutrients from the diet. People with coeliac disease must adhere to a strict gluten-free diet to prevent this from happening.

10.3.4 Oral health and chewing

Another important consideration when supporting the nutritional needs of older people is their oral health. If the person cannot chew safely, they may be at risk of choking or aspirating food and fluids. Painful gums and other dental conditions can also affect the person's ability to eat properly or routinely. Oral health considerations include the following.

- The person may require assistance with fitting their dentures before they eat.
- Dentures may be ill-fitting or missing.
- Missing teeth can make chewing unsafe; people need time to chew properly before they swallow.
- Mouth and tooth infections can decrease taste and cause pain, making people reluctant to eat.
- People with dementia may not be able to verbalise that they have a painful mouth.
- Some behaviours of concern can result in people not chewing food properly, increasing the risk of choking or aspiration.
- People with Down syndrome chew differently and may have a higher risk of choking or aspiration.
- The older person may have a dry mouth, a condition called xerostomia. Artificial saliva may be required before eating.

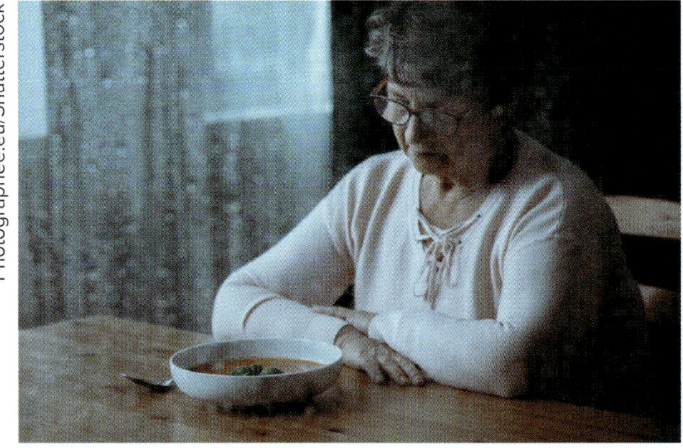

Photographee.eu/Shutterstock

Older people lose their appetite for many reasons

10.3.5 Loss of appetite

Older people lose their appetite for many reasons, including illness, medication side effects, depression and cognitive changes. The person may also have a dental issue or mouth issue that prevents them from wanting to eat. A lack of routine, or an existing routine, may not align with the person's preferences, or they may not like someone they sit with at the dining table. It is important for care workers to notice when older people lose their appetite so that the issue can be identified and addressed. Older people may eat less, but they need a lot of nutrients in the food they do eat. Always report and document your concerns about the person who appears to be losing their appetite.

10.3.6 Dementia-friendly design

Eating and drinking are generally social and pleasurable experiences. Because dementia causes progressive changes in a person's ability to function cognitively, to make decisions and to plan, it can challenge the senses of someone with dementia and alter their perception of the eating experience.

Mealtimes can be designed to provide an environment that reduces challenges for the person with dementia and increases their enjoyment and social connections. The following may be effective strategies:

- A loud and noisy environment can be difficult for people with dementia to cope with. Reduce excessive or loud noise by turning off the television and playing simple music at a low volume that is conducive to creating a relaxed atmosphere.
- Lighting is important, too, as bright fluorescent lighting can add to sensory overload and increase confusion. On the other hand, room lighting should not be so low that it poses a falls risk. Finding a balance is important.
- Some people with dementia will have difficulty with perception of colour, shadow and depth, so the crockery that is used for meals should not be over-patterned or be of a colour that makes it difficult to see the food. For example, it may be difficult for some people with dementia to properly see vanilla ice-cream if it is served in a white bowl. Research indicates that colours that contrast with the food, are helpful, as they improve the visual perception of the food. Plain colours such as blue, yellow and red may also help the person to focus on the food and make it look appealing.
- Dining in a communal area in an RACF can be challenging for people with dementia. Some people may not know what to do and may feel embarrassed, and others will be overwhelmed by the environment. People with dementia are more likely to eat and socialise when the environment is uncrowded, such as in a small dining area or when seated at a table for four.
- Organise or serve meals simply. The person with dementia may not know what to do with a meal tray as their brain has difficulty planning and organising. Care workers should set out the tray for the person in a way they can manage. The care worker might pour the milk onto the cereal or butter the toast, or open packets that the person cannot manage. People eating in dining rooms need adequate time to complete one meal component before another is introduced.
- It is a basic human right to have choice over what we eat, and people with dementia also have this right to choose. Having many menu options can be overwhelming, however. A choice of just two or three options can limit the person's distress and maintain their dignity and sense of inclusion.

The care plan will direct how to support the person. Meal support is never a one-size-fits-most approach for people with dementia, because while the signs, symptoms and stages of progression of the disease are predictable, every person will experience it differently.

10.3.7 Managing contingencies

FOOD REFUSAL

Older people may refuse food for many reasons other than loss of appetite. Strategies to encourage the person to eat include offering frequent snacks instead of meals, changing their routine to encourage socialisation, and supporting them to have a health check-up with their doctor to rule out physical causes for their refusal to eat.

Older people with a life-limiting illness, including dementia, may refuse to eat at end of life. Palliation ensures the person is supported to be comfortable at the end of their life journey and this includes management of symptoms such as nausea and vomiting. At end of life, it is not unusual for an older person to stop eating and drinking. This can be distressing for their family and friends; however, the person's advanced care directive can offer information about their wishes.

FOOD REQUESTS

Have you ever felt like having a late-night snack or maybe changing your usual meal choices? Older people who receive aged care services can feel like this, too, and all attempts must be made to accommodate these requests. Food requests made by people in an RACF need to follow the guidelines of the facility's food safety plan. As a care worker, you may occasionally be required to assist an older person to order a takeaway, or to make them a midnight snack.

Sometimes, food requests are not able to be supported. When they can cause harm to the person or they don't align with their care plan, a different approach is needed. Dignity of risk is aways balanced with duty of care, and careful and considerate conversations may need to occur between the person, their family and the nursing staff.

The following are examples of food requests that have a risk of causing harm to the person:

- People with diabetes may want to eat lollies, desserts and sweet biscuits. This may be manageable occasionally; however, if the person includes these foods as a regular part of their diet, they will become unwell.
- A person who is at risk of choking and aspiration, such as a person with Huntington's disease, may request toast and sandwiches. The risk of choking and death is very high with these foods.
- A person may display behaviours of concern that involve eating constantly and quickly and becoming agitated when they cannot access food. This person will have management strategies in their behaviour support plan to minimise their distress.

Care workers should refer any food requests to the RN or supervisor before acting upon those requests, to determine if it is safe to proceed.

10.3.8 Malnutrition in aged care

Many older people receiving aged care services are malnourished. Malnourishment occurs when the body doesn't receive the nutrients, vitamins and minerals that are essential for optimal health and wellbeing. Older people who are malnourished are prone to illness, take longer to recover from illness, and will progressively have decreased ability to function with their activities of daily living (ADLs). This means that untreated malnourishment can increase the person's dependence on care services and have long-term effects on their physical and emotional wellbeing.

Adequate hydration is also essential to enable bodily processes to occur to sustain health and life; however, many older people are chronically dehydrated and this can contribute to constipation, resulting in the need for aperients. Good nutrition and adequate hydration are essential for older people.

INCIDENCE

While the true number of older people who are malnourished is difficult to quantify, research indicates that malnutrition is very high in RACFs and is also prevalent in the community. Approximately 8 per cent of older Australians living in the community are malnourished, and it is estimated that of those living in RACFs, between 22 and 50 per cent are malnourished (Liotta 2019).

DEFINITIONS

It is important to understand the terminology that may be used around poor nutrition in older people so that you can appreciate the contents of medical reports, and instructions in the care plan by the RN or allied health professionals such as dietitians and speech pathologists. Table 10.3 defines common words used to relate to poor nutrition in older people.

TABLE 10.3 Common terminology used to describe poor nutrition in older people

Term	Definition
Malnutrition	Malnutrition is the term used to describe a condition in which the body hasn't received sufficient nutritional content to optimally maintain health. Malnutrition can also occur in obese older people when the food they consume doesn't contain nutritional value for health.
Undernutrition	The term "undernutrition" is sometimes used interchangeably with "malnutrition". It is a form of malnutrition where the person's intake of protein and kilojoules is insufficient (i.e. they are not eating enough for their body's needs).
Frailty	Malnutrition leads to a medical condition called frailty. A decrease in muscle mass, strength and energy from malnourishment can spiral an older person into a state of frailty. Frailty requires dependence on others for ADLs, and predisposes the person to experience falls, poor healing, pressure injuries and frequent longer hospital stays.
Sarcopenia	Sarcopenia is now recognised in Australia as a disease. It is a musculoskeletal disorder characterised by rapid loss of muscle and muscle function due to the ageing process but accelerated by contributing factors such as malnourishment. Sarcopenia predisposes the person to falls and is associated with frailty.

RISK FACTORS FOR MALNUTRITION

Older people are at high risk of malnutrition for several reasons, and those who live in RACFs are at even higher risk. Many factors that cause malnutrition in older people are preventable; however, some medical causes of malnutrition are unavoidable. The following are some medical risk factors for malnutrition:

- The person's medication may cause nausea, vomiting, vertigo or absorption issues.
- The person has difficulty in swallowing (dysphagia).
- The person has a chronic disease that affects the absorption of nutrients.
- The person has a life-limiting illness with associated symptoms.
- The person is cognitively or psychologically unable to identify when, what and how to eat independently or nutritionally (e.g. due to dementia, grief or depression).

The following are physical and social reasons that put an older person at risk of malnutrition:

- The person is geographically isolated, which can make accessing food difficult.
- Mouth and dental issues such as ill-fitting dentures, missing teeth or painful abscesses make eating difficult.
- The person relies on others to access food and for feeding.
- Staff fail to feed the person or to provide appropriate access to meals (e.g. food trays are left out of reach or are unprepared).
- Water isn't offered throughout the day or extra water isn't accessible on hot days.
- Servings of thickened fluids are not completely consumed.
- Physical disability prevents the person accessing or preparing foods independently.
- The person cannot afford to purchase healthier food items.

THE CONSEQUENCES OF MALNUTRITION

INCREASE IN MORBIDITY

In the context of aged care, **morbidity** refers to chronic or age-related diseases and conditions that can affect the older person's quality of life and life expectancy. Examples of morbidities include heart disease, stroke, depression and lung diseases such as emphysema. "Co-morbidities" refers to the health status of having more than one chronic disease or condition simultaneously. Older people who are malnourished often have co-morbidities such

Niels Kiim/Alamy Stock Photo

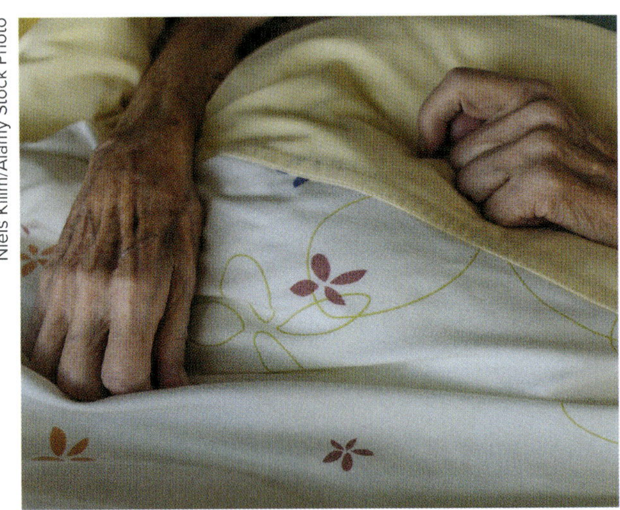

Fatigue and lethargy are common symptoms of malnutrition

as diabetes and obesity. Fatigue and lethargy are common symptoms of malnutrition, as the individual is not receiving precious energy-fuelling nutrients from their diet. The lack of energy can result in falls and a gradual loss of mobility.

INCREASE IN MORTALITY

Mortality refers to death, and morbidity is directly related to mortality. Malnutrition is a risk factor for chronic diseases and conditions such as heart failure, atherosclerosis, stroke and diabetes. Malnutrition also affects the immune system, and the older person has difficulty fighting infection. This can leave them susceptible to chronic and acute infections that may lead to death. A weak cough reflex can also increase the risk of the person developing serious respiratory complications that can result in acute illness and death.

DECREASE IN QUALITY OF LIFE

The person who is malnourished has decreased energy and is prone to infection and illness, as the body loses strength, dexterity and the capacity to fight infection effectively. Over time, the person may lose their mobility, which affects their quality of life. With decreased mobility, they may become incontinent of urine and faeces if they cannot make it to the toilet on time or require assistance to get to the toilet. Poor mobility also leads to pressure injuries, obesity and vascular issues.

Malnutrition leads to increased dependence on others to attend to ADLs, and to the loss of independence and wellbeing. The individual's mental health is also affected by malnutrition, and depression and anxiety may evolve as a consequence of the lack of energy, the development of morbidities, and the loss and grief associated with losing one's ability to care for oneself.

SIGNS OF MALNUTRITION

Some signs of malnutrition in older people may be obvious, while others may be more subtle. As a care worker, your observations are very important in preventing a health issue from evolving into a health crisis or a chronic health condition. Signs of malnutrition that are more obvious may include ill-fitting dentures, loose clothing, unexplained weight loss and dysphagia. Other signs that are related to poor nutrition include fatigue, depression-like symptoms, confusion, pale skin, disinterest in food or eating only small amounts, muscle loss and other changes that are new to the person. Changes in the person's usual bowel regimen can also indicate malnutrition, and ongoing severe constipation may indicate dehydration.

It is important to understand that while malnutrition can contribute to illness, it can also develop as a result of illness. An older person who experiences depression may become malnourished due to their lack of interest in food. Malnourishment can cause fatigue and tiredness, resulting in a low mood that can compound their depression. This can result in a cycle that causes the person's overall physical and mental health to spiral into a loss of independence.

Anna Lurye/Shutterstock

Depression may contribute to malnutrition due to a lack of interest in food

SCREENING

There are validated assessment tools that can assist in determining the person's risk of malnutrition. These tools are helpful in determining a baseline of information about a person's nutritional status and in monitoring their nutritional status over time.

FIGURE 10.4 The Mini Nutritional Assessment Tool

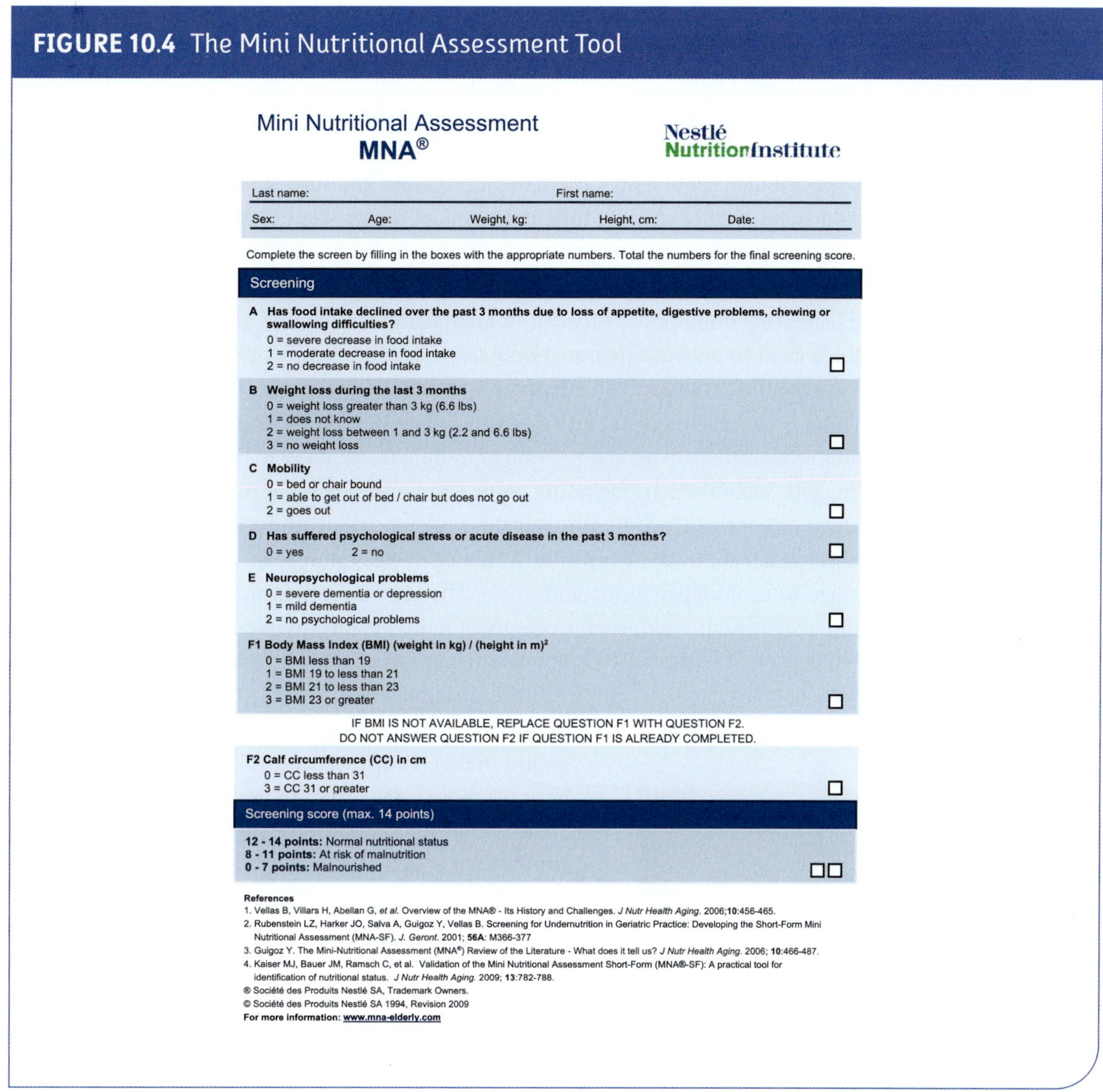

Mini Nutritional Assessment
MNA®

Nestlé
NutritionInstitute

Last name: First name:

Sex: Age: Weight, kg: Height, cm: Date:

Complete the screen by filling in the boxes with the appropriate numbers. Total the numbers for the final screening score.

Screening

A Has food intake declined over the past 3 months due to loss of appetite, digestive problems, chewing or swallowing difficulties?
0 = severe decrease in food intake
1 = moderate decrease in food intake
2 = no decrease in food intake ☐

B Weight loss during the last 3 months
0 = weight loss greater than 3 kg (6.6 lbs)
1 = does not know
2 = weight loss between 1 and 3 kg (2.2 and 6.6 lbs)
3 = no weight loss ☐

C Mobility
0 = bed or chair bound
1 = able to get out of bed / chair but does not go out
2 = goes out ☐

D Has suffered psychological stress or acute disease in the past 3 months?
0 = yes 2 = no ☐

E Neuropsychological problems
0 = severe dementia or depression
1 = mild dementia
2 = no psychological problems ☐

F1 Body Mass Index (BMI) (weight in kg) / (height in m)²
0 = BMI less than 19
1 = BMI 19 to less than 21
2 = BMI 21 to less than 23
3 = BMI 23 or greater ☐

IF BMI IS NOT AVAILABLE, REPLACE QUESTION F1 WITH QUESTION F2.
DO NOT ANSWER QUESTION F2 IF QUESTION F1 IS ALREADY COMPLETED.

F2 Calf circumference (CC) in cm
0 = CC less than 31
3 = CC 31 or greater ☐

Screening score (max. 14 points)

12 - 14 points: Normal nutritional status
8 - 11 points: At risk of malnutrition
0 - 7 points: Malnourished ☐☐

References

1. Vellas B, Villars H, Abellan G, *et al.* Overview of the MNA® - Its History and Challenges. *J Nutr Health Aging.* 2006;**10**:456-465.
2. Rubenstein LZ, Harker JO, Salva A, Guigoz Y, Vellas B. Screening for Undernutrition in Geriatric Practice: Developing the Short-Form Mini Nutritional Assessment (MNA-SF). *J. Geront.* 2001; **56A**: M366-377
3. Guigoz Y. The Mini-Nutritional Assessment (MNA®) Review of the Literature - What does it tell us? *J Nutr Health Aging.* 2006; **10**:466-487.
4. Kaiser MJ, Bauer JM, Ramsch C, et al. Validation of the Mini Nutritional Assessment Short-Form (MNA®-SF): A practical tool for identification of nutritional status. *J Nutr Health Aging.* 2009; **13**:782-788.

For more information: www.mna-elderly.com

Source: © Société des Produits Nestlé SA 1994, Revision 2009, see for further information: www.mna-elderly.com

When observations are made about the older person that might indicate they are becoming malnourished, a nutritional screening tool can help to identify the person's level of risk in the context of malnutrition. An example of a malnutrition screening tool is the Mini Nutritional Assessment Tool illustrated in Figure 10.4.

MANAGEMENT OF MALNUTRITION

The ultimate management of malnutrition is prevention, by ensuring that older people have access to nutritious foods such as proteins, to adequate kilojoules (for energy), and to vitamins and minerals. However, malnutrition in the older population is common, and treatment and management must take an individualised approach based on how malnutrition affects the particular person. Malnutrition may be managed using a combination of the following strategies:

- Chronic health conditions that can contribute to malnutrition, such as diabetes and obesity, are managed to ensure stability of a healthy diet and exercise. Meal plans that are suitable for specific chronic health conditions are documented in the person's care plan to ensure that everyone involved in supporting them knows what their dietary needs are.

- Supplements are used in aged care organisations and in the community aged care sector to provide added sustenance to the diet of older people who are experiencing, or are at risk of, malnutrition. These supplements are prescribed by the dietitian and include drinks, shakes and puddings that are enriched with the specific dietary boosters the person requires. The supplements are monitored like medications and some require specific measurements of the product to be taken. Information about the amount and type of dietary supplements used can be found in the person's care plan and/or medication chart.
- Food fortification is another component of treating malnutrition. Vitamins and minerals can be added to the person's meal to increase its nutritional density. For example, vitamin D drops can be added to foods to ensure the person has an adequate vitamin D intake.
- Any older person who is observed to be at risk of malnutrition should be referred to a dietitian. Dietitians are health professionals who can provide comprehensive assessments and relevant plans to support a person with malnutrition, including older people with feeding tubes.
- Addressing social and functional issues that place older people at risk of malnutrition is important to ensure the person has access to healthy foods. Assistive devices should be offered to the person for trial to assist them to eat independently and safely. Social aspects that increase the risk of malnutrition should also be addressed, such as respecting the person's request to eat alone or to join others in a dining area. If a person doesn't enjoy the company of others, alternative options must be considered.
- It is important to encourage older people to exercise within the realm of their abilities. Exercise can improve movement, strength and dexterity, which are essential for maintaining independence. It also contributes to effective management of chronic diseases.
- Monitoring food and fluid intake provides an important overview of the contributing factors that lead to malnutrition and identifies the person's risk of developing malnutrition. Monitoring may involve documentation such as fluid balance and food intake charts, or it can be informal, such as reporting your own observations about the person's eating and drinking practices that indicate they are not eating or drinking safely, and in the correct amount to provide their body with the nutrients it needs.

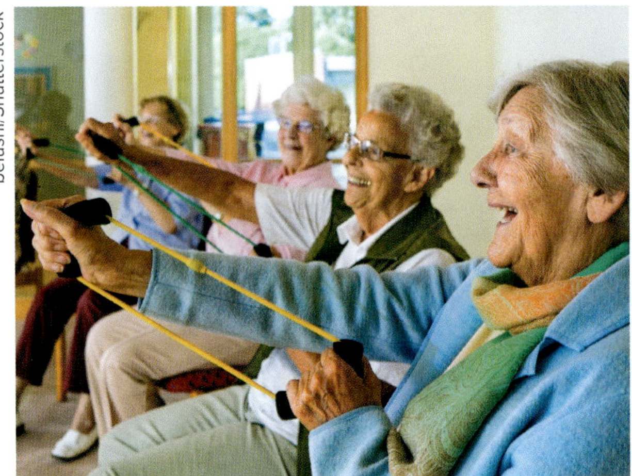

belushi/Shutterstock

Exercise contributes to the effective management of chronic diseases

THE LANTERN PROJECT

In 2013, an experienced practising dietitian, Dr Cherie Hugo, founded The Lantern Project. The aim of the project was to increase the quality and enjoyment of eating for older people living in RACFs, and to ensure their nutritional needs were met. The vision of The Lantern Project is: "To improve the quality of life of older Australians through good food and nutrition" (The Lantern Project 2015).

In collaboration with aged care services and industry bodies, The Lantern Project works towards several objectives, including research, education and sharing information that can improve the eating and dining experience for people using aged care services. Collaboration occurs through a network of members who share The Lantern Project's vision and philosophy.

WORKPLACE SCENARIO

Responding to a person who is refusing food

Margaret, who has end-stage dementia, lives in an RACF, where she is confined to her chair or bed. For the past couple of days, she has been refusing to eat or drink; at most, she will eat small amounts of custard. One of her care workers, Himari, has noticed that Margaret has refused her lunch again today, as she did yesterday. Himari checks Margaret's progress notes and notices that other staff have also documented her food refusal this past week.

Himari reports her concerns to the RN, who tells her to follow Margaret's end-of-life plan and continue to offer her the foods she enjoys while being aware that, as part of any life-limiting disease process, Margaret's desire or ability to eat and drink may come to an end.

Margaret's end-of-life plan reflects her advanced care directive, where she has requested that she be made comfortable in the event she is no longer able to eat or drink. She has expressly requested there that she not be fed artificially, and her family are very supportive of her decisions. Margaret's doctor is aware of her palliative plan.

Himari continues to offer small amounts of sweets and custard to Margaret, which she accepts from time to time.

CHECK YOUR UNDERSTANDING

1. What is dysphagia, and how can it occur?
2. List four reasons why an older person may lose their appetite.
3. What is malnutrition?
4. What are three signs of malnutrition?
5. Why are nutritional screening tools important?

SUMMARY

- Hazards and risks related to food include air-borne and food-borne pathogens that can cause serious illness in older people. Bacteria, viruses and parasites are some of the pathogens that cause food-borne illnesses. Practising effective infection control procedures can minimise contamination and prevent an outbreak in an RACF. PPE and hand hygiene are imperative for safe food handling.
- Food safety is important in aged care services, and RACFs are required under a regulatory framework to have a food safety plan. The food safety plan ensures that all matters related to food ordering, storing, preparation and consumption are supported by policies and procedures that take a risk-based approach to food handling.

- Older people need a diet that is rich in nutrients to ensure their body's nutritional requirements are being met. Malnutrition is a common condition among older people and can lead to loss of independence and poor mental health outcomes. It is essential that care workers report their concerns about the quantity and quality of foods the older person consumes.
- The role of the care worker in meal support for older people includes observing and reporting concerns, ensuring the environment is conducive to eating, and providing hands-on support in a way that minimises risk of harm and upholds the concepts of dignity, respect and self-determination of the older person.

REVIEW QUESTIONS

10.1 What aspects of food service are covered by food safety guidelines in aged care?

10.2 Outline how, as a care worker, you can encourage a person to eat.

10.3 **(a)** What are the general signs of dysphagia?

(b) List measures to help the person with dysphagia.

10.4 What is the purpose of providing adaptive devices to assist with eating and drinking? Provide two examples of adaptive devices.

BIBLIOGRAPHY

Australian Government, *Eat for Health: Australian Dietary Guidelines*, 2013, https://www.eatforhealth.gov.au/sites/default/files/content/The%20Guidelines/n55a_australian_dietary_guidelines_summary_131014_1.pdf, accessed 16 January 2022.

Food Standards Australia New Zealand (FSANZ), *Food Safety Standards: Health and Hygiene: Responsibilities of Food Handlers* (factsheet), February 2008, https://www.foodstandards.gov.au/consumer/safety/faqsafety/Documents/Technical_Fact_Sheet_Food_handlers_Feb_2008.pdf, accessed 2 January 2022.

Food Standards Australia New Zealand (FSANZ), *Standard 3.3.1: Food Safety Programs for Food Service to Vulnerable Persons*, February 2014, https://www.foodstandards.gov.au/industry/safetystandards/service/pages/default.aspx.

Food Standards Australia New Zealand (FSANZ), *Temperature Control* (factsheet), 2021, https://www.foodstandards.gov.au/consumer/safety/faqsafety/pages/foodsafetyfactsheets/charitiesandcommunityorganisationsfactsheets/temperaturecontrolma1477.aspx.

International Dysphagia Diet Standardisation Initiative (IDDSI), *The IDDSI Framework*, https://iddsi.org/framework, accessed 8 January 2022.

Klemm, Sarah, *Special Nutrient Needs of Older Adults*, 21 May 2020, https://www.eatright.org/health/wellness/healthy-aging/special-nutrient-needs-of-older-adults.

Liotta, Morgan, "Aged Care Facility Food Allowances 'Cutting Corners'", *The Royal Australian College of General Practitioners News GP*, July 2019, https://www1.racgp.org.au/newsgp/professional/aged-care-facility-food-allowances-cutting-corners.

Mental Health Foundation, UK, *Food for Thought: Mental Health and Nutrition Briefing Policy Briefing*, 2017, https://www.mentalhealth.org.uk/sites/default/files/food-for-thought-mental-health-nutrition-briefing-march-2017.pdf.

NSW Government, NSW Food Authority, *2-Hour/4-Hour Rule*, July 2021, https://www.foodauthority.nsw.gov.au/sites/default/files/202107/2_hour_4_hour_rule.pdf, accessed 10 January 2022.

Nutrition Australia, *The Healthy Eating Pyramid*, https://nutritionaustralia.org/fact-sheets/healthy-eating-pyramid/.

The Lantern Project (Australia), *About the Lantern Project*, 2015, https://thelanternproject.com.au/about-the-lantern-project-australia/, accessed 18 January 2022.

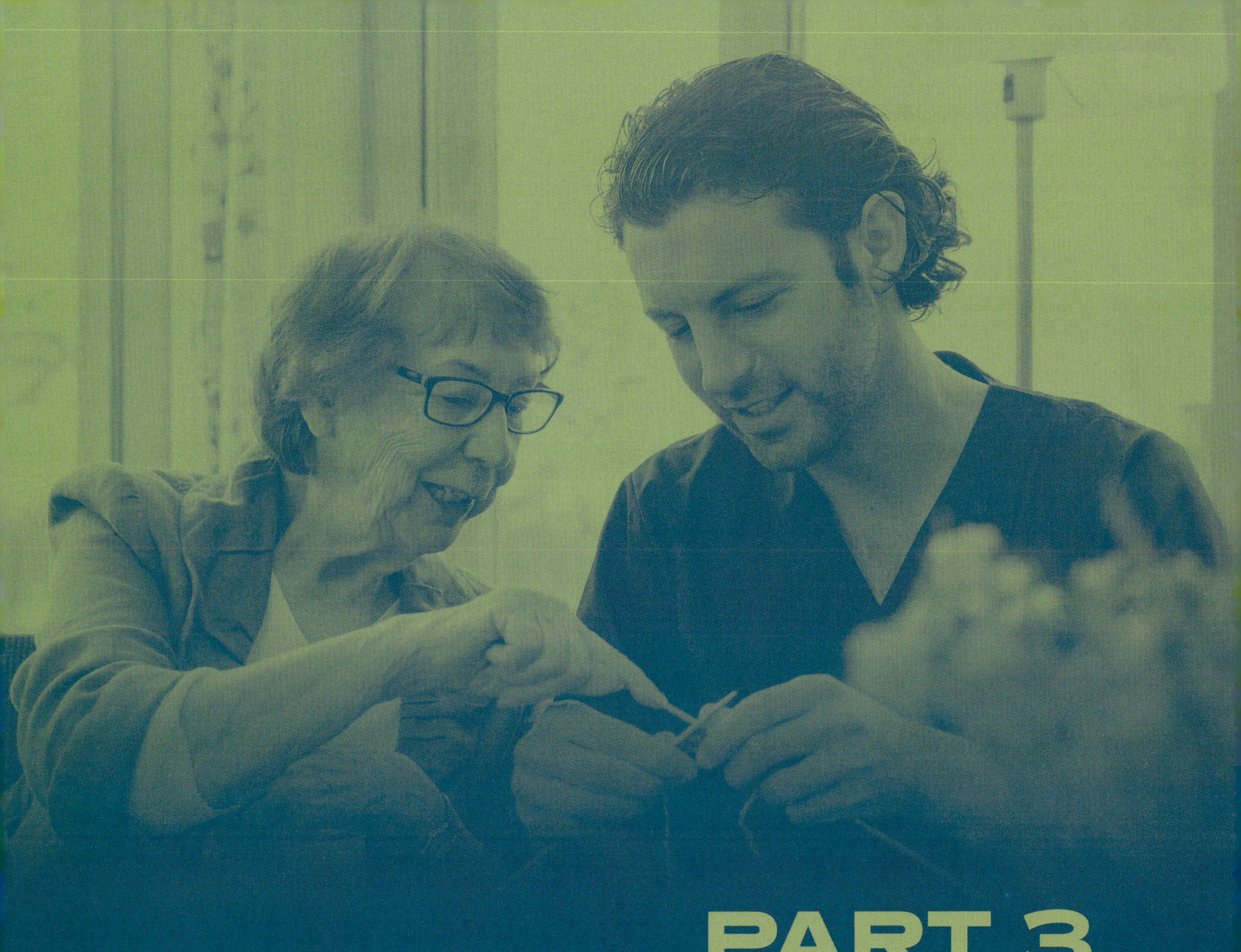

PART 3
Special care

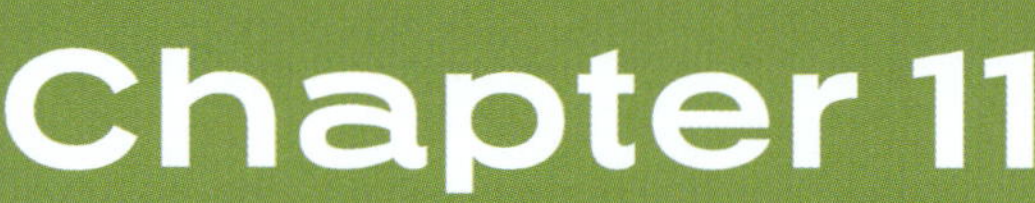

Chapter 11

Providing person-centred care to a person with dementia

LEARNING OBJECTIVES

11.1 Prepare to support a person with dementia

11.2 Use communication strategies

11.3 Maintain the person's dignity, skills and health

11.4 Understand distressed behaviours

11.5 Prepare documentation

11.6 Follow self-care guidelines

INTRODUCTION

THIS CHAPTER LOOKS AT THE SYNDROME OF DEMENTIA, and at the skills and knowledge required to provide person-centred care and support to people living with dementia by following an established individualised plan. Working with people living with dementia requires discretion and judgement. A care worker is supervised, either directly or indirectly, in this role, which they may carry out in the context of a residential aged care facility (RACF), a community or a family home.

This chapter introduces the condition of dementia, its related complications, and strategies to use when caring for and supporting those with dementia, their families and carers. There are various types of dementia with differing signs and symptoms, age of onset, severity and longevity. This chapter addresses the most common types and the recommended care strategies and support mechanisms available to implement person-centred holistic care.

INDUSTRY IN FOCUS

The basis of person-centred care: Personhood, relationships and the environment

The Australian health-care system is consistently faced with challenges as the population ages and lives longer. The progressive, degenerative neurological health condition known as dementia is particularly challenging and requires patience and understanding along with a caring, supportive, individualised approach known as the person-centred approach.

With a person-centred approach and individualised care planning, caring for someone with dementia can be very rewarding and fulfilling. The concept of personhood in relation to dementia, introduced by Kitwood (1997), has allowed for the relationship between individuality and person-centred care to develop and be applied holistically and thoroughly while developing relationships and considering environments and how they can be adapted or modified during care and support.

According to Kitwood, **personhood** focuses on the status of being a person with individual physical, mental, cognitive, social, emotional, religious, cultural and financial characteristics, likes, dislikes, needs and wants. It is natural to assume that one's personhood determines the types of relationships and environments we encounter during our lifetime. Relationships are formed in a variety of ways and for various reasons, often sustaining or diminishing personhood, which is particularly important in caring for someone with dementia. Environments in which we socialise, learn, function and live also play a role in determining our individual personhood and its characteristics. Therefore, the basis of person-centred care is the link between personhood, relationships and environment.

11.1 PREPARING TO SUPPORT A PERSON WITH DEMENTIA

11.1.1 What is dementia?

Dementia is an umbrella term for more than 100 diseases affecting memory, other cognitive abilities and behaviour that interfere significantly with a person's ability to function day to day. Diseases that cause dementia are Alzheimer's disease, vascular dementia, alcohol-related dementia and others. Dementia is a diagnosis feared by many because of its debilitating nature and unpredictability. It is one of the most challenging, draining and emotional medical conditions faced by everyone affected, including family, friends and care workers. Dementia is not a normal part of ageing; however, dementia predominantly affects people over the age of 65.

Supporting those affected by dementia requires patience and understanding and often takes place in a variety of settings. It is essential for a care worker to possess the skills and knowledge to be able to interpret and analyse the person's needs and wants, as well as to maintain stability, routine and familiarity by adopting a person-centred approach. Dementia care and support involves more than just the person diagnosed with dementia. For those diagnosed with the condition, care and support can be applied in many forms to meet their needs and preferences, such as physical, social, emotional, cultural and financial.

11.1.2 The effects of dementia on the brain and body

An area of the brain called the cerebrum is divided into two hemispheres, containing temporal, parietal, occipital and frontal lobes (see Figure 11.1). The temporal lobes are involved in hearing and understanding language, and memory. This area is often the first part of the brain to be affected by Alzheimer's disease.

The parietal lobes process sensory information, reading and writing, spatial orientation and attention. The right parietal lobe is analytical and logical, while the left parietal is the spacial centre. When these parts

FIGURE 11.1 Functional areas of the cerebral cortex

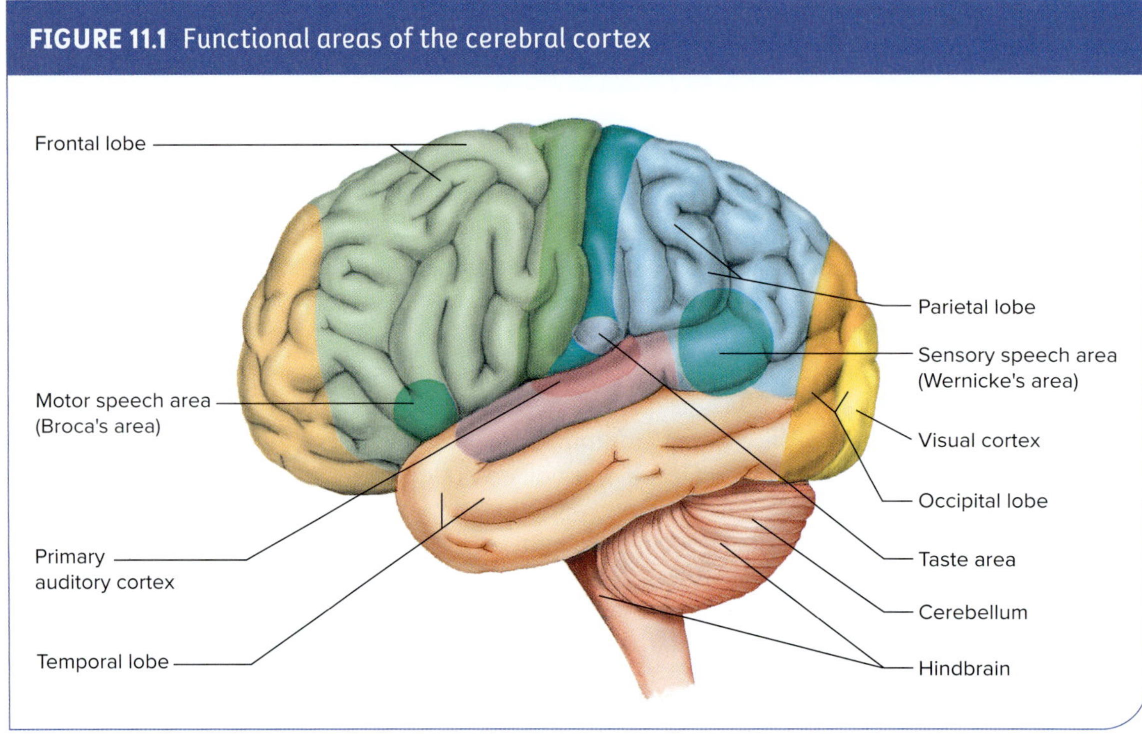

Source: © McGraw-Hill Education

of the brain are affected, the person may have word-finding difficulties along with other language difficulties, or they may have difficulty orientating themselves to where they are, and not be able to find their way home.

The frontal lobes of the brain, known as the control centre, are where actions are planned, social behaviour is adjusted and things get organised. When damage occurs in this area, people behave inappropriately, may appear to be unmotivated, and may repeat actions, stories, questions and behaviours over and over. This is called **perseveration** and isn't under the person's control.

Agnosia is the inability to recognise things and to know how to use them. So, you might ask a person with damage in the parietal lobes to pick up their fork and eat their lunch, but they can't see the fork in front of them. When a person living with dementia picks up their drink and tips it into their meal, they are not "being naughty" or trying to be defiant. They are genuinely trying to do what they have been asked to do, but the damage in their brain is preventing them from acting appropriately. When caring for a person with dementia, you will need to be kind and understanding, and to know that they are doing the best they can.

Apraxia is the inability to sequence tasks or to complete a task from beginning to end. It is no good correcting the person, or demonstrating to them how they should perform the task (e.g. setting the table); instead, we need to modify the parts of the task they can't achieve. We also work with their strengths, supporting them to do what they can (e.g. spreading the tablecloth over the table), but they might not be able to place the knives and forks out in the right order, so we support them appropriately with that part of the task. We try never to take over the task, and always promote the person's independence and success wherever possible. Apraxia will also present as putting on clothes in the wrong order or leaving out items of clothing altogether. It is important that the care worker promotes the person's dignity and provides sensitive care when this occurs.

The diagnosis of dementia has psychosocial implications, both from the beginning and as the disease progresses. Many people have insight into their condition and recognise that something is wrong. Some are relieved to have a diagnosis reveal they have a medical condition to explain what is happening to them. There are implications and things to consider, such as where they will live, how they will manage their finances, and who will be able to help them as the condition progresses.

11.1.3 Assessment and diagnosis

The sooner signs and symptoms are recognised, and a diagnosis is formed, the sooner treatment and management can be implemented. A formal dementia diagnosis can often take time and sometimes isn't official or substantiated until an autopsy is performed. Assessment and diagnosis occur primarily by using four specific tools.

- *Personal medical history:* Signs and symptoms are collated via discussion with a medical professional, the person, family and friends.
- *Physical examination:* A top-to-bottom and back-to-front physical examination involves blood and urine tests, and consideration of whether there are treatable conditions that could be causing the person's signs and symptoms or exacerbating a behaviour.
- *Neuropsychological tests:* Often used to monitor the progression of dementia, these tests involve memory testing, assessment and evaluation of problem-solving skills, language skills and cognition, as well as concentration and the ability to follow instructions and direction.
- *Radiological testing:* Often performed before an official diagnosis of dementia is made, this involves procedures such as an X-ray of the brain, computerised tomography (CT) scan, positron emission scan (PET), magnetic resonance imaging (MRI) and/or single photon emission computerised tomography (SPECT). These tests provide images of what the dementia looks like, where it is occurring and how much of the brain has been affected.

11.1.4 Treatment and management

There is currently no cure for dementia; however, some signs and symptoms can be medically treated to achieve relief, and in some cases the dementia can be slowed in its progression if diagnosis is made early. Therefore, the main goals of treatment are to maintain and maximise function, quality of life and a safe environment, as well as to promote social engagement and orientation. The care worker needs to understand the possible effects dementia can have on the person. This understanding will help everyone involved in their care and support to develop the most effective approaches for the person. The care worker can observe, monitor, record, trial new and different approaches, and talk to the team about any changes to ensure the best care and support are given.

PHARMACOLOGICAL INTERVENTIONS

The term "pharmacological interventions" refers to the use of medications to manage aspects of the dementia trajectory and to support the behavioural and psychotic symptoms of dementia. Pharmacological interventions often cause side effects, including dizziness, lethargy, weight gain, increased agitation, constipation, hypertension, headache and muscle cramps. When a person living with dementia is receiving medication, they need to be reassessed regularly, using standardised tests, to measure the effectiveness of the medication. The person's doctor will review their medications regularly and empower the person and the carer with knowledge so that they can make informed decisions about their own health and the use of medication.

NON-PHARMACOLOGICAL INTERVENTIONS

Non-pharmacological management of dementia involves principles of holistic person-centred care, empathy, patience, understanding, and thoughtful, appropriate communication strategies. The following are examples of non-pharmacological interventions.

- *Cognitive behavioural therapy:* May be helpful at the time of diagnosis to help with forward planning and related depression, by helping the person to understand the way they think and to behave in a certain way.
- *Psychotherapy and psycho-educational interventions:* Assists carers and the person with dementia by empowering them with knowledge, coping strategies and psychological support.

- *Behavioural management therapy:* Based on principles of conditioning and learning theories, this therapy uses strategies aimed at suppressing or eliminating challenging or difficult-to-manage behaviours.
- *Environmental approaches/modification:* This therapy creates an environment that is non-stressful, constant and familiar for the person living with dementia. Home adaptation therapy involves the home being modified after careful thought and consideration have been given to the person's needs and wants. Home adaptation allows the person to remain independent and safe in a familiar environment for longer, with help to ensure they retain a sense of control.
- *Dementia support groups and carer support groups:* Support groups can help people to develop networks and to realise the amount of support services available.
- *Memory training:* Using external memory prompts early in the disease process can maximise existing cognition and promote independence.

STAGES OF DEMENTIA

Table 11.1 demonstrates the stages of dementia as a set of signs and symptoms often observed during the stages. The strengths that remain throughout the disease process are the person's sense of touch and hearing, and their ability to respond to emotion. Emotions don't change in dementia. People living with dementia still have, and express, emotions.

11.1.5 Types of dementia

There are varying types of dementia.

ALZHEIMER'S DISEASE

Alzheimer's disease is the most common and most frequently diagnosed dementia in Australia. In Alzheimer's disease, sticky beta-amyloid fragments clump together in the brain and form the basis of amyloid plaques. Also, in the brain cells of people with Alzheimer's disease, tau proteins cease to function properly and, instead, form protein tangles inside the cell. This leads to a breakdown in the brain cell's ability to communicate with other brain cells, loss of connection between cells and cell death. It is a progressive, cognitive, neurological disease that exhibits signs and symptoms of memory loss, forgetfulness and lack of personal care of varying degrees.

It is the plaques and tangles in the brain of a person with Alzheimer's disease that are responsible for the person's actions, behaviours and state of being. As the condition progresses, the person loses the ability to care for themselves, to process information and to maintain safety. Inevitably, they become so debilitated that they require care and support with all aspects of daily living. Figure 11.2 demonstrates the pathophysiological effect of Alzheimer's on the brain.

VASCULAR DEMENTIA

Vascular dementia, or **multi-infarct dementia,** is the term used to describe a dementia occurring due to circulation problems whereby blood flow and oxygen supply to the brain are interrupted, which may be due to a clot or restriction to the flow via conditions such as atherosclerosis and arteriosclerosis. This type of dementia is the second most common dementia worldwide and affects 15–20 per cent of all diagnosed dementia cases in Australia (Dementia Australia 2022). When the blood flow is interrupted intermittently, it can damage blood vessels across the entire brain, causing damage over time as each episode contributes to an accumulation of brain injury. This is known as multi-infarct dementia. Signs and symptoms of vascular dementia include changes in learning, memory and language. Hypertension, lethargy, difficulty walking, emotional highs and lows, and more specific short-term memory loss, lack of concentration, inability to plan and follow instructions, and difficulty with managing finances are also indicators of vascular dementia.

TABLE 11.1 Stages of dementia

Early dementia	Moderate dementia	Advanced dementia
Often this phase is only apparent in hindsight. At the time, it may be missed or may be put down to old age or overwork. The onset of dementia is usually very gradual, and it is often impossible to identify the exact time it began.	At this stage, the problems are more apparent and disabling.	At this third and final stage, the person needs total care
Appears apathetic, with less sparkle	Memory for the distant past is generally strong, but some details may be forgotten or confused; more forgetful of recent events	Unable to remember occurrences for even a few minutes
Loses interest in their usual hobbies and activities	Confused regarding time and place	Loses their ability to understand or use speech
Is unwilling to try new things	Becomes lost if away from familiar surroundings	Incontinent
Has trouble adapting to change	Confuses one family member with another or forgets names of family or friends	Shows no recognition of people they know
Poor judgement and makes poor decisions	May leave gas unlit or forget that the stove or oven is on	Needs help with eating, washing, bathing, toileting and dressing
Takes longer to complete routine jobs and is less able to grasp complex ideas	Wanders around streets, perhaps at night, with the possibility of becoming lost	Fails to recognise everyday objects (agnosia)
Blames others for “stealing” lost things	Behaves inappropriately (e.g. goes outdoors in nightwear)	Becomes disturbed at night
Is less concerned with others and their feelings; more interested in self	Sees or hears things that are not there	Restless, perhaps looking for a long-dead relative
Forgetful of details of recent events	More repetitive	Easily upset, especially when feeling frightened
More likely to repeat themselves or to lose the thread of what they are talking about	Neglectful of hygiene or with eating	Has difficulty walking, eventually perhaps becoming confined to a wheelchair
More irritable or upset if they fail at something	Becomes angry, upset or distressed through frustration	Has uncontrolled movements
Has some difficulty in handling money	–	Has permanent immobility, and in the final weeks or months will be bedridden

LEWY BODY DEMENTIA

Lewy body dementia, or **dementia with Lewy bodies,** is a rapidly progressive and degenerative cognitive disease that more commonly affects men and often results in death approximately seven years after diagnosis. Lewy bodies are abnormal round structures that form in the neuron (the brain cell) and cause the death of the neuron in several areas of the brain, including:

- the cerebral cortex, where functions such as processing new and old information, perception, thought and language occur
- the limbic cortex, which is primarily responsible for emotions and behaviour

FIGURE 11.2 The pathophysiological effect of Alzheimer's on the brain

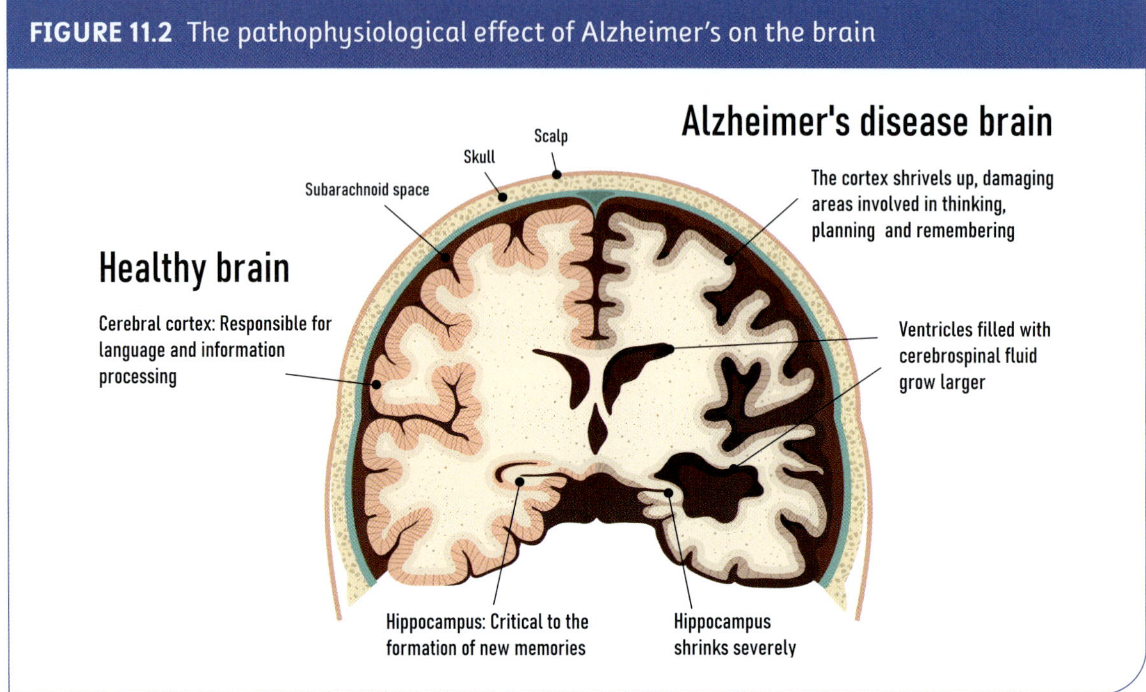

Source: logika600/Shutterstock.com

- the hippocampus, which is primarily responsible for forming new memories
- the midbrain and basal ganglia, which are involved in movement and coordination
- the brain stem, which plays an important role in the regulation of sleep and the maintenance of alertness
- olfactory pathways, which are the regions of the brain important in recognising and interpreting smells.

WERNICKE-KORSAKOFF SYNDROME

Wernicke-Korsakoff syndrome is a dementia type attributed to excessive alcohol intake over a prolonged period of time. High chronic intake of alcohol causes an inhibition of thiamine absorption and, hence, a thiamine deficiency. Thiamine (vitamin B1) is required for the brain to develop certain neurotransmitters that allow for specific actions and behaviours to occur. If suspected or diagnosed early and treated with thiamine injections, a five-food group diet and abstinence from alcohol, there is a chance of reversing or slowing the process of the disease.

"Wernicke" describes the inflammatory process that occurs, and "Korsakoff" describes the progression to brain matter damage–especially the section responsible for memory. During Wernicke-Korsakoff syndrome, it is common for the person to experience involuntary, jerky, uncoordinated movements of the limbs and eyes. Confusion, drowsiness, poor balance and a staggering gait, as well as short-term memory loss, are also common signs and symptoms observed throughout the syndrome. As the disease progresses, the person tends to exhibit behaviours of lying, confabulation and exaggeration, with poor social skills that often result in personality changes, and may be confrontational. Some people develop amnesia of fixation, which is the inability to remember the events of the previous few minutes.

FRONTOTEMPORAL LOBE DEMENTIA

Frontotemporal lobe dementia (FTLD) or frontotemporal lobar degeneration, which is also known as Pick's disease, affects the frontal and/or temporal regions of the brain. FTLD occurs over several years, is progressive and degenerative in nature and, like all dementing illnesses, shortens a person's life expectancy. FTLD progression is variable and the exact influence on mortality is unknown, but the early signs and symptoms can be managed to enable the person diagnosed to live as full and effective a life as possible. FTLD commonly affects the under-65 age group and hence can mean a very long life of signs and symptoms for some. Common symptoms include language and speech abnormalities, along with emotional ups and downs with inappropriate emotional responses to various situations. Apathy and disinhibition are also symptoms of FTLD, along with inappropriate actions, lack of interest in or enthusiasm for activities, neglect of personal hygiene and self-care, compulsive behaviours, difficulty in speaking or understanding speech, language recall problems, sometimes loss of reading and writing skills, and often difficulty with social interactions

HUNTINGTON'S DISEASE

Huntington's disease is an inherited, degenerative, progressive, neurological disorder that is diagnosed primarily in 30–50-year-olds; however, it has been diagnosed as early as two years of age. It is caused by a single defective gene. Primary symptoms include distinct disturbances with movement that are characterised by irregular and jerky movements; changes in cognition, judgement, planning and concentration; as well as emotional changes and short-term memory loss. The pathophysiological changes observed in the brain tissue, primarily the central area, of someone with Huntington's cause alterations in mood, especially depression, anxiety, and uncharacteristic anger and irritability. Obsessive-compulsive behaviour, leading a person to repeat the same question or activity over and over, has also been noted as a common symptom.

PARKINSON'S DISEASE

Parkinson's disease is a progressive neurological condition where the level of dopamine is affected to the extent that movement, balance and coordination are affected. Parkinson's disease doesn't cause the usual signs of dementia until much later in its progression compared with other dementias. Parkinson's typically causes tremors, a stiffness or rigidity to the limbs, a shuffling gait and a stooped posture. The intensity of the symptoms varies from person to person; however, the eventual outcome is always the same.

YOUNGER ONSET DEMENTIA

Younger onset dementia (YOD) is a set of signs and symptoms detected earlier in life and interferes with a younger person's activities of daily living (ADLs) sooner than when detected in an older person. The age group for YOD is commonly under 65 but chiefly between the ages of 40 and 50. Some people in their thirties are diagnosed with younger onset dementia. The progression of YOD may need to be managed differently, as the person may still be working in the early stages or have a young family. YOD may have the manifestations of any of the dementia illnesses. A full medical assessment is essential to rule out other potential diagnoses, especially mental health conditions and psychiatric disorders that may mimic early dementia signs. Symptoms can often be consistent with other conditions such as depression, vitamin and hormone deficiencies, and infections.

It is difficult to receive a diagnosis of life-limiting illness at any stage of life, but it is particularly difficult as a younger person to receive a dementia diagnosis. Dementia has been stereotyped and labelled as an older person's disease for so long that it is difficult for a younger person who may be still working, raising a family and mixing in various social settings to accept the diagnosis and initiate support and assistance. However, it is critical, regardless of age, that the person initiates getting support and assistance in the early stages of the disease so that they can maintain a high quality of life for a prolonged period.

CREUTZFELDT-JAKOB DISEASE

Creutzfeldt-Jakob disease (CJD) is a rare, degenerative disease of the brain. It is fatal. It is one of a group of diseases known as the transmissible spongiform encephalopathies. In CJD, the structure of a normal brain protein changes, forming prions, or misfolded proteins. The build-up of these prions damages brain cells and causes the neurological symptoms of CJD. Unlike bacteria or viruses, prions resist normal methods of heat and chemical sterilisation and, very rarely, prions can be transmitted to others. These people develop blindness, weakness and behavioural change, and become uncoordinated in walking. The have difficulty with speech, and early confusion develops into dementia. People with CJD live only for weeks, or perhaps months, after the onset of symptoms. There is no specific treatment. Rigid infection control strategies prevent the transmission of these prions. There is a support group network for CJD in Australia.

11.1.6 Conditions similar to dementia

Dementia is difficult to diagnose early and can quite often be masked or mistaken for other conditions that exhibit similar characteristics. Delirium and depression are two conditions commonly mistaken for dementia, and vice versa.

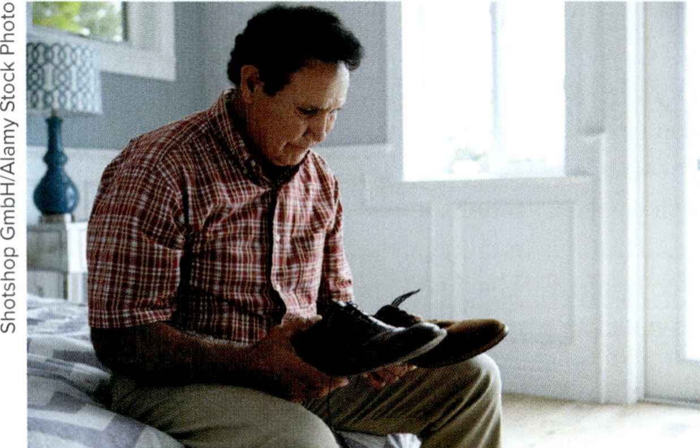

Shotshop GmbH/Alamy Stock Photo

Dementia may be mistaken for other conditions that exhibit similar characteristics

DELIRIUM

Delirium is a set of signs and symptoms that occur suddenly and is often a result of an infective process occurring. Delirium can occur at any age, yet it often occurs in the older population who display symptoms of sudden confusion and disorientation, sometimes with lethargy and drowsiness. Strategies for identifying, treating and managing delirium involve having a therapeutic relationship with the person and being able to quickly identify sudden changes and possible causes of changes. It is crucial that the care worker is familiar with the person's behavioural patterns and is invested in providing them with the best possible care. Once a suspicion of delirium exists, a process of assessment and elimination of causes should occur, followed by prompt and correct medical and nursing care. For example, if it is suspected that a person is suffering from a urinary tract infection, a urine sample should be collected and analysed and the doctor would prescribe the correct antibiotics, while the care worker would encourage the person to drink water, stay active and practise regular, correct personal hygiene (including the regular changing of incontinence aids).

Although infection is the most common cause of delirium in the older person, there are other conditions that could cause delirium, such as pain, low oxygen levels in the body, vitamin B1 deficiency, low blood sugar, alcohol consumption, hormonal imbalances and even electrolyte imbalances; therefore, the treatment will always be related to the cause.

DEPRESSION

Depression is another condition often mistaken for dementia; however, there are distinct differences between the two. With depression, the person remains orientated as to date, time, place and person, and can reason, justify actions and behaviours, and recall events. Depression is a mood disorder that causes constant feelings of sadness, worthlessness and loss of interest. It is not uncommon for a person with dementia to experience depression, yet it is extremely important to identify them as separate diagnoses so that the appropriate treatment and management can commence early. Just like when diagnosing dementia, there are specific screening tools used to assess and diagnosis depression, especially during dementia. The most frequently used scale in Australia is the **Cornell Scale for Depression in Dementia (CSDD).** As illustrated in Figure 11.3, the CSDD examines and assesses many aspects of physical and behavioural characteristics in order to diagnose depression during dementia.

Treatment and management of depression during dementia involve consideration of both pharmacological and non-pharmacological strategies. The use of antidepressants is popular, but it is also important to incorporate into a person's care successful strategies such as modifying environments, encouraging social engagement, setting realistic goals and maintaining routines.

FIGURE 11.3 Sample Cornell scale for depression in dementia

Name: ______ Age: ______ Sex: ______ Date: ______

Cornell Scale for Depression in Dementia

Ratings should be based on symptoms and signs occurring during the week before interview. No score should be given if symptoms result from physical disability or illness.

SCORING SYSTEM

a = Unable to evaluate   0 = Absent   1 = Mild to Intermittent   2 = Severe

Score greater than 12 = Probable Depression

A. MOOD-RELATED SIGNS	a	0	1	2
1. Anxiety; anxious expression, rumination, worrying				
2. Sadness; sad expression, sad voice, tearfulness				
3. Lack of reaction to pleasant events				
4. Irritability; annoyed, short tempered				
B. BEHAVIORAL DISTURBANCE	**a**	**0**	**1**	**2**
5. Agitation; restlessness, hand wringing, hair pulling				
6. Retardation; slow movements, slow speech, slow reactions				
7. Multiple physical complaints (score 0 if gastrointestinal symptoms only)				
8. Loss of interest; less involved in usual activities (score 0 only if change occurred acutely, i.e., in less than one month)				
C. PHYSICAL SIGNS	**a**	**0**	**1**	**2**
9. Appetite loss; eating less than usual				
10. Weight loss (score 2 if greater than 5 pounds in one month)				
11. Lack of energy; fatigues easily, unable to sustain activities				
D. CYCLIC FUNCTIONS				
12. Diurnal variation of mood; symptoms worse in the morning				
13. Difficulty falling asleep; later than usual for this individual				
14. Multiple awakenings during sleep				
15. Early morning awakening; earlier than usual for this individual				
E. IDEATIONAL DISTURBANCE				
16. Suicidal; feels life is not worth living				
17. Poor self-esteem; self-blame, self-depreciation, feelings of failure				
18. Pessimism; anticipation of the worst				
19. Mood congruent delusions; delusions of poverty, illness or loss				

Notes/Current Medications:

Assessor:

Score

Instruction for use: (Cornell Dementia Depression Assessment Tool)

1. The same CNA (certified nursing assistant) should conduct the interviewed each time to assure consistency in the response.
2. The assessment should be based on the patient's normal weekly routine.
3. If uncertain of answers, questioning other caregivers may further define the answer.
4. Answer all questions by placing a check in the column under the appropriately numbered answer. (a=unable to evaluate, 0=absent, 1=mild to intermittent, 2=severe).
5. Add the total score for all numbers checked for each question.
6. Place the total score in the "SCORE" box and record any subjective observation notes in the "Notes/Current Medications" section.
7. Scores totaling twelve (12) points or more indicate probable depression.

Alexopoulos GA, Abrams RC, Young RC, Shamoian CA. Cornell scale for depression in dementia. *Biol Psych* 1988;23:271-284.

Provided courtesy of CME Outfitters, LLC

Available for download at www.neuroscienceCME.com

Source: Alexopoulos, Abrams, Young, Shamoian. Cornell scale for depression in dementia. Bio Psych 1988, Volume 23, Issue 3.

Care and support should always be holistic and person centred, which includes organising activities at a time that the person prefers and when they are most alert and active, not when it suits the care worker alone. Older people tend to participate more in activities when they choose the activities themselves or are familiar with them. Being positive and offering praise also encourage participation and engagement; in turn, this builds self-esteem and feelings of self-worth, which can often be lacking in someone experiencing depression.

DELIRIUM AND DEPRESSION IN DEMENTIA

Delirium and depression can both occur during dementia, and both can occur at the same time, making the care and support of a person particularly challenging. It is crucial that the care worker is familiar with and aware of the whole person and is focused on them as an individual rather than a diagnosis. Many people may have the same diagnosis yet have different signs and symptoms along with varying strategies for care and support. Remember that delirium occurs over hours to days, depression over weeks to months, and dementia over months to years.

11.1.7 Supporting a person with dementia using person-centred care

Person-centred care (PCC) is respectful of, and responsive to, the preferences, needs and values of the individual. It is understanding what is important to the person, building trust, establishing mutual respect, and working together to share decisions around the plan of care. The concept and practice of person-centred care proposed by British psycho-gerontologist Tom Kitwood (1997) concentrates on three main principles:

- *Human rights:* Every individual has human rights that encompass all aspects of physical, social, emotional, religious, cultural, spiritual and financial needs.
- *Personhood:* At the centre of the principles is the reality that all human beings have their own identity and individuality, with specific needs and wants regardless of their diagnosis.
- *Environment:* A person's social environment impacts on their personhood and ability to adapt to the ever-changing pathway of dementia.

No matter where a person is in their journey of a dementia diagnosis, they are entitled to a quality of life that is of the highest standard; to have their individuality recognised; and to be treated with respect. Supporting a person with dementia using person-centred care has become more prominent and commonplace in health and community services, particularly over the last decade, thanks to advocacy, government policy and a shift in perception and understanding of dementia (Kitwood 1997). Person-centred care can be expressed using a simple equation: PCC = **V + I + P + S (VIPS)** (Brooker 2007) where:

- *V: Valuing* people with dementia is the beginning point of care regardless of age and cognitive ability, recognising that there is worth or value in each person no matter their circumstances.
- *I: Individuality* overlaps valuing and emphasises that each being is an individual and unique, despite their diagnosis, and should be treated as such while considering personal history, personality, belief systems, physical and mental health status, financial resources and social support systems.
- *P:* The person's *perspective* centres around having the ability to look at the world and environment through someone else's eyes (the person living with dementia) and perspective.
- *S:* Prompts the care worker to include the *social* aspect of someone's life and to create and encourage a positive environment when designing a plan of care.

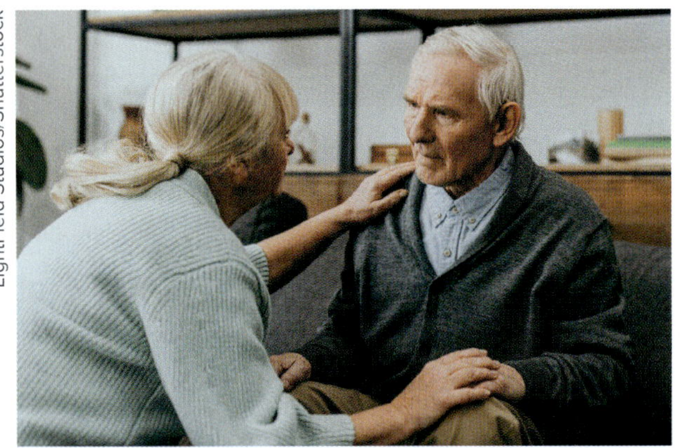
LightField Studios/Shutterstock

People with dementia need to feel valued

MORE ABOUT UNDERSTANDING ANOTHER'S PERSPECTIVE

The needs and wants of a person living with dementia are at the core of holistic, person-centred care. The most effective way to find out what such needs and wants are, as well as to get to know someone living with dementia, is to compile a physical, medical and social history of them. This history will form a documented account of some of the person's life. During this process, biographical information is gathered from the person with dementia and their family, friends and carers, including information about the person's childhood and midlife and up until the present day. Information should include what makes them happy or sad, their likes and dislikes, interests and hobbies, former employment, and significant life events.

Information about the person gathered from their family, carers and friends that is honest, accurate and significant can be documented and incorporated into care planning that reflects the needs, wants, likes and dislikes of the person with dementia. Such care planning is essential in providing the most appropriate care and support to those affected by dementia, but it also helps the care worker to perform their role without conflict and to comply with their organisation's policies and procedures.

Previous trauma will impact on the person living with dementia, and links are being found to exist between past trauma and the development of dementia. A trauma-informed model of care can also be useful. By understanding the person's history and looking at life through their eyes, the care worker acknowledges the person's existence and their reality, valuing their perspective and needs regardless of their cognitive ability– in other words, their personhood.

11.1.8 Recognising abuse and neglect

Elder **abuse** is the mistreatment or exploitation of an older person often by someone they know and trust. It is a complex issue and sometimes difficult to detect in someone with dementia as some of the symptoms of dementia may also be symptoms of abuse. For example, a person may be anxious and withdrawn or avoid people to whom they were previously close. These behaviours can be signs of both dementia and abuse. People with dementia have a heightened vulnerability to abuse and exploitation.

As a care worker, there is a duty of care to report any signs of distress in an older person and to leave the relevant health professional to make a diagnosis after a thorough investigation of the situation. It is much better to report and to be mistaken than to wait and find someone is injured and suffering. Care workers are deemed mandatory reporters and have a moral and legal obligation to report any suspicion of or actual **neglect** or abuse. Duty of care when caring for someone with dementia, with respect to abuse and neglect, also includes self-management and recognition of one's own circumstances that may impact on the delivery of care. The care worker has a duty of care to dismiss themselves from caring for someone, especially someone with dementia, if they have any doubt about their ability to care for them effectively.

11.1.9 Supporting carers

THE NEEDS OF CARERS

People affected by dementia include the person's carer, who is their primary support person. Carers of people living with dementia may be living with them in the community or assisting them from a nearby location. It is important that the care worker understands that the primary carer is likely to have many things to cope with. The types of stressors can be environmental and accumulated or cumulative. This refers to a common experience for people who work in chronically stressful situations. It results from an accumulation of various stress factors such as a huge workload, poor communication, frustration, coping with situations in which they feel powerless, and an inability to rest or relax. As you can see, these are all possible stressors for carers in this very demanding role.

MORE ABOUT STRESS FOR CARERS

Carers in the community may be experiencing a huge range of stressors:

- *Grief:* They may be grieving for the person as they were before their diagnosis, and grieving for the skills, abilities and understanding that their person living with dementia has lost.
- *Fatigue:* Caring for someone constantly brings fatigue and challenges. Carers can become exhausted looking after someone 24 hours a day, 7 days a week.
- *I can do it better...:* Many carers believe they are best placed to look after the person with dementia. Sometimes it goes back to promises they made to each other earlier in life. Carers can get very embarrassed by the person's behaviour and so conclude that it is easier and less trouble to do the work of caring themselves.
- *Guilt:* Many carers feel guilty if they are having difficulty managing all aspects of the person's care and behaviour. They may feel unprepared in their new role and that what they are doing isn't enough. They may also feel that they should never be angry or frustrated, which is unrealistic given the situation they are in.
- *Reduced self-esteem:* There is little worth or value attached to the carer role. This can make carers feel unappreciated and may start to erode their own sense of worth.
- *Social isolation:* Friends may no longer call by, and going out anywhere become much more complicated, so social connections drop away.
- *Compromises with employment:* If the carer is still working, then they have to combine their employment with the caring role. This is becoming more usual as more children care for their elderly parents. It is also an issue in younger onset dementia, as the partners of these people are often employed and their children may even be school aged yet still be involved in caring.
- *Uncertainty:* It isn't known how long the carer role will continue. Many carers don't know where to go for help or what to do if they feel they can no longer cope.
- *Fear:* Carers are fearful and worried about what might happen to the person if they themselves fall sick.

Carers who have placed a person in residential care may experience incredible guilt and shame. They may feel guilty because they believe they should have managed or that they made a promise to keep their family member at home. They may also feel guilty as they are now feeling relief at not having to manage the care themselves. Placing a loved one in care may increase the carer's sense of failure if they believe they should have managed for longer and done more. Carers can sometimes feel that the staff won't know the person as well as they do and so they won't be able to care for them properly. Surrendering the care of a loved one can also contribute to the loneliness of the carer, who might feel they have lost their purpose in life.

The care worker needs to consider the needs of the carer and ensure that the services and support organised don't increase the carer's stress levels. It is the care worker's job to assist the primary carer and to form a supportive, respectful, professional relationship with them. The carer and the family are part of the support team for the person living with dementia. The care worker should assess and acknowledge the importance of the carer's role and work in partnership with the carer and other family members in a manner that recognises the support they provide to the person.

WORKPLACE SCENARIO

A person with dementia has delirium... What do you do?

Penny (67) has been observed talking to herself intermittently and appears confused about where she is at present. She was recently diagnosed with early dementia, yet she has remained oriented to time and place. Talking to herself, and her disorientation, are sudden unexpected observations noted by the care worker, Jan. Jan also notes that Penny is visiting the bathroom more often than usual. Jan performs a urinalysis that detects abnormally high leucocytes and protein in Penny's urine, as well as an offensive smell and cloudy appearance. Penny is reviewed by the doctor, who suspects a urinary tract infection and commences her on antibiotics. The doctor also asks staff to encourage Penny to increase her water intake and to pay particular attention to her personal hygiene. Jan doesn't dispute Penny's current reality when they talk, because Penny's confusion is very real to her during delirium. Thanks to the timely observation, diagnosis and treatment, Penny makes a full recovery from the urinary tract infection and is no longer experiencing the delirium. She is reorientated to date, time and place and is no longer talking to herself.

CHECK YOUR UNDERSTANDING

1. What are the main symptoms of any dementia?
2. What are the main types of dementia?
3. Why do we need to understand dementia?
4. What other conditions are similar to dementia?
5. How is dementia diagnosed?

11.2 COMMUNICATION STRATEGIES

Communication is crucial to any therapeutic relationship, but it is more so when caring for and supporting those affected by dementia. Communication is the key to engagement, cooperation and successful person-centred care. How you respond to and communicate with someone with dementia can make the difference between gaining their trust and cooperation or alienating them. It is necessary to remember that, even though their cognitive abilities are declining, people with dementia have feelings and emotional reactions despite being unable to understand or express them.

For someone with dementia, communication can be challenging, frustrating, annoying, confusing and debilitating, just as it can be for a care worker attempting to communicate with the person with dementia. Therefore, the best approach is to consider and utilise various methods of communication. Communication isn't just the spoken word; it involves non-verbal, written, visual, auditory, body language and tactile aspects, particularly for those with dementia. People with dementia haven't lost the ability to communicate; they just need to find different ways to do it. It is the care worker's role to assess and utilise strategies that allow for the person to express themselves and be involved in their care for as long as possible.

11.2.1 Changes to communication that occur due to dementia

As dementia progresses, several changes may be apparent in the way a person communicates. The type and level of communication will vary depending on the type of dementia, the location of the damaged brain tissue and the stage of the dementia. In many cases of dementia, changes in communication occur slowly yet significantly. As the disease progresses, cognitive abilities decline; however, the person still has emotions and feelings to express, albeit inappropriately at times. For example, a person may have difficulty forming words or putting words together logically in a sentence, or they may have lost the ability to choose the correct word to use, so they use another word. With cognitive decline, the person may not understand fully what is being said, asked or requested of them and so misinterpretation and frustration occur.

Key changes in communication observed in those with dementia include:

- They may have difficulty in finding words.
- They misinterpret the intended message.
- Their speech is fluent but doesn't make sense (sometimes called word salad).
- Their ability to read and write may be affected, but they may be able to read the care worker's name badge! In Parkinson's disease, a notable symptom is micrographia (where writing gets smaller, the more is written).
- Normal social conventions and behaviours are forgotten, which may lead to interrupting, speaking over and even ignoring someone who may be speaking.
- The person may be able to converse about distant past events but not in the present context.
- The person's speech may deteriorate to muttering sounds or grunting and may cease altogether.
- As has already been discussed, remember that emotions don't change in this syndrome called dementia; just the ability to express them.

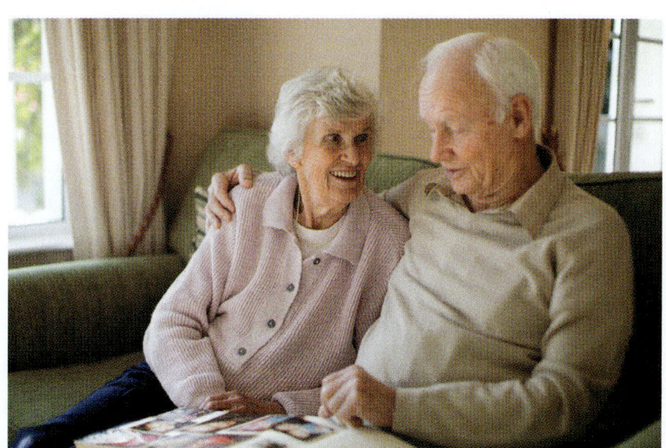

Blend Images/Image Source

Use reassuring words, phrases and body language to communicate with a person who has dementia

11.2.2 Communication strategies

Methods used to engage with the person with dementia include:

- verbal and non-verbal communication strategies
- using reassuring words, phrases and body language
- accepting the person's reality
- acknowledging and accepting their expressions of distress.

CULTURALLY SENSITIVE AND SAFE COMMUNICATION STRATEGIES

Before attempting to communicate with a person with dementia, it is helpful to consider physical, cognitive and cultural aspects, how they are feeling, and how the communication will be interpreted. Be patient and flexible by giving the person time to think and respond. If the response is difficult to understand, try to patiently determine what it is they are trying to communicate. For example, a person may get up regularly at 2.30 am and become combative when you try to assist them back to bed. However, this behaviour might be understandable if you consider the person's social history. If they were a baker for 45 years, they would normally have risen very early. In this case, this is what the person remembers, not the fact that they are in supported accommodation, and you are on a night shift. It is the care worker's role to adjust care to the person's needs and to communicate acceptance of their perspective.

The person with dementia may be experiencing changes in vision, hearing and/or cognition related to dementia itself or other illnesses, so it is essential to include these considerations in methods of communicating. Language and culture also play a vital role in caring for someone affected by dementia. Using medical terminology isn't conducive to effective communication with relation to dementia, and so it is best to use language and context that the person relates to and understands. For example, the words "faeces" and "urine" wouldn't make sense, so perhaps "poo" and "wee" would be used and better understood.

As dementia progresses, those people from non-English-speaking backgrounds tend to express themselves better or more effectively by using their first language. In these instances, care may involve the use of an interpreter or translator to ensure effective communication is achieved. Some words may exist in both English and another language but with a different meaning in the different cultures. For example, in Australia "kiss" means to touch lips, while in Sweden it means urine; hence, this can cause even further confusion for the person with dementia, or for the person caring for someone with dementia. Consideration, understanding and acceptance of culture and cultural context are just as important in dementia care as with any type of care. In some cultures, dementia is deemed embarrassing and shameful, while in other cultures it is accepted and expected as a normal ageing process. Cultural thought processes can change the way someone is cared for and the way they respond to a diagnosis of dementia; therefore, it is the care worker's role to support varying cultural needs and experiences.

As a care worker, it is vitally important to be aware of your own attitudes, values, beliefs and non-verbal communication during care because what we perceive as a normal part of our culture, or what we consider to be right or wrong, or acceptable or non-acceptable, someone else with their own attitudes, values and beliefs may see very differently. Care workers should anticipate, not assume, and be encouraged to be aware and always on guard for behaviours and challenging situations, some of which may be exacerbated by assumptions. For example, if a care worker was to assume that a person with dementia couldn't hear or understand what was being said in front of them and commented, "Oh, the poor thing. He's disgraced himself again", the person could interpret this as meaning he is being a burden and is a disgrace and an embarrassment. Such comments don't aid self-esteem or feelings of self-worth and hence are discouraged. Non-verbal cues such as hand gestures and eye contact are communication aids, but they can also inhibit or confuse communication between people from different cultures or backgrounds. For example, the thumbs-up gesture could be interpreted either as an offensive gesture or as a positive "Well done!" gesture.

ATTITUDE AND NON-VERBAL COMMUNICATION

Your attitude will affect the person with dementia and can dictate how they will respond to you. If you shout instructions and make demands of them, they might respond to you in the same manner. It is better to approach them quietly, gain their attention and negotiate the next step in a calm manner. Your body language will send a strong message. If it is open, inviting and non-threatening, this will contribute to your effective communication.

When the person living with dementia starts to have communication difficulties, they can experience intense frustration. They don't mean to make situations difficult, and they are trying to do what they can.

At this point, your non-verbal communication becomes even more important. Much can be gained by communicating non-verbally. Non-verbal communication includes:

- use of gestures
- tone of voice
- eye contact
- facial expressions
- body language, including posture and personal space
- spending time with the person
- paying attention to and interacting with the person.

Just being with the person, sitting alongside them, not talking, and perhaps using touch (if deemed appropriate) can create a deep bond of connection, acceptance and inclusion.

EMPATHY

A core component in care and support for people living with dementia is empathy, which is the ability to understand another's point of view, their thoughts and feelings, and the place they find themselves. Empathy can be expressed with effective communication techniques that show support and acknowledgement.

PROMPTING

A strength-based approach is the best way to work with people living with dementia. This involves working with what people *can* do, rather than concentrating on the things they find difficult. Care workers can involve them in conversations, tasks and activities where they can achieve success. This approach will build self-esteem and help the person feel comfortable in their world.

ACCEPTANCE AND ACKNOWLEDGEMENT

The care worker needs to be able to acknowledge and empathise with the person's feelings and their realty. There is no reason to argue with the person or to try and get them to understand the truth. This is sometimes referred to as "entering their world" and this will allow the care worker to meet them where they are. This approach demonstrates respect and will validate what is real for them. Care workers can:

- acknowledge the person's feelings in a warm, non-judgemental way
- show empathy and understanding
- read verbal and non-verbal clues
- provide verbal, non-verbal and physical reassurance.

DISTRACTION

Distraction will only work when the care worker first acknowledges and validates the person's current situation. Once the care worker has shown that they understand what is worrying the person, the person will be happy to have a cup of tea, for example, or to engage in something the care worker knows they like doing.

11.2.3 The environment

People living with dementia need an environment that is stable and familiar and supports their wellbeing. Creating a stable environment is necessary because of the impact of memory loss and disorientation as the person's dementia progresses. Memory loss and disorientation can cause agitation, anxiety, frustration and anger; therefore, the care worker is required to create and maintain a stable environment. People with dementia are cared for in a variety of settings, and sometimes in many settings, during their dementia journey. Settings for care can begin at home, with home assistance, respite and day care, residential care, acute care and palliative care all being accessed at some time during their lifetime:

- Home care with in-home services to supplement the family's care is popular when first diagnosed. However, as the diagnosis develops, respite and day care become utilised more as a way to begin the transition to full-time care.

- Respite and day care are also programs designed to assist older, frail persons to stay living at home longer with the help of support services. Day centres and community care services offer time away from home, socialisation, and activities that offer stimulation and maintenance of skills.
- Residential care is designed to provide the person with dementia with full-time care and support using an empowering approach to help the person develop their own living environment.
- Acute care is accessed when sudden and urgent care is required. Things such as surgical intervention for a fractured hip after a fall will require acute admission. Acute care can be very disorientating and distressing for a person living with dementia, as the acute environment is busy, unstable and unpredictable, with unfamiliar people. These factors make it very difficult for the person with dementia to be able to negotiate and orientate themselves to this unfamiliar environment, and many people will experience delirium as a result of hospital admissions.
- Palliative care is for people with life-limiting illness, and dementia is indeed a life-limiting illness. Palliative care principles encourage dignity, respect, trust, honesty, symptom management and person centredness, especially during the latter stages of the person's illness. Regardless of the environmental setting, holistic person-centred care forms the basis of all care interventions and encourages the care worker to consider and evaluate how the person is experiencing their illness, their support and services provided. Palliative care can be provided in a variety of settings, from home to the hospice and many places in-between.

IMPACT OF THE ENVIRONMENT ON SUPPORTING A PERSON TO INTERACT AND ENGAGE

The following are some ways that can assist in creating a supportive environment for someone with dementia. However, it is essential to be aware that different people will respond differently.

- Maintain routines.
- Keep familiar items such as photos and trinkets visible.
- Use notes in strategic positions as reminders.
- Avoid shiny floors and rich patterns, as they can cause confusion.
- Ensure lighting is adequate; neither too bright nor too dim.
- Label cupboards and rooms so that the person can feel they know their environment.
- Hide items that may cue certain behaviours. For example, car keys left visible may trigger a desire to drive, or hats and coats on a rack near the front door may entice someone to try to leave the premises.
- Minimise conflicting noises. For example, turn the TV off if you are telling the person it is time to go to the dining room for lunch.
- Avoid rearranging the furniture and the person's personal belongings.
- Disguise exits if appropriate.

CREATING A SUPPORTIVE SOCIAL ENVIRONMENT

Creating a calm, soothing, simple, yet functional environment nurtures a person living with dementia. It may be the one thing during care that they find familiar and relaxing. A dementia-friendly environment is a well-designed space that considers the person holistically and individually, while creating opportunities for social interaction, safety, a sense of wellbeing, and opportunity to use skills and increase feelings of self-worth, achievement and purpose. In a supportive environment, independence and autonomy are supported and the person develops a sense of control. Activities to provide meaning and purpose are provided. The atmosphere of a supportive environment is non-threatening and pleasant, with reduced distracting stimuli. Highlighted helpful stimuli and orientation cues are provided. It is safe and secure, adaptable, and provides areas for wandering. In general, an environment should be as home-like and visually pleasing as possible.

MUSIC THERAPY

It has been shown that intervention with music can improve cognitive function in people living with dementia, as well as their quality of life following long-term depression (Moreno-Morales et al. 2020). Music therapy, both listening to music and singing, is therefore used as a treatment or strategy for the improvement of cognitive function in people with dementia. Some organisations use individual headphones and playlists that have been tailor-made for the individual. Sometimes people who have no language have been heard to sing, and evidence implies that the music pathways in the brain often remain functional, even long into dementia.

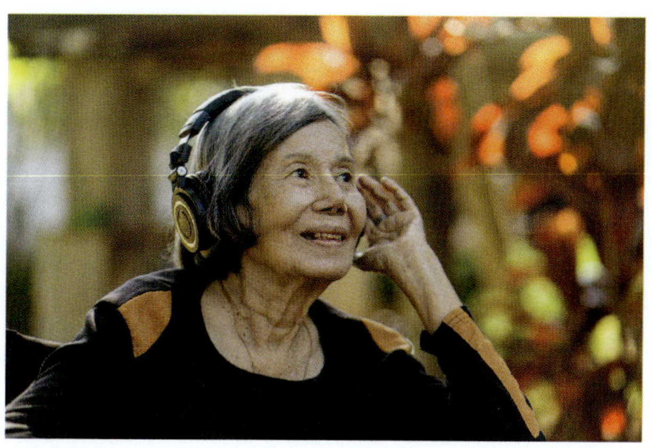

Toa55/Shutterstock

Music therapy can improve cognitive function in people with dementia

PET THERAPY

Studies in animal-assisted therapies (i.e. pet therapy) have shown that interacting with animals has many benefits, including physical, social, emotional, motivational and cognitive function. Animal-assisted therapies, or pet engagement, also aims to provide pleasure and relaxation while helping to reduce mental health conditions such as anxiety and depression. There are many well-documented benefits from pet therapy for people living with dementia, and it is easy to see why this therapy is becoming more popular. In one trial that involved dog-assisted therapy for 60 people living with dementia, all the participants increased their pro-social behaviour and reduced behavioural disturbances while interacting with the dog.

Some of the known benefits of pet therapy include increased verbal communication, increased willingness to exercise, improved interactions with others, improved joint movement and motor skills, improved independence or assisted movement, increased self-esteem, improved social skills, increased willingness to take part in activities, decreased depression, decreased isolation and loneliness, reduced boredom and reduced anxiety (Scalabrini 2022).

MULTISENSORY STIMULATION

The following senses can be used in the care and support of people living with dementia:

- visual (seeing)
- auditory (hearing)
- tactile (touching)
- gustatory (tasting)
- olfactory (smelling).

People with dementia may benefit from multisensory stimulation such as hand massage, walking outdoors, cooking, exposure to familiar smells from the kitchen (e.g. cinnamon or lemongrass) and touching familiar things such as knick-knacks or photos. It is easy to overstimulate someone with dementia, so it is best to incorporate just one stimulant at a time into the care and support of people living with dementia. It has been noted that sensory and multisensory stimulation interventions (e.g. art therapy, music therapy, bright light therapy, activity therapy and aromatherapy) allow the person with dementia to communicate and express their feelings, desires and needs when they struggle to do so verbally. Stimulation in this manner can also assist with desire to eat, encouragement with medications and supporting behaviours.

THERAPEUTIC RELATIONSHIPS

Therapeutic relationships are those that are built on trust and honesty and have the specific aim of providing benefit and support to the person with dementia. Acceptance and acknowledgement are the first step in building a therapeutic relationship and in communicating to the person with dementia that they are the centre of care and have meaning and purpose. Appropriate verbal and physical reassurance during the relationship sets the tone for the ongoing success of communication and the relationship.

VALIDATION THERAPY

Validation therapy is a concept developed by gerontological social worker Naomi Feil between 1963 and 1980 as a way of communicating with people with dementia by acknowledging, and empathising with, their feelings and reality. The principles behind the concept mean that there is no correcting a person or arguing about the truth of something; instead, it is about the care worker stepping into the person's world of reality and respectfully acknowledging and validating their feelings and what is real for them.

Validation therapy suggests that all behaviour has meaning, no matter how inappropriate it may be. A core component of validation is empathy–the ability to understand another person's circumstances and experience. By picking up non-verbal cues exhibited by the person with dementia and naming the feelings being expressed, the hope is that the person's anxiety will be reduced, which in turn reduces the stress for the care worker and loved ones.

REALITY ORIENTATION

Another therapy that has been useful in communicating with people with dementia is reality orientation. This is a process whereby the care worker tries to orient the person with dementia by presenting information about time, place and/or person. Reality orientation can be used by providing:

- reminders of the day and time
- reminders of events
- reminders of relationships
- reassurance.

Some people respond to constant prompting throughout their day to orientate them to place, time and person. This may help keep them engaged in a particular task and can be achieved through verbal and non-verbal communication. For example, holding out your arm to Val and saying, "Val, it's time for lunch" may prompt her to walk with you to the dining area. A care worker may use photos as a reminder of events and special occasions in a person's life, such as weddings and birthdays. A person may forget an important occasion, so having a photo to refer to is useful. Other people may experience an increase in frustration and sense an even greater loss of control, and such prompts may make them aware of what they have forgotten.

One of the most advanced signs of dementia is when a person forgets the name of someone who has been close to them–for example, a husband, sister or son. This is very distressing for both the person and their loved ones. One solution to this problem may be to have photos with the person's name written underneath and, perhaps, the relationship the individual has with the person. You may also like to talk with the person about their family, thereby encouraging them to reminisce.

REMINISCENCE

Reminiscence uses long-term memories to connect with the person who has dementia. It is based on the understanding that the person will have short-term memory loss but that their long-term memory remains active. Reminiscing is more than merely recalling memories; it is a tool for communicating that relies on the care worker having an in-depth knowledge of the person's history so they can converse about topics and activities they are interested in.

Another way of eliciting memories is to use the senses, as mentioned earlier: touch, taste, sight, smell and sound. For example, the smell of bread or of lavender may bring back childhood memories; classical music may soothe by bringing back pleasant memories of occasions when they heard the music or saw it performed. It is wise to be mindful that not all memories are happy ones and that certain music or aromas, or reminders of events, may actually increase distress.

A memorabilia (or keepsake or rummage) box is another concrete and creative way to encourage communication. The box can hold things from, or that make reference to, the person's past, such as a piece of lace, a concert program, a pair of gloves, a brooch or a tobacco tin. These items can be obtained from second-hand shops or from relatives who may have kept some keepsakes from the person's life.

If a person is reminiscing, they may become agitated or distressed if they start thinking about or looking for someone who is no longer there or ask about an activity or a household chore they routinely undertook. The care worker can offer relevant reassurances, such as: "Tell me more about that person" or "It's okay, the chickens were fed this morning".

Validating reality or encouraging reminiscences may not always have a positive outcome. If the care worker suspects that unpleasant memories have been evoked, they should listen to the person, be aware of their feelings and change the subject or the setting. This is called distraction and is used to divert the person into another more pleasant area of interest. Before distracting the person, acknowledge their feelings and then move onto something that will calm them. The choice of activity depends on the behaviour being modified and the person's needs and interests, as well as the environment. Cognitive and emotion-oriented interventions such as reminiscence, reality orientation and validation therapy use laughter, pleasant associations and praise along with acknowledgement and validation of feelings and emotions.

THE MONTESSORI APPROACH

The Montessori approach is a relatively new and innovative philosophy of care where support is provided for people living with dementia by creating a prepared environment filled with cues and memory supports that enable individuals to care for themselves, others and their community. The Montessori approach aims to develop communities that care for individuals with respect and dignity, and honours their choices, so they live as independently as possible. It enriches lives through the engagement in roles, routines and activities that foster a sense of belonging and purpose for the person with dementia. Environments that have proven to be successful include storytelling times, group activities and dementia-friendly gardening clubs.

SIMULATED PRESENCE THERAPY

The use of simulated presence therapy (SPT) during dementia care is emotion orientated and relies on the individual responding positively to a video or audiotape recording of family or friends, particularly during episodes of agitation or behaviours of concern. SPT has also been shown to be effective during episodes of confusion, anxiety, depression and loneliness.

WORKPLACE SCENARIO

The importance of positive relationships

James experiences episodes of confusion and frustration where he becomes angry and confrontational with unfamiliar staff. He verbalises his lack of trust of strangers and unwillingness to share his feelings with them. Although Shelly is a care worker who regularly cares for James, he often forgets who she is and that she has cared for him previously. Shelly always introduces herself to James and encourages him to discuss his feelings by asking him regularly: "What would you like ...?", "How would you like ...?" Shelly finds that this approach empowers James in decision making, gains his trust, and allows for a positive relationship to develop between herself and James, who is then more likely to remain calm and non-confrontational if he doesn't feel rushed or confused.

Another care worker, Michelle, doesn't use Shelly's positive approach. Instead, she is dominating, makes many decisions for James without consulting him, and always hurries him. As a result, James becomes confused, frustrated and confrontational. Michelle then feels vulnerable and anxious, and considers it is unsafe to continue to care for James.

Shelly's approach demonstrates a positive relationship, which has beneficial impacts on the delivery and receipt of person-centred care, compliance, safety, teamwork and time management.

CHECK YOUR UNDERSTANDING

1. What strategies can be used to gain maximum engagement with someone with dementia?
2. What is reality orientation?
3. How can communication barriers interfere with delivering care needs to someone with dementia?

11.3 MAINTAINING THE PERSON'S DIGNITY, SKILLS AND HEALTH

A diagnosis of dementia doesn't mean that a person's dignity, respect, life skills and health are lost. Instead, it means that a care worker is tasked with the role of creating or modifying activities that maintain these qualities for as long as possible. It is important to consider that activities need to meet functional needs but also needs for independence, socialising, connectedness and purpose.

11.3.1 Independence and autonomy

One of the main aims in supporting someone with dementia is to promote their dignity and independence. Remember that the person with dementia has been independent for many years; therefore, maintaining their independence is necessary for their health and wellbeing.

Promoting and maintaining independence are also reliant on being familiar with the person's social history, cultural background, routines, habits and preferences. Knowledge of a person's social history and cultural background can provide the carer with information on how to meet their needs and promote their independence, but it can also highlight situations of risk and cultural misunderstanding. Supporting the person to practise their regular routines, to maintain old habits and to express their personal preferences enables the carer to become familiar with the person, encourages the person's autonomy, and limits their challenging behaviours and non-compliance with care.

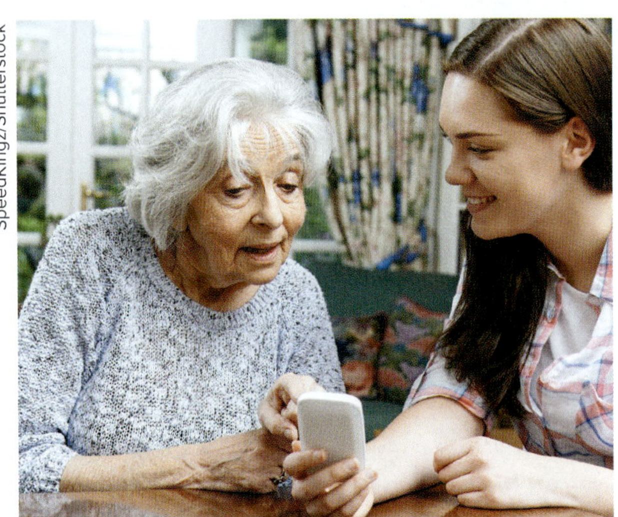

SpeedKingz/Shutterstock

Assistive technologies such as mobile phones may help people living with dementia

ASSISTIVE TECHNOLOGIES

Assistive technologies include hardware, software, tools and equipment, as well as everyday mobile phones, tracking devices and electronic tablets (see Table 11.2). Some of these technologies can assist people living with dementia, enabling inclusion and participation in life activities; however, many of them are not commonly available or used. As the person's dementia progresses, these things may become too complicated for them and for their carer at home.

An example of the use of assistive technology in RACFs is movement sensors, where a sound or light signal is sent out from the room when the person gets out of bed in the dark to go to the toilet. Movement sensors pick up the activity, and the lights might come on automatically to notify the care workers that the person might require assistance. The technology is used in this instance as a risk management strategy to prevent falls.

TABLE 11.2 Examples of the uses of assistive technologies to support the person living with dementia

Assistive technology	Use
Clocks Communication aids In-home cameras Medication management Prompts can be recorded on a device in the home and then played back out loud at the appropriate time	Self-care
Home monitoring devices Houses can be programmed to respond to internet setting commands (e.g. ovens can be turned off remotely, lights turned on and blinds opened)	Home and other environments
Clocks Prompts	Eating and drinking
Pressure-relieving mattresses	Pressure area management
Electrical appliances used for monitoring GPS location and tracking devices Home-care robots Home monitoring devices	Daily living activities
Prompts can be recorded on a device in the home and then played back out loud at the appropriate time Home monitoring devices (e.g. sensors that pick up when the bed or chair is wet, or turn the lights on when movement is sensed)	Continence and hygiene
Scooters and mobility aids Injury prevention and safety mats Low-to-the-ground beds for falls prevention	Mobility and transferring
Reminder messages recorded on a device in the home and then played back out loud at the appropriate time	Cognition and memory loss
Picture phones, large print, colours used to highlight important structures	Vision and hearing
Prompts can be recorded on a device in the home and then played back out loud at the appropriate time	Daily living activities
Electronic books, podcasts, television, streaming	Recreation and leisure
Spell checkers, visual search engines, recorders, text to speech	Education and employment

11.3.2 Dignity of risk and safety

Dignity of risk refers to the legal right of every person, including those with dementia, to choose to take risks in order to learn, grow and have a better quality of life. As the brain deteriorates in dementia, it is up to carers and others involved in care, including the care worker, to balance safety with dignity of risk. For example, if the person wishes to walk but constantly falls over, dignity of risk can be balanced with safety by the person wearing protective padding, or even a soft helmet, so if they fall, injuries will be minimised. Dignity of risk increases personhood.

11.3.3 Promoting comfort

Pain or discomfort can affect the person with dementia. It can even trigger difficult behaviour, where the person cannot explain how they are feeling. Confusion and disorientation are common when there is underlying pain or discomfort. It is the role of the care worker to observe and monitor the person. The care worker can help reposition them, using extra padding or pillows, and ensure they are in a well-ventilated space and in a comfortable setting. The care worker can check the temperature of the room and the temperature of the person and assist them accordingly. A person who is non-verbal may have a grimace on their face or clench their fists if they are in pain, and it will be the care worker who documents this and reports it to the supervisor. Medication may be required to ease the pain. The person needs the care worker to advocate for this to the supervisor, as they are unable to do it themselves.

11.3.4 Activities

Activities are done on a day-to-day basis. Some activities are the practical aspects of living, while others meet a psychological need. Activities for people with dementia are not only about functional need; they are also a way of connecting and interacting with others and provide a wonderful opportunity to participate in something that has purpose and meaning. In any one day, a range of activities can be offered. They can be structured, or less so, and should include tasks across all domains. For example:

- *Activities of life:* the role in life that has helped to define the person–such as their occupation, leisure activities and creative activities.
- *Basic activities of daily living:* eating and drinking, personal hygiene and grooming, mobilising, transferring, changing position, maintaining personal safety, communication, attending to the spirit, expressing sexuality.
- *Instrumental activities that allow a person to live independently:* using a telephone, accessing finances, shopping, socialising, preparing a meal, doing the housework and laundry, carrying out home repairs, taking medications, paying bills, performing spiritual activities, travelling in private or public transport, leisure and sport.

Wherever the person with dementia lives, it is important to support them to be as independent as possible. This will help to maintain their residual skills, enhance their physical and cognitive wellbeing, and increase their self-esteem. Strategies for promoting independence in activities for the person with dementia include:

- breaking down tasks into steps and presenting them one step at a time
- prompting and modelling the task
- modifying the environment to suit and to increase safety
- taking a strengths-based approach–for example, focus on what they can do, even if they can only do part of the task. They may be able to place the pillow on the bed but not tuck in the sheet. Thank them for what they have done and encourage them to keep helping.

DESIGNING ACTIVITIES

The care worker may be involved in supporting people with dementia to become engaged in activities. Investigate their social history, talk to the family, and develop an understanding of who they are and what might be a suitable or enjoyable activity for them. Remember: not everything will suit everybody. Activities should be dignified and appropriate to the age of the person. They should not be hurried and should be carried out one step at a time. Activities should not set the person up to fail, so they must be suitable, achievable and of interest to them (see Table 11.3). Cognition is often better in the morning, so more complicated tasks might be attempted then; but remember: they should be failure proof! Supporting cultural needs is also important when considering suitable activities, taking into account that the person with dementia will revert to old behaviours, old teachings and old beliefs. If they learnt to speak English as a second language, they may lose it and revert to their first language. When they are doing the activity, try to build on their strengths and to support them only when they indicate they require it.

TABLE 11.3 Aims and types of activities the care worker can initiate

Aim of activity	Type of activity	A few examples
To increase self-esteem	Encourage activities where the person may feel helpful	Carrying groceries Feeding pets Washing dishes Sweeping
To create a sense of purpose	Daily living skills	Eating independently after you have cut up their food (as needed) Holding a washcloth in the shower to attend to what they can do Passing their clothes to them in sequence to avoid them getting mixed up (apraxia)
	Activities related to their occupation	Painting an old bookshelf Rebuilding an old radio Stacking books
	Relaxation and pleasure	High tea and conversation Cards (can be modified to suit the players—anything from playing games, to sorting them, to talking about the pictures on them) Happy hour
To re-establish past roles	A routine or habitual activity they performed in the past	Playing a musical instrument Folding the washing Sorting socks Raking leaves Collecting the mail Polishing shoes or utensils Knitting may become too hard as the dementia progresses, but many things can be done with a basket of different-coloured balls of wool (e.g. sorting them by colour)
To provide emotional release	Recreational activities	Playing music Listening to music Painting Being with children Being with animals
To encourage participation in group activities	Belonging, inclusion and social interaction	Watching live entertainment Having picnics Walking Playing board games (e.g. Scrabble)

WORKPLACE SCENARIO

Promoting self-esteem through meaningful activity

Graham has alcohol-related dementia and has problems with memory loss, apathy and planning. Care worker Leonard has been supporting Graham for some time and has noticed that his motivation has decreased and his social skills have declined. He is concerned about Graham's overall health and wellbeing. He asks some colleagues and Thong, the nurse practitioner, about implementing the broader aspects of person-centred care to give Graham a greater sense of self and normality.

(Continues)

In consultation with Graham, his wife Esther and Thong, the care team identifies further examples of what Graham's "normal" life was like prior to his illness. Thong points out that this is especially relevant in Graham's case, as skills he had developed prior to the onset of this type of dementia are often maintained and may be masked by depression.

Esther explains that Graham enjoyed listening to music and playing the piano, that he doesn't like to get up before 8 am, and that he loves her very much and enjoys playing with his dog.

Based on this information and Graham's existing social history, Thong explains that staff will make efforts to create an environment that is more familiar to Graham, including playing the music he enjoys and giving him an opportunity to play the piano, to spend more time with Esther and to visit his dog.

In a staff meeting, Thong outlines that the aim of these more personalised arrangements is to convey that Graham is known, that his family is welcome to visit him, that his interests are meaningful and that his environment reflects his preferences.

Graham's mood soon improves and he is more engaged socially, indicating an overall increase in his self-esteem.

CHECK YOUR UNDERSTANDING

1. Provide some examples of assistive technologies and how can they be used to support a person with dementia.
2. What strategies can promote independence for the person with dementia?
3. How can you design activities for an individual living with dementia?
4. What activities can help to increase self-esteem for a person living with dementia?
5. What activities can create a sense of purpose for the person living with dementia?

11.4 UNDERSTANDING DISTRESSED BEHAVIOURS

11.4.1 The causes of distressed behaviours

People with dementia can develop behaviours that are difficult for those around them. These behaviours are sometimes referred to as challenging behaviours or behaviours of concern but the correct name is behavioural and psychological symptoms of dementia. Most people think of these behaviours as concerning and difficult. Examples might include:

- social withdrawal
- resistance to care
- verbal disruption
- repetition of speech or actions
- disinhibition
- eating problems
- social or sexual inappropriateness
- wandering and intrusiveness
- absconding
- sleep disorders.

The person with dementia is trying to make sense of their world and can sometimes misinterpret cues or stimuli. For example, someone who experienced trauma as a result of a bushfire might become very frightened when a match is lit to light candles on a birthday cake. This way of understanding people's behaviour overlaps with trauma-informed practice, where past events have had an impact and now, as understanding diminishes, they become more fearful and troubled. It is good for the care worker to know and understand the person's past and to deliver care and support with that in mind.

The environment and immediate surrounds can impact on a person's behaviour. Relationships with the people they are interacting with, whether their communication is clear to others and whether they can understand what is being said, will impact on the way they behave. Their physical health and wellbeing, their nature and their temperament can also impact on their behaviour. The normal channels of communicating have been disrupted, so they will search for other ways to get their message across. Their cognition deficit causes the behaviour; the person is not "acting out" or "being naughty"—they are just searching for a way to meet an unmet need. In summary, predisposing factors to behaviour during dementia are often identified as either:

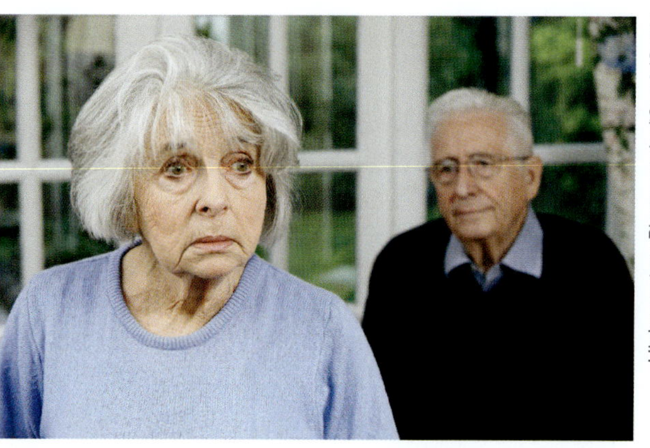

Highwaystarz-Photography/iStock/Getty Images Plus

The person with dementia can become confused about their environment

- *environmental:* e.g. bright lights, noise, unfamiliar surrounds or people
- *physical or biological:* e.g. pain, discomfort, constipation, hearing or visual impairments, hunger, thirst, dehydration
- *emotional:* e.g. fear, anxiety, depression, happiness, sadness, loneliness.

Behaviour is the way a person acts or performs physically, socially and emotionally. It is the way we communicate and express ourselves in any given situation, offering meaning and purpose. Behaviour is personal, open to interpretation by others, and can change in response to various factors. Each person with dementia is unique and therefore responds uniquely to their own circumstances or to changes in their circumstances. During dementia, not all behavioural changes are challenging, of concern or distressing; yet many offer information about underlying pathology and needs. New behaviours may be an indication of pathological changes in the brain, or of environmental changes and the need to communicate an unmet need.

Sometimes it is difficult to identify the reason or trigger behind changed behaviour, but well-planned and appropriately designed activities and environments have been found to limit the occurrence of challenging and distressing behaviours of concern. As dementia progresses and cognitive abilities decline, normal channels of communication are disrupted and, as a consequence, the person with dementia needs to find another way to communicate.

It is important to note any predisposing factors and to communicate them to the team, both verbally and by using documentation such as behavioural charts and incident reports. These actions will ensure consistency and continuity of care in a safe and effective manner.

11.4.2 Predisposing factors and triggers for behaviours

It is important to identify what might have caused a behaviour of concern. It isn't always easy to identify triggers; some may not be obvious, but it has become widely believed that difficult behaviours are an attempt to communicate an unmet need. The care worker needs to learn to respond to the person in a person-centred way to determine what message may be trying to get through. This may minimise or eradicate the behaviour. Activities we have spoken about earlier are a way to manage the behavioural and psychological symptoms of dementia. While people are engaged in an activity that is meaningful to them, they are less likely to be agitated and unsettled. Because the person living with dementia cannot change the way they respond, the care worker should adapt their own behaviour, language and communication with them, in an effort to understand what has triggered the behaviour.

11.4.3 Behavioural and psychological symptoms of dementia

The **behavioural and psychological symptoms of dementia (BPSD)**—also known as behaviours of concern, challenging behaviours or distressed behaviours—are often highly subjective in their interpretation. Distressing behaviours are those behaviours that cause distress of any description to the person with dementia or to another person, no matter how small or big the impact. In relation to dementia care, such behaviours may distress a care worker, the person with dementia, family, friends, the general public, or other visitors to and residents of a facility.

THE PROBLEM OF LABELLING

It is unfortunate that the negative behaviours of people with dementia are reported more often than their positive behaviours, because these observations cause bias, prejudice, discrimination, stereotyping and labelling of people with dementia. In turn, this can lead to inaccurate descriptions and interpretations of a behaviour and its triggers, as well as to poor choices of care provided.

SPECIFIC BEHAVIOURS WITH DE-ESCALATION PROCESSES

AGITATION

Agitation includes behaviours of wandering, rummaging, pacing, yelling, screaming, repetitive questioning and hoarding. Triggers for these behaviours are very individual; hence, it is important to get to know the person with dementia in order to better understand their particular triggers.

AGGRESSION

Aggression expressed verbally and/or physically is often stimulated or triggered by frustration and physical symptoms of pain and discomfort. Grieving has also been noted to cause anger and aggression. In all instances, the safety and wellbeing of all persons close by are of the utmost importance. Therefore, it is common practice not to attempt to intervene to stop the aggressive behaviour but, instead, to remove oneself and others from the immediate area and out of harm's way if it is safe to do so. Sometimes it is best to physically direct the person displaying the behaviour to a private area using a calm and sensitive approach.

Validation of the person's feelings is helpful, as it may show them that you acknowledge and understand their emotion. This is empathy. Sometimes the person may benefit from having the opportunity to express their feelings safely. Distraction is another strategy that may be helpful in de-escalating the person's feelings and expression; however, it doesn't deal with the cause of the behaviour. Medical reviews are important for eliminating potential causes of the behaviour, and all medications should be reviewed frequently.

Your safety is essential. If you are threatened by someone's confrontational behaviour, maintain a safe distance from them and implement the following strategies:

- Don't turn your back on the person.
- Avoid being backed into a corner.
- Keep a solid article (e.g. a bed or a table) between you and the person.
- Know the locations of the exits and have a clear pathway to one.
- Know how to use distress alarms.
- Communicate clearly with colleagues about the whereabouts of the situation before it escalates.

The important thing to remember is that aggression is a communication method. The person is trying to communicate a message in probably the only way they know how.

SUNDOWNING

Sundowning is where the person with dementia becomes agitated and restless, wanders off, and becomes anxious, confused and disorientated in the late afternoon or early evening. No definitive cause for sundowning has been established; however, it has been suggested that it may be linked to the person being tired or in pain or having memories relating to familiar events that occurred at this time of day. For example, for many people it is a time when family members returned home from work or school, so theory suggests that the person with dementia is wandering around, looking for them and anticipating their return.

Strategies used to manage sundowning include ensuring the person's safety by arranging the environment so they cannot wander out into traffic and validating what is occurring for the person by asking them questions and responding appropriately without escalating the behaviour. For example, if the person says they are looking for someone, ask them about the person and what they do. This often calms, reassures and validates the person, while safely managing the situation. Other strategies could include organising activities for that time of the day to distract the person. For example, the person could assist with setting the table for dinner or be asked to fold linen, or it could be a time for napping or resting. When new instances of sundowning occur, a medical review should be done and triggers monitored.

APATHY AND WITHDRAWAL

Apathy, where there is a lack of interest or concern, and withdrawal are also specific behaviours commonly observed in the later stages of dementia. These behaviours may be indicators of depression or grief, or feelings of loneliness and of not fitting in. In these situations, strategies require thought and creativity to engage the person and keep their attention. Successful strategies always focus on the person themselves and on understanding what is occurring for them. Knowledge of their social history, and consideration of their cultural background and of information gathered from family and friends, can be helpful in designing activities and strategies to re-engage them and encourage interaction in new environments, in particular. It is essential that these behaviours are investigated by a medical professional to ensure they are not linked to a clinical issue such as depression or hypoactive delirium.

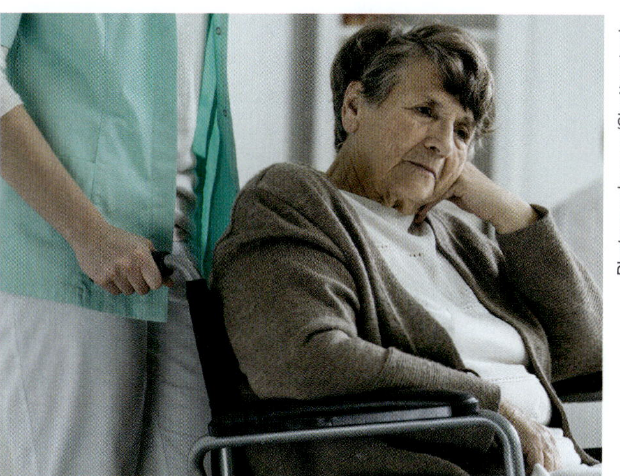

Photographee.eu/Shutterstock

Apathy and withdrawal are commonly observed in the later stages of dementia

CATASTROPHIC REACTIONS

Catastrophic reactions are reactions where the person with dementia overreacts to a stimulus and often results in undesirable, or what may be deemed inappropriate, behaviour. Examples include uncontrollable and often inappropriate laughter, crying, screaming, yelling, agitation and anxiety. Catastrophic reactions may occur suddenly or can follow a slow build-up. As they can initiate or escalate the behaviours of others in group settings, the care worker needs to pay particular attention to this possibility and seek assistance as required so as to ensure the safety of all.

Strategies the care worker may use to avoid or limit such reactions include:

- being aware of moods and what triggers behaviours
- being aware of group dynamics
- speaking slowly, calmly, quietly and appropriately
- acknowledging feelings and behaviours
- avoiding confrontation
- providing the person time to express their feelings and to calm down alone if it is safe to do so
- following policies and procedures.

Regardless of the type of behaviour the person is experiencing, they are trying to communicate something. As Nathaniel Hawthorne wrote, "He deemed it essential, it would seem, to know the man before attempting to do him good" (1850). The key to successful behaviour management is knowing someone well and understanding what further behaviours or actions will escalate or de-escalate a situation for that individual.

THE ROLE OF THE CARE WORKER

Ultimately, the care worker's goal is to understand and prevent behaviours of concern, and this may be achieved when you have a deeper understanding of the individual. However, even the interventions and proactive strategies noted below for addressing identified behaviours are not guaranteed to work every time.

- Keep a record of the behaviour.
  - Identify the behaviour. Who is it a problem for?
  - Is there a medical reason for the behaviour? (For example, it is common for a person with a urinary tract infection to feel confused and disoriented.)
  - When does it happen?
  - How often does it happen?
  - How long does it last for?
  - What happened before the behaviour? (This is identifying the triggers.)
  - Was that a trigger for the behaviour?
  - What happened during and after the behaviour?
  - Review the environment. Is there a trigger in the current environment?
  - Are the person's routines and activities meeting their needs?
  - Are their psychosocial needs being met?
  - Do they feel valued? How is their self-esteem?
  - What are possible ways to minimise this behaviour?
  - Use what you know about this unique person to implement strategies.
  - Consult and collaborate with other staff for consistency and more information.
  - Trial and evaluate any new strategy that is implemented.
- If everyone is safe, then the behaviour isn't really causing any distress. If the behaviour needs to be reduced, try the following:
  - Let your supervisor know that the person might need a medical check-up to exclude illness or pain.
  - Ask your supervisor if the person's medications could be causing this behaviour.
  - Remove triggers such as keys from view.
  - Ensure the environment is secure (e.g. use murals to disguise exits).
  - Ensure the person has identification on them at all times.
  - Engage them in movement and physical activity during the day to promote sleep at night.
  - Place familiar items from home in their environment (e.g. their own bed quilt or small, significant objects).
  - Schedule activities that are meaningful to them to promote engagement and keep them busy.
  - Adjust the environment to suit the individual.

ANTECEDENT BEHAVIOURS CONSEQUENCE (ABC) MODEL OF BEHAVIOUR SUPPORT AND MANAGEMENT

The **Antecedent Behaviours Consequence (ABC) model** identifies the behaviour, looks at the triggers that may have caused it and evaluates the consequences of the behaviour. This information is used to guide staff and carers in preventing or minimising the behaviour in future. Always remember that the behaviour originates from the pathological changes in the brain and is not intentional or malicious.

WORKPLACE SCENARIO

Managing distress

Olek yells for up to three hours a day and most of the care staff say that he is "a selfish nuisance". He is on a substantial dose of antipsychotic medication that the staff complain makes no difference to his behaviour, and they avoid going into his room apart from when they must provide him with personal care and assistance with meals.

The causes of Olek's behaviour lie in his traumatic past and in his current physical discomfort in the care environment. The following factors are contributing to his distress:

- He doesn't know that he yells and has apologised for being a nuisance, suggesting the staff have conveyed their feelings to him.
- He is socially isolated.
- He is a survivor of internment in Krakow, Poland, during the Second World War, and the use of a German-speaking interpreter caused him to experience flashbacks.
- The staff are unaware of his past.
- He is unable to change his position and is often uncomfortable and in pain.

Zac holds a staff meeting and explains what is happening to Olek and why. Mary, the RN, and Sony, the team leader, review the schedule for repositioning Olek, and Mary discusses his medications with the doctor, who cancels all antipsychotics. The care staff now respond quickly to Olek's screams, comforting him and offering reassurance rather than rebukes. They also assess his pain and report any changes to Mary and Sony. Olek is also provided the opportunity to be in the lounge area, where he can interact with staff and see other people. He is now having fewer outbursts and his relationships with staff have improved.

Helping all care staff to understand the meaning of Olek's behaviour is sufficient to change their attitude and responses, thus improving Olek's quality of life and creating a better work environment for themselves.

CHECK YOUR UNDERSTANDING

1. Provide six examples of challenging or difficult behaviours that may be present when a person is living with dementia.
2. What causes challenging behaviours?
3. What is your role when supporting a person with challenging behaviours?
4. What is the problem with labelling a person as having challenging behaviours?
5. What does BPSD stand for? Describe what it means.

11.5 DOCUMENTATION

Review and evaluation are important for the continuity of safe and effective care and the management of behaviours of concern. Dementia is progressive; the brain is constantly changing, affecting the person's behaviours over time. This means the review and evaluation of their needs and preferences is ongoing, and these processes involve communication, collaboration and consultation. Communication should occur in collaboration and consultation with all involved in the care and welfare of the person with dementia, including family and friends.

Evaluating care interventions and reviewing outcomes takes place daily, before and after new interventions, and as required or indicated by changes in behaviours, deterioration, or further diagnosis of a medical condition. Reviewing processes may also be indicated by funding arrangements and be directed by the policies and procedures of a given facility or service. It is everybody's role and responsibility to review and evaluate care and management in response to the individual's needs as a method of ensuring the safety and wellbeing of everyone involved. Documentation has to be accurate, objective and appropriately detailed.

11.5.1 Organisational policies and procedures

Reporting and documenting requirements may differ from setting to setting, especially where reporting and documentation are directly linked to funding. Some organisations will have policies and procedures in place that direct the frequency and format of documentation and records, as well as the circumstance when various types of documentation are to be implemented.

Behavioural charts are commonly used to document, analyse and monitor BPSD as a way of identifying triggers for behaviours and of communicating when and why behaviours occur. It is also essential to complete documents and forms specific to the individual, as well as other assessment tools such as falls risk assessment tools, pressure area care charts, wound charts, pain scores, etc. As a requirement of government funding, forms such as these may need to be completed and updated with any changes in order to secure the funding.

Verbal reporting is just as important as written documentation. All reporting should be professional, honest and in the best interests of the person receiving care while providing information to be used during care provision. Verbal reporting is often used between shifts to ensure the care delivery is consistent and information is shared for continuing safety and wellbeing of the person with dementia. This verbal exchange is often referred to as handover. Verbal reports are also used in other circumstances, such as reporting to the registered nurse or supervisor, or to other health professionals and the person's carer and family.

Language used should be universal and able to be understood by all receiving the verbal report, with only relevant information shared that is non-judgemental, non-discriminatory and free of stereotypes, bias and prejudice. Derogatory comments, assumptions or accusations are uncalled for and disrespectful and breach the care worker's code of conduct; therefore, they should not be verbalised at any stage.

Some facilities use an acronym–**ISBAR**–to describe the content of a verbal report on each person who is receiving care from shift to shift. The acronym ensures that all relevant information is reported systematically and in an organised format. ISBAR is interpreted as:

- *Introduction/identify self:* Identify yourself, who you are talking to and who you are talking about.
- *Situation:* What is the current situation, concerns, observations, behaviours, etc.?
- *Background:* What is the relevant background? This helps to set the scene to interpret the situation accurately.
- *Assessment:* What do you think the problem is? This requires the person making the verbal report to interpret the situation and the background information and to form an opinion on what is going on.
- *Recommendation:* What do you need them to do? What do you recommend should be done to correct the current situation? What strategies could be used that are in compliance with duty of care and the need for safety?

11.5.2 Restraint and restrictive practices

Restraint is the forcible restriction of movement of a person to prevent injury to themselves or others. It may be necessary occasionally for limited periods of time when a person is severely restless, confused or confrontational. The use of restraints is causing more and more concern because it can violate a person's right to free movement. To restrain inappropriately may lead to charges of false imprisonment and is ethically unsound. The use of restraints should be viewed as a temporary solution to behaviours, and only ever as the last resort, when all other alternatives have been considered. The least-restrictive form of restraint possible must be used and should be ordered by the doctor after discussion with the person's family. Restraints can only be used when people are harming themselves or others, where they are causing damage to property, or they are severely disrupting the lives of their family or friends.

TYPES OF RESTRAINT

Physical restraint is the intentional restriction of the voluntary movement of a person by the use of a device, removal of a mobility aid or the use of physical force without the consent of the person. *Chemical restraint* is the use of medication, such as prescribed antipsychotics, or over-the-counter or complementary medications, to control a person's behaviour. Other types of restraint include environmental restraint, extreme aversive practices, and person-to-person restraint, which can be hands-on, verbal or psychological.

ALTERNATIVES TO RESTRAINT

Various environmental, physical and psychological strategies can be used as an alternative to restraint. An environment that is well lit, quiet and free of clutter will help the person to stay safe. By lowering the bed, for example, bed rail restraint won't be required, as the person cannot fall far from a bed that is close to the floor. Creating safe spaces for the person to wander in, both inside and outside, with activities set up to catch their attention, will deter people from exit seeking and intrusive behaviour. There are many more environmental factors that can minimise the need for restraints.

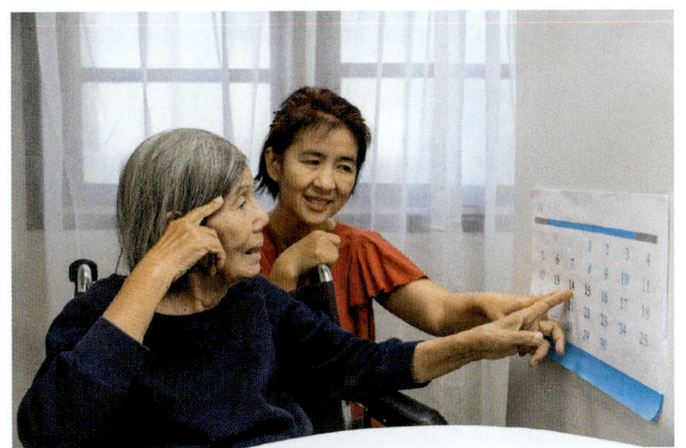

Toa55/Shutterstock.com

Having dedicated staff to support people living with dementia can contribute to a restraint-free environment

Physical assessment, medication review and pain management are among the physical strategies that can minimise the use of restraints. Meaningful activities, social programs, leisure, gardening and hundreds of other ideas can be considered as an alternative to restraint.

Alterations to care, such as having dedicated staff to support people living with dementia and maintaining routines, can contribute to a restraint-free environment. Most organisations across disability and aged care have committed to a restraint-free environment.

LEGISLATIVE AND REGULATORY REQUIREMENTS REGARDING RESTRAINT

Restraint must be, by law, the least-restrictive form possible. It needs to be ordered by the doctor. After discussion with the doctor, the family must approve of this intervention. Sometimes a guardianship tribunal may be involved. The type of restraint must be documented and time limits for application and release recorded, and the person must be observed closely at regular intervals and their safety maintained. Staff need to be educated in these legal requirements and educated in the policies and procedures around restraint. The decision to use restraint must be recorded in the person's individual plan and be re-evaluated constantly and consistently.

As stated above, the use of restraints must adhere to legal guidelines, which include the requirement to monitor and document observations of the restrained person and the times of application and release of restraints. This recording may be within the scope of the care worker.

The use of restraint is governed by the compliance requirements of the Aged Care Quality and Safety Commission, and failure to use restraint appropriately can be a reportable incident under the Serious Incident Response Scheme framework.

11.5.3 Reporting

Regardless of employment location or environment, the care worker has a role and responsibility to observe, report, communicate and document behaviours. It is through comprehensive, accurate and honest observation and reporting that behaviours can be identified, monitored and managed effectively and consistently. It is also integral to the assurance that individual needs are met appropriately and legally within the Aged Care Quality Standards.

Legally and ethically, care workers involved in the care of someone with dementia have a role and responsibility to report and document their observations about the person, such as changes to behaviour that may have an impact on the next person involved in care. This is essential for ongoing support for the person and also for the safety of other people. Reporting should occur in a timely manner and not be left until the person reaches a point where they become so distressed they are potentially at risk of causing harm to themselves or others.

WORKPLACE SCENARIO

Using an ABC chart

Edna (93) is experiencing mild symptoms of dementia. She has recently been admitted to a residential aged care facility for full-time care and management after episodes of unsafe wandering at her usual place of residence, her lifelong home. Last night, Edna was found to have wandered into another resident's room. She became angry when the care worker tried to direct her back to her own room. She shouted that she was looking for her children, who needed to go to bed. Using the ABC approach, the care worker was able to target interventions aimed at modifying the consequences.

The **A**ntecedent was identified as an unfamiliar environment, while the care worker validated and respected the **B**ehaviour of wandering by ensuring Edna's personal space and using a calm tone when talking with her and redirecting her back to her room. The **C**onsequence of the behaviour and interaction allows Edna to continue to wander safely, but she can be easily redirected back to her room without her becoming angry or yelling. Further strategies may be used in scenarios similar to this, including using role modelling and offering explanations of where her children are.

CHECK YOUR UNDERSTANDING

1. What are the types of restraint?
2. What is the role and responsibility of the care worker where restrictive practices are used?
3. What are the legal ramifications when restraint is used?
4. What is the ABC approach to managing challenging behaviours?
5. What methods can be used instead of restraining someone?

11.6 SELF-CARE

Working with people who are experiencing dementia can be challenging and stressful, and these feelings can accumulate over time and affect care workers' personal lives. Recognising the need for self-care interventions is critical to the care worker's health and wellbeing, but it is also crucial to the longevity and safety of the care being delivered. Self-care needs are directly related to stress levels and experiences.

Under work health and safety (WHS) legislation, each workplace should have a system in place that is focused on identifying self-care requirements and then implementing strategies to support self-care. This means:

- Supervisors are supportive and responsive when care workers are feeling stressed.
- Managers recognise that stress is a WHS issue and develop prevention strategies.
- Managers provide training and staff development activities to reduce stress.
- Support staff are involved in decision making around care strategies, especially for managing difficult behaviours.
- Procedures and policies are in place for managing conflict, confrontation and violence.
- Post-incident support is in place.
- A review system is in place.

Care workers should be given the opportunity to raise concerns and issues and be encouraged to be part of a problem-solving approach. This benefits everyone, as it has an effect on workplace culture and initiates change for the better.

11.6.1 Stress

Stress is essentially a very individual illness described as anything that causes an interruption to a person's ADLs, including physically, mentally, socially, emotionally, religiously, culturally, spiritually, sexually or financially. There are many causes of stress, and each individual experiences it in an individual way. Caring for someone with dementia has been recognised as a particularly stressful task for the care worker, family, friends and caretakers.

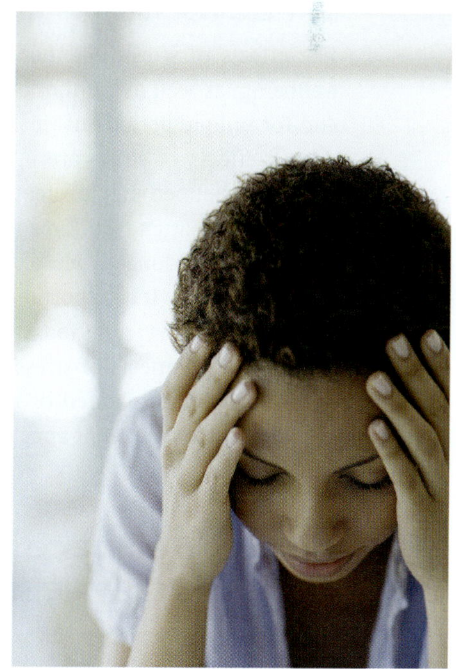

Caring for a loved one with dementia can be a particularly stressful task for family members

CAUSES

Causes of stress for someone caring for a person with dementia are related to fear, frustration, repetitiveness, lack of patience and the emotional drain associated with observing the decline in cognitive and physical function of someone with dementia. When caring for someone with dementia, it is common to develop a fear associated with the unpredictability of the person's behaviours. Frustration and a lack of patience may develop as a result of the repetitiveness of care activities and the constant need to repeat instructions or conversations, while emotional drain can occur when observing the deterioration of a once physically and cognitively active person. As well as work-related stress, there can be trauma and vicarious trauma.

Vicarious trauma results from empathetic engagement with trauma survivors. Anyone who engages empathetically with survivors of traumatic incidents and with material relating to their trauma is potentially affected, including care workers, RNs, doctors and other health professionals. This can increase the stress felt in the workplace. Shift work, time management and teamwork may also contribute to a care worker's stress levels in any given situation.

SIGNS

It is reasonable to expect that the signs and symptoms of stress may vary quite widely from person to person. A person with dementia may experience similar signs and symptoms of stress as a person not diagnosed with dementia. Table 11.4 lists common signs and symptoms of stress.

TABLE 11.4 Common signs and symptoms of stress

Physical	Cognitive	Behavioural	Psychological or emotional
Headache	Memory loss	Alcohol use	Anxiety
Chest pain	Inability to organise	Drug use	Inappropriate emotional expression
Sudden weight gain	Inability to plan	Isolation	Crying
Sudden weight loss	Disorientation	Increased socialisation	Yelling/outbursts
Interrupted sleep patterns	Confusion	Attention seeking	Anger
Acne	Misunderstanding/lack of comprehension	Excessive spending	Lack of motivation
Dishevelled appearance		Changes in sexual activity	Thoughts of paranoia

EFFECTS

The effects of stress, whether short or long term, can have a significant effect on a person's health and wellbeing, as well as on the longevity of a care worker's career. Each person experiences stress differently and for unique periods of time; however, the overall effects are somewhat similar. The personal and work-related effects of stress are intertwined and often coexist. For example, a person who is feeling stressed and overwhelmed may overeat, which can lead to obesity, low energy levels and poor motivation. Loss of motivation to attend work may result in increased sick leave. With long-term stress (also known as burnout), a person is no longer able to function effectively or to capacity, on a personal or professional level and sometimes both. It is important to recognise that burnout doesn't happen suddenly; it is the result of chronic levels of stress over a period of time.

Short-term effects of stress can be overcome or remedied more effectively and more quickly than long-term effects. Unexplained or increased absences from work, poor work performance, missed or extended meal breaks, an unkempt appearance and inappropriate verbal responses are common signs that someone is experiencing stress at work.

11.6.2 Self-care strategies

MANAGING STRESS EVERY DAY

Self-care is about recognising your own needs and taking whatever action is required to care for yourself physically, emotionally, culturally, religiously, spiritually, socially and financially. Self-care doesn't have to be complicated or time-consuming, but it does need to be done daily to ensure holistic health and wellbeing is maintained.

Self-care strategies that can be used daily to prevent stress escalating, and to manage stress before it reaches burnout, include eating well, getting enough rest and sleep, and socialising with friends and family as often as required. Planning, being organised and time management are also daily self-care strategies that work for most people. The important thing to remember is that self-care is exactly what the person who requires self-care wants it to be, because self-care is based on individual needs.

As an individual, you can manage everyday stress by:

- keeping things in perspective and prioritising tasks
- being well informed about your role
- setting yourself realistic goals
- practising relaxation techniques (e.g. going for a walk during meal break)
- sharing your worries with colleagues, family and friends (when appropriate)

- eating healthily and exercising regularly
- finding time to have fun with family and friends and trying something new.

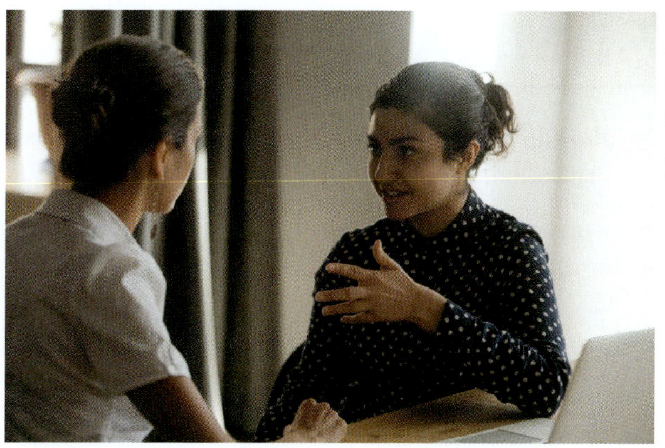

fizkes/Shutterstock

Debriefing with colleagues can be helpful in addressing stress

RESOURCES FOR CARE WORKERS

All workers have a right to a safe workplace under the WHS Act, and this includes minimising the risk of the worker suffering harm or an injury. The employer has a legal responsibility to do everything reasonably practicable to prevent psychological harm to employees and will have policies and procedures in place that support employee wellbeing.

Debriefing with colleagues is helpful in addressing stress or stressful events, and many organisations will organise group debriefing sessions to provide support to staff.

Most organisations have accessed the services of an independent organisation to provide counselling and psychological support for employees who require it. Such employee assistance programs (EAPs) are private and confidential and are available free of charge to all staff members.

WORKPLACE SCENARIO

Managing personal stress

Sandra has been a care worker for several years. For the past several months, she has worked in the dementia support area. Sandra has always taken pride in her work and displayed a happy manner when interacting with the people she supports. However, her colleagues are noticing that she has been taking a lot of sick days recently, and that when she is at work, she keeps to herself. They have also noticed that she seems uninterested in supporting the residents with activities, which is something that she used to enjoy.

Marie, the team leader, invites Sandra for a coffee catch-up. After explaining to Sandra the concerns the other staff members have, she asks her how she is feeling. Sandra bursts into tears. She tells Marie that she feels she isn't coping with work because she is exhausted. Her marriage isn't doing well, she says, and her father has been diagnosed with dementia. She says she doesn't want to imagine what his future might look like. Seeing people with dementia every day at work is stressing her out.

Marie and Sandra come up with a plan that will help Sandra with her stress while she processes what is happening in her own life. The plan includes having a regular coffee catch-up with Marie to debrief, taking some time off work immediately, and returning to work on different duties for a while. Marie also gives Sandra contact details for the organisation's EAP if she chooses to access it.

CHECK YOUR UNDERSTANDING

1. Define self-care.
2. Define stress.
3. How can we self-care?
4. What resources are available for self-care as a care worker?
5. Why can caring for someone with dementia cause stress?

SUMMARY

- Providing care to someone with dementia and supporting a person affected by dementia is a complex task requiring dedication, patience and understanding.
- Currently, there is no cure for dementia; however, signs, symptoms and behaviours encountered with dementia can be managed via holistic, person-centred care.
- This chapter has discussed the requirement to develop skills and knowledge in:
  - preparing to provide support to those affected by dementia
  - using appropriate communication strategies
  - providing activities for maintenance of dignity, skills and health
  - implementing strategies that minimise the impact of behaviours of concern
  - completing documentation
  - implementing self-care strategies.
- Persons living with dementia are worthy of a high standard of care and a quality of life that allows human rights and personhood to be respected and dignified.

REVIEW QUESTIONS

11.1 How does dementia affect the functioning of the body?

11.2 How is a diagnosis of dementia made?

11.3 What are the two types of treatment or management for dementia? State the purpose of each.

11.4 What are the principles underlying designing activities for someone with dementia? Provide one example of each principle to support your answer.

11.5 What actions can you take to minimise the frequency and reduce the impact of behaviours of concern on the person living with dementia and others?

BIBLIOGRAPHY

Aged Care Quality and Safety Commission, *Serious Incident Response Scheme*, https://www.agedcarequality.gov.au/sirs, accessed 20 March 2022.

Australian Institute of Health and Welfare (AIHW), Dementia, 23 July 2020, https://www.aihw.gov.au/reports/australias-health/dementia/, accessed 20 March 2022.

Brooker, D., *Person-centred Dementia Care: Making Services Better*, Jessica Kingsley Publishers, 2007.

Dementia Australia, *Types of Dementia*, 2022, https://www.dementia.org.au/information/about-dementia/types-of-dementia/, accessed 20 March 2022.

Dementia Australia, *Vascular Dementia*, 2022, https://www.dementia.org.au/about-dementia/types-of-dementia/vascular-dementia, accessed 15 April 2022.

Dewing, J. & McCormack, B. "Editorial: Tell me, how do you define person-centredness?", *Journal of Clinical Nursing* 26(17–18), 2017, pp. 2509–10. doi:10.1111/jocn.13681.

Emerson, E., *Challenging Behaviour: Analysis and Intervention in People with Severe Disabilities*, Cambridge University Press, 2001.

Hawthorne, N., *The Scarlet Letter*, 1850.

Kitwood, T., *Dementia Reconsidered: The Person Comes First*, Open University Press, 1997.

Moreno-Morales, C., Calero, R., Moreno-Morales, P. & Pintado, C., "Music therapy in the treatment of dementia: a systematic review and meta-analysis", *Frontiers in Medicine* 7, 2020, p. 160. https://doi.org/10.3389/fmed.2020.00160.

My Aged Care, Short-term care, https://www.myagedcare.gov.au/short-term-care, accessed 19 April 2022.

Orgeta, V., "Post-traumatic stress disorder linked to increased risk of dementia–new research", *The Conversation*, September 2020, https://theconversation.com/post-traumatic-stress-disorder-linked-to-increased-risk-of-dementia-new-research-146325/, accessed 31 March 2022.

Scalabrini, *The Benefits of Pet Therapy for People Living with Dementia*, 2022, https://staging.scalabrini.com.au/the-benefits-of-pet-therapy-for-people-living-with-dementia.

Stokes, G., *Challenging Behaviour in Dementia: A Person-Centred Approach*, Taylor & Francis, 2017.

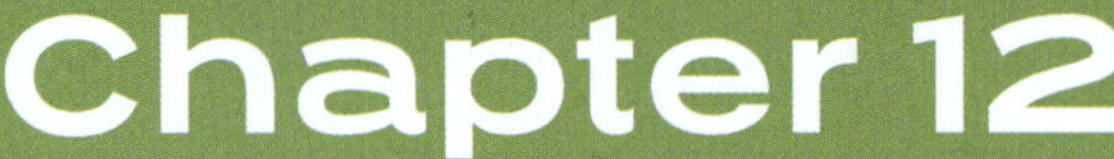

Caring for people with a life-limiting illness

LEARNING OBJECTIVES

12.1 Understand the principles and aims of a palliative approach

12.2 Respect the person's preferences

12.3 Follow advance care directives in the individualised plan

12.4 Respond to signs of pain and other symptoms

12.5 Follow end-of-life care strategies

12.6 Manage your own emotional responses to dying and death

INTRODUCTION

PALLIATIVE CARE IS HOLISTIC, person centred and aims to improve quality of life, to maintain respect and dignity, and to address physical, social, emotional and psychological issues, including pain and discomfort, from the beginning of diagnosis to death. The principles of palliative care form the basis of a person's ongoing care plan, regardless of where they reside and the stage they are at in their life-limiting illness.

This chapter discusses the requirement to develop skills and knowledge in:

- applying the principles and aims of a palliative approach when supporting individuals
- respecting the person's preferences for quality-of-life choices
- following the person's advance care directives in the care plan
- responding to signs of pain and other symptoms
- following end-of-life care strategies.

INDUSTRY IN FOCUS

The importance of advance care planning

An advance care plan (ACP) is a plan of care ahead of the time of need, for example on admission to residential aged care, so that the person's wishes and expectations are communicated to all concerned. It is ideally developed in consultation with the person, family and significant others. The importance of advance care planning is that it allows for the person's individual wishes to be documented, respected and upheld while also relieving the burden on family members to make choices on behalf of the person when they don't feel comfortable making such decisions. ACPs can also sometimes assist family members in resolving conflict over opinions and decisions associated with care. Often the person will voice their wishes, requests and concerns to the care worker, rather than to family or friends. The care worker is then responsible for recognising and reporting any needs or issues disclosed by the person to appropriate others so that these can be documented and included in the individualised person-centred care plan. It is imperative that the care worker understands and accepts the person's ACP without bias, prejudice or discrimination, so that their own personal opinions, beliefs and attitudes don't influence the care they provide. ACPs form part of the person's records and are usually stored with their day-to-day records for ease of access, review and update by the multidisciplinary team.

12.1 UNDERSTANDING THE PRINCIPLES AND AIMS OF A PALLIATIVE APPROACH

Palliative care aims to provide the best quality of life through a holistic approach which supports the physical, emotional, social and spiritual aspects of the person and their family. The WHO (2020) defines palliative care as follows:

> *Palliative care is an approach that improves the quality of life of patients (adults and children) and their families who are facing problems associated with life-threatening illness. It prevents and relieves suffering through the early identification, correct assessment and treatment of pain and other problems, whether physical, psychosocial or spiritual.*
>
> *Addressing suffering involves taking care of issues beyond physical symptoms. Palliative care uses a team approach to support patients and their caregivers. This includes addressing practical needs and providing bereavement counselling. It offers a support system to help patients live as actively as possible until death.*

Applying the principles and aims of palliative care can be complex and physically and emotionally exhausting.

12.1.1 Definition and core values

Palliative care is the care provided to a person and their family and friends where a life-limiting illness exists and there is no cure. A palliative care approach also ensures that a holistic, person-centred care plan can be developed and implemented according to the person's wishes.

Palliative care has been available in Australia since the 1980s, when hospices were introduced. Since then, there has been much development in the area of palliative care, including increased government funding and universal recognition that palliative care is a professional model of care that requires guidelines, policy and leadership for it to be successfully implemented.

The psychological and emotional impact on the person, family, carer and others following a diagnosis of a life-limiting illness will be influenced by the person's emotional, cultural, religious and spiritual values in relation to death and dying. Palliative care services are not just for the person with cancer or for someone who is aged. They can also occur in neonatal units, paediatric units and general practitioner clinics.

Palliative care differs from curative care (see Table 12.1). **Curative care** is the care provided to a person which aims to extend the life span by diagnosing and focusing care on the person and implementing active treatment whereby the health problem is resolved by curing the illness. Curative care is generally delivered in an acute care setting. In palliative care, the focus is on improving the person's quality of life where there is no cure.

TABLE 12.1 Comparison of palliative and curative care

Palliative care	Curative care
Aims to improve quality of life where there is no cure	Aims to extend life span
Manages pain and other symptoms	Involves more active treatment
Recognises psychological and spiritual concerns and supports these as well as the physical symptoms	Includes diagnosis and treatments such as medication or surgery
Can be delivered at home, in a hospital or hospice, and in other locations	Primarily delivered in an acute hospital setting

In your studies around palliative care, you will come across some other terms that will help you to clarify the types of care that you may be applying:

- A *palliative approach to care support* works towards improving the quality of life for those living with a life-limiting illness or who are dying. The aim is to reduce suffering by early diagnosis, assessment and holistic intervention for pain and other symptoms. The person's physical, psychological, cultural and social needs are considered with them and their families.
- A **life-limiting illness** is any illness that restricts, limits or cuts short a person's abilities and of which death is a direct consequence. When someone is diagnosed with a life-limiting illness, it is expected that at some stage during that illness palliative care will be accessed. It is an individual's choice as to when they access palliative care, and each person's experience with palliative care will vary. Examples of life-limiting illness include cancer, dementia and heart disease.
- *Specialised palliative care* involves referral to the palliative care team, a multidisciplinary team of professionals who provide advice, education and support for the complex nature of the person and their family. These professionals may include specialists, doctors, registered nurses (RNs), physiotherapists, social workers, pastoral care workers and others.
- **End-of-life care,** also known as **terminal care**, follows the principles of respect, dignity and comfort with a focus on incorporating family, friends and significant others during the last few weeks of a person's life. The person's care plan and decisions are reviewed and changed more frequently during this stage to ensure their wishes are met as they experience changes associated with their illness and their needs change. Terminal care focuses on the provision of care during the last days of a person's life, when the person is recognised as imminently dying, and focuses on principles of delivering care that is respectful, maintains dignity, and promotes comfort, including addressing their physical, emotional, spiritual, religious and cultural needs, while including family and friends appropriately during death and bereavement.

A holistic approach, which provides support that looks at the whole person, is extended over time and not just at end of life. The support should also consider physical, emotional, social and spiritual wellbeing. Each person will have a different experience influenced by their age, culture, heritage, language, faith, sexual and gender identity, relationship status, life experience, medical conditions and beliefs. A holistic approach focuses on a person's wellness and not just their illness, diagnosis and condition. The holistic approach continues into end-of-life care.

The care worker will support the person, carer, family, and others identified by the person, to express their needs and preferences and report this information to their supervisor. They will also communicate with the person, carer, family and others identified by the person, and report to their supervisor information gained, in relation to the person's quality of life, pain and comfort. Communication strategies to build trust, show empathy, demonstrate support and empower the person, carer, family and others are important aspects of care during palliative or end-of-life care. Organisational policies and procedures provide for the provision of both a palliative approach and palliative care.

The care worker will adjust communication techniques to meet the individual needs of the person and their carer, family and others. Communication techniques need to demonstrate respect and to identify the individual needs of the person and their carer, family and others. The care worker needs to support them to express their needs and preferences and again report information to the supervisor. The person, the carer, family and others are an integral part of the care team and require information and support.

12.1.2 Resources

There are many resources available for consultation and assistance during the stages of palliative care for the person, family, friends, the care worker and significant others to access. It is important to consider all members of the care team and to provide local and national resources, information and support systems for them.

NATIONAL PALLIATIVE CARE STRATEGY 2018

The National Palliative Care Strategy 2018 was developed and implemented with the purpose of guiding governments, organisations and individuals in continually improving the palliative care received in Australia. The strategy provides guidance, authority and a shared direction for the continual improvement of palliative care services via six guiding principles:

1. Palliative care is person-centred care.
2. Death is a part of life.
3. Carers are valued and receive the care they need.
4. Care is accessible.
5. Everyone has a role to play in palliative care.
6. Care is high quality and evidence based (Australian Government, Department of Health and Aged Care, 2018).

PALLIATIVE CARE AUSTRALIA

Palliative Care Australia (PCA) is the peak national body for palliative care in Australia, representing all who work towards high-quality palliative care for all Australians. PCA aims to improve access to, and promote the need for, palliative care by working closely with consumers and member organisations and the palliative care workforce. PCA believes quality palliative care occurs when strong networks exist between specialist palliative care providers, primary generalists, primary specialists and support care providers and the community. PCA's vision is quality palliative care for all, while its mission is to influence, foster and promote the delivery of quality palliative care for all. See https://palliativecare.org.au.

PALLIAGED

palliAGED is an online palliative care evidence-based and practice information resource for the Australian aged care sector, in particular. The site provides support and trustworthy information for health-care practitioners, older Australians, their families and friends, as well as resource developers, and focuses on the palliative care of aged persons. See https://www.palliaged.com.au.

DEMENTIA AUSTRALIA

Dementia Australia is the peak body in Australia for people with living with dementia and their families. It supports people living with dementia to access the care and support they choose and works to elevate their voice. Dementia is the leading cause of death for women in Australia and the second leading cause of death for Australians generally (Dementia Australia 2022). See https://www.dementia.org.au.

WORKPLACE SCENARIO

Applying the principles of person-centred care to a palliative approach

Joan (80) was diagnosed with multiple sclerosis when she was 55. She has been living with this life-limiting illness aided by home support services and wishes to remain at home with care until she dies. She wishes to die at home with her family around her. Although Joan has verbalised this wish to friends, she hasn't formally developed an advance care plan or directive.

Lisa, a nurse, visits Joan at home weekly to monitor her pain relief and activities of daily living (ADLs). One day, Lisa hears Joan verbalise her wishes to her best friend, who suggests that two of Joan's daughters wouldn't agree with the idea of her being cared for at home until her death. Lisa encourages Joan to develop an ACP and directive with the multidisciplinary team. She suggests that these plans would reduce her family's decision-making burden. Lisa also explains that having an ACP would enable her family and friends to plan ahead and be better prepared with services, support mechanisms and resources to assist Joan with the end stage of her life.

Joan agrees and commences the process with the assistance of her general practitioner (GP). Lisa visits Joan at home two weeks later, when the process is finalised, and learns that the family members have met with Joan to discuss her wishes and plans and have agreed to them all. Lisa explains to Joan's daughters the principles of palliative care and person-centred care. She listens to their concerns around analgesia and other measures being available to provide Joan with pain relief and comfort and reassures them that their mother will be treated in a way that respects the family's cultural practices, both before and following Joan's death, as set out in the relevant documentation. All members of the multidisciplinary team involved in Joan's care are aware of this documentation, Lisa says.

Joan dies peacefully, and with dignity and respect, two months later at home with her family by her side.

CHECK YOUR UNDERSTANDING

1. Define palliative care.
2. Where can palliative care occur?
3. Name three resources available to assist palliation.
4. How can the care worker involve the person's family and friends in their palliative care?

12.2 RESPECTING THE PERSON'S PREFERENCES

12.2.1 Quality of life

The measure of quality of life is determined by the individual person and is a term used to describe how people see themselves and their lives. A person's perception of quality of life is influenced by their attitudes, values, beliefs, past experiences, and expectations, including having relationships, physical things and experiences.

The WHO defines quality of life as "an individual's perception of their position in life in the context of the culture and value systems in which they live, and in relation to their goals, expectations, standards and concerns" (WHO 2022). It is a broad-ranging, complex concept, incorporating the person's physical health, psychological state, level of independence, social relationships, personal beliefs, and relationship to salient features of the environment.

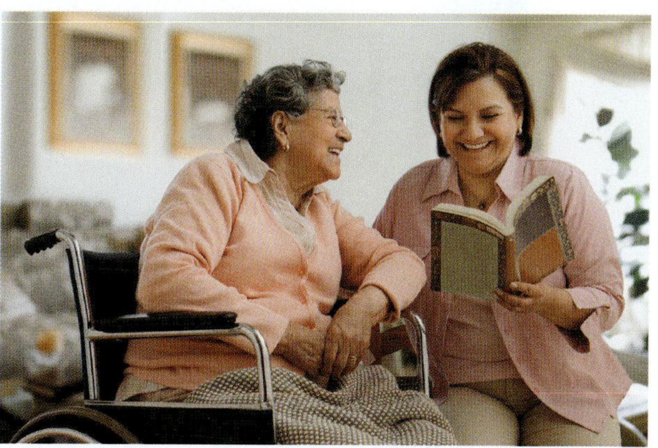

Jose Luis Pelaez Inc/Blend Images LLC

Quality of life is an individual measure

Respecting a person's choices regarding their quality of life can be challenging when their choices may not be the same as yours or as expected. It is important to have a non-judgemental attitude and to understand that quality of life is an individual measure, and not impose your own ideas, beliefs and measures on the person. It is appropriate to offer suggestions and ideas by way of providing information, and inappropriate and non-respectful to impose or influence decisions. Your ingrained biases or preconceived ideas can have negative impacts when providing palliative care. As a care worker, you may feel uncomfortable talking to someone about their beliefs and quality of life measures, especially when it is obvious they have made choices that differ from yours. Sensitivity and active listening, combined with privacy and confidentiality, provide them the opportunity to voice their beliefs and to feel supported by you regardless of your differences.

During palliative care, there could be a conflict of values whereby the care worker may feel inadequate and unable to attend to the care and follow the care plan as intended. When this occurs, the care worker has a duty of care to openly disclose this to their supervisor and remove themselves from the situation at the earliest opportunity. Occasionally, the care worker gathers the courage and strength to continue to provide care, although they will dismiss themselves from certain activities or parts of care that don't meet their own values and beliefs. A care worker is not expected to compromise their own values and beliefs when providing care, but they *are* responsible for disclosing a conflict of values and beliefs where this may compromise care.

12.2.2 A supportive environment

During the delivery of palliative care, it is important to create and maintain a supportive environment where the dying person, family, friends and significant others feel comfortable and able to express themselves honestly and freely without feeling embarrassed, intimidated or subjected to judgement, discrimination or racism.

The physical environment itself can create a welcoming, calm and friendly atmosphere by being private, spacious (but not too spacious) and personalised, rather than being sterile, clinical and non-personal. The person's family and friends could be encouraged to provide belongings and personal items of significance to the dying person for them to have close by. Even a pet might be considered here! Other examples might be a well-loved soft toy, a favourite perfume or piece of music, a special religious token, or other meaningful items. It is comforting to have familiar items and smells around, to feel secure and able to reminisce.

Information is much more easily transferred when the environment is comfortable and welcoming, private, and without noise and clutter. Palliative care and palliative service are accessible in a variety of settings,

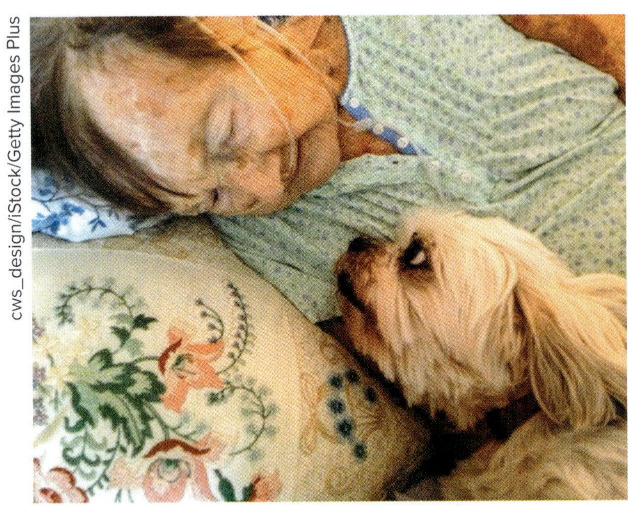
cws_design/iStock/Getty Images Plus

A beloved pet can form part of a supportive environment

including during respite, hospitalisation and at home, whether it is a residential aged care facility (RACF) or a long-standing family home.

In addition to the external environment, you can create space within you, to create a healing presence which calls for both intimacy and separation. Be willing to connect with the person, to offer them your empathy and unconditional positive regard, to accept them exactly as they are, at this moment. Relate to them in a gentle, non-judgemental way. Stay within your role by feeling your own feelings, listening to your heart and making your own decisions, and letting them do the same. This type of self-care strategy is discussed later in the chapter.

12.2.3 Respecting individual choices

It is best practice and essential to professional care that a non-judgemental approach and respect for autonomy and individualism is evident during palliative care. It is important to be open minded, flexible and culturally sensitive, and aware of any potential conflict of values. Palliative care requires a non-judgemental approach that allows the dying person and their family and friends to feel free and able to express their own personal and unique feelings, beliefs, values and practices with regard to palliative care. Personal choices and preferences underpin all palliative care, including preferences relating to culture and spirituality; therefore, it is essential to discuss spirituality and culture with the dying person and their family and friends. Open, non-judgemental and honest discussion leads to effective, respectful and culturally appropriate palliative care and understanding of one's values and beliefs.

Care workers may find it difficult or uncomfortable to discuss such aspects of care when there are differing values and beliefs. It is important, therefore, to access resources and services that assist the conversation to be informative and person centred. Resources and services available will vary; however, commonalities exist where access to a person of religion and spirituality can facilitate the conversation or access to interpreters and translators may be beneficial. Often, family and friends aid the conversation by advocating for the dying person and verbalising specific spiritual and cultural needs. The care worker has the responsibility to not assume or impose particular religious, spiritual or cultural beliefs, values and practices during care. They are encouraged instead to learn from the dying person and their family and friends what practices are important to implement.

12.2.4 The role of the care worker

Organisations will have their own guidelines for the care worker to follow. These will be around legal and ethical requirements, care policies, job role procedures and documentation. The person, the carer and the family are all involved in the role of the care worker and the supervisor. The care worker will be assisting to provide holistic care, including attending to the person's physical, psychosocial, cultural and spiritual needs. They will be part of the team involved in all aspects of care.

PROVIDING EMPATHY AND EMOTIONAL SUPPORT

The care worker's role during palliative care involves providing empathy and emotional support at every stage of the dying process. Empathy is having the ability to appreciate and understand what another person is feeling at any given time; sympathy is feeling sorry for or pitying someone's situation; and compassion is the ability to have an extended understanding or awareness of someone's suffering and wanting to relieve such suffering. Each individual will experience death and dying in their own personal way, but it is important to remember the common theories of grief and dying. The care worker needs to be able to offer emotional support, empathy and compassion without trying to control the person's grief. By providing an appropriate environment where the person's emotions and feelings can be expressed freely, honestly and without judgement, they will be demonstrating empathy and compassion.

A LITTLE MORE ABOUT GRIEF

Grief is a natural reaction to loss; however, not all people grieve in the same way or for the same duration. Elizabeth Kübler-Ross identified five common stages of grief (1969):

1. *Denial:* This is generally the stage where the person denies being unwell and tries to hide it.
2. *Bargaining:* This is the stage where the person begins to bargain with self and others by suggesting "If I ..." or "What if I ... ?"
3. *Anger:* Often the third stage of grief, where the person gets angry and starts to question "Why me?". This is the stage where behaviours may escalate.
4. *Depression:* This stage is observed when the person begins to isolate and become socially withdrawn.
5. *Acceptance:* The final stage is where the person begins to make changes, take charge of their destiny and begin planning their last stages of life.

There are many other models and theories about death and dying, including those proposed by Sigmund Freud, Ernest Becker, Adrian Tomer and Grafton Eliason. Freud stated that whatever one fears cannot be death, since, as one has never died, no fear can be associated with the experience of dying. Becker believed that anxiety is so complex and intense that it generates fears and phobias of everyday life. He felt that the impact can result in fear of being alone and that much of a person's routine behaviour involves attempts to deny and avoid the possibility and inevitability of death, thus keeping their anxiety under control. Tomer and Eliason's regret theory focuses on the premise that people rate their worth and quality of life, and that they generally feel more anxious if they haven't accomplished what they wished to achieve during their life, which creates an environment whereby they consider how to live more fully in the present moment.

Researchers McKissock and McKissock (1999) proposed the following basic principles for understanding grief:

- Grief is very important in healing wounds that have resulted from loss.
- The bereaved may feel a wide range of feelings, from sadness, shock, anger, guilt and despair to hope and acceptance.
- It is healthy to express the pain and intensity associated with loss.

The process of grief can be experienced psychologically, physically, behaviourally and emotionally, and this is part of the healing process

MONITORING AND REPORTING NEEDS TO YOUR SUPERVISOR

The care worker's role and scope of practice during palliative care is determined by their qualification and the policies and procedures of the facility or service. It is the care worker's responsibility to work within their scope of practice and to understand and recognise needs and issues outside their scope of practice. It is then the care worker's responsibility to report, document and refer these needs or issues to the appropriate person for intervention. It is important for the dying person and their family and friends also to be professionally and respectfully informed that an intervention may not be part of the care worker's scope of practice. Working within a given scope of practice is a legal and ethical requirement. Whenever there is doubt over scope of practice, there is a duty of care to consult policies and procedures, but also the manager or supervisor, for further clarification. The care worker should never attend to a care intervention without being sure that it is within their scope of practice. If a care intervention, skill or knowledge has not been taught, demonstrated or practised, it is assumed it doesn't belong to the care worker's scope of practice at that particular time.

REPORTING CHANGING NEEDS AND ISSUES

As with all care in any given situation, it is important to recognise, report and document changing needs and issues as they arise. During end of life, changes will inevitably occur and impact on care delivery and implementation.

PRACTICE POINT

Not all deaths are predictable, and many people don't experience dying over a trajectory of time. Some deaths occur suddenly and take staff and family by surprise. It is important when this occurs to remain a source of stability and comfort to the family and to acknowledge the experience with them. It is also important to be aware of your own needs surrounding the death of the person and to consider accepting support, such as a debriefing session with colleagues.

EVALUATING CARE

Regular, detailed and thorough assessment and evaluation is crucial in providing consistent, holistic, person-centred palliative care. Evaluation at regular intervals and after significant changes in someone's condition is best practice in identifying effective and non-effective care. It is through regular and structured assessment and evaluation that care workers become aware of the person's priorities and needs as their condition changes. Care can be evaluated via close observation and by recognising verbal and behavioural responses. Specific formal tools such as pain assessment tools, fluid balance charts and mini mental status exams can be utilised to provide universal and objective methods for evaluating care. It is important to document findings of evaluations via the care plan and notes to ensure that communication between each member of the multidisciplinary team is ongoing, clear and accurate.

12.2.5 Communication

It is important for the care worker to have effective and appropriate communication skills that encourage discussion, expression, inclusiveness and collaboration, along with teamwork and professionalism. Both empathy and compassion encourage communication and a trusting therapeutic relationship. Empathy can be provided by actively listening and communicating the emotional needs of the dying person and their family and friends. Being patient and taking time to sit and converse with the person shows compassion and interest in their emotional needs while building that therapeutic relationship. Sound communication skills, professionalism and respect are essential in supporting the conversation and expression of needs.

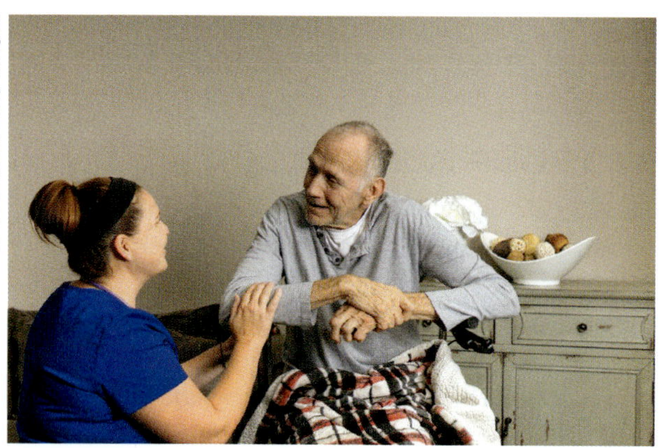

Regular evaluation is crucial in providing holistic, person-centred palliative care

Communication strategies to build trust, show empathy, demonstrate support, and empower the person, carer, family and others are important aspects of care during palliative or end-of-life care. It is important to communicate with the person, carer, family and others as appropriate, in relation to the person's quality of life, pain and comfort, and to report any information to your supervisor. Your communication techniques need to identify the individual needs of the person and their carer, family and others, and you need to support them to express their needs and preferences and again report information to your supervisor. The person, carer, family and others are an integral part of the care team and require information and support.

WORKPLACE SCENARIO

Spirituality and culture in palliative care

Mark is a 63-year-old member of the Aboriginal community who has been transferred to the palliative care unit where you are working. You have noted that Mark doesn't want to participate in care activities and is reluctant to converse with others. He shows very little engagement with the staff and often has verbal outbursts. His family and friends visit him regularly and have voiced their concern that his Aboriginal culture isn't being respected or considered in his care, especially now that he is receiving palliative care. You spend some time with Mark's family and friends learning about Aboriginal culture and the spiritual practices that are commonly observed during the dying phase of life, known as passing on, in the Aboriginal community. You understand that these practices are complex, very meaningful and purposeful. As a result, you approach the supervisor, report your findings and request that traditional Aboriginal spiritual practices be included in Mark's care. These practices include:

- supporting as many visitors as possible at any given time, including overnight stays, until the whole family ceases all communication with the service
- understanding that it would be respectful and expected that, after Mark passes on, his name won't be mentioned and photos of him won't be openly displayed, out of respect for the belief that this would call his spirit back and prevent his safe passage to the spirit world of the ancestors.

Mark's care plan is updated and communication begins about the practices to be included during his end-of-life care. Once these are implemented, it is noted that Mark is more comfortable with care provision. Two weeks later, he passes on peacefully with family and friends beside him. Photos of him are removed from view and Mark becomes known as "Room AG1" during communications such as handovers among staff.

Note: It is essential never to make assumptions about cultural practices. Every Aboriginal and Torres Strait Islander person may have differing beliefs, values and practices. The diversity found within Australia's states and territories results in there being many different cultural beliefs and practices. The key to any successful interaction during care is open, honest and clear communication and asking the sick person and their family what their wants and needs are.

CHECK YOUR UNDERSTANDING

1. Define quality of life.
2. How would you discuss spirituality and culture with a dying person?
3. Name strategies to assist with providing empathy and compassion.
4. What should you do if a care need is outside your scope of practice?
5. Name and discuss the five common stages of grief identified by Kübler-Ross.

12.3 FOLLOWING ADVANCE CARE DIRECTIVES IN THE INDIVIDUALISED PLAN

12.3.1 Legislation and regulations

When someone is diagnosed with a life-limiting illness, it allows for preparation and planning to occur with regard to end of life, dying and death itself. Processes to develop advance care directives and advance care plans are initiated and communicated to the multidisciplinary team so that care is followed according to the person's personal and individual wishes. The advance care directive informs the care plan, and the care plan informs the care worker and multidisciplinary health-care team. The following ethical principles relating to advance care directives and advance care plans apply to care workers:

- The individual has the right to determine their care, including the right to receive or refuse treatment.
- Care staff will act in the individual's best interests in determining whether the service has the capability to provide care appropriate to their needs.

Care workers are responsible for consistently following advance care directives in the person's care plan, in line with their work role and following organisational guidelines. Providers are legally obliged to follow the person's wishes. If you are asked by a person, their family, friends, significant others or a colleague to do something you don't feel comfortable with, you should check the organisation's policies and discuss the situation with your supervisor. It is not expected that the care worker has an obligation to perform a task that goes against their own ethical principles or religious and cultural beliefs and values. The care worker has the right to declare a conflict of interest in such circumstances and to be reassigned other duties.

12.3.2 Advance care directives and the advance care plan

An **advance care directive (ACD)**, also known as a **living will**, is a legal, formal, individualised document that is developed with the aim of communicating a person's wishes for care during their life-limiting illness and, more specifically, at the end stage of life when death is imminent (see Figure 12.1). In most states of Australia, an ACD is a legally binding document and must be followed by the multidisciplinary health-care team without alteration. In addition, people who are cognitively competent and over the age of 18 have the right to appoint a **substitute decision maker** to make informed, accurate and trusted decisions on their behalf about their medical care. Substitute decision makers may be appointed legally as a power of attorney, an enduring power of attorney and/or guardian. In some states, substitute decision makers may be known as agents or attorneys, among other terms.

The **advance care plan (ACP)** is a plan of care formulated and documented according to the person's perception of what they feel is appropriate care that will provide respect, comfort and dignity during the end stage of their life. The care plan is unique and individualised so as to inform care workers with regard to potential care needs, religious and spiritual practices, and cultural and emotional needs. Following and monitoring the care plan ensures that the person's wishes are respected and upheld.

All states have guidelines about end-of-life care in relation to documenting a person's wishes and the authority given to others to make decisions regarding medical treatment. While the terms differ, the intention is to record a person's wishes and support them when they lose their capacity to make decisions for themselves regarding treatment. These guidelines are part of common law legislation.

12.3.3 End-of-life decisions

When it comes time to make end-of-life decisions and to plan ahead in anticipation of death, the palliative care team will be available with a wide range of skills, knowledge and expertise to help a person manage a

FIGURE 12.1 Sample advance care directive

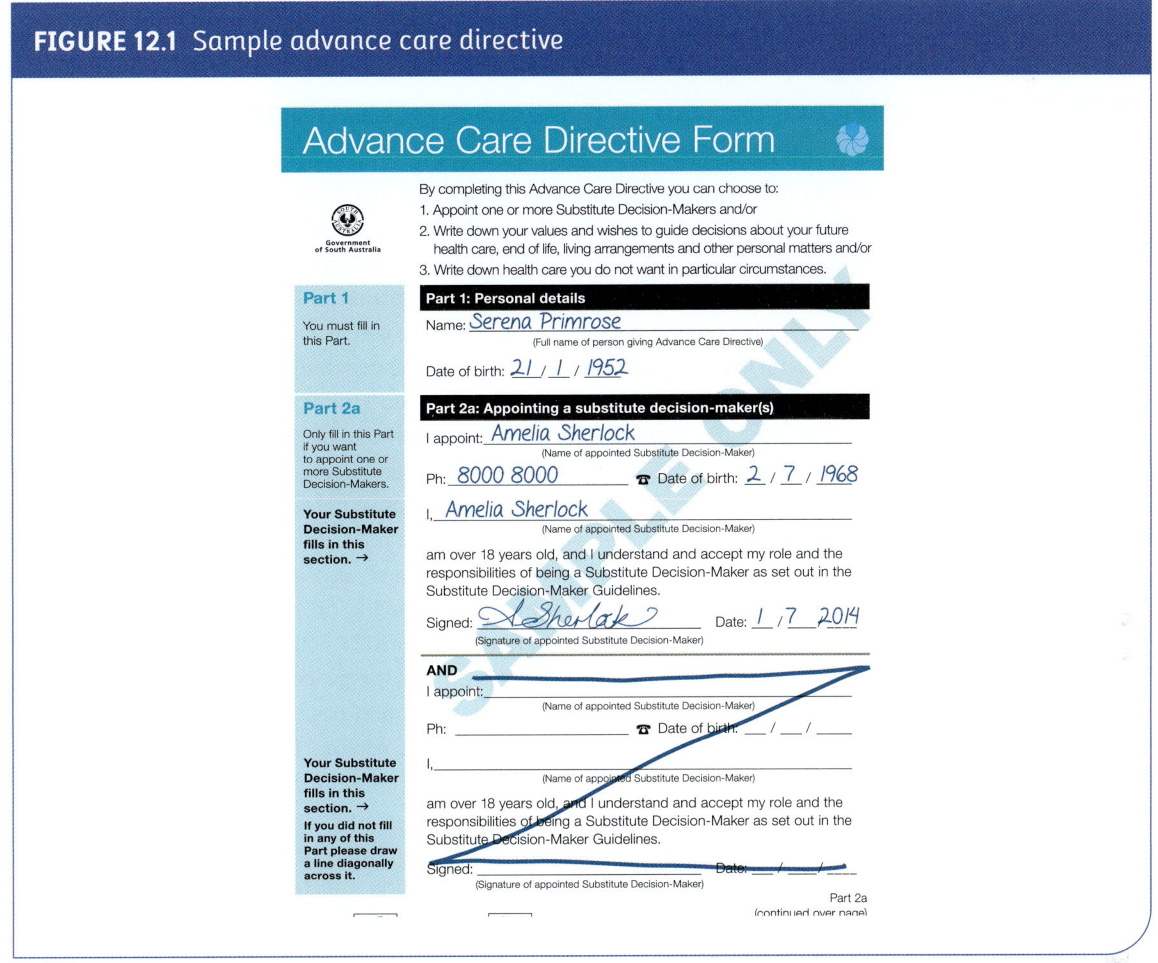

Advance Care Directive Form

Government of South Australia

By completing this Advance Care Directive you can choose to:
1. Appoint one or more Substitute Decision-Makers and/or
2. Write down your values and wishes to guide decisions about your future health care, end of life, living arrangements and other personal matters and/or
3. Write down health care you do not want in particular circumstances.

Part 1
You must fill in this Part.

Part 1: Personal details

Name: Serena Primrose
(Full name of person giving Advance Care Directive)

Date of birth: 21 / 1 / 1952

Part 2a
Only fill in this Part if you want to appoint one or more Substitute Decision-Makers.

Part 2a: Appointing a substitute decision-maker(s)

I appoint: Amelia Sherlock
(Name of appointed Substitute Decision-Maker)

Ph: 8000 8000 ☎ Date of birth: 2 / 7 / 1968

Your Substitute Decision-Maker fills in this section. →

I, Amelia Sherlock
(Name of appointed Substitute Decision-Maker)

am over 18 years old, and I understand and accept my role and the responsibilities of being a Substitute Decision-Maker as set out in the Substitute Decision-Maker Guidelines.

Signed: A Sherlock Date: 1 / 7 2014
(Signature of appointed Substitute Decision-Maker)

AND

I appoint: ____
(Name of appointed Substitute Decision-Maker)

Ph: ____ ☎ Date of birth: __ / __ / ____

Your Substitute Decision-Maker fills in this section. →

If you did not fill in any of this Part please draw a line diagonally across it.

I, ____
(Name of appointed Substitute Decision-Maker)

am over 18 years old, and I understand and accept my role and the responsibilities of being a Substitute Decision-Maker as set out in the Substitute Decision-Maker Guidelines.

Signed: ____ Date: __ / __ / ____
(Signature of appointed Substitute Decision-Maker)

Part 2a
(continued over page)

Source: The Government of South Australia, Advance Care Directive Form, sourced on 17 February 2022, https://advancecaredirectives.sa.gov.au/forms-and-guides. Please check https://advancecaredirectives.sa.gov.au/forms-and-guides for the most current version of this form.

life-limiting illness. The palliative care team works together in a holistic, individualised and person-centred manner to meet the physical, psychological, social, emotional, spiritual and cultural needs of the dying person and their family and carers.

12.3.4 The rights of the older person at the end of their life

As a care worker, it is important to understand the rights of the older person at the end of their life. The older person is more vulnerable to death, yet this doesn't mean they don't have rights that they once had. Our rights don't change as we grow older. The rights of older people are embedded in international human rights conventions on economic, social, civil and political rights. Unfortunately, what does change is that older populations are considered to be inherently less valuable to society. Increasingly, they encounter barriers to participation and often older people become more dependent on others and lose some or all of their personal autonomy. It is these changes and threats to dignity that make the elderly more susceptible to issues such as neglect, abuse and, ultimately, violation of human rights.

In addition, the older person has the right to be afforded the opportunity to accept, or to refuse or decline, care and treatment. Principles of self-determination and dignity of risk apply, upholding the right of an older person at the end of life to express their wishes, values and beliefs through an ACD and advance care planning. Older persons also have the right to choose where and, in some cases, when to die. In summary, the older person has the same rights as all other people, including the right to non-discriminatory, non-judgemental and non-prejudicial care at the end of life regardless of their age, gender, sexual preferences, life circumstances, and religious, cultural or spiritual values and beliefs.

12.3.5 Reporting changing needs and issues

This process ensures that the best possible care is delivered in a respectful and timely manner during the most challenging time of a person's life; it also ensures that family, friends and significant others feel supported and acknowledged. It is important to report the holistic changing needs of the person, family, friends and significant others via the care plan and the person's medical notes so as to ensure that communication among the multidisciplinary team members is accurate and documented for guidance. Processes for reporting and documenting will vary from service to service, yet the aim of providing holistic person-centred palliative care will not.

It is particularly important during the palliative care experience to respect and support carers and family. They form part of a network that offers vital information, solutions and strategies to be incorporated into holistic, person-centred care. It is often the family, friends and carers who express, on behalf of the person, their needs and preferences without realising how they themselves are being affected by the situation. Supporting family and carers during palliative care ensures that the palliative person is reassured that grieving will be supported. It is important to include and involve family, friends and carers in the care and decisions for the palliative person so as to deliver holistic, person-centred care, but also to ensure the experience of palliative care is a positive one and has the desired outcomes. The grieving process for family, friends and carers will commence from diagnosis and continue until after death, which could be months or years. By involving family, friends and carers in palliative care from the beginning, the process of grieving will be easier to navigate, and the dying person will feel reassured and find comfort and ease with the process of dying. Family, friends and carers also offer a role of advocacy for the dying person. Respecting and supporting family, carers and significant others is best achieved by being patient, offering reassurance and empathy, and being collaborative rather than controlling.

Respect is characterised by considerate concern for the feelings of others and implies that support will be given despite individual differences in age, gender, values and culture, and that communication will be inclusive, open and honest. It is imperative that the person and their family, friends and significant others know that care workers and other members of the care team will be reliable and consistent. Additionally, a relationship with the person and their family that is underpinned by trust and respect will enable a positive exchange of information and a feeling of full support.

12.3.6 End-of-life locations

Deciding on where to reside during end of life is a hard decision, yet it can be empowering to have some control over where death occurs and is often considered a key factor in dying well. If we look back through history, care of the dying and their death commonly happened at home; then, as medical knowledge developed and improved, death became more of a clinical event. There is currently a move towards a less clinical approach to dying, connecting with the uniqueness of the person and responding to their needs and wishes. There is an even stronger connection developing to the individual, holistic approach to care, facilitating more choice and control for the individual. Death is a natural process, yet many people are uncomfortable with the idea of dying because they haven't had experience with caring for a dying person or with planning ahead.

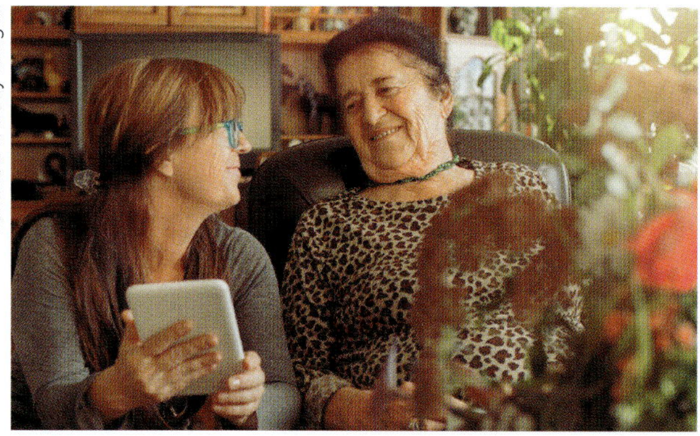

nemke/E+/Getty Images

Palliative care at home is only possible if the person has sufficient support among family and friends

There are varying options of end-of-life locations to choose from. Choice is the key principle to follow, along with the principle of individuality, which enables each person to choose differently according to their particular preference.

The options are to end one's life at home, in a palliative care unit, hospice or hostel, in a hospital, or in an RACF. Despite most people wishing to die at home, it is more common to die in a medical-type environment. Some people may choose this medical-type environment as they don't want to be a burden on their family, or for other reasons. There are times when choice is limited for reasons such as: the person has medical needs that only a hospital or palliative care unit (hospice) can meet; remote living may not allow for home visits, or housing may be unsuitable; or family or friends may say they feel unable to cope caring for the person at home.

It is imperative to talk to the palliative care team about concerns and to find out what options are available for effective planning to occur. The choice of palliative care at home is only possible when the person has sufficient support among family and friends to provide ongoing care every day. Care at home is supplemented by visits from the community team who provide the medication, help and support required by the person and their carers. In community care, it is important to ensure the person and family are safe and able to cope until the care worker's next visit. Contact phone numbers should be provided so that services can be reached in the event of a crisis.

If a person's symptoms can no longer be managed at home, they may be admitted to an acute facility. Most of the help at home is provided by family, friends and significant others, who may all also need to be cared for to prevent physical and emotional exhaustion, especially if the person's illness is long and/or difficult.

Terminal care in a hospital may have the following features:

- Care may be less personal.
- The person may feel isolated from their family and friends.
- The needs of people in an acute care environment may limit the delivery of holistic care.
- People dying in a hospital are more likely to die alone.
- Medical and nursing staff may lack specific palliative and end-of-life care expertise.

Palliative care is provided to people in aged care facilities to the extent that this has become one of the main "models of care" in RACFs. For conditions such as cancer, dementia and emphysema, people are supported and made comfortable as their condition deteriorates. Standards and guidelines for aged care address palliative care, identifying that the comfort and dignity of terminally ill people is the expected outcome.

Hospices provide specific, holistic care for the terminally ill. Hospice care:

- recognises death as "normal"
- focuses on the relief of symptoms
- maintains quality of life as far as possible
- involves family and friends in care and support
- regards the whole family as the "unit of care"
- provides a home-like environment with special medical facilities and resources.

As a person's situation changes, the choice of where to die may change and this is to be expected and encouraged with respect and without judgement. There may be a need to have ongoing conversations with the person, their carers and the medical team about the best place for end-of-life care due to the person's changing circumstances and needs. It is important to encourage conversation around death and dying, symptom management and maintaining dignity, along with planning ahead to increase the likelihood of receiving end-of-life care in the place of choice. End-of-life **doulas** (non-professional trained companions/supporters) and other allied health professionals can assist the medical team in these varied locations, and advocate for the person and their wishes where appropriate.

12.3.7 Voluntary assisted dying

Voluntary assisted dying is often referred to as **euthanasia;** yet, when analysed more fully, it is the action of an adult person asking for medical help to end their life in a humane and dignified manner. The primary principles behind voluntary assisted dying are accessing medication and enabling a person legally to choose the time and manner in which they die. Voluntary assisted dying emphasises the voluntary nature of the person's choice and their ongoing legal ability to make this decision without being coerced or influenced by others.

It is not yet legal to voluntarily assist a death in all Australian states and territories, however that is changing. On 29 November 2017, Victoria became the first state to pass legislation to enable voluntary assisted dying to become an available choice, and since then other states have followed, including Western Australia and New South Wales. A person's decision to request voluntary assisted dying in Australia must be:

- voluntary without influence from another or via coercion (i.e. it is the person's own decision); and
- consistent (the person makes three separate requests for voluntary assisted dying during the process); and
- fully informed (the person is well-informed about their disease, and their treatment and palliative care options).

WORKPLACE SCENARIO

Implementing advance care directives

James is a 53-year-old at the end of his life after a diagnosis of motor neurone disease. He has developed his ACD (also known as a living will) with his GP and supplied a copy to his adult children. The family have read the ACD and have mixed feelings and emotions about their father's wishes. James wishes to have his wake, or celebration of life, before he dies and doesn't wish to be resuscitated in any way. Specifically, he has requested no oxygen or cardiopulmonary resuscitation measures, yet the family feel this is inappropriate and too heart-breaking for them. The care worker refers the family and James to a counsellor and the palliative care team social worker, who facilitate a discussion where each person can share their feelings and point of view. James voices his feelings without hesitation, yet the family are hesitant to join in the discussion. It is obvious that they feel very sad and are unable to comprehend that their father has accepted he is dying and that it could happen any day. Finally, the family voice how they are feeling and express their fears. James begins to understand why they are so upset with the ACD and decides to alter the care he wishes to have implemented to include having oxygen applied during the last stages of life. The family feel more comfortable with this and say they understand their father's wish to have the ACD implemented, although it isn't what they would want for him themselves.

While under the care of the palliative team, James and his family hold a ceremony to celebrate James's life. Friends and family attend and spend time sharing stories and paying tribute to James and his life achievements. James feels satisfied that he has had a chance to say goodbye to his family and friends and to settle any differences with them. He also feels very honoured and humbled that he had the chance to hear what people will remember about him and what impact he has had on people's lives. Three weeks later, James dies peacefully at home in the company of his family.

CHECK YOUR UNDERSTANDING

1. What is an advance care directive?
2. Who develops the advance care directive?
3. When should an advance care directive be formulated?
4. Can the family disagree with the advance care directive and change the care?
5. Define voluntary assisted dying.

12.4 RESPONDING TO SIGNS OF PAIN AND OTHER SYMPTOMS

Life-limiting illnesses can cause many symptoms and often much pain. Symptoms are what the person tells us about what they are feeling and experiencing during their illness. As the illness progresses, symptoms may become more frequent, intense and obvious. The most debilitating symptom for many illnesses is pain and the concept of total pain. Pain is whatever the person says it is; it is unique, individual and specific to the person experiencing it. The concept of total pain holds that physical pain is experienced when physical, psychological, social and spiritual components interact. Pain is an unpleasant sensation (whether throbbing, aching, stabbing, burning or shooting) that is transmitted via the nervous system and occurs as a consequence of an illness, disease or injury. Pain has both physical and emotional or psychological components and can range from mild to severe. Regular assessment should include the person's and their family's understanding of what is happening. The organisation's particular assessment tools should be used whenever possible.

Table 12.2 summarises some common signs, symptoms, assessment types and management strategies that a palliative person may experience.

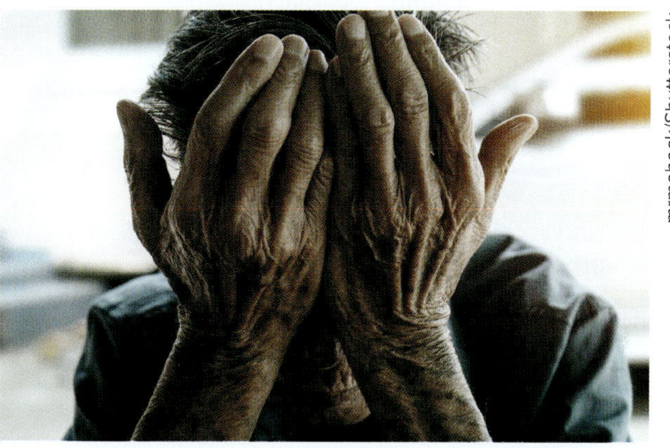

mrmohock/Shutterstock

Pain is the most debilitating symptom for many illnesses

TABLE 12.2 Common signs, symptoms, assessment and management

Signs/symptoms	Assessment	Management
Pain	PQRST assessment or Abbey Pain Scale Verbal questioning Observation of vital signs Observation of body language and behaviours	Reposition for optimal comfort Offer complementary therapies Use distraction therapy Provide medications Provide aids (e.g. splints)
Nutrition	Verbal questioning Observation Identification of reversible malnutrition factors Use of fluid balance chart	Offer a variety of foods (alternatives), including different textures, colours, smells, quantities Offer supplements, vitamins, minerals Provide percutaneous endoscopic gastronomy (PEG) feeding at person's request
Hydration/ dehydration	Observation of the signs: dry skin and mucous membranes; thickened secretions; decreased urine output; headache; cramps; constipation; drowsiness; disorientation Use of fluid balance chart	Offer supplements Attend to mouth care by moistening mucous membranes Offer ice blocks or small sips of water, Provide nasogastric tube feeding (NGT) and intravenous therapy at person's request Manage constipation with aperients
Loss of appetite	Observation Verbal questioning	Offer variety of smells, colours, textures Offer oral care Provide snacks Encourage social interaction during mealtime Treat nausea before mealtime

(Continues)

TABLE 12.2 Common signs, symptoms, assessment and management (continued)

Signs/symptoms	Assessment	Management
Dyspepsia	Verbal questioning Observation	Offer small quantities of food/fluid frequently Limit spicy foods Avoid foods that cause indigestion pain Raise head of bed Offer subcutaneous omeprazole or other medication
Nausea and vomiting	Verbal questioning Observation of change in eating habits and behaviours	Offer antiemetics before mealtimes Avoid causes if known
Constipation	Verbal questioning Observation Daily assessment (including history of bowel habits)	Determine and treat the cause Encourage fluids, gentle exercise Apply abdominal massage to stimulate peristalsis Offer aperients, laxatives, suppositories
Diarrhoea	Verbal questioning Observation Daily assessment	Determine and treat the cause Ensure correct hygiene practices Use safe food handling practices
Dyspnoea and coughing	Verbal questioning Observation	Determine and treat the cause (e.g. with antibiotics) Position for optimal comfort and breathing Raise bed head, elevate with pillows Use relaxation techniques Offer physiotherapy
Oral discomfort	Observation for thrush, ulcers or other	Determine and treat the cause Offer regular oral care Provide dental care as required Remove ill-fitting dentures
Urinary discomfort	Verbal questioning Urinalysis Observation of characteristics	Encourage fluids Determine and treat the cause (e.g. antibiotics for UTI) Ensure personal hygiene is adequate Provide medications as required
Skin irritations	Observation Verbal questioning	Determine and treat the cause Moisturise skin Attend to personal hygiene regularly Cover wounds
Confusion and delirium	Observation Verbal questioning Use of cognitive assessments	Determine and treat the cause Reorientate the person Encourage reminiscence Encourage familiar visitors/persons
Fatigue	Verbal questioning Observation Piper Fatigue Scale (revised)	Determine and treat the cause Encourage adequate sleep, rest, nap periods Set realistic goals

12.4.1 Promoting comfort

It is essential when delivering palliative care to understand that not everyone will experience pain. It isn't always present. When it *is* present, it is experienced differently by each individual and most pain can be relieved. It can also often change with different activities and moods and emotions.

Managing pain and promoting comfort are closely linked. However, the absence of physical pain isn't always sufficient to provide comfort. Comfort exists when there is freedom from both pain and emotional distress.

There are various factors to consider when promoting comfort during end-of-life care. They include:

- the disease process and progression
- self-esteem
- positioning
- cultural, religious and spiritual needs
- the approach and attitudes of care staff
- the environment
- the feelings of family, friends and significant others and the impact the palliative person's life-limiting illness has had on them.

Developing strategies to promote comfort is achieved by:

- having regular conversations with the person and their family, friends and significant others
- making regular observations of the person, using the service/facility's assessment tools, and noting behaviours such as restlessness, irritability, facial grimaces and tense muscles.

12.4.2 Evaluating care

The care worker will monitor, record and report the effectiveness of pain management strategies by means of:

- regular reporting using assessment tools, the person's individual care plan, notes, case conferencing
- regular documentation using assessment tools, individual care plan, notes.

12.4.3 Complementary therapies

Conventional medicine may not always be desirable or effective in managing pain, discomfort or various symptoms; therefore, it is reasonable for the use of complementary therapies to be considered. Complementary therapies are a set of diverse medical and health-care systems, practices and products that are not presently considered a part of conventional medicine. Many specialist palliative care services in Australia offer complementary therapies during care, including pet therapy, massage, hypnotherapy, aromatherapy, relaxation techniques, meditation, acupuncture, music therapy and art therapy.

Complementary therapies have been found to offer support, comfort and symptom relief by:

- managing pain
- encouraging social interaction
- being culturally sensitive and appropriate
- being able to improve functional capabilities (e.g. walking)
- being beneficial in improving a person's sense of control.

Regardless of their benefits, all complementary therapies require monitoring and careful consideration especially when used in conjunction with traditional interventions to ensure adverse effects and interaction are minimised.

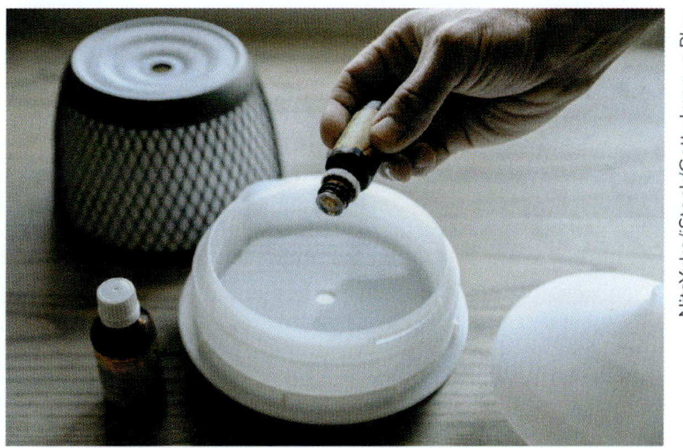

NitaYuko/iStock/Getty Images Plus

Complementary therapies may be used to help manage pain

12.4.4 Medications

Medications are used during palliative care to treat various signs and symptoms—primarily, pain and nausea—towards the end of life. Before medications are introduced, it is essential to complete a thorough medical and physical assessment of the person to determine their individual needs and wants, as some people don't wish to have medications incorporated in their care. The palliative person has the right to use—or refuse to use—medications at any stage of their illness.

TYPES OF MEDICATIONS

Common types of medications used during palliative care are generally those used for pain relief, nausea and management of secretions. Paracetamol and ibuprofen are likely to be used to manage temperature control, inflammation and pain, while morphine and prednisolone are likely to be used for difficulty in breathing, management of secretions and pain control. Nausea is often managed with medications such as omeprazole and maxolon. Occasionally, sedatives and antianxiety medications such as midazolam and haloperidol may be used to decrease anxiety and restlessness. Other medications may be used to manage conditions such as constipation.

The correct dose of pain relief is the dose at which the person reports relief of pain, not the dose the health-care professional assumes is adequate. It is best practice to commence with the least-invasive method of analgesia and lower-level analgesics initially, increasing the level of medication until pain is absent. During palliative care, and particularly at the end of life, avoid judging a person's pain and its characteristics. Pain is unique and is exactly what the individual says it is.

Regardless of which medications are used, it is essential to be aware of any side effects, adverse effects and contraindications that may also need treatment and management to ensure the palliative experience is acceptable, dignified and respectful.

PRACTICE POINT

As a care worker, you are in a valuable position to observe the effects of end-of-life medication. In the final days to hours, medications will often be gradually increased to maintain the dying person's comfort and dignity. If they appear to be sleeping and comfortable, the medications might be working for them.

Unpleasant symptoms can return quickly when prescribed medications are missed or omitted. You can be an advocate for effective pain management at end of life by reporting your observations to the RN or supervisor.

MISCONCEPTIONS AROUND THE USE OF MEDICATIONS IN END-OF-LIFE AND PALLIATIVE CARE

Problems with pain management usually arise when staff lack observation skills, avoid reporting and documenting responses to pain medication, and misunderstand pain management. Misconceptions about pain and pain management are addressed by communicating with all staff and having consistent tools and documentation procedures. In a palliative care environment, staff are obliged to know as much as they can (consistent with their role) about pain and to provide support to relieve people's distress. Common misconceptions around pain management are listed in Table 12.3.

TABLE 12.3 Common misconceptions around pain management

Myth	Truth
Pain is an expected part of dying.	Pain relief should be given regularly, and no one should be expected to have untreated pain.
People should not receive analgesics until symptomatic relief is achieved.	Unrelieved pain is not acceptable. If pain continues, pain relief becomes more difficult.
There is no reason for pain when there is no physical cause.	Pain can arise for numerous reasons, including emotional distress.
Pain never killed anyone.	Chronic pain has serious side effects, such as lowering the immune system, which can lead to further deterioration in the person's condition.
Pain relief should only be given when the pain is present.	It is kinder and much more effective to give pain relief in anticipation of pain.
Analgesics are addictive.	Analgesics such as morphine, when prescribed and used properly, are not addictive

WORKPLACE SCENARIO

Pain relief in palliative care

Rami has bowel cancer and has recently been diagnosed with metastatic disease (secondary spread of a primary tumour) in the pelvic bones and the lungs. He has been coping with an increased level of pain for some months; however, it has become clear to care staff that the pain is now taking all of Rami's attention and affecting his motivation and capability.

In assessing Rami's pain, care workers Sally and Anna have noticed that he is:

- restless
- unable to sleep
- holding his chest
- curling into a ball
- grimacing when assisted to move.

They share this information with their colleagues Jim and Carol at handover, and it is decided to use the FACES pain rating scale and to consult the palliative care team about pain management. Jim assesses Rami's pain during the shift and observes that his pain becomes more intense as the day progresses, despite regular pain relief.

The palliative care team arrive the next day. In consultation with Rami and his partner Beena, the team encourages Rami to describe the pain, its level of intensity and what brings relief. It becomes clear that he is experiencing breakthrough pain. The team explain that medication needs to be taken regularly to keep pain relief levels stable in the body. They also decide to prescribe a combination of paracetamol and/or ibuprofen plus small doses of morphine, such as codeine. Jim reassures Rami and Beena that stronger pain relief will be available if it is required or requested. Beena expresses concerns about the side effects of medications, such as constipation, nausea and vomiting, drowsiness and confusion. Jim explains that these side effects can be managed using laxatives and antiemetics. Any drowsiness will probably last a few days, he says, but if it persists, especially in the presence of confusion, the medication schedule will be reviewed immediately.

CHECK YOUR UNDERSTANDING

1. How can the care worker promote comfort?
2. Name five common symptoms experienced during end of life.
3. What complementary therapies may be used in palliative care?
4. Why is it important to evaluate care?
5. How should medications such as morphine be administered?

12.5 FOLLOWING END-OF-LIFE CARE STRATEGIES

End-of-life care can be identified as care provided when a person is in the final stages of life. The time leading up to death can be anywhere from days to hours. The goals of care are focused on the person's physical, emotional and spiritual needs, and on supporting the family and loved ones. The care team will ensure the following:

- pain relief is maintained
- complications are prevented or managed
- medications not essential for controlling symptoms are ceased
- symptoms are minimised
- quality of life is maintained as much as possible
- medication delivery methods are changed if necessary
- carers have adequate support
- planning is in place to meet the last wishes of the dying person and their family, friends and significant others.

Services, health professionals and support workers can be organised to allow a person to decide on the location of their end-of-life care, depending on:

- the person's needs
- the resources and the needs of the family, friends and significant others.

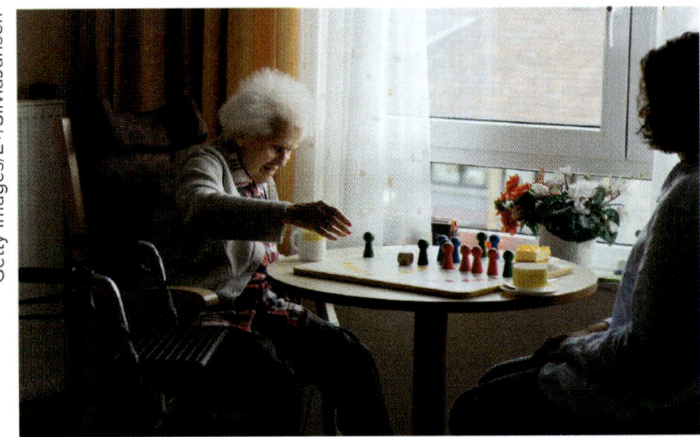

Getty Images/E+/SilviaJansen

The care team will ensure that the person's quality of life is maintained as much as possible

12.5.1 Provide a supportive environment

It is important to provide a supportive environment to the person, carer, families and others involved in end-of-life care. The days leading up to death are generally quite peaceful, with a gradual decline and sometimes a drift into a state of unconsciousness before breathing and circulation stop. Regardless of the physical and cognitive state of the person at end of life, a consistent focus on their dignity and comfort, and on the comfort of their family, friends and significant others, is paramount. End-of-life care continues to involve physical care, personal hygiene, wound care as required, and further care as indicated by the person's condition.

Those nearing end of life may also have spiritual and cultural needs, which are just as important as physical care. Spiritual needs may include finding meaning in one's life, ending arguments or conflict with someone where possible, and finding peace in knowing that things have been settled adequately.

Studies have shown that sometimes there are barriers to sound end-of-life care. Barriers can include the person's or their family members' avoidance/denial of death, the influence of managed care on end-of-life care, and lack of continuity of care across settings where end-of-life care occurs.

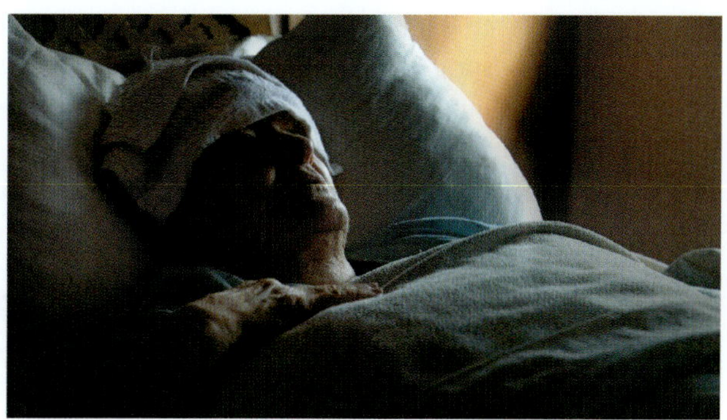

NicolasMcComber/E+/Getty Images

As death approaches, the person may exhibit increased lethargy and tiredness

12.5.2 The signs of deterioration and imminent death

As death approaches, you can demonstrate respect for and support the person's preferences and culture when providing end-of-life care according to their individualised plan and within the scope of your job role. There is no accurate method for identifying that death is imminent, but there are specific signs and symptoms that develop that indicate deterioration, which should be documented in the care plan. Not all aspects mentioned below will be seen in every person, nor will they occur in any particular sequence. Sometimes these physical signs appear a few hours before death, sometimes a few days. They are part of the normal, natural process of a person's body gradually slowing down.

Although signs of deterioration and imminent death may vary, death is likely to be imminent in the following instances:

- There is a gradual cooling of the skin and changes in colour. It can become pale and bluish.
- The person displays increased anxiety, restlessness and confusion (terminal restlessness). If this restlessness does occur, it can be treated.
- The person's appetite and thirst may decrease, and they may have little desire to eat or drink. This concerns many carers, but it is a natural process and is not painful for the person. Sips of water or a moist mouth swab and oral care will help provide comfort. Attempting to feed someone who is unable to swallow may make them distressed and cause harm. Sometimes even the smell of food can increase nausea, and this can increase distress. Weight loss is common as death approaches.
- There is a gentle winding down that may take several days as the body starts to "let go" of life.
- The person exhibits increased lethargy and tiredness. Changes in their body mean that they may spend a lot of time asleep, may be drowsy or difficult to wake up. A decreasing level of consciousness will follow.
- They may experience periods of pausing in breathing, and other breathing changes including rattling.
- Their pulse may become fast, irregular and weak.
- The person will have low blood pressure.
- They may produce a decreasing amount of urine due to their reduced intake of fluid. The urine may become stronger smelling and darker in colour. Many carers are concerned that the person will lose control of their bladder and bowels. This doesn't always happen, but pads, easy-to-use equipment and special absorbent sheets can help to enhance comfort and hygiene if the person becomes incontinent.
- Out-of-body or near-death experiences and death-bed visions or dreams may feature in some people's end of life. These "doorways to the unconscious" (Barbato 2013) experiences are often joyful and comforting to the dying person, and the care worker may hear about some of these types of experiences. It is essential that care workers don't dismiss these experiences, as they are real to the person who experiences them.

When signs and symptoms that indicate death is close are observed, it is essential to report to your supervisor or the appropriate member of the care team, according to organisational policies and procedures, so that family, friends and significant others (as per the person's wishes) can be notified.

Apart from the signs described above, you may notice other changes that worry you. The palliative care team can assist you by providing information and support. Ask for help at any time. Your supervisor and the palliative care team expect to have increased contact with you in the last stages of the person's life.

PRACTICE POINT

We know that you can bring enormous benefit to the person you are caring for simply by sitting with them, holding their hand, and speaking to them in a calm and reassuring manner. Even if the person doesn't respond, they can probably hear you. Don't underestimate the value of these simple things. "Being with" can be more important than "doing for" at this time.

12.5.3 Signs of death

Death has occurred when the following signs are present:

- Breathing has stopped.
- The heartbeat and pulse have ceased.
- The person cannot be roused.
- Their pupils are fixed. (The eyelids may be half open.)
- There may be a leakage of urine or faeces and the sound of fluids moving in the body.
- The facial muscles relax, so the face may take on a peaceful expression.

After death occurs, the specific actions that must be taken include:

- declaration by a doctor that the person is deceased
- physical care of the deceased according to policies, procedures and cultural practices
- care and support of the family, friends and significant others, including staff
- arrangements for the deceased to be transported to the funeral home or mortuary.

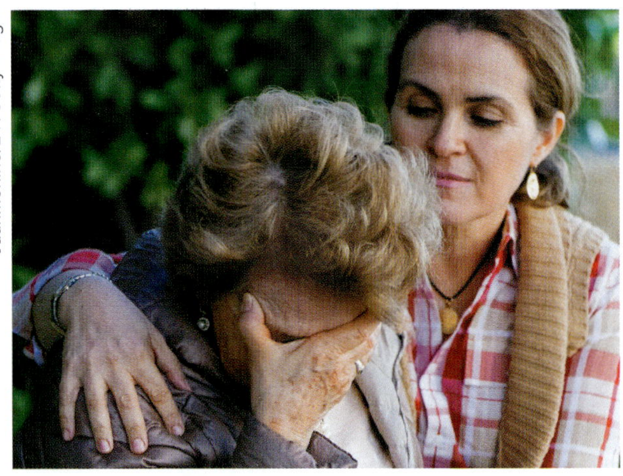
Juanmonino/E+/Getty Images

After the person dies, the care worker continues to provide emotional support to their family

12.5.4 Provide emotional support

When a death has occurred, the care worker continues to provide emotional support, within the scope of their own job role, to the person's family, carers and others. The family should be encouraged to sit with their loved one as long as they wish, and to perform any practices and rituals associated with their faith and culture.

As a guide, the person's body should be straightened, as limbs will stiffen over time and stay contracted in a set position, and their eyes closed and dentures replaced. Heating should be turned off and the funeral home contacted. Before after-death care is provided, a doctor must confirm the death and sign a death certificate. The person's wishes about what is to happen after death should be followed, which may include religious beliefs about how they want their body to be cared for. If an advance care directive exists, it should be followed exactly.

Personal hygiene, dressing and grooming should be carried out respectfully, in a way that preserves the person's dignity and with the same attention and care as if they were alive. Standard precautions and safe manual handling techniques should be employed. Some family might choose to be involved in after-death care, such as helping to wash the person, brushing their hair or massaging their hands if they wish. If the person's death is a coroner's case (when it must be investigated), it is essential to follow specific organisational policies and procedures.

WORKPLACE SCENARIO

The last few days

Bernadette has end-stage liver failure because of fatty liver disease due to diabetes and high blood pressure. She has been assessed as dying and her family have been notified. For some time, Bernadette has commented on increasing fatigue, loss of appetite and itchy skin. The care staff have observed that Bernadette's legs and abdomen are swollen and that she has lost weight. In the last two weeks, she has become confused, disorientated about time and place, and sometimes hasn't recognised care staff who have supported her since her admission three years ago. She has also developed wounds on her lower legs due to excessive swelling.

When Bernadette's family arrive, they are distressed to see her restless, anxious and moaning. The RN Carol explains that this may be a sign of liver failure or of a condition known as terminal restlessness. She discusses other signs and symptoms that indicate death will occur soon. These include:

- loss of interest in eating and drinking
- increased periods of lethargy
- prolonged periods of sleep
- changes in breathing
- a gradual cooling of the skin and change in colour.

Carol outlines what will be done to manage these signs and symptoms, incorporating pain management, personal care, repositioning for comfort and wound care.

Bernadette's family are reassured that being with her as she dies is their choice and that at no time will they be pressured or hurried. Carol explains that the family's needs are important and that they will be supported to take breaks, that food and drink will be provided for them and that emotional support is at hand. They are also reminded that when Bernadette dies, they will have the opportunity to be involved in the physical after-death care that will be provided. The care staff tell Bernadette's family that they are available for whatever the family needs, whether that is listening, or just being present or providing them with privacy.

CHECK YOUR UNDERSTANDING

1. Why check for changes in the care plan?
2. What are signs and symptoms of imminent death?
3. Why is it important to consider culture and religion when caring for a body after death?
4. What is a coroner's case?
5. Should an advance care directive be followed after death?

12.6 MANAGING YOUR OWN EMOTIONAL RESPONSES TO DYING AND DEATH

Bereavement is the feeling of grief and mourning after the death of someone you were close to. Support should be made available to members of the multidisciplinary health-care team, as well as to the person's family, friends and significant others. Support may include:

- talking to a close colleague
- counselling and debriefing
- stress management training
- social interactions with other staff
- access to the employee assistance program (EAP).

Rituals can help at this time. Some RACFs support staff to form a guard of honour as the deceased person is removed from the building. Other strategies could include signing a remembrance card for the person's family, and/or holding a formal remembrance ceremony to assist staff to farewell the person. A simple ceremony in a quiet, communal area of the RACF can also provide an opportunity for the person's family members to acknowledge their death. Members of the multidisciplinary health-care team may be invited to attend the funeral, celebration of life or other ceremony, in which case it is essential that they follow their organisation's policy and procedure.

12.6.1 Reflecting on your own responses to dying and death

Although you may regularly have the experience of caring for someone who is dying, it is not possible to "get used to" death or to cease to feel sad when someone dies. Some deaths will have more impact on you than others. Reflection may bring up memories of the death of a loved one or someone you looked after. You may visualise your memories of them and experience certain feelings. As difficult as this is, it is important to understand your personal reactions to death so that you can readily identify how you might react in the future. This will help you to manage your reactions and seek support if necessary. It will also help you to focus on supporting family and other colleagues as they experience loss and grief.

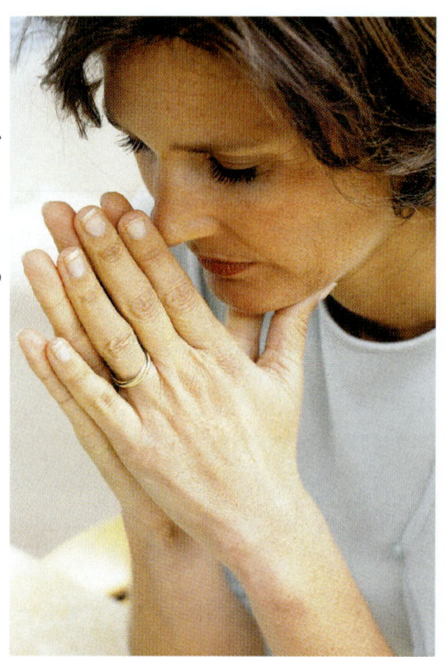

Image Source/Alamy Stock Photo

Care workers need to understand their own reactions to death and seek support if necessary

12.6.2 Ethical concerns

Supporting someone in a palliative care setting often raises ethical issues. Ethical issues are those that bring into question morals, principles, beliefs and values whereby a decision needs to be made as to whether something is right or wrong. Some of these issues include:

- decisions regarding medical treatment
- personal values that conflict with those expressed by the family
- when to initiate or cease procedures
- requests for assistance to die.

It is very important to seek support from your supervisor when you feel conflicted about someone's treatment or management. Occasionally, counselling and further support may be required to be able to ethically continue to care for someone where there is a conflict of morals, beliefs, values and principles. The care worker has a duty of care under the code of ethics to notify their supervisor of any conflict that may interfere with or interrupt the quality of care of a person.

12.6.3 Self-care strategies

Self-care is knowing when you need assistance or support and how to access it. The act of actually accessing it means that you can self-care effectively and appropriately. Self-care involves understanding your own strengths, weaknesses, beliefs, values, thoughts, motivations and emotions. Deciding on ways to care for yourself is necessary when dealing with dying and death, especially if you deal with it on a regular basis. Self-care will include:

- eating properly and regularly
- getting enough sleep
- connecting with friends and doing things you enjoy
- spending time exercising and relaxing
- identifying mentors and trusted colleagues who you can talk to when you feel stressed
- taking a day off as required for own mental health care.

Self-care is essential in preventing the accumulation of stress so that it becomes overwhelming and interrupts normal ADLs. When stress accumulates, you are at risk of "burnout". This term refers to long-term exhaustion and reduced interest in work or ability to do one's job. Burnout can be avoided by employing the strategies listed above and by developing realistic expectations about the degree of support you can provide to dying people and their families, friends and significant others.

12.6.4 Accessing support

Deciding when to access support is difficult and individual to each person, as we all have varying degrees of coping mechanisms. Within workplaces, regardless of the type of service or facility, policies and procedures exist, as well as employee assistance programs or schemes for ensuring employees are taken care of. EAPs or EASs are designed to offer support in a confidential manner and are free to access. Sometimes a workplace will offer assistance via private counselling for an agreed number of sessions free of charge by negotiation.

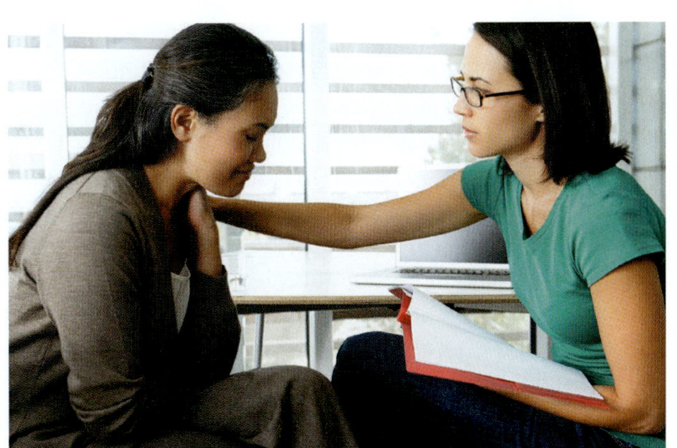

Shutterstock

Care workers can access employee assistance programs if they need support

In addition, there may be local support groups available online, via phone or in person, to debrief and discuss feelings, emotions and reactions to various issues. Support groups aim to provide a forum for emotional, practical and moral support. For example, the bereavement support groups at the Australian Centre for Grief and Bereavement (ACGB) are a therapeutic, inclusive and supportive space in which to share common grief experiences.

Spiritual advice and care can be accessed by consulting personal chaplains or spiritual care advisers as required. Attending church or spiritual services or ceremonies and talking with elders or significant figures within spiritual and cultural groups can also assist with advice and care. Spiritual support doesn't have to relate to a specific religion or scripture. Spirituality can be a person's connection with another person, with nature, or with anything that gives meaning and purpose to their life.

Private counselling may be available through your GP or medical centre.

12.6.5 Organisational policies and procedures

Organisations will have policies about how grief and loss will be managed by and for their employees. Ideally, an organisational policy will:

- implement training and support to improve the occupational experience of direct care workers and allow them to provide better palliative care in residential aged care facilities and in-home care
- provide a foundation on which a supportive response to grieving employees can be developed
- show that the organisation takes grief experienced by its staff members seriously.

WORKPLACE SCENARIO

When staff are grieving

Michelle has been a care worker for 10 years, working primarily in a palliative care environment. Recently, she cared for a person of her own age, and with similar family characteristics, who passed away suddenly and without family and friends close by. Other staff have noted that Michelle has become quiet and withdrawn and is spending a lot of time in the facility's chapel before going home after her shifts. When questioned by her colleagues, Michelle denies she is grieving and insists she is okay. Staff don't have the opportunity to attend the funeral service and a debriefing session hasn't occurred.

For the next few weeks, Michelle continues to isolate. She is skipping meals and declines offers to socialise with colleagues she used to spend a lot of time with outside of work. During a performance appraisal meeting, Michelle voices her feelings of non-closure with regard to the death of the woman she had cared for. As a result, the manager organises a debriefing session for Michelle and others. He also suggests that Michelle access the EAP for confidential counselling and grief support. Michelle attends the debriefing and accesses the EAP, where she is able to express herself freely, openly, honestly and without feeling judged. Strategies are offered for Michelle to gain closure and be able to move on so that her everyday life isn't impacted. A few more weeks pass and Michelle has used the strategies, attended counselling and begun to socialise with her colleagues again.

Grief among staff can take many forms, with varying characteristics and durations. Yet, with policies and procedures available and accessible, it can be overcome successfully and appropriately.

CHECK YOUR UNDERSTANDING

1. What is an ethical issue?
2. What is self-care?
3. Why is self-care important?
4. Discuss what you understand about spirituality.

SUMMARY

- Palliative care is the holistic person-centred care provided to a person nearing the end stage of their life and the care and support given to family, friends and significant others.
- Grief and bereavement are individual and may have detrimental effects on a person so that they require support and assistance.
- Providing palliative care to someone, and supporting a person affected by a palliative diagnosis, is a complex task requiring dedication, patience, understanding, empathy and self-care.
- People receiving palliative care are worthy of a consistent, high standard of care and quality of life that enables them to reflect on and feel satisfied with the respect and dignity afforded them during the end-of-life phase.

REVIEW QUESTIONS

12.1 Outline the differences between a palliative approach and specialised palliative care.

12.2 What constitutes a supportive environment in a palliative setting?

12.3 Outline the differences between an advance care directive and an advance care plan. Provide an example of each to support your answer.

12.4 List strategies to promote comfort.

12.5 List ways to support the experience of loss and grief for:

- **(a)** the person who is dying
- **(b)** carers and families.

BIBLIOGRAPHY

Advance Care Planning Australia, *Understand Advance Care Planning*, https://www.advancecareplanning.org.au/understand-advance-care-planning, accessed 1 December 2020.

Australian Centre for Health Law Research, *Voluntary Assisted Dying*, QUT, https://end-of-life.qut.edu.au/euthanasia.

Australian Government, Department of Health, *What We're Doing about Palliative Care*, https://www.health.gov.au/health-topics/palliative-care/about-palliative-care/what-were-doing-about-palliative-care, accessed 11 December 2020.

Australian Government, Department of Health, *Implementation Plan for the National Palliative Care Strategy 2018*, https://www.health.gov.au/sites/default/files/documents/2020/10/implementation-plan-for-the-national-palliative-care-strategy-2018_2.pdf, accessed 20 October 2020.

Australian Government, Department of Health and Aged Care, *National Palliative Care Strategy 2018*, https://www.health.gov.au/resources/publications/the-national-palliative-care-strategy-2018, accessed 20 October 2020.

Barbato, M., *Care for the Living and the Dying*, 2nd edn, Michael Barbato, Rochester, NY, 2010.

Barbato, M., *Midwifeing Death*, Michael Barbato, Rochester, NY, 2013.

Corr, C.A., "Should we incorporate the work of Elisabeth Kübler-Ross in our current teaching and practice and, if so, how?" *Omega–Journal of Death and Dying*, 31 July 2019, https://journals.sagepub.com/doi/10.1177/0030222819865397.

Dementia Australia, *Statistics*, https://www.dementia.org.au, accessed 23 April 2022.

Horwood, G. (ed.), *Individual Support in Australia: Ageing, Disability, Home and Community Care*, Vocational Education & Training Resources (VETRes) by TAFE NSW, 2016.

International Council of Nurses, *The ICN Code of Ethics for Nurses*, revised 2012, https://www.icn.ch/sites/default/files/inline-files/2012_ICN_Codeofethicsfornurses_%20eng.pdf.

Kübler-Ross, E., *On Death and Dying*, Macmillan, New York, 1969.

McKissock, M. & McKissock, D., *Coping with Grief*, ABC Books, Sydney, 1999.

Miller, J.E. & Cutshall, S.C., *The Art of Being a Healing Presence: A Guide for Those in Caring Relationships*, Willowgreen Publishing, Fort Wayne, IN, 2012.

My Aged Care, *Palliative Care*, https://www.myagedcare.gov.au/search?keys=palliative+care, accessed 23 December 2020.

NSW Health, *What is a Holistic Approach?*, 27 January 2005, https://www.health.nsw.gov.au/mentalhealth/psychosocial/principles/Pages/holistic.aspx, accessed 6 March 2022.

palliAGED, https://www.palliaged.com.au/.

Palliative Care Australia, *Voluntary Assisted Dying in Australia*, https://palliativecare.org.au/wp-content/uploads/dlm_uploads/2019/06/PCA-Guiding-Principles-Voluntary-Assisted-Dying.pdf, accessed 1 December 2020.

World Health Organization (WHO), *Palliative Care*, 5 August 2020, https://www.who.int/news-room/fact-sheets/detail/palliative-care?msclkid=ca6b5a85c37611ecb63c704d2ba50157, accessed 24 April 2022.

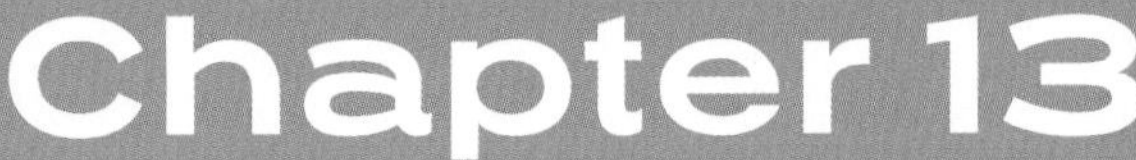

Chapter 13

Recognising falls risks

LEARNING OBJECTIVES

13.1 Understand the importance of falls risk assessment

13.2 Identify risk factors and falls prevention strategies

13.3 Report risk of falls

INTRODUCTION

FALLING IS A MAJOR CAUSE OF INJURY, COMORBIDITY (the existence of more than one medical condition or disease) and death among the older population. In fact, according to the World Health Organization (WHO), adults 60 years and older suffer the greatest number of fatal falls. Understanding some of the risk factors for falling can help us to implement strategies to prevent falls for those in our care. This is a collaborative approach to risk minimisation, and the care worker has an integral role in this process.

There are several factors that can increase the risk of falling for older people, and your ability to recognise and report these risk factors will contribute to the safety and wellbeing of the people you care for. A risk factor is anything that increases a person's chance of having a fall. The more risk factors a person has, the more chance they have of falling. As a person ages, their risk factors increase. The ageing process can have a direct impact on the ability to balance, mobilise safely and react quickly when a trip or fall occurs. Other factors that increase a person's risk of falling include the type and quantity of medications they are prescribed, the environment they live in, and some physical and mental health conditions.

Risk factors can be considered as physical/emotional and environmental in nature. We will look closely at these in this chapter, as well as at how medications may impact an older person's falls risk.

INDUSTRY IN FOCUS

National Aged Care Mandatory Quality Indicator Program

All residential aged care facilities (RACFs) that are approved providers of residential care services are required to be involved in the National Aged Care Mandatory Quality Indicator Program (QI Program). Approved providers are RACFs that receive Commonwealth funding to support care provision for consumers. They are required to demonstrate that they are compliant by providing services that are in line with government legislation and regulations. The three main objectives of the QI Program are:

- to compile a national database that can be used to provide aged care information across the residential aged care sector and to influence policy directions on a government level
- to provide, on a facility level, information and data that can be used to improve services and care outcomes through a quality improvement lens
- to enable transparency of services for potential and actual consumers of aged care providers to assist in decision making regarding quality care service provision.

The program has been functioning since July 2019 and all approved providers must participate as a compliance requirement. The Aged Care Quality and Safety Commission (the Commission) oversees the program. Approved providers are required to collect and report information about quality indicators across five components of care provision, under the guidance of the program. Reporting occurs quarterly (every three months). Assessments and measurements within each component are used to collect information. These components are:

- physical restraint
- unplanned weight loss
- falls and major injury
- pressure injuries
- medication management.

With regards to falls and major injury, for each quarter approved providers must report on how many consumers experienced a fall at the service, how many consumers experienced a fall at the service resulting in a major injury, and how many consumers were assessed for falls and major injury. Major injury in this reporting context includes bone fractures, joint dislocations and closed head injuries with changes to consciousness and/or subdural haematoma. In other words, RACFs collect information about falls their consumers have experienced and send the data to the QI Program. The information is then placed into a report for facilities to use in their quality improvement activities. It is also made available to consumers and potential consumers.

The information collected is used to identify areas in care provision that can be improved in a way that benefits consumers and improves practices within the organisation. The QI Program is not a disciplinary process; rather, it is a transparent method for improving care quality outcomes for consumers. However, non-reporting may result in compliance and enforcement actions by the Commission.

13.1 UNDERSTANDING THE IMPORTANCE OF FALLS RISK ASSESSMENT

13.1.1 The consequences of falls

The physical and emotional impact of falls on an older person can be life changing. Head injury from falling can have catastrophic outcomes. People die from serious falls that result in trauma to the brain. Any person who suffers a fall where a high risk of a closed head injury is present should have medical imaging to rule out bleeding or swelling within the cranial cavity, including the brain. This may include older people, especially those who take blood-thinning medications.

Older people who fall are more likely to fracture bones such as the wrist, hip and pelvis due to decreased bone density. These fractures not only take time to heal but can also have a direct impact on the person's quality of life and level of daily functioning. Tasks that were easier to achieve prior to falling, such as dressing, showering and meal preparation, are often compromised due to pain or limited mobility and dexterity. Consequently, many older people will require some type of personal care support after a fall involving a fracture. This affects people living in RACFs, as well as community dwellers.

Often, care is provided by family members. In this instance, the carer can be impacted by the person's fall, too. Their own routine will need to change to accommodate the needs of their loved one. Carers can also be impacted financially, as they may need to take time off work to look after their family member.

Falls can affect the emotional wellbeing of older people and their carers. Older people who experience falls can be affected psychologically if they become extremely fearful of another fall. Injury sustained from falling, or having multiple falls, can lead to anxiety and depression in older people. Loss of independence and functionality due to falling can impact the mental health of an older person. Chronic pain can also impact mental health in a negative way.

Carers, too, are affected emotionally when supporting a loved one after a fall. As the person loses their independence, carers can experience changes to their own lifestyle that can inhibit their availability to interact with their peers on a social level. Caring for a person with significant disability because of injury, whether temporary or permanent, is exhausting physically and emotionally. Sleep is often disturbed and relationships with other family members and friends will change due to time demands on the carer. Many carers may experience depression as a result of providing care and support to a person who has disability after a fall.

Care workers need to be mindful of what older people and their carers may be experiencing and show empathy throughout their communications with them.

13.1.2 Recognising risk of falls

Recognition of the risk of falls within your role as a care worker can occur through both informal and formal observations. Informal observations include those that come to your attention during your interactions with the older person and others in the workplace. In the course of your work, you might notice that someone is unsteady on their feet, or that they complain of feeling dizzy when they move, or that their new shoes don't fit them correctly. The older person or their carer may tell you that they have almost fallen over once or twice, and they can often identify the reason why. It could be a loose paver on the pathway to the clothesline, or maybe they struggle to step over the hub in the shower recess. It is

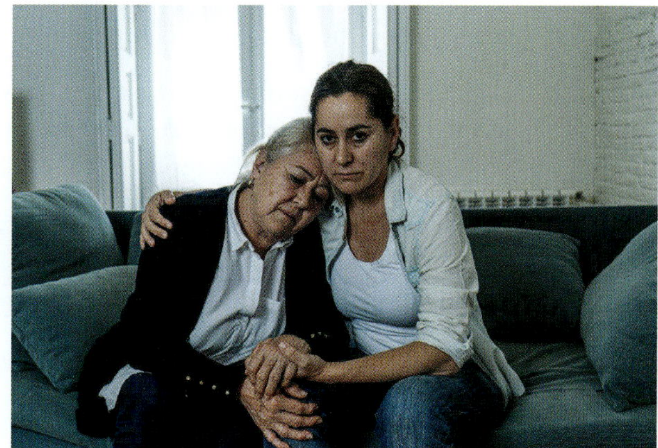

SB Arts Media/iStock/Getty Images Plus

Supporting someone after a fall is important

very important to act on these informal observations and to report them to the supervisor to ensure the person is offered support to minimise falls.

The person may not be aware of the help that is available to prevent them from falling. When you report your observations, you are fundamentally the first step in the falls prevention process. Your report may result in the person obtaining assessments for mobility aids or home modifications such as grab rails or bathroom redesign. The person may benefit from a referral to a health professional such as a physiotherapist to help with muscle strength or with an occupational therapist to assist with provision of suitable assistive devices (e.g. raised toilet seats, non-slip bathroom mats, and grabrails next to stairs).

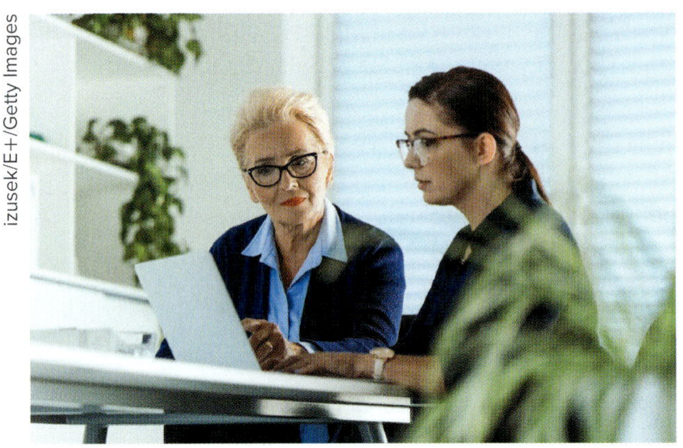

izusek/E+/Getty Images

The care worker should collaborate with a health professional to determine that they can undertake a falls risk assessment within their scope of practice

When risks are identified, strategies to minimise them are developed in consultation with the older person and their carer into a plan that is reviewed and changed according to the person's ongoing needs. The planning stage of a falls management plan may not be within your scope of practice; however, you may be asked by a health professional or organisation to implement the falls risk assessment tool. The first step in the formal assessment process is that you have collaborated with the health professional, such as a registered nurse (RN), to determine that you can undertake the assessment within your scope of practice. Consent to undertake the assessment must be obtained from the older person, who has the right to include–or not include–their carer.

13.1.3 Risk assessment tools

Formal observations that identify risk of falling include prescribed assessment processes. These processes include the use of a validated assessment tool (forms) that can assess the risk of falling for an older person. Commonly, these tools involve asking the older person questions about their physical and mental health, their environment, their medications and their falls history. Most falls screening tools use a scoring algorithm to determine a grouping of risk factors.

The following are some of the assessment Tools used to recognise the risk of falls for an older person:

- Falls Risk Assessment Tool (FRAT): https://www2.health.vic.gov.au/about/publications/policiesandguidelines/falls-risk-assessment-tool
- Falls Risk for Older People (FROP)–community setting: https://fallsnetwork.neura.edu.au/wpfd_file/falls-risk-for-older-people-community-setting-frop-com-guidelines-2/
- Modified Falls Efficacy Scale (MFES): http://geriatricphysio.yolasite.com/resources/falls%20efficacy%20scale.pdf

The type of risk assessment tool used will depend on the context of care–that is, residential or community–as well as on the preferences of the organisation or service provider. Some tools are tailored for use within the community and others for residential aged care.

WORKPLACE SCENARIO

Reporting observations

Lucy is 82 years old and lives at home alone. She is quite healthy and independent, but she needs some personal support to help her shower. Ella, a community care worker, is rostered to visit Lucy. When she is assisting Lucy to undress for her shower, Ella notices dark bruising on Lucy's left thigh and upper arm.

She is also moving more slowly than usual and is breathless. When Ella asks her about the bruising, Lucy says she fell while watering her garden.

After the shower, when Lucy is comfortable, Ella asks if she is in pain and whether she has fallen before. Ella then contacts her supervisor and reports the incident, including her observations about Lucy's bruising and breathlessness.

CHECK YOUR UNDERSTANDING

1. How might fractured bones sustained in a fall affect an older person?
2. Describe how falls can affect an older person's emotional wellbeing.
3. What is the difference between informal and formal observations in the context of falls risk minimisation?

13.2 IDENTIFYING RISK FACTORS AND FALLS PREVENTION STRATEGIES

13.2.1 Physical factors that contribute to the risk of falls

As a worker who provides services to older people, it is important to understand the physical indicators that increase the risk of falls. When you can recognise these risk factors, you are better placed to report your concerns to the appropriate health professional or supervisor. Your knowledge will also allow you to have safe and comfortable conversations with older people and their carers about falls risks, within your scope of practice.

There are many physical factors contributing to the risk of falling for an older person. These include the physical process of ageing, gait and balance problems, medication use and the presence of one or more chronic diseases. Acute physical conditions such as delirium and pain are also key contributors to falls in older people.

THE AGEING PROCESS AND HOW IT MIGHT AFFECT THE RISK OF FALLS

The ageing process is a risk factor for falling, and older people have a high rate of morbidity and mortality due to falls. As we age, gradual physical change is inevitable. We become aware of this when we look in the mirror and notice a little wrinkle here or there, or maybe some strands of grey hair. But the ageing process is far more dynamic than what we may notice and affects every body system. Ageing affects everyone, but it will affect individuals differently. There are many factors that contribute to how well people age, including genetics, lifestyle and health conditions.

On an organic level, we are made up of cells. Cells form tissue and tissue forms organs. Organs are specific to body systems. These body systems start to physically deteriorate from around age 30. However, it isn't until approximately our late 40s that we really start to notice early age-related physical changes.

Consider the body systems and their role in **homeostasis**. The systems work in harmony with each other, so that when one system isn't functioning to full capacity, it can affect the other systems. This capacity of body systems to work effectively and in harmony with each other decreases as we age.

It is important to note that chronic health disorders cause more functional decline than the ageing process. However, it is the ageing process, along with genetics and lifestyle, that can predispose us to chronic health conditions. The relationship between chronic health conditions and falling will be discussed later in this chapter.

For the purpose of understanding the risks of falls associated with the ageing body, we will look at the body's various systems, all of which are affected by ageing.

CARDIOVASCULAR SYSTEM

The following changes occur in the heart and blood vessels as a result of ageing:

- Blood vessels narrow and lose elasticity. Blood flow to vital organs can be reduced—for example, to the kidneys. This can result in changes to the ability of the kidneys to filter blood adequately of toxins, including leftover medication. An accumulation of circulating medication in the body can contribute to falls in older people.
- The body can automatically adjust the blood pressure when needed, although this ability can be affected by changes in the blood vessels. If a person's blood pressure drops suddenly when they stand, they can become dizzy and unsteady, which can cause them to fall.
- The heart's "natural pacemaker" can change the heart's conduction rhythm, and this can affect blood flow to the body. Changes to the heart's natural rhythm (**arrythmia**) can affect blood pressure and cause acute anxiety, both of which will increase the risk of falling.

Healthy living practices for heart health, including in older populations, may include eating a nutritionally balanced diet, exercising under a doctor's advice and having regular health check-ups.

CENTRAL NERVOUS SYSTEM

As we age, our brain reduces in size and our cognition is affected. It is important to note that diseases of the brain such as dementia and other neurological disorders often affect older people but are not a normal part of ageing.

The following changes can occur to our nervous system as a result of ageing:

- Multitasking can become more difficult and may increase the risk of falling when concentration requires more effort. For example, an older person may have a higher risk of falling if they are trying to have a conversation with someone while carrying grocery bags and climbing stairs at the same time.
- The depression that many older people experience will increase their risk of falling, due to the shift in mindset that depression produces and the person's inability to assess possible hazards and to exercise due caution. People who take medication for depression may have an increased risk of falling due to the intended and unintended effects of such drugs on the brain.

MUSCULOSKELETAL SYSTEM

The muscles, joints and bones are essential for movement, dexterity and mobilisation. The following changes to our musculoskeletal system as a result of ageing can increase our risk of falling:

- Bones become porous and are more likely to fracture from falling when we are older. Our bones are constantly going through changes throughout our life. This is called remodelling. The process progressively slows down as we get older and the bone tissue, along with mineral content, decreases. Bone density is lost due to osteoporosis. This condition is the reason many older people fracture bones when they fall. Hip fractures are most common. Ligaments become less elastic and more rigid, and the cartilage in the joints tends to lose fluid, resulting in arthritis.
- Ageing causes a reduction of muscle mass. The fibres in the muscles decline in number and functionality, and this has a direct effect on the ability of our muscles to react. The tendons that attach our muscles to our bones lose flexibility as their fluid content decreases with age. These changes to our muscles can be minimised by remaining active. Sedentary living hastens the loss of muscle mass and flexibility. The decline in muscle functionality contributes to serious injury

due to falling as a result of slower muscle reaction times, having less strength and dexterity, and the rapid deconditioning that can occur during times of prolonged immobility, such as a hospital stay.

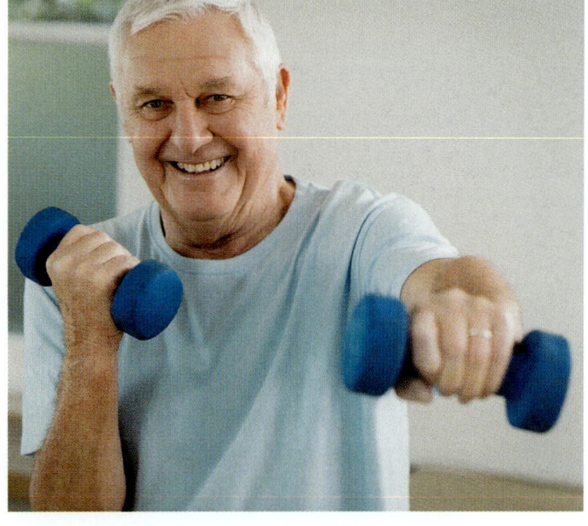
wavebreakmedia/Shutterstock

Changes to our muscles as we age can be minimised by remaining active

URINARY SYSTEM

The urinary system (also sometimes known as the renal system) includes the kidneys and bladder. The kidneys filter blood of waste and create urine. Urine is stored in the bladder until it is excreted. The kidneys are also important organs for the regulation of fluids, salt and other electrolytes.

The following changes to our urinary system are due to ageing:

- By approximately age 80, our kidneys have lost almost 20 per cent of their mass, which includes the loss of almost half of the functional units of the kidney, the nephrons. This loss can affect the elimination of medications from the body, and how efficiently some body processes occur, which may increase the risk of falling in older people.
- The bladder can lose elasticity as we age, which may make complete emptying of it difficult. Residual urine in the bladder can contribute to urine infection in both men and women. An older person with a urine infection is at higher risk of falls due to their need to urinate frequently, and sometimes falling can occur if the person is experiencing a sense of urgency to get to the bathroom. Incontinence is not a normal part of ageing; however, the urinary sphincter and the muscles that support urination may become weaker, especially for women with a weak pelvic floor. It is important to note that a urine infection is a common cause of delirium, which in turn is one of the most common causes of falls in the older population.

PRACTICE POINT

Ensuring the person has access to the toilet according to their care plan is important to prevent episodes of incontinence. They may be able to use the toilet independently or may require assistance with mobility to get to the toilet. If a person is incontinent frequently, ensure the RN or supervisor is made aware. Many types of urinary incontinence are preventable and reversible.

VISION

While not a body system, vision as a special sense is important to note in regard to falls risk. Good vision is essential for safety within our immediate environment. Our vision changes with age and this increases our risk of falling.

The following changes to our vision are associated with the physical ageing process:

- The lens in the eye can become dense and rigid, making focusing difficult, especially close up or in dim light.
- Depth perception can become compromised due to nerve changes, and this can exacerbate a falls risk. The pupil may have slower reaction times to changes in lighting, and this will add to the changes in depth perception. For example, a person may misjudge depth and overstep the guttering on the roadside when walking.

GAIT AND BALANCE

The word **gait** is used to describe the way a person walks. Walking occurs when a series of movements follow on from each other. Normal gait requires strength, balance and coordination. The central nervous system (the brain and the spinal cord) works closely with the musculoskeletal system to enable us to walk and run. The normal gait has a cycle that includes all movements between one heel strike and another heel strike. In other words, one stride is a gait cycle. Our normal gait can be affected by disease processes, substances and trauma. It is essential that you recognise different gaits so that you can understand the risk of falls they present.

Table 13.1 illustrates the most common types of gaits you may witness within your role as an aged care worker.

TABLE 13.1 Abnormal gaits that result from injury or disease

Gait	Characteristics	Considerations
Ataxic	This gait affects people with cerebellar disease or injury. It should be noted that people who are extremely intoxicated with alcohol have a similar gait. The person has exaggerated and awkward movements and will sway from side to side when standing still. Movement includes a wide and staggering base, and the person cannot walk using heel to toe as in the normal gait.	The person cannot walk in a straight line and will sway around markedly when standing still. Risk of falling is high, as is risk of injury due to their wide base of mobility.
Choreiform (hyperkinetic gait)	This gait is seen in people with Huntington's disease and other **dystonia**-related diseases. The person will experience highly irregular, jerky and involuntary movements when mobilising and at rest. All extremities are affected by these movements.	People with these conditions are at extreme risk of falls with catastrophic outcomes due to the involuntary movements that are exacerbated with walking. Some people benefit from a forearm support frame, while many people opt to continue to walk independently despite knowing they will fall. Some people will wear protective body wear or head gear as an injury minimisation strategy. Dignity of risk must be balanced with duty of care when providing care for people at such high risk of harm.
Diplegic (scissors gait)	This gait may be seen in people who have or are experiencing brain injury or cerebral palsy. Hips and knees are slightly flexed with an abnormally narrow base. Legs are dragged when walking occurs, and the toes often scrape the ground. The legs can cross over each other tightly when walking due to abnormal hip muscles. This may resemble scissors.	People may choose to have surgery to the abnormal hip muscles to assist with mobility. Many people will use supportive devices such as leg braces and in-shoe splints. Some medications may be prescribed to assist with muscle cramping and muscle over-activity. Ensure that the person has adequate time for activities due to falls risk.
Hemiplegic	Commonly seen after a stroke has caused physical changes to one side of the body. **Unilateral** weakness on the affected side. The arm on the affected side is often held by the person or supported in a sling when walking. The affected leg is straight with flexion of the foot and toes. When walking, the affected leg is dragged in a semicircle (circumduction).	People with this type of gait are often supported with physiotherapy and the use of a quad stick when mobilising. High falls risk.

TABLE 13.1 Abnormal gaits that result from injury or disease (continued)

Gait	Characteristics	Considerations
Myopathic (waddling gait)	People with muscular dystrophy and other **myopathy** may have this gait. The muscles around the hips are called the hip girdle and are important for normal mobilisation. When the person experiences weakness in one or both hips, the hips will become uneven, and the person will drop lower on one side when walking. If both hips are affected, the person may appear to be waddling.	It is important to support quality of life for people with myopathy and to understand that they have a high risk of falling due to progressive weakness of their muscles. Be aware that fatigue from walking can also contribute to falls risk.
Neuropathic (steppage gait)	Seen in some people with uncontrolled diabetes and other peripheral nerve diseases. This gait is characterised by foot drop (toes downward) whereby the person is unable to lift the foot at the ankle. Therefore, the person will step higher than usual to ensure the foot clears the ground. Can affect one or both sides of the lower body.	This gait increases falls risk due to the extra effort the person has to make to step higher in order to mobilise. They may overstep on some surfaces or fall when moving from a lower surface to a higher surface such as steps.
Parkinsonian (propulsive gait)	More common in the later stages of Parkinson's disease. The person has shorter and shuffling steps and appears stooped forward.	The person may have difficulty initiating and stopping movement. High incidence and risk of falls in late Parkinson's disease. Remember dignity of risk.

Changes to a person's gait indicate a neurological problem and can be temporary or permanent. Acute illness, low blood glucose levels, and states of delirium can change the way we walk. These conditions may last for minutes, days or weeks. Permanent changes to gait occur due to injury to the brain or limbs, and to progressive neurological diseases.

MEDICATION AND FALLS

The types of medication an older person may take will increase their risk of falling and, due to the ageing process, people are more likely to experience health conditions that require medications. This may be due to the physical ageing process, a disease or illness, or both. Medications are prescribed by a medical professional to assist an individual with a specific problem or problems. All medications have intended effects, but they all also have unintended effects. These effects may include dizziness, vertigo, changes to the heart rhythm, changes in mobility and visual perception, and many more.

The use of five or more medications by a person is referred to as **polypharmacy** and these medications can include prescribed medications, over-the-counter medications and complementary drugs. The more medications an older person uses, the higher is the risk that they will experience a fall. It is the unintended effects of medications that can increase their risk of falling and the more medications taken, the more unintended medication effects will exist. Most best-practice guidelines recommend a comprehensive medication review as part of a falls prevention plan.

Some groups of medications place the older person at higher risk of falling than others. These include medications that affect the brain, blood pressure, movement and pain.

MEDICATIONS THAT AFFECT THE BRAIN ("PSYCHOACTIVE" MEDICATIONS)

Psychoactive medications are designed to influence the way the brain works. There are many reasons a person will require these types of medications, including epilepsy, neuropathic pain, dementia and behaviours of concern. Despite the intended effects of these types of medications, many unintended effects are common and will increase the risk of an older person falling.

- *Psychotropics:* This group of medications is designed to support psychosis and other symptoms of conditions such as schizophrenia, bipolar disorder and other mental health illnesses. Psychotropic drugs are also used for behaviour and psychological symptom management in the treatment of dementia. Research indicates that the use of psychotropic medication increases the risk of falls in the older population. These medications can cause changes to perceptions of space and depth and affect a person's mobility and acuity. Long-term use can cause rigidity of the musculoskeletal system and impaired reaction times to falling. There is documented evidence that some antipsychotics used for management of dementia can have a direct influence on the circulatory system of older people, resulting in stroke and arrythmias.

- *Benzodiazepines:* This group of medications is often prescribed for their sedative effects to combat insomnia and support anxiety, among other reasons. They are medications that are best prescribed for short terms such as several weeks, as clinical dependence can occur with long-term use. People who are taking long-term benzodiazepines must be weaned off them, and not cease taking them immediately, to avoid complications from dependence. Some benzodiazepines tend to be short acting but can hang around in the body for a couple of days, so any risks associated with them are prolonged. The risks of falls from the use of benzodiazepines in older people include changes to perception of depth and of the space around them. For example, a person may walk down some steps and not consider the last step and subsequently fall, or they may not step up onto the gutter when crossing a road because they don't acknowledge it is there until they fall. The sedative effects of these drugs make people less aware of their environment and can influence their judgement regarding safety. These medications also increase drowsiness and have been linked to the development of dementia. Much research supports the fact that benzodiazepines should not be used in the older population, as statistically they have been found to cause falls, fractures, car accidents and death in this population.
- *Anticonvulsants/mood stabilisers:* Some medications have a dual effect. Anticonvulsants work to control seizures in epilepsy but are also therapeutically used as mood stabilisers in the management of mental illnesses such as bipolar disorder. Some anticonvulsants have a third therapeutic use as an agent to relieve neuropathic pain (nerve pain). Unintended effects of these drugs that increase the risk of falling in older people include drowsiness, confusion, depression, impaired balance, changes to reaction times and gait changes, to name just a few.
- *Antidepressants:* Research indicates that many antidepressants have side effects that may increase an older person's risk of falling. These effects include **ataxia** (changes to balance or coordination), confusion, slower reaction times and hypotension (low blood pressure). There are different groups of antidepressants; however, many of the side effects are the same. Older people should be prescribed the lowest dose possible when they initially start to take these medications, combined with effective psychotherapy.

MEDICATIONS THAT AFFECT BLOOD PRESSURE (ANTIHYPERTENSIVES AND DIURETICS)

Hypertension is the medical term for the condition of having high blood pressure. Constant high blood pressure can place stress on the heart, the blood vessels and other body systems. The group of medicines that are designed to lower blood pressure are called antihypertensives.

There is not a lot of research that claims this group of medications contributes to falls in the elderly when taken correctly for a long period of time. The risk of falling from taking long-term antihypertensives usually arises from the interaction between multiple medications the person may be using. Remember the term "polypharmacy"? If a person is taking antihypertensive medication to lower their blood pressure, they may be taking another medication for a completely different reason that has the unintended effect of reducing blood pressure. So, in this example, both drugs lower blood pressure. One does it intentionally and the other does it unintentionally.

Diuretics are a group of medications that support the heart and kidneys by managing the fluid status of the body. They are commonly known as fluid tablets and are prescribed for several reasons, including high blood pressure and heart failure. When the heart is struggling to work effectively, the blood pressure is affected in a way that influences the body's ability to circulate blood around the body efficiently. This can lead to stroke, kidney and heart failure, and excessive fluid build-up in the tissues and lungs. Doctors will often prescribe diuretics to remove excess fluid and salt from the body. When excess fluid is removed, the heart and kidneys don't have to work as hard. Diuretics can also have unintended effects such as dehydration, dizziness, high blood glucose, and changes to potassium and sodium levels that can affect how the heart works. Severe dehydration in an older person can lead to confusion and heart arrythmias. These are all risk factors for falls in older people. Older people who take diuretics will urinate more frequently as the medication encourages the kidneys to produce more urine. This can be a falls risk if the person must get up quickly to use the toilet, especially at night when they are more likely to trip over objects.

MEDICATIONS THAT AFFECT INVOLUNTARY MOVEMENTS (ANTICHOLINERGICS)

Acetylcholine is a chemical messenger or neurotransmitter that is responsible for movement just about everywhere in the body. Its functions include muscle contraction, blinking, and involuntary movements of smooth muscle found in the bladder, stomach, heart and other body systems. Acetylcholine also functions to support our memory, learning and cognition, and research suggests that a change in acetylcholine levels can be linked to Alzheimer's disease. Anticholinergic medications are used to block or inhibit acetylcholine when a problem exists. This may be for muscle spasms or tremors in Parkinson's disease, for a motility issue with the digestive system or an allergy issue with sedating antihistamines.

Anticholinergics as a group of medications are not suitable for older people, especially those with comorbidities. The side effects of these medications include drowsiness, confusion, sedation, memory loss and delirium, all of which increase the risk of falling.

MEDICATIONS USED FOR PAIN

Opioids are a group of medications that are prescribed for pain that doesn't respond to other pharmacological interventions. Common opioids include morphine, fentanyl, oxycodone, hydromorphone and tramadol. These medications are used with extreme caution and are very potent. There are conflicting reports that opioid use in older people contributes to falls; however, side effects of opioids–including drowsiness, dizziness and sedation–increase the risk of falling.

Cohorts of older people who are at risk of falling due to the use of opioids are those who are newly prescribed these types of medications. People who are opioid naïve (in other words, their body is not used to the effects of the medication) are more likely to fall as a result.

Medication use is a leading cause of falls in older people. Polypharmacy increases the risk of falling and of drug-to-drug interactions. One risk can be the catalyst for another risk. For example, a medication that causes dehydration can cause delirium. Delirium can cause a fall.

Unfortunately, older people may be prescribed medications by more than one doctor. This is true when the person may see other doctors apart from their own general practitioner (GP). Other doctors may include specialists, after-hours doctors, emergency department doctors and other treating practitioners in the hospital setting. The more people prescribing, the higher the risk of polypharmacy and the associated unintentional effects of medications. The effects of a medication can accumulate in the body and thereby have more intensity. This occurs to older people who take medications, especially several medications, and whose body doesn't clear the medications efficiently. This is because the ageing urinary system has a vastly reduced ability to filter drug metabolites into urine, resulting in more medication in the person's system.

It is very important that any older person who takes medications has their list of medications reviewed by a doctor or pharmacist at least annually. Some medications may be de-prescribed, some may have changes to doses, and others may be tapered off. A medication review is best practice as a falls minimisation strategy.

Part of your role may be to report your concerns about the number of medications someone takes and the risk of falling that this presents. If you are working in the residential aged care facility environment, you can refer your concerns to the RN; and if you work with older people in the community, you can encourage the person to seek a medication review from the pharmacist. Always be aware of your policies and procedures about confidentiality, privacy and working within your scope of practice.

MEDICAL CAUSES OF FALLS

The reasons older people fall are multifaceted and can be complex. Many risk factors for falls can overlap or exacerbate each other. For example, a person with a hemiplegic gait who takes medication to lower their blood pressure and has dementia has multiple risk factors for a fall. This person may feel dizzy (due to low blood pressure), not realise they need to rest (effects of dementia) and try to walk quickly down the corridor (with a hemiplegic gait).

There are many medical reasons that cause older people to fall. Some of these affect blood pressure, some affect cognition and alertness, and others affect functional ability. The following paragraphs describe some of the more common medical causes of falls and how they can impact the risk of falling for older people.

POSTURAL HYPOTENSION

Postural hypotension is a sudden drop in blood pressure when a person changes their position, such as standing up quickly. The causes of postural hypertension can be age related, induced by medication effects, induced by underlying health diseases such as heart failure or induced by an adverse health status such as dehydration.

Monitoring blood pressure for people with postural hypotension is essential as part of a falls management plan. A blood pressure measurement is taken when the person is lying in bed and is then repeated three minutes after they sit up. (Sit to stand is also another way this measurement can be taken.) If there is a significant change between the readings, the person may have postural hypotension. Older people with postural hypotension are at a higher risk of falls than those who have a normal blood pressure.

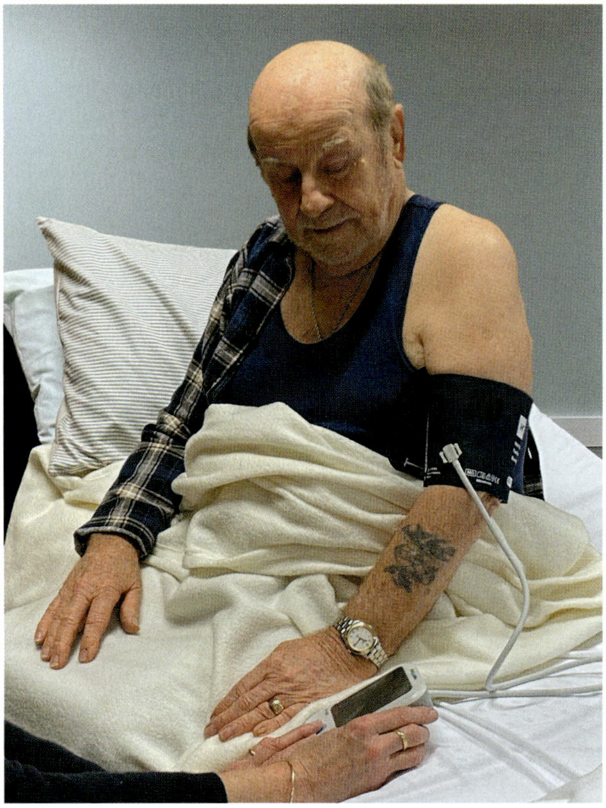

For people with postural hypotension, a blood pressure measurement is taken when the person is lying in bed and then repeated three minutes after they sit up

You may be the person who notices that a person is dizzy when they stand or sit on the edge of the bed after waking. You may also notice they are unsteady when they stand up from the dining table and then they seem okay after a few minutes. These observations that you make are clinical indicators of postural hypotension and other medical issues. It is essential that you report these observations immediately to the appropriate person within the context of your work role, after you have ensured the person is safe to be left alone. Never assume that nursing and medical staff are aware of every medical problem a person has. New signs and symptoms present themselves at any time. Remember: when you make a verbal report to a supervisor or health professional, you should always follow it up with a documented version, too. Follow your organisation's policies and procedures regarding documentation and privacy processes.

OSTEOPOROSIS

It is known that the ageing process causes our bones to lose density and become more porous over time. This is osteoporosis (*osteo* [bone] *porosis* [state of being porous]). Other disease processes and some medications can also contribute to a decrease in bone density.

Calcium is needed for bone and teeth health. Our body also uses calcium for muscle contraction and blood clotting processes. The body will always take from the bones if it needs more calcium, which is detrimental to bone health. Vitamin D is needed for calcium to work effectively in the body, and we get most of our vitamin D from sunlight. It can be difficult to get enough vitamin D from food, and many older people, especially women, will be prescribed vitamin D and calcium supplements by a health professional.

Osteoporotic bones are more likely to fracture when a fall occurs. The main bones affected by osteoporosis include the femur, the wrists and the spine. Fractures result in pain and potentially deconditioning and functional decline if the older person has poor health and comorbidities at the time of the fracture occurring. According to a 2017 Australian study, "older individuals with hip fracture are more than 3.5 times more likely to die within 12 months compared to non-injured counterpart" (Lystad, Cameron & Mitchell 2017).

DIABETES MELLITUS

Another chronic condition that increases a person's fall risk is diabetes mellitus. Diabetes mellitus occurs when glucose levels in the blood are unable to be used by the body for energy. This may be because the person doesn't produce enough of the hormone insulin, or the body cannot use the available insulin properly. Insulin is a hormone produced by the pancreas and its role is to allow glucose to get inside cells where it is needed to work effectively.

Many people with diabetes will require insulin injections to regulate their blood glucose levels. Older people with diabetes are at a higher risk of falls based on the following manifestations of the disease:

- Chronic high blood glucose levels (hyperglycaemia) can cause damage to the microscopic and small blood vessels in the feet. Over time, the sensory ability of the skin to inform the brain of pain and discomfort can decrease. Blood flow becomes impaired and, once injured, diabetic feet are very difficult to heal. Many diabetics undergo amputation of part or both lower extremities. Decreased sensation is called neuropathy, and this can increase the falls risk for an older person with diabetes as they lose sensation when walking.
- Acutely high blood glucose levels can increase thirst and increase fluid loss from frequent urination. The body will try to offload the extra glucose in the blood by sending it to the kidneys to be filtered into the urine. The kidneys assist with fluid balance, so they will also create large volumes of urine in response. This, in turn, may lead to falls risk with the frequent getting up and down to use the bathroom, with a sense of urgency, especially at night. Dehydration is also a possibility due to the fluid loss and may trigger a delirium that increases falls risk.
- When blood glucose levels are very low (hypoglycaemia), the risk of falling is very high. The brain needs glucose to function, as do most organs. Without enough glucose in the circulation to feed the brain, a person can show signs of hypoglycaemia that include extreme confusion, a very unsteady or ataxic gait, a loss of balance and coordination, and a declining level of consciousness. Hypoglycaemia is a medical emergency and should be treated immediately as per the person's care plan. Left untreated, the person will become comatose rapidly.

VESTIBULAR DISORDERS

The vestibular system of the human body is complex and is designed as a sensory system to promote balance, spatial awareness and equilibrium. Anatomically placed within our inner ear, this system also contributes to eye movement and our coordination. The vestibular system communicates with other body systems continually. It can be said that any vestibular disorder affects mobility, balance and coordination, and results in dizziness and nausea–all strong risk factors for falls.

PAIN

Poorly controlled pain and pain within the joints can be indicators of an increased falls risk in the elderly. Conditions such as arthritis, muscle pain and chronic back pain can have a direct effect on mobility and balance.

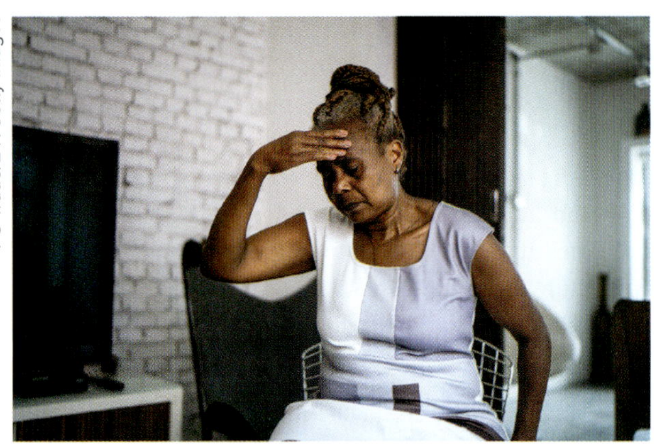

FG Trade/E+/Getty Images

Vestibular disorders affect mobility, balance and coordination—strong risk factors for falls

Some medications that are used for pain can have unintended effects that include sedation, blurred vision, sleep disturbance and depression. All these effects are risk factors for falling in the elderly.

Pain can also mask undiagnosed conditions such as fractures and osteoporosis. Activities of daily living can be disrupted due to pain. Older people may have trouble showering or dressing and undressing independently due to pain, and their risk of falling during these activities will be increased.

Pain also prevents people from mobilising and moving like they did before experiencing pain. This can in fact promote deconditioning of muscle mass, which also increases the risk of falls. Effective and safe pain management is essential to minimise falls in people with chronic or poorly controlled pain.

It is within your scope of practice to report your observations that indicate a person is experiencing pain. The older person you support may tell you directly that they are in pain, or you may notice changes in their functional abilities or their routines that indicate pain is an issue. No one should be in pain, and interventions can be initiated when health professionals are informed.

COGNITIVE RISK FACTORS FOR FALLING

Our cognition is our mental ability to process and understand information. This includes making decisions, judgements and plans, and using memory effectively. There are many reasons why a person's cognition may change. Cognitive impairment can occur due to injury, physical and mental illness, delirium or disease processes such as dementia. Cognitive impairment can be temporary or permanent.

When brain cells are damaged, message systems can become compromised. That is, our ability to translate and understand the message can be reduced when brain cells are damaged. Therefore, we see changes to a person's behaviours and abilities when they have dementia or an acquired brain injury.

Falls risks are increased for older people with impaired cognition. Damage to the brain can make it more difficult to move safely and to use planning to enable the body to navigate high-risk areas such as stairs, broken footpaths and gutters. Changes to vision due to brain damage can also involve significant changes to perception of depth, and this can increase the risk of falling. For example, depth perception can affect how a person interprets black-and-white chequered tile flooring. The black tiles are perceived as deep holes and the person will step cautiously around them. Clearly, depth perception can increase the chances of a loss of balance.

A person who has cognitive impairment may also lack insight into safety. We need judgement to be able to make decisions that will keep us safe. For example, we know not to walk into traffic. Poor judgement can place older people at risk of falling as well as placing them in harm's way.

DELIRIUM

Delirium is a sudden and new onset of confusion and can be experienced by a person of any age; however, older people are the most vulnerable to delirium. Delirium is often triggered by an infection, but other triggers are pain, constipation, hunger and thirst, or a lack of oxygen in the blood, just to name a few.

Delirium can co-occur with depression and dementia, which presents the risk of misdiagnosis for determining delirium. It can also affect a person without dementia. Delirium will recede when the cause is reversed. For example, a urinary infection may cause delirium in an older person until the infection is successfully treated. The cause for delirium isn't always isolated, and this is cause for concern because the person may succumb to illness or, in the event they survive the incident, they will experience some functional decline upon recovery.

Delirium can be hypoactive in nature, whereby the person appears to have depression-like symptoms. This is not actually depression but is often misdiagnosed as such. A person with hypoactive delirium may be sluggish and lethargic, show apathy and not be able to participate in usual self-care activities. This increases their risk of falls.

Hyperactive delirium is the opposite of hypoactive delirium; it can present like psychosis and is often misdiagnosed as a psychotic symptom of dementia. In this state of delirium, the person may be constantly moving around, sometimes erratically. They may climb or move items of furniture to reach heights. Their balance and coordination are impaired. Clearly, people in this delirious state are at a high risk of falling.

The most common form of delirium is a mixed delirium where a person experiences both hypoactive and hyperactive symptoms. These episodes ebb and flow and are marked by hallucinations and other indicators of sudden confusion. This type of delirium is often misdiagnosed as dementia. Again, the person's risk of falls is very high.

It is important to get treatment for the older person with delirium. If you observe a new and unusual behaviour from an older person you care for, ensure that you report it immediately and document your observations as per your organisation's policies and procedures. Any concerns about delirium must be reported in a timely manner, as it can signify a worsening infection.

PRACTICE POINT

If you notice signs that the person has a sudden or new confusion, or a new behaviour, they may be experiencing one of several health issues. Don't rule it out as dementia immediately. Consider the conditions that can affect the ability of the brain to function correctly, such as infection, low blood glucose levels, dehydration, stroke, low oxygen levels, medications and trauma. People with and without dementia can experience any of the signs and symptoms of the conditions that affect the way we behave and think. Always report your observations about behaviour changes in older people, as the change means something isn't right.

FEAR OF FALLING

Fear of falling affects some older people after they have experienced a significant fall, although not all people who experience this fear have had an actual fall. The phenomenon can have adverse and detrimental effects on an older person if it isn't recognised and supported with a therapeutic approach. Fear of falling causes people to have an exaggerated fear of having a fall. This fear goes far beyond the expected fear that can occur after a fall and can become a disability. Fear of falling will increase the person's risk of falling.

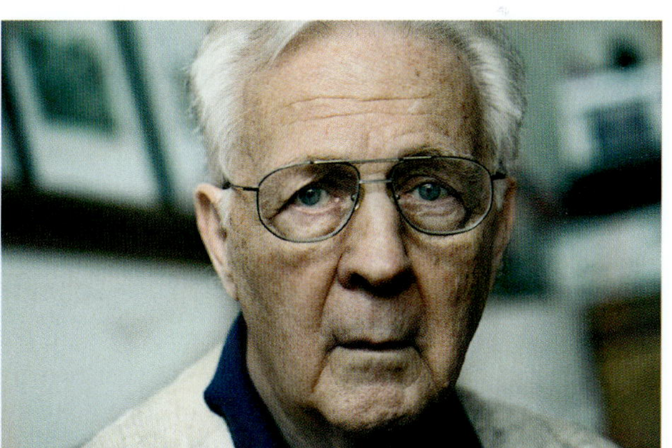

Image Source/Alamy Stock Photo

The most common form of delirium is marked by indicators of sudden confusion, greatly increasing the person's risk of falls

The following are characteristics of fear of falling:

- The person is reluctant to mobilise. They will minimise their chance of falling by limiting their mobility. This results in further deconditioning of the muscles and joints and contributes to risk of falls.
- The person will use a walking cane or a walker earlier than they need to.
- The person will use furniture, doors and benchtops as a walking aid (known as furniture walking). They touch these items as they mobilise as if to reassure themselves that they have some support in case they fall.

- The person is reluctant to participate in activities they enjoy. This has the potential to socially isolate them from social networks such as friends and family.
- Depression and anxiety often coexist in a person with a fear of falling. These mental health conditions can contribute to falls and will exacerbate fear of falling symptoms.
- The person may be over-cautious, in an attempt not to fall, and this will in fact increase their chance of falling. Slow, careful and methodical movements will result in a changed gait. Changed gaits are an indicator for falls.

Validated screening tools such as the Falls Efficacy Scale (FES) are used to help identify if a person is experiencing fear of falling. The FES is designed to determine a person's level of concern about falling while carrying out particular tasks such as shopping, cleaning or walking. Other tools are also used to determine depression and anxiety as contributing factors to a person's fear of falling. Older people have the lowest recognised diagnosis of depression and often go untreated.

As a care worker, you are in the best position to notice changes in the older person's behaviour that may indicate fear of falling, or depression. It is acceptable to question why they are no longer interested in participating in activities they usually enjoy. The person may be mobilising differently, they may request a walker, or they may not want to leave their room. These could be signs that they are avoiding walking and may be experiencing fear of falling. If you are a community worker, you may notice changes in the person's routine. For example, they may request you check their mailbox when usually they take a walk outside to check it themselves. As a one-time event, this may not draw your attention; however, if it is an ongoing request, then it is worth reporting it to your supervisor.

Fear of falling can increase risk of falls, increase deconditioning of muscles and functional decline, and lead to social isolation of the older person.

THE ROLE OF THE CARE WORKER IN MINIMISING FALLS RISK

While it can be said that the risk of falling increases because of the physical ageing process, it is important to note that many older people experience chronic disease processes that also compound their risk of falling. Many elderly people therefore have comorbidities that make healthy ageing very difficult to achieve. Regardless, as a care worker, you can promote healthy ageing among the people you provide support to. In the course of your work, you may notice some changes in the person's usual physical abilities that can put them at risk of having a fall. It is essential that you report your concerns to the appropriate person within your organisation. Always ensure you follow the person's service delivery plan and collaborate with health professionals about any concerns you have about the person's risk of falling.

13.2.2 Environmental risk factors for falls in older people

It has been identified that many physical factors increase a person's chance of having a fall as they age, but it is also important to consider the environmental risk factors for falling. Once referred to as extrinsic factors, environmental risks are those that influence an individual's chance of falling because of mechanisms, situations and processes that are not from within the body.

UNEVEN FLOORS AND OTHER SURFACES

Many falls occur when an older person, especially one who lives in the community, trips or slips over on an uneven floor or other surface. Uneven surfaces or flooring include broken or chipped pathways in the person's yard or the public footpath. Inside the home, the older person may trip on a floor mat or where two surfaces, meet such as carpet and linoleum. Many people who live in the community reside in a home that was built in a time when falls minimisation wasn't a consideration. Of these homes, many have had renovations over the years by owners with no building experience, at a time of little regulation. Therefore, many homes older people live in have flooring that isn't consistently level throughout the house.

Outdoor laundries and toilets are still in use today, which add to the risk of falls when the older person navigates to these outbuildings at night.

Slippery and wet floors present an extremely high risk of falling for older people. Many falls occur in the bathroom during or after a shower, and a loose bathmat can also add to the risk. A fall in the bathroom can have catastrophic outcomes such as head injuries, fractures and even death, as a result of falling onto the hard tiled environment.

Floors and other surfaces within an RACF are designed to minimise falls. They are on one level and tend to be of a uniform colour that doesn't challenge depth perception. If there are steps, they are marked with high-visibility non-slip tape, with signage that indicates the steps are present. Corridors are wide and well-lit and have handrails along the walls.

Bathrooms within an RACF are designed to minimise falls. They are fitted with grab rails in the shower recess and around the toilet that offer support to the older person to sit and stand safely. Flooring in these bathrooms is slip resistant but not slip proof. Care workers must always be vigilant when assisting an older person with personal care in the bathroom.

The older person who lives in the community will have higher risks of falling in their own bathroom, as not all private dwellings have safety modifications. Modifications in the bathroom include handrails in the shower and by the toilet to assist the person to sit, stand and remain steady when showering. A bath board can assist the person to use the bathtub safely, and non-slip floor mats prevent slips.

Risks of falling on uneven or unfamiliar surfaces outside of the person's usual residence are also present. Shopping centres offer challenges to safe mobility for older people, too. Using escalators safely can be a challenge, and an older person may experience anxiety when stepping on and off the escalator due to the quick-thinking coordination of movement that is needed. This can cause a fall.

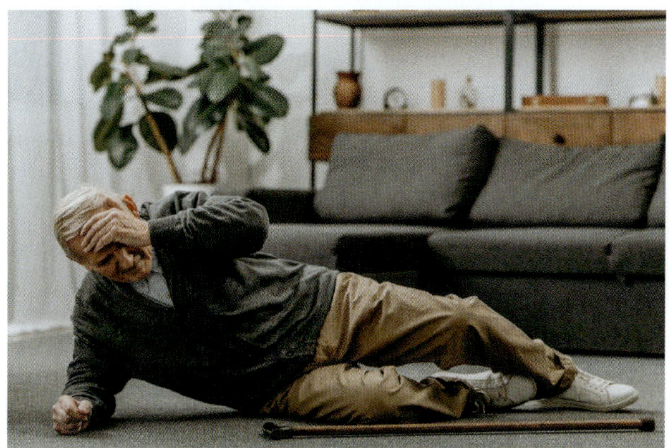

LightField Studios/Shutterstock

Many falls occur when an older person is reliant on a mobility aid such as a walking stick

INADEQUATE LIGHTING

Many older people are challenged by vision changes that occur due to the ageing process or a disease process, and inadequate lighting can contribute to a high falls risk. Poorly lit environments, including familiar ones, can make it difficult for a person to see hazards such as an upturned floor mat or a pair of shoes left in the hall. Dimly lit staircases, both indoor and outdoor, can challenge the person's perception of depth and space, causing them to overstep and fall. Good lighting is essential to minimise falls in both familiar and unfamiliar environments.

CLUTTER

Any clutter in walkways will increase the risk of falling or tripping. In the person's own home, clutter may consist of anything that obstructs a clear and safe walkway–for example: extension cords across the floor, piles of magazines, baskets of washing on the floor, and so on. In an RACF, walkways and corridors can become cluttered with equipment such as trolleys, hydraulic lifters and wheelchairs, especially during busy times of the day. Individuals' rooms can be cluttered with personal belongings, too.

While it is important to clear obstructed walkways and areas, you must always maintain the dignity of the older person. It is not acceptable to move a person's belongings out of your way or to tell an older person to clear up their home or room. The concept of home is essential to belonging and wellbeing, and older people can live the way they choose. Dignity of risk is important in this context. If the older person is aware that clutter can increase their risk of falling and still chooses to live in a cluttered environment, that is their choice. However, under workplace health and safety (WHS) laws and regulations, you have a responsibility to keep *yourself* safe in the workplace, as does the organisation you work for, so compromise may be the solution.

PRACTICE POINT

People can become very comfortable in their own environment, and they may not notice the potential hazards that can lead to a fall. It is good practice to quickly scan the environment for environmental hazards when you initially enter the person's home or room, and to politely minimise the risk of falling by removing or changing the hazard. Always ask permission before changing the environment in any way—for example, moving a cord that is lying across a doorway. Make it a habit to scan for hazards; it will become second nature in no time!

SUPPORTIVE EQUIPMENT AND CLINICAL DEVICES

The aged population often have at least one chronic disease or condition, and many people have more than one. These comorbidities require treatment and management strategies that may include the use of equipment and clinical devices. There may be some risk factors for falling attached to the use of equipment and devices that include tripping over tubing and incorrect use of the equipment.

Walking frames, wheeled walkers, canes and hydraulic lifters will place an older person at risk of falling if used incorrectly. If the person doesn't use their walking aid correctly or omits to use it for short distances, their risk of falling increases. Hydraulic lifters pose a risk of catastrophic falls, or falls with severe injuries and outcomes, when they are used incorrectly. Lifters have a weight limit to be used safely and care workers should ensure that they are using the correct lifter for the person's weight. The "sling" that supports the person during the transfer must also be the correct size for the weight of the person and be fitted correctly. A smaller person can slip through a sling if it's the wrong size or is fitted incorrectly. When the lifting device is at a standstill, the brakes must be placed on to prevent the lifter rolling away from the stationary person. Any worker who is expected to use hydraulic lifting devices must be trained to do so competently by the organisation they are employed by. This is an expectation under the *Work Health and Safety Act 2011* (Cth) (the WHS Act).

Urinary catheters and oxygen tubing are often used to treat chronic conditions, and therapy can occur in the home or in an RACF. Regardless of where the person resides, the risk of tripping over tubing is high. Catheter bags are attached to the catheter with tubing and can fall to the ground if care isn't taken or if the person has a cognitive impairment and doesn't recognise what the catheter is. Home oxygen also presents a high falls risk, as the oxygen tubing that is attached between the oxygen concentrator (the machine) and the person (the mask) is designed to allow the person to walk from room to room. Lots of tubing on the floor poses a high risk of falling. Older people who require long-term oxygen therapy can do so in their own home or in an RACF.

Any older person who is prescribed eyeglasses should be encouraged to keep them clean and to wear them. Part of the care worker's job is to ensure that the person has clean glasses, and that they wear them as prescribed. Of course, the person has the right to refuse to wear them; however, poor vision is a falls risk in older people.

Other environmental factors that increase the risk of falling include inappropriate footwear and clothing, pets, overgrown gardens, and anything else the person can trip or fall over. Footwear should fit correctly and snugly. Velcro straps are preferable to shoelaces. Wearing socks, floppy slippers, high heels and oversized shoes all increases the risk of slips, loss of balance and falls. Similarly, clothing that is too big can contribute to falls. Long pants, dressing gowns and dresses that sweep the ground can cause a trip and fall. When an older person trips, they will often over-correct in an attempt to regain their balance, which can cause them to fall, due to the physical factors that have been discussed earlier.

WORKPLACE SCENARIO

Working as a team to reduce the risk of falls

Rodney (78) has resided at The Havens for two years. He has many friends there, and he loves to read books and call the bingo numbers on Friday nights. Three days ago, he returned from a stay in hospital, where he had an operation to repair a hernia. Jae, a care worker at the facility, has noticed that, since Rodney's return, he is unsteady on his feet when he stands up and he grabs at chairs when walking around the dining area. When Jae asks him about this, he says he is fine and doesn't want to talk about it. He spends a lot of time in his room and says he doesn't want to attend bingo anymore. His daughter tells Jae when she visits that Rodney had a fall in the hospital and she is worried about him. Jae considers the indicators of Rodney's fall risk as age, fear of falling, social isolation, depression, and possible new medications or changes to medications. She talks to her supervisor about a formal assessment using a collaborative approach involving other health professionals and practitioners, as well as a validated falls risk assessment.

CHECK YOUR UNDERSTANDING

1. List four physical risk factors for falling among older people.
2. Why does impaired cognition increase the risk of falling?
3. Delirium increases the risk of falling. Why do older people experience delirium?
4. List three characteristics that explain how the fear of falling can increase the risk of falls.
5. List three environmental risk factors for falls in older people.

13.3 REPORTING RISK OF FALLS

13.3.1 Scope of practice

All health workers and health professionals have a scope of practice. The term "scope of practice" refers to the skills and knowledge a worker has and how that is applied in the workplace. Each position has its own scope of practice. For example, a registered nurse will have a different scope of practice than a doctor or a care worker.

Your scope of practice can be determined by your qualification, the policies and procedures of your organisation, and your job description. To work outside of your scope of practice can place the consumer at risk of harm and yourself at risk of litigation. If you are requested to perform a task that is outside your scope of practice, it is within your right to refuse and to ask for training or guidance.

Your scope of practice within recognising and reporting the falls risks of the older people you support will include having the skills and knowledge to identify when a person is at risk of falling. You are required to report your concerns to your supervisor or the RN, depending on where you work. It is you who may notice that the person is dizzy when they stand up, or that they seem to lose balance when they try to get dressed. These observations are invaluable and are the first step in developing and implementing a falls management plan.

It is the scope of practice of the team leader, the supervisor or the RN to act on your observations. It may not be within your scope of practice to make referrals for the person to other health professionals, to complete assessments with the person, to make clinical judgements about medications or to develop the falls management plan. Your organisation's policies and procedures and your job description will identify what you can and cannot do within your scope of practice at a particular workplace.

13.3.2 Legal and ethical considerations

Workplace compliance with legal and ethical frameworks exists to ensure people's safety and wellbeing. Within the role of care worker, there are several considerations to keep in mind when recognising and reporting the falls risk of an older person. These considerations include balancing dignity of risk and capacity with duty of care, understanding informed consent and supporting the rights of older people.

DIGNITY OF RISK, CAPACITY AND DUTY OF CARE

The term "dignity of risk" describes the absolute right of all people to take risk within the choices they make. To have choice is a basic human need that no one should be denied. We all have the right to take risks, and this is important for our sense of self-worth. Self-determination and empowerment are key elements of dignity of risk as they support the principle of independence. We take risks every day. Drivers take a risk when they use the roads, smokers take a risk when they smoke cigarettes, diabetics take a risk when they don't follow a diabetic diet, and so on. Older people may have lived experience, but they, too, take risks when they make decisions.

"Capacity" describes the ability of an individual to understand information and to make an informed decision based on that information. Capacity allows us to identify possible risks within our decision-making process. All individuals are deemed to have full capacity under the law, unless stated otherwise by a health professional based on medical and psychological assessment. People with dementia and other conditions that affect judgement and decision making may have an impaired capacity to make safe decisions. This doesn't mean that individuals with impaired capacity cannot make decisions about what they want. When we support an older person with impaired capacity to make decisions, it is essential that we balance their dignity of risk with our duty of care.

The term "duty of care" describes the care worker's legal obligation to do what is reasonably practicable to prevent foreseeable harm to those they provide support to. In other words, you have a legal responsibility to minimise risk of harm to the older people in your care. Older people with capacity to understand information have the right to make an informed decision that may or may not have elements of risk attached. Offering ways to minimise risk is an important part of your role and you have a duty of care to do so. For example, an older person with Huntington's disease may refuse to use medication and safety equipment to minimise their risk of falls. They may choose to walk unaided and to remain mobile as a quality-of-life decision. If the person has capacity to understand that their risk of having a catastrophic fall is extremely likely without these interventions, they have a right to refuse them. Workers can support the person by offering less intrusive safety measures, such as elbow and hip protectors, and by encouraging them to take rest breaks.

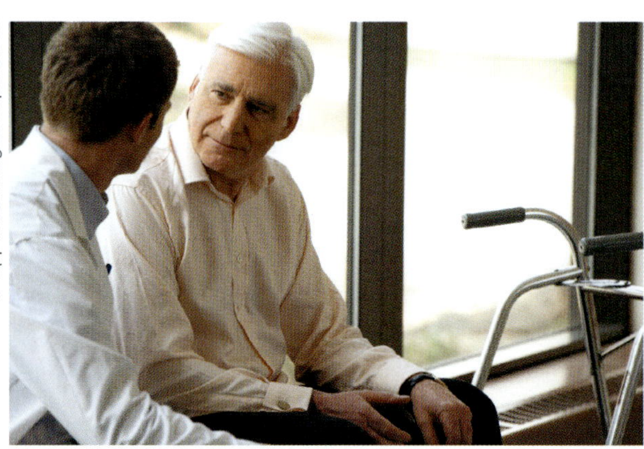

Offering ways to minimise risk is an important part of your role and you have a duty of care to do so

Older people with impaired capacity to understand information and to mitigate risks will require more support with decision-making processes. It is essential to involve the person as much as possible, as well as their substitute decision maker if they have one. For example, an individual with dementia may choose to leave their walking frame inside when they go outside. A worker can encourage the person to use the walker outside but cannot force them to. Risk of falling can be minimised by supervising the person when outdoors, by ensuring the environment is as safe as possible and by encouraging the person to wear suitable footwear when outdoors. This is balancing dignity of risk with duty of care.

You should always document any decisions the older person makes, regardless of their capacity, where there is risk attached. Documentation is essential to ensure that everyone involved in the support of the person understands the rights and responsibilities associated with the person's choices. In the event that a person in your care refuses to participate in a previously agreed strategy to minimise falls, you should report this verbally as soon as possible to the appropriate person within your organisation and document the event according to policy. This ensures that discussions around risk minimisation with the individual can occur in a timely manner with the appropriate health worker.

Workers have a legal obligation to minimise risk and to prevent possible harm; however, this should be balanced with supporting the decisions the person makes.

HUMAN RIGHTS

Human rights are entitlements that exist for all individuals regardless of age, ability, ethnicity, race or religion. Fundamental to human rights are the principles of dignity and respect. With regards to recognising falls risk and reporting falls, you uphold a person's rights by:

- reporting your observations and concerns about their falls risk
- providing information to them and their carers in a way that supports self-determination
- encouraging and proactively participating in a safe work environment
- supporting dignity of risk and upholding duty of care responsibilities
- following organisational policies and procedures
- recording and documenting fall-related information as per the organisation's protocols.

POLICIES AND PROCEDURES

All services and organisations have policies and procedures. Legislation (laws) can be specific to an industry, or some are shared over many industries. For example, the WHS Act is a law that tells businesses how to keep workplaces safe. Many organisational policies and procedures stem from this Act and may cover areas related to manual handling and falls management.

PRIVACY, CONFIDENTIALITY AND DISCLOSURE

All health workers are bound to work within the laws that govern privacy and confidentiality, and consumer privacy is paramount to a trusting and professional rapport between workers and the people they care for. These individuals and their families have the right to take legal action against an organisation and/or an individual worker if information about their health and other sensitive matters is shared without consent. Breaching privacy laws is a breach in duty of care, and all workers must recognise and implement all policies and procedures, confidentiality agreements and other documents that reflect the law.

Consent must be obtained before any health information can be shared. For example, if an individual is required to be referred to a physiotherapist for a falls prevention program, written consent should be obtained from the person before information is shared in the referral process.

WORK HEALTH AND SAFETY

To be able to recognise and report risks of falls, workers need to have a good understanding of WHS policies and procedures. Safety is key to minimising falls, and WHS knowledge will enable workers to identify hazards and risks associated with falls. Take opportunities to become involved in WHS matters within the workplace, such as joining the WHS committee or taking part in a safety inspection. Active participation will contribute to your skills and knowledge and ultimately benefit the people in your care. Recognising the risk of falls relies on your ability to identify hazards.

13.3.3 Completing documentation

Documentation within the aged care industry is not only a legal requirement; it is also an effective way to ensure the continuum of care for older people. Types of documentation that are relevant to recognising and reporting falls may include assessments and checklists, progress or case notes, referrals and incident report forms.

Any documentation must be written or typed in a legible manner and the content must be clear and concise. Documents that are used or created for the purpose of providing care for individuals may be used in a court of law for litigation or coronial purposes. It is essential that documentation contains facts, not your opinion. All documentation must be dated and signed.

Incident reports are documents that are used to record details of an incident where harm may or may not have occurred. They are considered legal documents and therefore must be completed correctly. As a care worker, you have a legal obligation to complete an incident report according to the policy of your workplace, and the information that you document must be concise and correct. If someone you provide support to has a fall, or almost has a fall, you must complete an incident form. It will contain critical details that can assist with the continuum of care for that person, as previously unidentified risks can come to light.

In accordance with privacy and confidentiality laws, all documentation must be stored in a safe environment. Paper-based documentation, such as client files, should be stored in a secure, locked area with limited access by staff. Client files must be immediately locked away when not in use, and not be left out on desks for people to access.

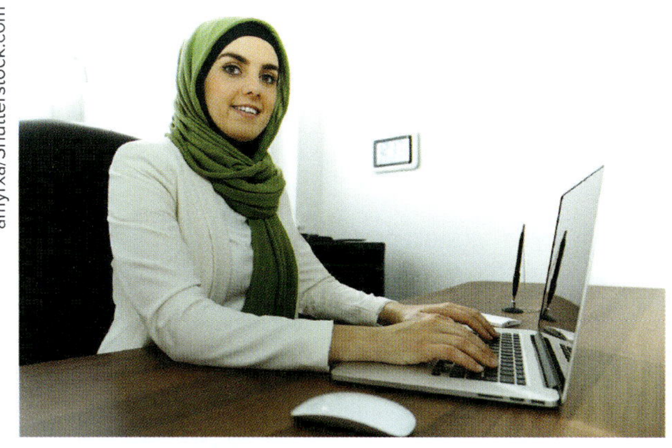

Incident reports are legal documents and must be completed correctly

Electronic documentation is securely saved or stored in cyberspace or on devices such as computers or external computer storage drives. Allocated passcodes act as an electronic signature for health-care workers. Don't share passcodes for documenting purposes, as you will be responsible for any breach of privacy under your passcode.

Always be factual and timely in completing documentation. In the event of a fall or near miss, timely documentation in the form of an incident form, case notes and handover reporting ensures that care support can be provided and assessment processes can be implemented to minimise falls for the older person.

13.3.4 Communication

Assessments that involve verbal communication will require a quiet place where the older person feels safe and comfortable to talk, at a mutually agreed time. It is important to reassure the person that any information they share with you for the purpose of the falls risk assessment will be managed according to the privacy policies of the organisation. Maintaining the privacy and confidentiality of the person's information is a legal requirement for all workers.

Opportunities must be provided for the person and their carer to clarify and ask questions throughout the meeting. Should you not know how to respond to a question, you will need to refer to your supervisor. For example, the person may ask you if they should use a walker. The person should be referred to a physiotherapist or an RN, who can assess and assist with the need for a mobility aid. You are not expected to have all the answers; some of these will come from a supervisor or nurse with a different scope of practice to yours. Reassure the person that you will ensure that the supervisor or nurse will contact them to answer their question.

Effective communication skills will support the assessment process. Non-verbal communication skills such as making appropriate eye contact, sitting with an open body posture, and using head nodding and relevant facial gestures will demonstrate to the person that you are genuinely interested in what they have to say. When using verbal communication, keep your voice at room volume and use your normal tone.

Of course, the older person may be hearing impaired, and you will need to adjust your volume accordingly. Good lighting will support communication with people who may have hearing or visual impairments. Don't use jargon or terminology that the person won't understand, as this will complicate the communication process unnecessarily.

There may be cultural considerations to recognise before communication can be effective. It is your responsibility to identify if you have the communication skills appropriate for the situation. In the event that you need an interpreter, your supervisor will support you to organise one. Be sure to talk to the older person, not to the interpreter. Family members can interpret; however, assessments for health purposes are best supported with an interpreter who doesn't know the person. This ensures the information they pass on is factual and alleviates the risk of it being intentionally or non-intentionally biased.

Remember that the questions you are asking are personal and require a sensitive approach. It is very important to show respect when having discussions with individuals and their carers. As individuals, we are our own experts–and older people are no different. Our aim is to empower, not to disempower. We can do this by providing valid information to assist decision making and by respecting the older person's rights to determine the outcomes for their own health and wellbeing. Any information that you provide must be approved by the health-care professional and supported by facts. It is not within the job role of the care worker to give advice, regardless of how well intentioned it may be.

When discussing falls with the older person and their carer, the use of inclusive language and open-ended questioning can support the person to contribute more to the discussion. Asking the person and carer for input also provides you with information you need to ensure the person's needs are identified. Open-ended questions may include, for example, "I can see that you are well and independent, but can you tell me the process you use to carry out the laundry?" or, "You have told me that you feel your risk of falling is higher at night because you need to use the bathroom more frequently. What do you find works well for you at the moment to prevent this from occurring?"

Providing opportunities for the person and their carer to have meaningful inclusion in all communications about their support demonstrates respect and reflects the person-centred approach in service delivery.

WORKPLACE SCENARIO

Balancing duty of care and dignity of risk

Lilly is 92 years old and still lives in her own home, independently. She loves to cook and makes amazing scones. She has home support to enable her to do her washing and to shower safely. Her daughter, Marion, visits on the weekend. Every Monday and Thursday, Lilly walks to the local community shopping centre as she has done for years. She uses a four-wheeled walker, and all the shop owners know her well. She makes scones for the butcher and the newsagent occasionally.

When Ro visits Lilly to help her do the laundry, he finds her upset. She tells him she had a fall on Thursday when she went to the shops and spent the night in the emergency department. Her daughter is furious with her, she says, and has banned her from walking to the shops ever again. Lilly tells Ro she would rather fall than be a prisoner in her own home. She asks Ro to have a chat with Marion and try to change her mind.

Ro understands that while he has a duty of care to prevent harm to Lilly, she also has the right to dignity of risk. She might have another fall if she continues her regular walks to the shops; however, if she cannot leave her house, she may become socially isolated and, possibly, depressed.

Ro explains to Lilly that she has the right to make her own decisions and that he can also understand her daughter's concern. He tells her he will ask his supervisor to organise a meeting with Lilly and Marion together to discuss the issue, if Lilly feels this will help. Lilly agrees this is a good idea.

CHECK YOUR UNDERSTANDING

1. What would your actions be if you were asked to do something that was outside your scope of practice?
2. Why is it important to complete an incident form when a person has a fall or near fall?
3. Explain why respectful communication processes are important when providing support for older people and their carers.
4. What is capacity, and why is it important?
5. What are four ways you can support the human rights of older people you care for?

SUMMARY

- Older people are more likely to suffer major injury or death from a fall due to several factors, including the ageing process, medical conditions, medication use and environmental influences.
- Recognising and reporting the risk of falls involves both informal and formal observations. Any concerns you have about a person's risk of falls must be reported to the RN or supervisor in a timely manner. Documentation of your observations can support the continuum of care for older people.
- Falls risk assessment is extremely important for the safety of the older person and contributes to the maintenance of independence and prevention of the loss of functional abilities. Falls and the fear of falling can limit an individual's capabilities and result in an increase in their dependence on others for activities of daily living and instrumental activities of daily living. Falls risk assessment is a collaborative approach that involves a multidisciplinary team.

REVIEW QUESTIONS

13.1 As a care worker, what do you need to be familiar with when considering falls prevention?

13.2 What are some common fears around falling among members of the older population?

13.3 **(a)** Define extrinsic factors associated with falls and provide an example to support your answer.

(b) Define intrinsic factors associated with falls and provide an example to support your answer.

13.4 Complete the table below, outlining how each product minimises falls risk.

Product	How does the product minimise falls risk?
Mobility aid	
Lifters	
Hip protectors	
Floor sensor mat	

BIBLIOGRAPHY

Australian Government, Department of Health, *National Aged Care Mandatory Quality Indicator Program Manual*, https://www.health.gov.au/resources/publications/national-aged-care-mandatory-quality-indicator-program-manual, accessed 29 August 2021.

Lystad, R.P., Cameron, C.P. & Mitchell, R.J., "Mortality risk among older Australians hospitalised with hip fracture: A population-based matched cohort study", *Archives of Osteoporosis* 12(1), 2017. DOI: 10.1007/s11657-017-0359-7.

ScienceDaily, "Hip fracture often deadly, study shows", *ScienceDaily*, 7 September 2017, www.sciencedaily.com/releases/2017/09/170907143003.htm.

World Health Organization (WHO), "Falls", https://www.who.int/news-room/fact-sheets/detail/falls, accessed 8 August 2021.

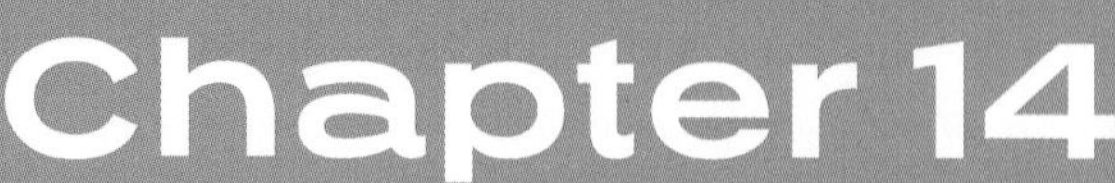

Chapter 14

Responding to signs of abuse and neglect

LEARNING OBJECTIVES

14.1 Identify abuse, neglect and exploitation

14.2 Support people experiencing abuse, neglect and exploitation

14.3 Prepare documentation

14.4 Manage the personal impact of support

INTRODUCTION

THE WORLD HEALTH ORGANIZATION (WHO) states that elder abuse is "a single or repeated act, or lack of appropriate action, occurring within any relationship where there is an expectation of trust, which causes harm or distress to an older person" (WHO 2021). The abuse of older people can occur within their own home or a community living environment, and in a residential aged care facility (RACF).

The perpetrator of the abuse is often an individual the older person relies on or trusts, such as their spouse, child, other family member or friend, and paid caregivers such as staff from aged care services.

The types of elder abuse include physical abuse, sexual abuse, psychological abuse, financial exploitation, emotional abuse and neglect. Abuse, neglect and exploitation can have serious outcomes for the older person's physical and psychological wellbeing. An important aspect of the care worker's role is to be able to recognise and report suspected, alleged or known incidents of abuse and to respond according to their organisation's policies and procedures.

INDUSTRY IN FOCUS

The incidence of abuse in aged care

It is difficult to state the extent of elder abuse in aged care because there are no available prevalence rates of this type of abuse in Australia. We can only estimate the rate at which older Australians experience abuse, using data from other countries around the world as a guide.

According to the WHO, a review of 52 studies from around the globe in 2017 estimated that one in six people aged over 60 years (living in the community) experienced some form of abuse. Also according to the WHO, another review of international studies on the abuse of older people in RACFs found that two in every three staff reported they had committed abuse within the previous year. Staff cited chronic staff shortages and poor time availability as the main reasons for the abuse occurring (WHO 2021).

Many incidents of elder abuse in aged care go unreported, either because older people who experience abuse choose not to disclose it or because staff are not confident of making a report. In 2020, the Office of the Royal Commission into Aged Care Quality and Safety (the Royal Commission) provided experimental estimates of elder abuse in aged care facilities in Australia, using data from a survey prepared by the National Ageing Research Institute. The estimates didn't include data for sexual, social and financial abuse; however, they did include data for physical abuse, neglect and emotional abuse. According to the Royal Commission, around 39.2 per cent of older Australians living in RACFs experience neglect, or physical or emotional abuse (Royal Commission into Aged Care Quality and Safety 2020).

For the purpose of understanding the potential prevalence of elder abuse in aged care in Australia, the prevalence of elder abuse in other countries around the world is considered. The Australian Institute of Family Studies claims that, based on the prevalence estimates of elder abuse in other countries, "between 2% and 14% of older Australians experience elder abuse in any given year, with the prevalence of neglect possibly higher" (Kaspiew, Carson & Rhoades 2016). While the data available provides estimates of elder abuse, it is important to recognise that, as stated above, many incidents are not reported at all.

People in Australia are living longer, with the proportion of older people in the Australian population expected to increase to between 21 and 23 per cent by the year 2066 (ABS 2018). The demand for aged care services will increase as the population ages, and hence it may be projected that the incidence of elder abuse will increase, too.

14.1 IDENTIFYING ABUSE, NEGLECT AND EXPLOITATION

14.1.1 Types of abuse, neglect and exploitation

EMOTIONAL ABUSE

Emotional abuse affects how a person feels about themselves and their life. When a person is emotionally abused, they can experience feelings of hopelessness and worthlessness and a sense of being devalued as an individual. The emotional abuse of an older person includes actions that are verbal and non-verbal and have the intent of damaging their self-esteem and changing the balance of power to the **perpetrator**'s benefit. Examples of emotional abuse include speaking to and acting in a condescending way towards the person, treating them in a derogatory manner and then in a positive way (causing them to be unsure of their worth to

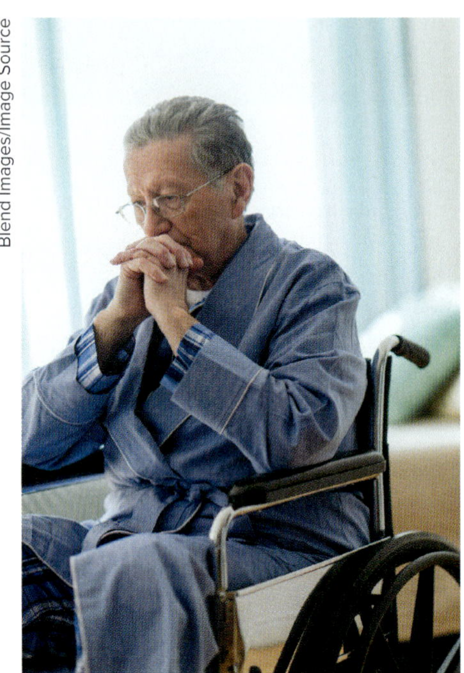
Blend Images/Image Source

Emotional abuse affects how a person feels about themselves

the abuser), harassment, belittlement, and the use of blackmail. Ongoing emotional abuse can lead to psychological abuse.

PSYCHOLOGICAL ABUSE

Psychological abuse can occur when an individual experiences ongoing, repetitive emotional abuse, and can lead to serious mental health conditions such as depression and post-traumatic stress disorder. The effects of psychological abuse lead a person to believe their abuser and to succumb to the abuse over time, as they come to believe they are worthless and don't deserve to enjoy a sense of purpose or to set goals for themselves. Victims of psychological abuse are at risk of becoming dependent on the abuser for many aspects of living, due to the control the abuser has over the person's ability to make decisions safely and effectively.

Examples of psychological abuse of older people include repetitive verbal and non-verbal actions that make the person feel insignificant and devalued as an individual in their own right. These actions may include excluding the person from activities or events that are meaningful to them, intimidation, the use of passive-aggressive language like that used in **gaslighting**, and threats of abandonment or isolation.

NEGLECT (DEPRIVATION)

Neglect occurs when an older person's basic and important needs are unmet by an individual or organisation that is responsible for meeting these needs. Neglect may also be referred to as deprivation, when needs such as medicines, food and fluids, personal hygiene, adequate living conditions and medical treatment are withheld for the older person. Neglect can be intentional or non-intentional. Intentional neglect occurs when the person responsible for the care of the older person knowingly withholds the basic needs of the older person; while non-intentional neglect occurs when the person responsible doesn't understand the level of care the older person requires, or they are physically or cognitively incapable of meeting the older person's needs.

Neglect occurs when a person, care worker or an organisation breaches the duty of care they have to the older person, and harm occurs to the older person as a result of the breach. An example of neglect in an RACF is the failure of care staff to report that an older person has had a fall, when they are required by their organisation's policies and procedures to make such a report. In the event the older person suffers harm as a result of the fall, such as a fractures, or even death, the care staff and the organisation may face litigation for neglect, based on breaching their duty of care to the older person. Neglect also occurs in the community, often by family or the person's carer. In severe cases, older people have been found with serious injuries such as fractures and maggot-infested wounds in both the community and within RACFs. Malnutrition can also be an indicator of neglect.

FINANCIAL ABUSE

Financial abuse occurs when the older person's money and property are obtained by another party (often a family member) through methods of coercion, deceit and/or physical abuse. Available literature suggests that financial abuse is one of the most common forms of elder abuse, and that it occurs across the aged care services industry in Australia and within the older population in the community who are not recipients of aged care services.

Financial abuse in aged care services includes efforts by staff to coerce the person to change their will, asking the person to buy items for them, using deceit and emotional abuse to convince the person to gift them an item (such as jewellery) and the direct stealing of the person's money or belongings. Older people who live in the community who don't receive aged care services can be financially abused by their carer or family; for example, the person may be held responsible for paying all of the household bills while the working adult children refuse to contribute. Older people may be forced or manipulated by family (often their adult children) to sell their property due to attitudes of entitlement of early inheritance; or they may have their pension taken from them or have their bank accounts fraudulently accessed by their **power of attorney**. Older people who are financially abused are often dependent on the perpetrator for support.

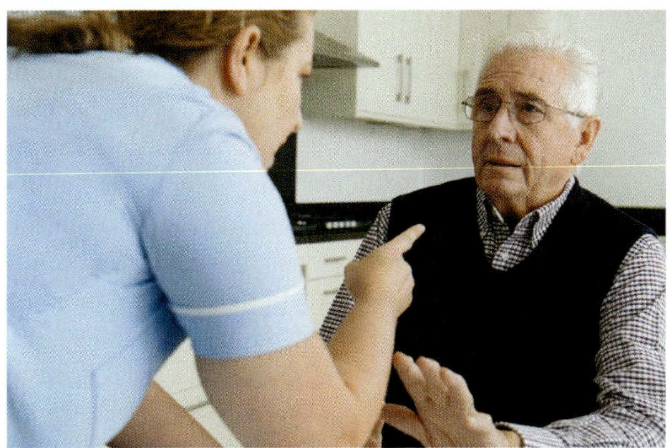

Ian Allenden/Alamy Stock Photo

Older people who experience abuse are often abused by a person in a position of trust such as aged care staff or a family member

PHYSICAL ABUSE

Physical abuse can be described as the actions inflicted by one person on another that cause them physical harm or suffering. Older people who experience physical abuse are often dependent on others for their activities of daily living (ADLs), and the abuser is most likely to be a person in a position of trust, such as a carer, family member or aged care services staff member.

Physical abuse includes harm caused to the older person as a result of physical contact such as hitting, punching, spitting, burning, kicking, scratching or pushing. It is important to note that physical abuse can also include the force-feeding of food, fluids and medications; threats of abuse; and inappropriate use of physical restraint, including isolation. Physical abuse commonly coexists with emotional or psychological abuse, as the older person is often threatened with more violence should they speak out.

SEXUAL ABUSE

Sexual abuse can be defined as abuse of a sexual nature, either explicit or implicit, that occurs without the person's consent or where the person lacks capacity to understand the intentions of the abuser. Examples of sexual abuse include sexual assault and touching the person inappropriately, showing them pornography without their consent, speaking in a sexual manner around them, taking intimate photographs of them, and discussing anything of a sexual nature with them. Sexual abuse commonly coexists with emotional or psychological abuse, and sometimes physical abuse, as the older person is often threatened with violence should they speak out.

GROOMING

Grooming describes a form of abuse that is a precursor to other forms of abuse, often sexual or financial. While it is most prevalent in the teen and child populations, grooming occurs in the older population, too. Grooming is a manipulative form of abuse that is based on a false relationship that develops between two people. The abuser will spend time building a relationship with the older person, developing a sense of trust, before gradually starting to isolate the person from their social support networks. This isolation from family and friends can leave the individual more vulnerable to the abuse that often occurs much later in the relationship.

It is important to remember that the person being groomed is unaware of the nefarious intentions of the groomer, who early in the relationship will give the older person extra attention, make them promises and give them special favours. These are all actions and behaviours that make the older person feel that the groomer is genuinely a nice person who looks out for them. In time, the groomer will start to ask for favours for themselves and this is the catalyst that starts the physical, sexual and financial abuse of the older person. An older person's wellbeing can be devastated by an abuser who uses grooming as a tool to get something they want.

UNDUE INFLUENCE

Undue influence is the legal term given to the incidence of a person obtaining benefit through deceit from within an existing relationship. When the balance of power isn't equal within a relationship, the person with the least power is vulnerable to **exploitation** by the other person. For example, an older mother who has three adult children may be convinced by one of them to change her will, in that child's favour, during a time when the mother is unwell. Undue influence can also be seen when someone close to the older person, such as a long-term neighbour, takes advantage of the person's diagnosis (such as dementia) and convinces the person to sell them their car for an excessively low price. Undue influence, similar to grooming, relies on trust within the relationship in order to manifestly breach that trust for the abuser's financial or sexual benefit. The outcomes of undue influence can be psychologically catastrophic for the older person and may include broken family relationships and depression.

SYSTEMIC ABUSE

Systemic abuse relates to the processes and procedures within aged care services that can have a negative impact on the wellbeing of older people who use the services. Models of service delivery have been undergoing transition from the institutionalised and medical models of care to more person-centred and rights-based approaches to care. This person-centred philosophy of care and support is still transforming today and is fuelled by the recommendations of the Royal Commission into Aged Care Quality and Safety. However, some practices and processes in service delivery for older people continue to be reminiscent of an institutionalised culture that can encroach on the rights and wellbeing of service users in a negative way. Staffing issues, time constraints, disproportionate funding and the task-focused model of care are all contributing factors to the "get the job done" culture in aged care, much to the frustration of workers in the industry.

Older people who receive government-funded care often have their services delivered in a time frame that doesn't support the person-centred approach. Many care recipients therefore have limited choice or input around their service provision, especially in RACFs where multiple people require intensive support. Choices that are limited include things such as the time of day when the person would prefer to have their shower and its duration, when and what they eat and with whom, and whether they share a room. The Aged Care Quality Standards (the Quality Standards) will ensure that the person-centred and rights-based approaches to care delivery will continue to improve, together with changes to staff ratios, staff training and skills mix.

14.1.2 Indications of abuse, neglect and exploitation

Understanding the types of abuse that can occur can facilitate understanding of the indicators of abuse, neglect and exploitation. Many older people won't disclose that they have been abused or are experiencing abuse. This may be because they are fearful of reprisal from the perpetrator or that they won't be believed, or they may have a cognitive disorder such as dementia and are unable to explain what has happened to them.

Specific observations about older people who have been abused, or are experiencing abuse, can provide valuable information that supports positive outcomes for the person and the prevention of further abuse. While some indicators of abuse are specific to the type of abuse, many indicators cover multiple types of abuse.

PHYSICAL INDICATORS OF ABUSE

Physical indicators of abuse include all observations that can be noticed about, or witnessed to be present on, the person who has been abused. Physical indicators are related to neglect and physical, sexual and psychological abuse. Physical indicators of abuse may involve the following unexplainable observations:

- scratches on the body–in particular, on the forearms (defensive injuries)
- bruising that is shaped oddly and is present on parts of the body that are usually hidden (such as the chest, upper and inner thighs, and back). Some bruises have patterns (such as those that

resemble grabbing marks of fingers around a person's wrist), and bruises change colour over time. Multiple bruises that are present and in various stages of healing (blue, black, pink, purple, green and yellow) can indicate repeated trauma to the skin over a period of time
- burns on the skin (cigarette and lighter burns) can be in different stages of healing if they are inflicted over a period of time
- unexplained fractures or joint issues (broken nose, fractured wrist, etc.)
- urinary tract infections that are unusual for the person
- bleeding or injury around the genitals or anus; blood-stained incontinence pads
- unexplained sexually transmitted infection (STI)
- newly broken or missing teeth
- changes to mobility
- new and undiagnosed pain
- unexplainable weight loss over a short period of time
- consistently poor hygiene.

BEHAVIOURAL AND EMOTIONAL INDICATORS OF ABUSE

All types of abuse create emotional pain and trauma for the person involved. Whether physical indicators of abuse are present or absent, the behavioural and emotional indictors of abuse can guide workers in the provision of safe support for the older person. It is important to note that behaviours that may indicate abuse are not necessarily the known behaviours of concern for which a person has support plans in place; rather, it may be a change in the person's "normal" behaviour that is indicative of abuse.

PRACTICE POINT

Remember that a sudden and new confusion is often associated with delirium, which is frequently a sign of infection, or other organic issues that the person may be experiencing. Always report your observations of sudden and new confusion in people to the registered nurse (RN) or supervisor, even if the person has dementia. In the context of abuse, delirium may indicate infection, pain, injury, or the trauma of abuse.

Some behavioural and emotional indicators of abuse include:

- mental distress
- sleep disturbances
- eating disturbances
- wanting to sleep with the light on
- shadowing staff, not wanting to be left alone
- new confusion
- withdrawal from activities and social engagements that are usually enjoyed
- fear around certain staff, family members or other people
- the person makes death statements, such as: "I won't be here much longer"
- attention-seeking behaviours, such as complaining excessively.

ENVIRONMENTAL INDICATORS OF ABUSE

Environmental indicators of abuse may identify that an older person has or is experiencing abuse. Community care workers will make observations about the older person's living environment that may require them to make a report to the organisation they work for, so that the potential risk of exploitation and neglect can be addressed within the realms of policy.

Environmental indicators of abuse in community care may include:

- overgrown gardens and weeds
- non-functioning or no smoke detectors
- little food in the home, or spoiled food, or food that is of little nutritional value
- unavailable medications or expired medications
- empty alcohol bottles
- drug paraphernalia in the home
- lack of electricity, heating and cooling, or refrigeration
- inappropriate bedding, or soiled bedding and furniture
- overloaded garbage
- unclean living conditions
- poor sanitary conditions
- home infestation of vermin or pests
- dangerous living conditions, such as broken glass, no ventilation around gas, rotting woodwork such as verandas and floorboards, exposed electrical wiring
- being forced to live in an external building on a property such as a shed, or a smaller room within the home, when family members move into the person's house.

Within an RACF, the environment is cleaned and modified by the provider; however, a person's environment is more than just their living space. Environmental indicators of abuse in RACFs may include:

- social isolation (the person refuses to interact with others for meals, outings, etc., or they may not want to see certain staff or family members)
- rushed practices, which may result from inadequate staff ratios
- resident-to-resident harassment and abuse (stalking, shadowing, intimidating)
- staff who are overly attentive to a person and overtly friendly
- deliberate and deceptive omission of tasks by staff (not changing soiled incontinence aids or bedlinen in a timely manner; not repositioning a person who cannot attend to their own pressure injury prevention; not feeding an entire meal to a person, etc.).

EXTERNAL INDICATORS OF ABUSE

External indictors of abuse are signs and signals that an older person is experiencing, or may experience, abuse. These indicators increase the vulnerability of an older person to abuse and are separate from the older person. The following are examples of external indicators:

- Carer stress. Fatigue, depression and carer burnout can lead to the carer feeling frustration and resentment towards the older person.
- The older person is a carer for someone who is cognitively or intellectually impaired who may physically or sexually abuse them.
- There is discord among family members.
- The person is dependent on someone who has a dependency on alcohol and/or other drugs.

- The person has lost their supportive social network (i.e. they are frequently absent from, or unable to attend, community events and social group activities).
- Family members restrict the person's decision making and speak for them even though they have capacity to decide and speak for themselves.

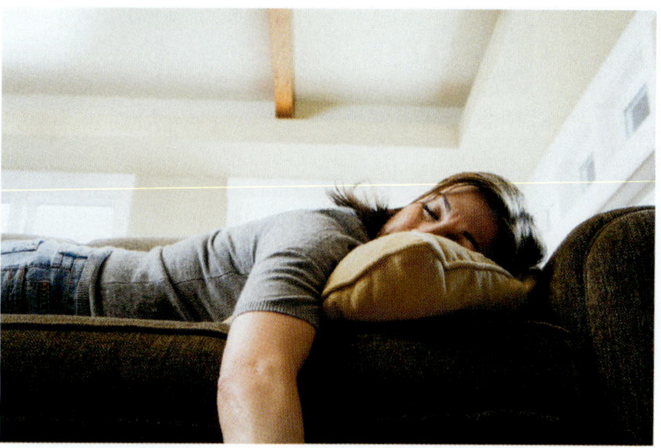
ColorBlind Images/Blend Images LLC

Carer burnout can lead to the carer feeling frustration and resentment towards the older person

The context of the indicators for abuse are important to understand in order to consider the outcomes for the older person. Care workers must report all observations about the people they support to the RN or their supervisor, regardless of the context. The abuse of older people is not always obvious and may be suspected or alleged. An older person who is an abuse victim may have one or more indicators to suggest the abuse occurred, while other older people may not have even a single indicator. In your role as a care worker, always report your observations about the person, or their situation, to the RN or supervisor. After reporting your observations, follow your organisation's policies and procedures for documenting your concerns about the person, remembering that not all indicators of abuse necessarily mean the person has been abused. Bruising and disturbed sleep may be present for other reasons, meaning that objective and thorough assessment is essential.

14.1.3 Risk factors for abuse, neglect and exploitation

Risk factors for the abuse, neglect and exploitation of older people exist within the community and within aged care services. Table 14.1 lists the elements that place older people at risk of abuse, both at home and within aged care services in Australia.

14.1.4 Consequences of abuse, neglect and exploitation

Older people experience life-changing consequences as a result of abuse, neglect and exploitation. Abuse affects their physical and psychological wellbeing and can lead to financial ruin, homelessness and social deprivation. *Devaluation* is the term used to describe the underestimation of the value or importance of something or someone. In society, older people are often viewed as:

- non-contributors to society
- potential victims of crime
- incapable of learning
- asexual
- too old to work
- incapable of driving
- always sick
- a burden on the health system
- unable to use technology.

These myths about older people are ageist. *Ageism* is discrimination against a person based on their numerical age and is perpetuated through the representation of older people in the media.

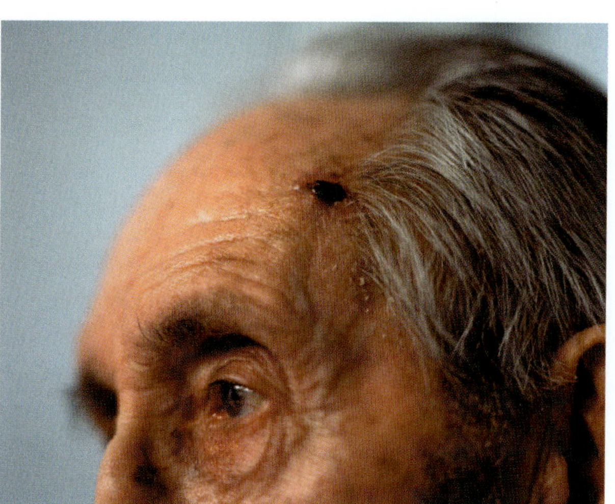
Image Source/Getty Images

Victims of abuse are more likely to experience depression

TABLE 14.1 Risk factors for abuse, neglect and exploitation

Risk factor	Explanation
Functional dependence	The ongoing and sometimes intensive care support of older people who are dependent on others such as care staff or family carers for their ADLs can lead to carer stress and frustration. Functional dependence also increases abuse by a perpetrator with nefarious intentions, as often the older person cannot physically defend themselves from the abuse.
Financial dependence	Older people who are reliant on others for financial support are at risk of abuse. Threats of financial separation or financial deprivation are components of psychological abuse and neglect.
Geographical isolation	Older people who live in a remote or rural location have little support to access help. Geographical isolation increases the vulnerability of the person as they are reliant on the abuser for support such as transport, access to shops and appointments, etc.
Social isolation	An older person can be socially isolated within their family, the community and an RACF. Reasons for social isolation include illness, dysfunctional relationships, diversity and culture. The lack of a social network increases the risk of harm to older people, as information about the person's rights and available support is more difficult to access.
Ethnic and cultural practices	Some cultural practices may view abuse as acceptable or necessary. Available support may not be appropriate for the person's culture. The subject of abuse may be taboo for some cultures.
Language barrier	The person cannot ask for help or understand how to access help. The person may not have information about their rights.
Gender	While both older males and females experience abuse, elderly women are more likely to experience physical and sexual abuse.
Dysfunctional relationships	Family history of dysfunction: the older person may live with the person who abuses them, often a son or daughter or grandchild.
Cognitive/intellectual impairment	Older people with dementia or intellectual disability are more likely to experience physical and sexual abuse, as they cannot report their experience to anyone. These people may be financially exploited because of their poor judgement and decision making.
Physical disability or impairment/frailty	Older people who have poor physical health have an increased risk of being victimised as they often don't have the physical capacity to fight back or escape the perpetrator. Poor physical health may increase the older person's dependence on others to meet their needs (functional dependence).

Stereotypical attitudes of society about the older population play a role in the relationship between abuse and devaluation. Devaluation can facilitate the abuse of older people through justification; for example, a family member may take money from the older person's bank account and justify their action as follows: "Mum's 76 years old. She doesn't need that much money."

Mental health can be seriously affected by abuse, neglect and exploitation, and can result in the degradation of the older person's sense of purpose and wellbeing. The older person may experience feelings of fear, guilt, shame, worthlessness and uselessness as a result of abuse.

Victims of abuse are more likely to experience psychological injury or anxiety disorders such as post-traumatic stress disorder and depression. It is important to note that depression is often undiagnosed in the older population and that older people in Australia have a statistically higher risk of suicide (Australian Institute of Health and Welfare 2022).

Physical injuries that result from abuse are more likely to be serious, with disabling outcomes for older people based on the ageing process and the presence of chronic health conditions. Premature admission into an RACF is a consequence of abuse, neglect and exploitation for some older people.

WORKPLACE SCENARIO

Assessing and acting on risk of abuse

Gabe works in a dementia-specific cottage within an RACF where he knows all the residents quite well. The past couple of weeks have been difficult, due to staff shortages, and the organisation has had to rely on staff from nursing agencies to fill the gaps in the roster.

On one evening shift, Gabe notices that a male care worker he hasn't seen before is speaking inappropriately to the older women in the cottage—in particular, to Susie, who has moderate dementia. He is complimenting Susie on her clothing and her figure. When Gabe approaches the worker and asks him to stop, the worker says he is just having fun and making "the old girl feel good".

Later that evening, Gabe hears Susie screaming for help. When he goes to her room, he finds she is clutching her unbuttoned blouse and shouting, "Don't touch me! Don't touch me!" The male care worker is also in the room and says, "I was just trying to get her into her nightgown."

Gabe asks the worker to leave the room and then sits with Susie until she feels calm enough to have a cup of tea. He has never known her to scream like that and she is usually very cooperative with her personal care. Gabe feels something isn't right about the way the care worker has behaved and he contacts the RN to discuss reporting his suspicions that Susie has been abused.

CHECK YOUR UNDERSTANDING

1. What are the six types of elder abuse?
2. What is neglect?
3. List five behavioural or emotional indicators of abuse.
4. List five physical indicators of abuse.
5. Why is someone with impaired cognition at risk of abuse?

14.2 SUPPORTING PEOPLE EXPERIENCING ABUSE, NEGLECT AND EXPLOITATION

14.2.1 Legislation and regulatory requirements

REGULATORY REQUIREMENTS

All aged care service providers have legal obligations to report known, alleged or suspected incidents of elder abuse, in alignment with industry regulation. However, in Australia responses to elder abuse can be complicated by the laws and policy frameworks that exists across the Commonwealth, state and territory levels.

Within the aged care services sector, certain types of abuse come under criminal laws, such as domestic violence and assault (common assault, assault occasioning bodily harm, unlawful wounding, grievous bodily harm, and sexual assault). Physical injury or contact doesn't need to be evident for the charge of assault to occur. Incidents of elder abuse where illicit drugs or weapons are involved may sit under the jurisdiction of criminal law. Some instances of abuse may involve physical or psychological crisis and require immediate intervention by emergency services such as police and paramedics.

The *Aged Care Act 1997* is supported by various principles that enable aged care providers (organisations that receive government funding) to meet their regulatory requirements, including supporting the rights of older people. Aged care services are aware of their reporting and legal obligations under the quality framework that is managed by the Aged Care Quality and Safety Commission (the Commission). The Quality Standards and the Charter of Resident Rights advocate for the rights of older people and the timely reporting of allegations of elder abuse as part of the compliance framework of the aged care services sector.

DUTY OF CARE

All workers within the aged care services sector have a duty of care to report suspicions or allegations of abuse to their workplace management, regardless of their job description. Reporting is a mandatory requirement in RACFs.

The term *duty of care* refers to the worker's legal obligation to do what is reasonable to prevent foreseeable harm to those they provide support to. A breach of duty of care, through actions or inaction, can cause harm to the older person. A care worker, and/or the organisation they represent, may face litigation for neglect if they wilfully breach their duty of care and cause harm as a result.

An example of breaching your duty of care is when an older person you support discloses to you that they have been abused by another staff member and you don't report it. Your duty of care is to ensure the older person is supported in their disclosure through the reporting process and, by doing so, to prevent further abuse. It is not your role to determine if the older person is telling the truth or not. Withholding disclosures of abuse is not only breaching duty of care; it is also putting the older person at risk of further harm.

14.2.2 Ethics and human rights

At the core of all elder abuse is the infringement of the person's human rights. Older people have the right to feel safe and not be exploited by others. The Universal Declaration of Human Rights, the United Nations Principles for Older Persons and the Charter of Resident Rights all support the rights of older people to live a life free from exploitation regardless of where they live.

Aged care services have a responsibility to the people using their services, and one of those responsibilities is to ensure that those people's rights are upheld. The Aged Care Quality Standards, which regulate government-funded aged care services (providers), also promote the rights of the individual receiving services and require organisations to demonstrate how the Standards are implemented. This includes how elder abuse is identified and responded to within the organisation.

Above all, care workers must work legally and ethically. The code of conduct that guides how all care workers are expected to practise ensures they understand what working ethically means. In the context of the abuse of older people, working ethically means the following:

- Report and document all suspicions or allegations of abuse according to workplace procedures.
- Maintain the confidentiality of the suspected or alleged incident of abuse.
- Make reports about abuse in good faith.
- Don't participate in gossip within the organisation about the incident. This is breaching privacy and confidentiality obligations.
- Document relevant information about the incident in a timely manner.

- Don't discuss incidents related to abuse with the media.
- Advocate for the rights of older people within your care.
- Follow your organisation's policy regarding consent.

When older people are unable to exercise their rights, they are vulnerable to exploitation and poor mental health. Many older people, especially those who have dementia, are not aware of their rights and part of the care worker's role is to protect and advocate for the rights of those they care for. Older people who have their rights breached can experience feelings of worthlessness and depression, and a sense of being devalued.

14.2.3 Mandatory reporting

In all aged care services, reporting abuse is mandatory. Mandatory reporting means that workers must report abuse, according to the law. In the context of aged care, mandatory reporting of abuse involves older people, but separate policies may also involve the mandatory reporting of the suspected or alleged abuse of children.

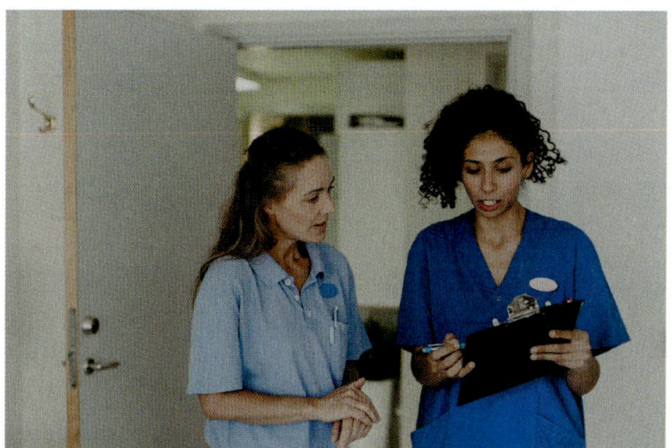

Maskot/Alamy Stock Photo

Reporting abuse is mandatory under the SIRS

In 2021, the Commission introduced the Serious Incident Response Scheme (SIRS) to encompass a broad reporting mechanism for alleged abuse of older people living in RACFs, with the aim of increasing awareness of elder abuse and preventing incidents of abuse. Under the SIRS, all RACFs (providers) are required to have an incident management system in place for the purpose of identifying, recording and preventing serious incidents. Providers must have evidence of the measures that have been implemented as a result of an incident.

According to the Aged Care Quality and Safety Commission (2021, p. 20):

> *Under section 54-3 of the Aged Care Act, a reportable incident is any of the following incidents that have occurred, are alleged to have occurred, or are suspected of having occurred to a residential care recipient (consumer), in connection with the provision of residential care, or flexible care provided in a residential setting:*
>
> - *unreasonable use of force against a consumer*
> - *unlawful sexual contact or inappropriate sexual conduct inflicted on a consumer*
> - *psychological or emotional abuse of a consumer*
> - *unexpected death of a consumer*
> - *stealing from, or financial coercion of, a consumer by a staff member of the provider*
> - *neglect of a consumer*
> - *use of a restrictive practice in relation to a consumer (other than in the circumstances set out in the Quality of Care Principles)*
> - *unexplained absence of a consumer from the service.*

It is mandatory for these incidents to be reported to the Commission. The process for making a report about any of the reportable incidents will be clearly documented in an RACF's policies and procedures, and reporting processes are also included in staff education.

PRACTICE POINT

You may be required to make a disclosure to your organisation about your suspicions of abuse against an older person. Under the SIRS, care staff and other workers who make a report in good faith are protected from civil and criminal liability that may arise from the disclosure. The law also provides protections for workers against potential litigations of defamation.

The SIRS initiative is a Commonwealth scheme that holds aged care providers accountable for preventing and managing a broader context of reportable incidents than previous mandatory reporting mechanisms. The SIRS takes a quality and regulatory approach to the management of incidents within RACFs and is due to be extended to in-home aged care services in late 2022. More information about the Serious Incident Response Scheme can be found at the Aged Care Quality website: www.agedcarequality.gov.au.

There are no mandatory reporting mechanisms for elder abuse in New South Wales and other states and territories, until the Commonwealth government incorporates SIRS into the community aged care sector. Current reporting processes within community aged care remain, while the reporting of the suspected or alleged abuse of older people who receive aged care services in their home will vary according to the legislation of the states and territories. In New South Wales, in-home aged care services have policies and procedures in place that assist care workers to identify and respond to suspected or alleged abuse of older people. These policies and procedures are written in alignment with the NSW Interagency Policy and the NSW Elder Abuse Toolkit. These two important documents provide guidance for organisations that provide in-home aged care services on how staff can identify and respond to abuse appropriately and safely. The NSW Elder Abuse Toolkit uses a five-step approach for identifying and responding to abuse:

Step 1: Identify abuse (suspected, witnessed or disclosed).

Step 2: Assess immediate safety.

Step 3: Provide support.

Step 4: Inform manager and document.

Step 5: Respond and refer.

The toolkit provides detailed information on each step to assist in policy development for organisations and to inform care workers. See https://www.ageingdisabilitycommission.nsw.gov.au/tools-and-resources.

14.2.4 Consent, privacy, confidentiality and disclosure

In the context of responding to suspected or alleged abuse of the older person, workers will need to ensure they have permission from the older person to do so. Consent must always be informed and be given freely without coercion. Information given to the person must be accurate and relevant to assist them in decision making around consent. The type of information and consent required will depend on the scope of practice of the worker.

The person must have the cognitive capacity to be able to process information and understand the potential consequences of giving consent. Some older people who have a cognitive impairment (such as dementia) will require a substitute decision maker to provide consent.

Care workers will be required to request consent as part of the process for supporting an older person who has experienced, or may be experiencing, abuse. The request for consent may include permission to report the incident; to share information about the incident to relevant health professionals; to provide information to the person about services that can provide them with further support and assistance; and to organise an appointment with said services on behalf of the older person.

Consent is not required in an emergency situation. Emergency situations may involve actual or imminent threat of harm to the person or others, such as when weapons are present or the person has harmed, or is threatening to harm, themselves or others (the older person or the alleged perpetrator). In the case of an emergency, the only actions are to keep yourself as safe as possible and to call emergency services in the first instance on 000. Workers may disclose information about the person and the incident to police and emergency services without consent.

Privacy and confidentiality laws ensure that all workers have a legal obligation not to share sensitive or personal information about the older people they provide support to. Workers must not share information about the incident involving the older person that is outside the scope of their organisation's policies and procedures, especially those related to the privacy and confidentiality of service users. Information about the suspected or alleged abuse of the older person is highly sensitive and is occasionally part of a criminal investigation. Sensitive information can only be shared with the informed consent of the older person or their substitute decision maker, unless the information is required under mandatory reporting obligations or is requested by a police officer or a subpoena under a court of law.

When abuse is suspected or alleged, the older person may not want to discuss it. Some older people who experience abuse may choose not to disclose the incident, for many reasons. It is important that the older person is supported to make informed decisions about the course of action they prefer to take in the context of reporting their experience. Table 14.2 illustrates some common barriers to disclosure.

TABLE 14.2 Common barriers to disclosure among older people who have experienced abuse

Barrier to disclosure	Explanation
Fear of reprisal	The person may be frightened that the perpetrator will punish them for disclosing. They may fear the perpetrator will harm them, their loved ones or their pets in retaliation.
Fear of being placed into a residential aged care facility	The older person may be fearful of losing their home or their independence.
Dependence	The older person relies on the perpetrator for daily living needs, so will be reluctant to disclose.
Legal implications for the perpetrator	The person may be worried that disclosure will affect the perpetrator legally and criminally.
Internal barriers	The person may have feelings of guilt or shame.
Cultural barriers	Disclosure of abuse may be taboo in some cultures; the person may be shamed by their community.

Ultimately, older people have the right to disclose and the right to choose not to disclose. All individuals have the right to make their own decisions, even if there are elements of risk attached to those decisions. Informed decision making allows people to weigh up the outcomes of the decisions they make. When abuse is suspected, alleged or known to have occurred to an older person, workers can provide them with information about disclosure, including the available options for support. The person is free to exercise their right to refuse the information, and the care worker should document and report this refusal.

Older people who have altered capacity may have difficulty in disclosing abuse. The person's substitute decision maker may be offered the information about processes for disclosure (if they are not suspected as the perpetrator) and the available support services. Care workers have a duty of care to report any concerns about the older people they care for in the context of suspected abuse, even within the older person's own home by their own family.

People who have disclosed that they have been abused, or are being abused, also have the right to retract their disclosure. This may occur for many reasons, not dissimilar to the reasons people don't disclose at all. It may be difficult to understand why an older person retracts their disclosure of abuse; however, a care worker's role is to respect the person's choice (dignity of risk), to keep the lines of communication open between the older person and the organisation, and to report and document their concerns.

14.2.5 Organisational policies and procedures

Policies and procedures are legal requirements that explain to workers what needs to be done and how it is to be done. In the context of recognising and responding to abuse, workplace policies and procedures provide staff with the actions they are required to take if abuse is suspected, alleged or known.

As noted previously, the process for reporting abuse within in-home aged care services will change in late 2022 when the sector joins residential aged care services in using the SIRS. This process will be influenced by the outcomes of the consultation sessions that occurred in 2021 between the government and the industry. Until then, policies and procedures in community aged care services will provide information to workers about recognising and identifying abuse, reporting abuse, escalating an incident to other services and referral to other services. Updated information regarding the transition of SIRS into in-home care services can be found at https://www.health.gov.au/initiatives-and-programs/serious-incident-response-scheme-sirs.

Policies about privacy and confidentiality, disclosure and documentation will be evident across all types of aged care services. Care workers can access information from policies and procedures that can help them to understand the processes and systems for managing suspected abuse, and how to access additional support for making a report. Remember: as a care worker, you have access to other staff members that include health professionals. The type of support you can provide to an older person may be limited by your scope of practice, and relevant policies and procedures will stipulate the roles, responsibilities and actions of different members of the multidisciplinary team.

14.2.6 Responding to and supporting the person

Recognising when an older person has been abused, or may be experiencing abuse, is the first step in facilitating support for them. How workers respond to and support the person is important in creating an environment in which the person feels protected, safe and believed. Acknowledgement of the impacts of the experience on the older person can have a positive influence on their physical and psychological healing processes in the long term.

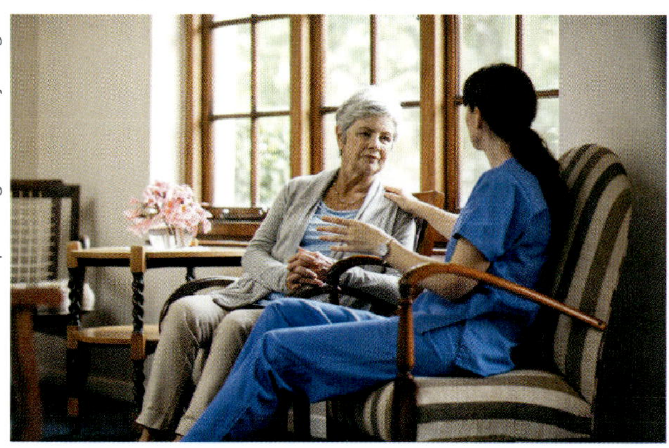

shapecharge/E+/Getty Images

Acknowledging the impacts of abuse on the older person can have a positive influence on their healing processes in the long term

It is essential to understand as much as you can about the person and their circumstances, and this information can be found in their individual care plan. The plan can provide important information that can assist the care worker to respond appropriately to the incident, including information about the older person's capacity, their usual behaviour and their communication needs. The plan provides a baseline of information that can assist the care worker to identify if anything is different about the person.

When responding to an allegation of abuse, it is important to ensure the person's immediate safety (as long as your own safety isn't jeopardised). Determine how urgent the situation is with regards to any help the person needs in that moment and seek support from others such as the RN or supervisor. If the situation is an emergency, call 000 immediately for emergency services. Don't touch any potential evidence such as clothing, cups, waste bins or used incontinence pads. If the abuse was physical or sexual in nature, encourage the person not to shower until advised to do so. Forensic evidence may be required from the person.

Provide reassurance and show empathy to the person when they speak to you and let them speak without interruption. Their account of the incident is important. Document it according to your organisation's policy. Explain the internal reporting process to the person and reassure them that they will be supported by management, staff and, possibly, external services throughout the process.

It is helpful to discuss with the person what the course of action should be, and it is essential to obtain their consent to move forward. Always report to the RN or supervisor (or other designated person) whether consent is granted or denied and ensure this is documented. Encourage the person to ask questions and seek clarification if you don't have the answer. Always acknowledge what the person is saying and validate what they are feeling.

PRACTICE POINT

The process for recognising and responding to abuse will be specific to the aged care service you work in. Government-funded RACFs report suspicions of abuse, neglect and exploitation according to the SIRS, while at the time of writing in-home aged care services report suspicions of abuse, neglect and exploitation according to organisational policies and procedures.

14.2.7 Additional support and assistance

Incidents of suspected or alleged abuse may require additional support and assistance from services that are external to the organisation you work for. It may, or may not, be in your scope of practice to provide information to the older person about services that can help them when an incident of abuse has occurred. Sometimes it can take the person a long time to want to access help. An aged care organisation should have information readily available to give to the older person that explains what the services are and how they can provide support. Workers may be required to make a referral to a service on behalf of the older person; however, consent must be obtained from the person, or their substitute decision maker, prior to referrals being made.

Additional support and assistance for the person may include services such as:

- the police
- emergency services
- domestic violence support
- sexual assault services
- counselling and psychology
- financial services
- other government services such as Centrelink
- housing
- advocacy services.

If the person refuses to engage with other services at the time of disclosure, information about the services, such as contact numbers and brochures, can be left with them, if it is safe to do so. In-home services can follow up and monitor the person's situation as services continue; however, the older person has the right to refuse any interventions or support regarding their experience.

WORKPLACE SCENARIO

Responding to allegations of abuse

Maeve is a care worker who provides personal care support to Jill, an older woman with multiple sclerosis. Jill lives in her own home with the support of Maeve's organisation, which assists with showering and house cleaning. Today, when Maeve arrives at Jill's house, she notices that Jill's son Rod is visiting. She hears him yell at his mother: "I'm telling you to sign it now!"

Maeve knocks on the door, which Rod answers. He is smiling and welcoming, but when Maeve enters the house she can see that Jill is shaken and upset. She asks her: "Are you okay, Jill?"

Rod replies: "She's just fine. Aren't you, Mum?" He then leaves the house, telling his mother he will return the next day.

During her shower, Jill tells Maeve that Rod wants her to sell her home because she will need to go into a nursing home at some stage. Jill says she doesn't want to leave her home. She asks Maeve what she should do. She doesn't feel safe around her son, she says, because he told her he could kill her in her sleep "and no one would know".

Maeve obtains Jill's consent to tell her supervisor of Jill's fears. The supervisor, on Jill's behalf and with her permission, refers the incident to the police. Maeve provides reassurance and empathy to Jill and ensures that she isn't left alone while waiting for the police to arrive.

CHECK YOUR UNDERSTANDING

1. What might happen if duty of care is breached in the context of abuse?
2. List four ways you can work ethically with regards to recognising and responding to abuse of older people.
3. What is the SIRS?
4. List three barriers to disclosure for older people who have experienced abuse.
5. What are three types of additional services that may be involved with the suspected or alleged abuse of an older person?

14.3 PREPARING DOCUMENTATION

Documentation is an essential component of all services that are provided to older people because it creates a record of important information about a person. Documenting information means to write it down, either on paper or digitally. All information that is documented about a person's health and other sensitive matters is protected by Australia's privacy laws, and care workers have a legal obligation to maintain the privacy and confidentiality of the person's information.

The type of information that is documented about the older person who receives aged care services will be expansive and occurs in many contexts. In the setting of reporting the suspected, alleged or known abuse of an older person, documentation requirements are essential and are specific to the type of aged care service.

14.3.1 Legal requirements: The Serious Incident Response Scheme

Reports (sometimes called notifications) of suspected or alleged abuse of older people who reside in RACFs are made using the SIRS. Reports are made electronically, via a portal that is used by approved providers (facilities that are government funded) called the My Aged Care service provider portal. Within the portal, the staff member will use the approved form to make the report of suspected, alleged or known abuse. It is mandatory to answer all questions contained in the form unless otherwise stated. The form requests information about the following:

- *SIRS portal user details:* information about the aged care facility and the person making the report.
- *Incident details:* information that is specific to the incident being reported, such as time; date; if death occurred as a result; the type of incident; and a detailed description of the incident and the people involved.
- *People involved:* information about the victim and the alleged offender.
- *Unexplained absence:* information is requested if the older person is missing from the facility.
- *Police:* information is requested about the details of police contact, if relevant.

All RACFs are required to have an incident management system (IMS) in place to support the prevention, management and notification of incidents that involve older people who receive care services. Apart from the reporting method used in the My Aged Care portal, the Commission requires facilities to document all incidents, whether they are reportable or not, as part of the IMS. Incident forms used internally as part of the organisation's IMS must be made available to the Commission on request and be kept for a minimum of seven years.

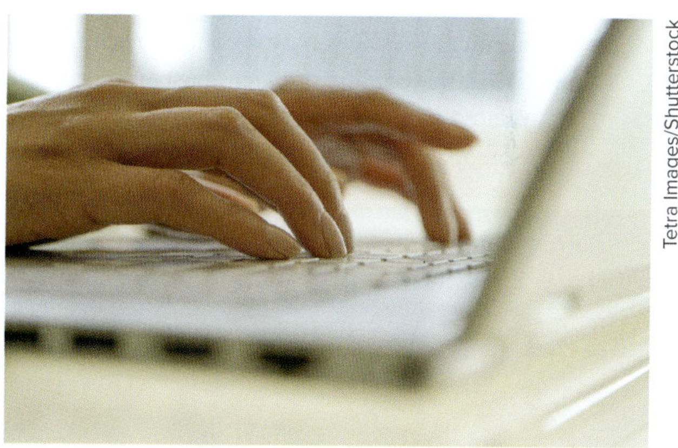

Tetra Images/Shutterstock

Reports of suspected or alleged abuse are made electronically, via the My Aged Care service provider portal

14.3.2 Organisational policies and procedures

All documentation must comply with the policies and procedures of the organisation, as they have been developed in alignment with legislation. This includes storing the person's information in a way that protects their privacy and confidentiality. The use of electronic passcodes can minimise the exposure of personal and sensitive information due to the limited access to records. Paper-based records are required to be locked in a safe place when not in use, such as a file room or lockable cabinet.

The following are some important principles of documentation and reporting:

- Document clearly and concisely.
- Be objective and state the facts. (Don't document your assumptions.)
- Always sign and date your documentation.
- Use quotation marks to document what the person said, if relevant.
- Document your observations–for example: "Alice started to moan like she was in pain."
- If documenting with a paper-based system, don't use white-out. Place a single line through the error and initial it.
- Document in a timely manner.

Many organisations will have a dedicated role for making reports about suspected, alleged or known incidents of abuse of older people. It is important to be aware of who undertakes this role in your organisation, and of what the process is for making a report in the organisation.

PRACTICE POINT

All documentation is classified as legal and can be used in a court of law. In the context of reporting suspected or alleged abuse, document honestly and factually. While your opinions and feelings are important, any documentation should only include the facts of the incident. Seek support from your manager if you need assistance with documentation.

14.3.3 Improving practice

Care workers have obligations to work legally and ethically. Implementing a duty of care and working with the policies and procedures of the workplace can ensure a safe and productive work environment. The continuous improvement of workplace practices and processes can facilitate positive changes in the way things are done. Continuous improvement is also known as quality improvement, and all government-funded aged care services have a continuous improvement plan.

In the context of elder abuse, the principles of open disclosure can assist in the prevention of incidents related to abuse and the prevention of repeated incidents of abuse. Open disclosure means the organisation accepts responsibility for the incident and works with the person and their family to make things right. Open disclosure facilitates transparent communication about areas of practice that have caused harm to the people who use the service and applies to all aspects of service delivery.

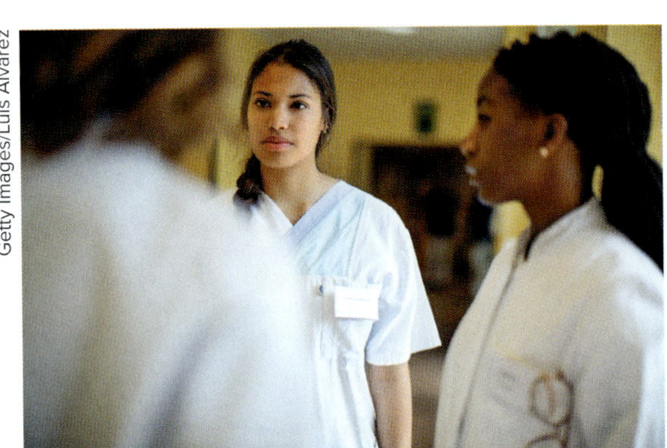

Getty Images/Luis Alvarez

The continuous improvement of workplace practices can facilitate positive changes in the way things are done

Care workers can participate in improving the practices of the workplace in the context of abuse by:

- attending education and training about the reporting process
- being a role model in working ethically and legally
- providing input aimed at changing the systems of the workplace through involvement in workplace meetings, committees and awareness activities
- proactively participating in and sharing public awareness campaigns for elder abuse and relevant services.

WORKPLACE SCENARIO

Contributing to improved practice

Moses works for a community care organisation. He recently attended an external education session about elder abuse and was shocked by what he heard. He realised that most of his colleagues probably didn't know much about it either. What concerned him the most was the fact that even though his organisation was a positive and caring workplace, it didn't have any information to offer older people who might be experiencing abuse.

At his organisation's next team meeting, Moses offered to collate some information about services that can help if an older person needs support regarding abuse. Another worker suggested they develop an information pack that can be left with anyone wanting more information about their options. By the end of the meeting, Moses and four other staff members had moved to create an Abuse Support Committee for their organisation.

CHECK YOUR UNDERSTANDING

1. What is the name of the system that all government-funded RACFs must have for recording incidents?
2. What is the name of the digital platform used under the SIRS to make a report?
3. In the context of documentation, how can the care worker ensure a person's privacy and confidentiality?
4. List three principles of documentation and reporting.
5. What is one way a care worker can contribute to the process of improving systems and procedures in the context of abuse?

14.4 MANAGING THE PERSONAL IMPACT OF SUPPORT

14.4.1 The impact of recognising and responding to abuse

The impact of recognising and responding to abuse can affect the care worker in a negative way. Workers who respond to the suspected, alleged or known abuse of an older person they support may experience distress, trauma and feelings of frustration. Workers can experience physical, mental and emotional impacts of recognising and responding to abuse. Poor worker mental health can result from impaired sleep, stress, anxiety and worry.

Care workers are often the first to become aware of incidents of abuse to older people and are often left wondering if they could have done more to prevent the person's experience. While all workers have a duty of care to do everything practicable to prevent foreseeable harm to older people receiving care, it is not reasonable to expect that workers can prevent all harm.

Following policies and procedures will ensure that workers do all they can to support the older person during a difficult time. It can be beneficial to reflect on the incident in a healthy and supportive way. Learning how to reflect on the incident can therefore be helpful in managing feelings that may linger after recognising and responding to abuse.

14.4.2 Self-reflection and debriefing

In the context of recognising and responding to abuse, self-reflection is the process of reviewing the event and our actions in order to understand the incident in a proactive way. Self-reflection is a skill that can be used for many aspects of your practice, and when done meaningfully it can provide a clear understanding of what went well and what didn't go so well.

The aim of self-reflection is not to self-punish, but rather to foster learning and development from the incident. Meaningful reflection enables the worker to think about the incident without placing judgement on themselves or others. A process for self-reflection may involve taking some time out in a quiet place and asking yourself some questions about the incident, such as:

- What are the feelings I am experiencing about the incident?
- What were my strengths during the incident?
- What could I have done differently?
- Are there external reasons that are contributing to my stress?
- What can I change about the incident?
- This incident has made me feel anxious and depressed. What can I do about that?

Self-reflection can expose the elements of the experience that may need further support. Other aspects of the job can add to the stress of responding to abuse and can amplify feelings such as shame, guilt and anger that the worker may be experiencing.

14.4.3 Professional support

Workplace stressors such as chronic staff shortages, the responsibilities and physical demands of the job, and bullying and harassment in the workplace all contribute to a negative impact on the worker's mental health and wellbeing. Work and life balance is a fallacy that requires workers to "switch off" their personal lives when they arrive at work, which isn't reasonable or logical. Workers of all delegations have stressors in their personal lives. The experience of recognising and responding to abuse can be a catalyst for the need to reach out to others for support.

Care workers can approach their immediate supervisor to debrief following an incident. A debrief is a discussion about an incident that can serve a similar purpose to self-reflection. It can be helpful to have the support of someone who is familiar with the incident and the reporting process, and to be able to talk with them about all aspects of the incident. Being able to openly discuss their feelings about the incident can also be helpful for the care worker. A debriefing session can include the worker and the supervisor, or it may include a group of workers. A debrief in the workplace offers support that can help workers to gain a perspective of how they may be feeling about the incident.

Workers can also access health professionals such as certified counsellors and psychologists for support. The workplace may have an employee assistance program (EAP), a private and confidential counselling service that workers can access at the employer's cost. The worker's privacy and confidentiality are maintained by the EAP, and the workplace is not privy to the information that is discussed in counselling sessions.

14.4.4 Strategies to protect wellbeing

While workplace stressors such as working short-staffed and heavy workloads are risk factors for stress, anxiety and other mental health issues, there are protective factors that can minimise this risk. Protective factors are strategies that workers can put into practice to minimise stress and anxiety and increase resilience, and they focus on self-care. Some of these strategies include:

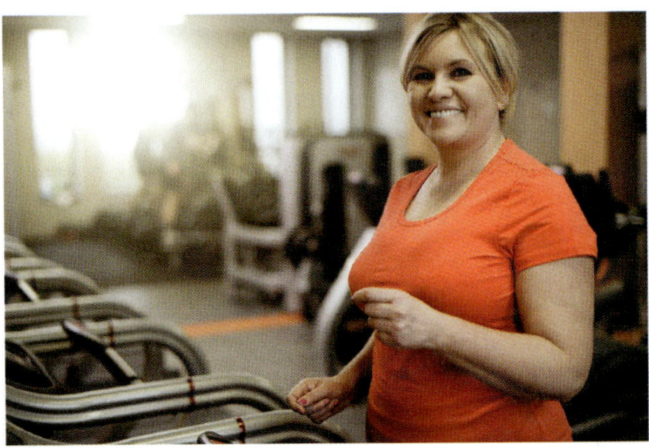

gpointstudio/Shutterstock

Protective factors such as exercising regularly can minimise workplace stressors for care workers

- eating a healthy diet
- exercising regularly
- taking a break
- requesting time off work
- engaging in debriefing with the workplace
- accessing other workplace supports such as the EAP
- seeking private counselling
- practising self-care activities such as meditation, walking, listening to music, reading, etc. (These activities are unique to the worker's tastes.)

Developing self-awareness of how incidents affect you as a care worker can provide insight to help you identify areas where extra support may be required. It is important that workers continue to monitor their own physical and mental health. The process of self-reflection can assist with this.

WORKPLACE SCENARIO

Managing the consequences of reporting a colleague for abusing an older person

A week has passed since Yvette made a report of the physical abuse of one of the older people in her care. She followed her organisation's policies and procedures when she made the report, but Yvette keeps replaying the incident over and over in her mind. She remembers walking into Mr Alby's room and seeing another colleague, Jane, hit Mr Alby across the face with a spoon. Jane was feeding Mr Alby his meal at the time of the incident. Yvette still can't believe that Jane would do that.

Yvette isn't sleeping properly, and she can't get the image of Mr Alby's anguished face out of her mind, even after debriefing with her supervisor. She feels she needs to see someone about her mental health and decides to access the employee assistance program that she has seen advertised on a poster in the staffroom.

CHECK YOUR UNDERSTANDING

1. What makes self-reflection meaningful?
2. List three questions you might ask of yourself when self-reflecting.
3. Why is debriefing with a supervisor helpful?
4. What is an EAP?
5. List four strategies that can protect your wellbeing.

SUMMARY

- The abuse, neglect and exploitation of older people in aged care is difficult to quantify but estimates of abuse are high.
- Older people may experience emotional and psychological abuse, neglect, financial exploitation, physical abuse, sexual abuse, grooming, undue influence and systemic abuse. The abuser is most likely someone the person knows and holds in a position of trust. The abuser uses their perceived power over the older person to control them.
- Care workers follow the policies and procedures of the organisation they work for when they recognise and respond to the suspected, alleged or known abuse of older people in their care.
- Responding to the abuse of older people can have a negative impact on the care worker's wellbeing. Self-reflection and debriefing with supervisors are helpful in protecting your wellbeing. Accessing professional external help is another option that you may consider.

REVIEW QUESTIONS

14.1 List three legislative, regulatory and ethical considerations relevant to reporting abuse.

14.2 Under the Serious Incident Response Scheme, there are eight reportable incidents. Name four.

14.3 How do you support a person who has allegedly been abused, neglected or exploited?

14.4 Identify techniques that can be used to manage your own response to witnessing and reporting an incident of abuse.

BIBLIOGRAPHY

Aged Care Quality and Safety Commission, *Serious Incident Response Scheme Guidelines for Residential Aged Care Providers*, Version 1.6, 1 October 2021, https://www.agedcarequality.gov.au/sites/default/files/media/sirs-guidelines-october-2021.pdf, accessed 13 December 2021.

Australian Bureau of Statistics, "Population projections, Australia", 22 November 2018, https://www.abs.gov.au/statistics/people/population/population-projections-australia/latest-release, accessed 28 April 2022.

Australian Institute of Health and Welfare (AIHW), "Older people; demographic profile", November 2021, https://www.aihw.gov.au/reports/older-people/older-australians/contents/demographic-profile, accessed 22 April 2022.

Australian Institute of Health and Welfare (AIHW), "Deaths by suicide over time", last updated 14 April 2022, https://www.aihw.gov.au/suicide-self-harm-monitoring/data/deaths-by-suicide-in-australia/suicide-deaths-over-time, accessed 14 July 2022.

Kaspiew, R., Carson, R. & Rhoades, H., *Elder Abuse: Understanding Issues, Frameworks and Responses* (Research Report No. 35), Australian Institute of Family Studies, Melbourne, February 2016, https://aifs.gov.au/publications/elder-abuse, accessed 11 December 2021.

Royal Commission into Aged Care Quality and Safety, *Elder Abuse in Australian Aged Care Facilities*, December 2020, https://agedcare.royalcommission.gov.au/news-and-media/elder-abuse-australian-aged-care-facilities, accessed 11 December 2021.

World Health Organization (WHO), *Elder Abuse*, October 2021, https://www.who.int/news-room/fact-sheets/detail/elder-abuse, accessed 11 December 2021.

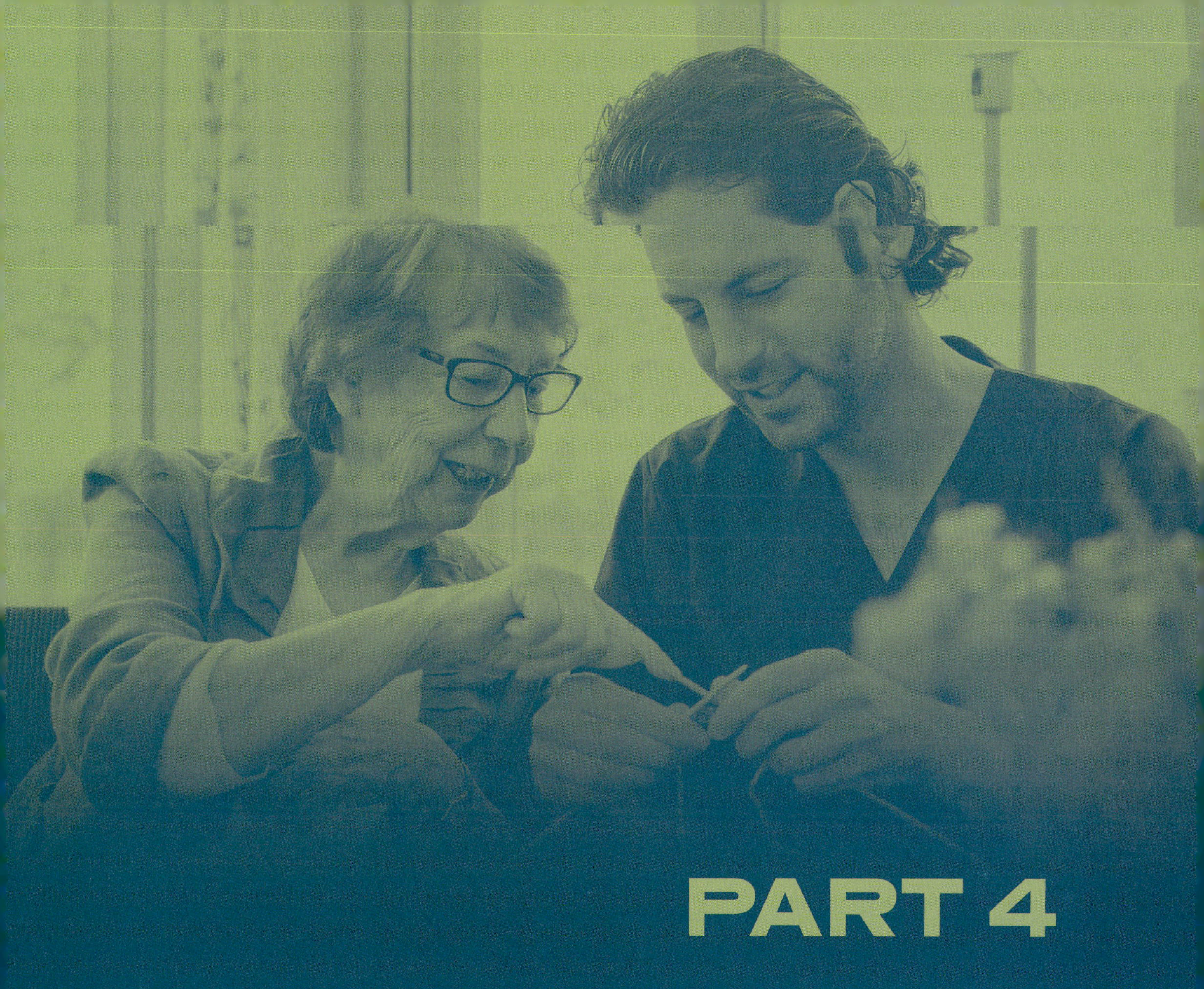

PART 4
Health

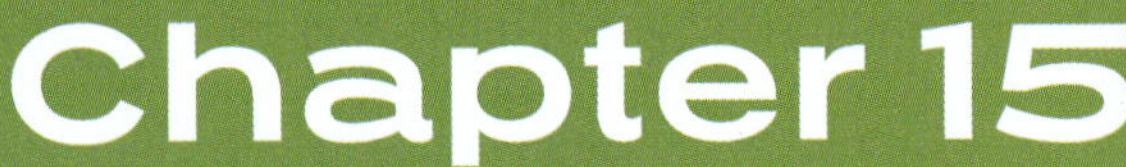

Chapter 15

Understanding the human body

LEARNING OBJECTIVES

15.1 Work with information about the human body

15.2 Recognise and promote ways to support healthy functioning of the body

INTRODUCTION

THE BODY IS A COMPLEX ORGANISM whose different systems work together to maintain healthy functioning. It is necessary for the care worker to understand the various components of the body and how they work together, as this knowledge will enable them to provide specific, ongoing care for individuals according to their assessed needs and to identify and report changes in functioning to their supervisor. A key element of reporting these changes in functioning is medical terminology, which is a language shared among health professionals that facilitates accurate reporting and documentation. Using correct terminology allows the care staff to share their observations and discuss their concerns with other members of the care team, thereby enabling potential and actual problems to be addressed in a timely fashion, thus promoting healthy functioning and contributing to wellbeing.

INDUSTRY IN FOCUS

The importance of understanding the human body and reporting changes to normal functioning

Over the last two decades, the profile of people in residential aged care has changed significantly. People live longer and remain in their homes for a greater length of time before moving to an aged care facility. Consequently, when people do move, they are less physically fit, and have more chronic health conditions and increasingly complex needs than their predecessors. They have experienced more cognitive changes and are frailer, plus they have fewer economic resources and fewer social opportunities.

There are many implications of this trend. In economic terms, ageing is seen as a "problem" as the population of older, ill and dependent adults increases and the tax revenue generated by those of working age decreases, making the cost of residential aged care less and less viable. On the other hand, if the incidence of illness and disability in the older population can be reduced due to education and medical and care interventions, then the contribution to society of healthy, older adults becomes a bonus. In this sense, care staff can have a significant impact in encouraging individuals to maintain their health, wellbeing and quality of life.

In terms of the workforce, the increasing complexity of care needs places more responsibility in the hands of care staff. This increased responsibility, together with greater accountability to government for providers and staff, requires all staff to have a sound understanding of both the physical and psychosocial changes the individuals in their care experience as they age. Recognising what is normal, interpreting information about the person's health, and deciding what should be reported and acted on, are essential skills all care staff require. Encouraging individuals to maintain their health—to undertake physical activity, to have adequate rest and sleep, to maintain a healthy weight, to socialise, to manage existing health conditions, and to avoid risks (such as being exposed to infection)—is also important, even within the confines of chronic health issues and frailty.

15.1 WORKING WITH INFORMATION ABOUT THE HUMAN BODY

15.1.1 Normal body structure and functions

Understanding about the human body is essential for care workers. This includes knowing about anatomy (the *structure* of the body) and physiology (the *function* of the body).

CELLS

Cells are the basic structural unit of the body. All cells require food, water and oxygen to survive and maintain their designated functions. The shape and size of cells vary according to their function; however, all cells in the human body have the following components (see also Figure 15.1):

- The *cell membrane* contains the structures within the cell. The membrane is semi-permeable, allowing for the passage of water, food and oxygen from the bloodstream *to* the cell plus the removal of waste *from* the cell back into the bloodstream.
- The *nucleus* controls the growth and functions of the cell. The nucleus contains genetic material that determines characteristics that are passed from one generation to the next, such as eye colour and vulnerability to certain diseases, such as breast cancer.
- *Cytoplasm* is a gel-like substance in which the components of the cell are suspended.
- *Organelles* are structures within the cell that have different functions, such as producing energy (e.g. mitochondrions), destroying toxins and building proteins (e.g. ribosomes).

FIGURE 15.1 The components of a cell

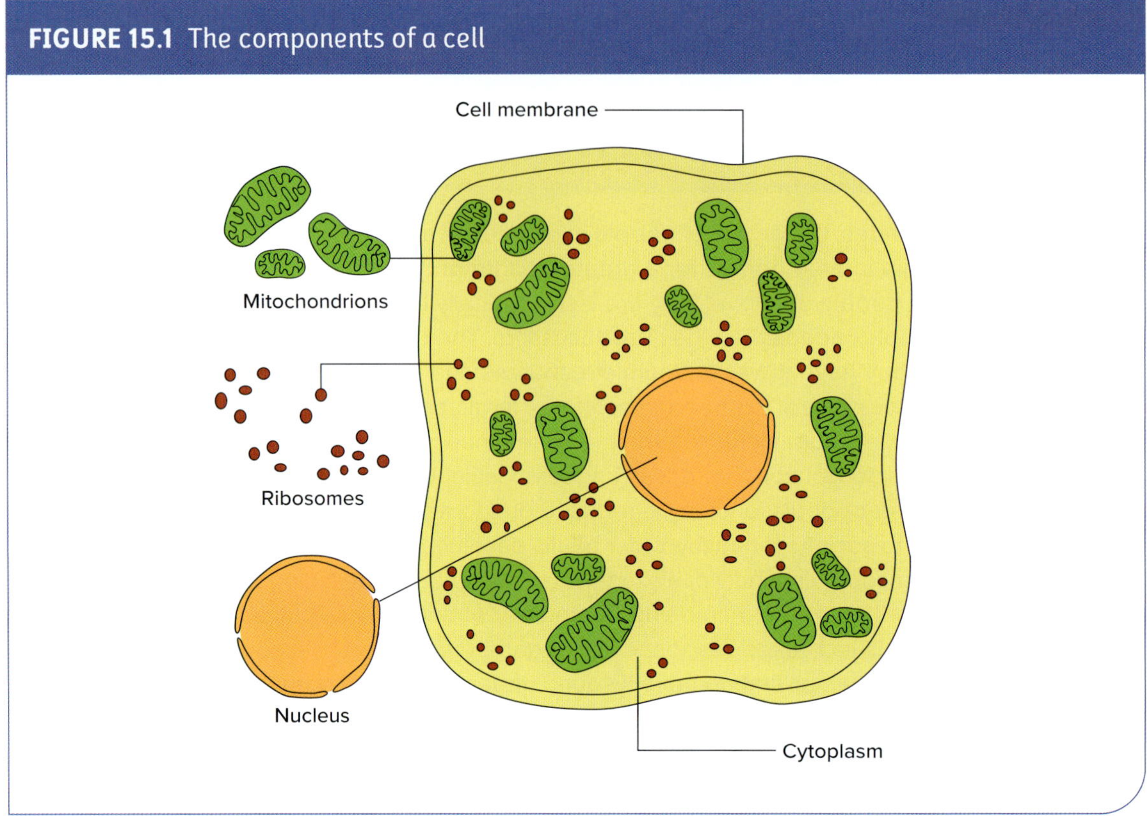

Source: July Store/Shutterstock

Cell types vary greatly in their size and shape, according to their different functions. For example, red blood cells are shaped like discs and carry oxygen around the body; fat cells are circular and provide protection to organs and other structures of the body. Normally, cells only multiply when required—for example, in wound healing.

Sometimes, cells change (mutate) and fail to die naturally. When this happens, they reproduce with no restrictions on their growth, causing them to invade other tissues. Cancer is a result of this uncontrolled growth.

TISSUES

Cells with a similar structure and functions group together to form tissues. There are four main types of tissue in the body, each with a specific function:

- *Epithelial tissue* covers and lines internal cavities and tubes, such as the glands in the gastrointestinal system that secrete juices to aid digestion.
- *Connective tissue* supports and frames the body (e.g. bone and cartilage).
- *Muscular tissue* can contract and relax, thereby aiding movement. There are three types of muscle: cardiac (heart), skeletal (attached to bones) and smooth (the organs).
- *Nervous tissue* receives and sends messages (impulses) via nerve cells and chemicals—for example, to muscles, causing them to contract and relax.

ORGANS

Organs perform specific functions in the body and comprise more than one type of tissue. For example:

- The heart moves blood around the body.
- The kidneys filter blood.

- The stomach digests food.
- The lungs exchange oxygen and carbon dioxide.
- The brain processes messages from the senses.

Figure 15.2 illustrates the human body, from a single cell to a complex human organism.

LUNGS
KIDNEYS
STOMACH
INTESTINES
BRAIN
HEART
SPLEEN
LIVER
Macrovector/Shutterstock
Human organs

SYSTEMS

The body's systems comprise groups of organs that work together to perform specific functions. No body system can perform alone; they all work together to maintain healthy functioning. There are 11 body systems, each performing a different function. Table 15.1 summarises the 11 systems, their main organs and their functions.

FIGURE 15.2 The human body—from a single cell to a complex human organism

Cellular level
Smooth muscle cell
Tissue level
Smooth muscle tissue
Serous membrane
Organ level
Smooth muscle tissue layers
Stomach
Epithelial tissue
System level
Oesophagus
Stomach
Liver
Pancreas
Gallbladder
Small intestine
Large intestine
Organism level
Digestive system

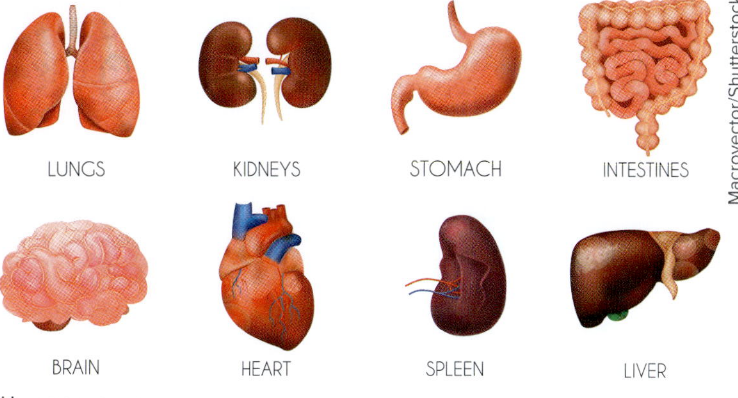

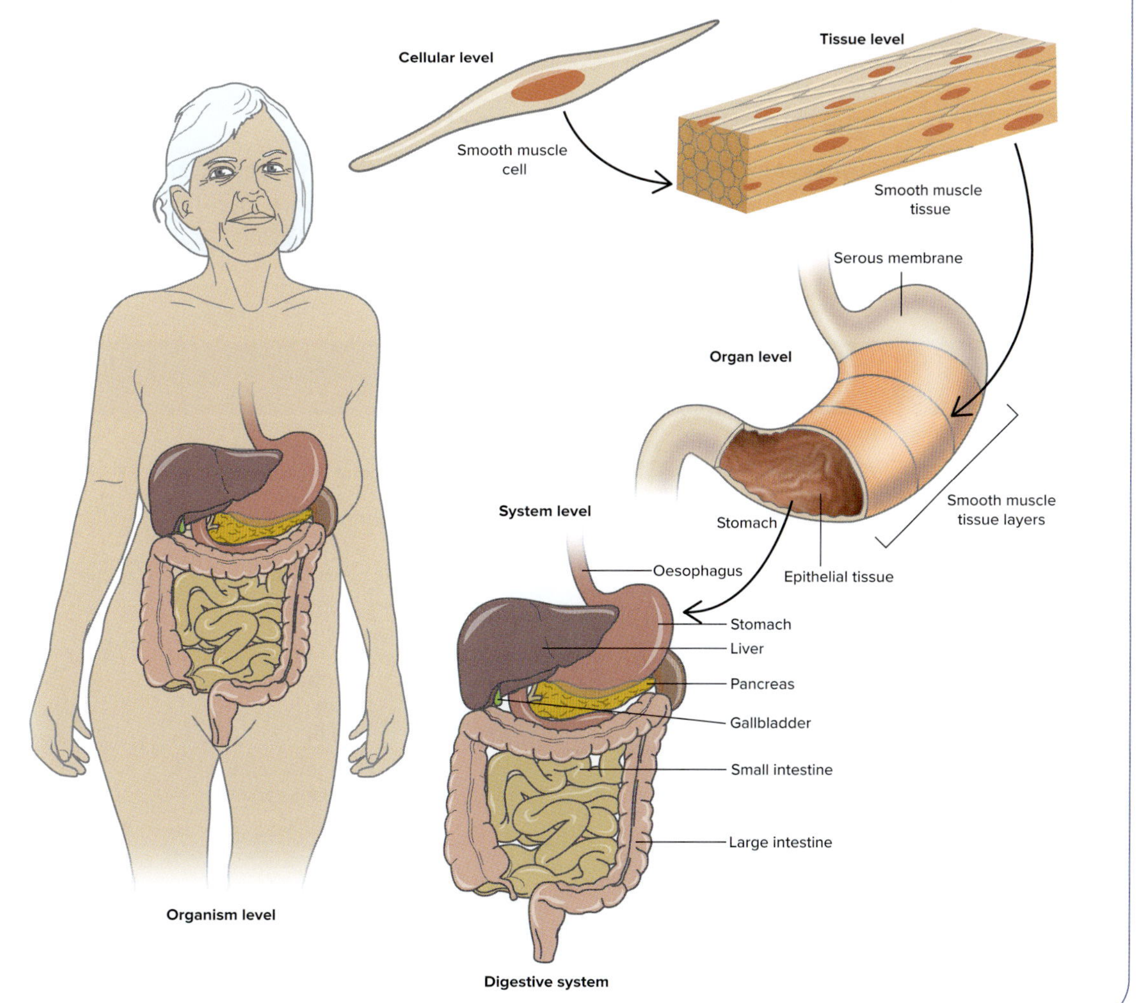

TABLE 15.1 The body's systems, involved organs and specific functions

Body system	Main organs	Function
Cardiovascular	Heart, blood, blood vessels	Moves gases, nutrients and waste to and from different parts of the body
Respiratory	Trachea, lungs, bronchioles, alveoli	Moves gases in and out of the body
Muscular	Skeletal muscles, smooth muscles, cardiac muscles	Assists movement
Skeletal	Bones, joints, cartilage	Supports and protects the body
Digestive (gastrointestinal)	Mouth, oesophagus, stomach, small and large intestines, anus	Ingests and digests food, absorbs nutrients and eliminates waste
Integumentary	Skin, hair, nails	Protects the body
Endocrine	Glands, hormones	Regulates various body functions
Urinary (renal)	Kidneys, ureters, bladder, urethra	Filters the blood of waste, creating urine
Nervous	Brain, spinal cord, nerves	Sends and receives messages
Lymphatic and immune	Lymphatic vessels, glands, cells	Filters the blood and fights disease
Reproductive	Uterus, ovaries, vagina Penis, testes	Performs functions relating to reproduction and expressing sexuality

15.1.2 The organisation of the body

The body has two main cavities or internal spaces that contain various organs, the ventral and dorsal cavities (see Figure 15.3). These two cavities are further divided into four smaller ones (see Table 15.2) and are separated from other structures by muscles, membranes and parts of the skeleton.

FIGURE 15.3 The body's two main cavities

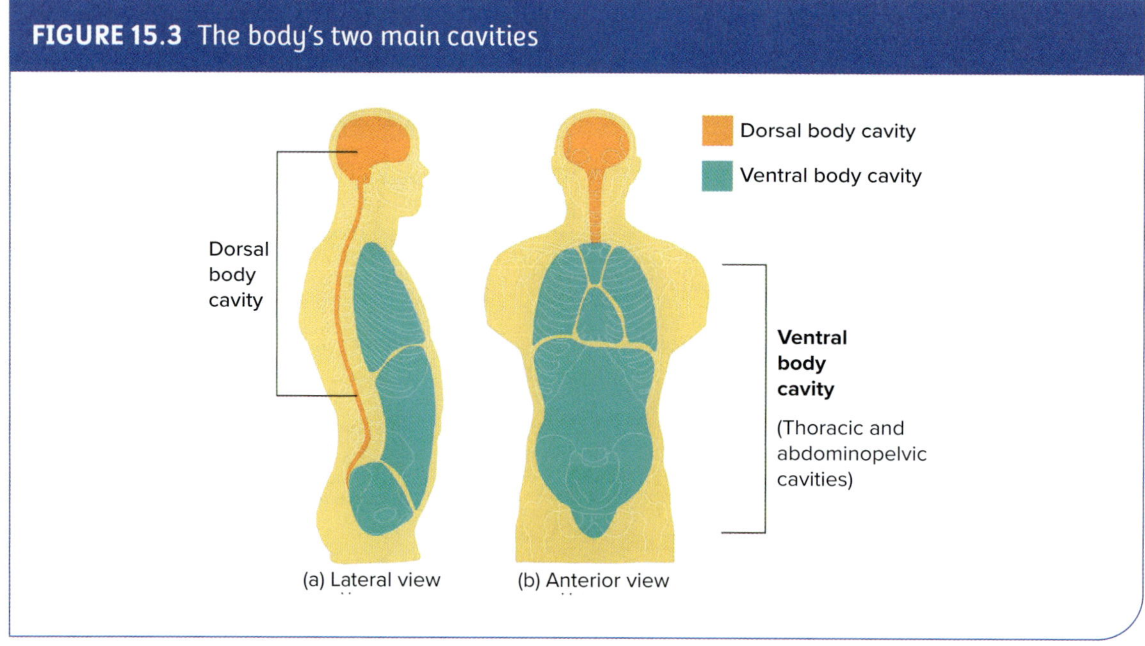

Source: Catherine Rappazzo/Shutterstock

TABLE 15.2 Body cavities and their organs

Main cavity	Smaller cavities	Organs
Ventral	Thoracic Abdominal Pelvic	Lungs, heart, large blood vessels Stomach, pancreas, liver, kidneys Uterus, ovaries, bladder
Dorsal	Cranial Spinal	Brain Spinal cord, vertebrae

Specific terms are used to describe the position of one part of the body in relation to another (see Table 15.3). These are known as *directional terms* and are especially useful when writing a report—for example, when describing the location of an individual's pain or the site of an injury.

TABLE 15.3 Directional terms

Term	Definition	Example
Superior	Uppermost or above	The skull is *superior* to the cervical spine
Inferior	Lowermost or below	The cervical spine is *inferior* to the skull
Anterior	Towards the front	The sternum is *anterior* to the spinal column
Posterior	Towards the back	The spinal column is *posterior* to the sternum
Medial	Nearest the mid-line of the body	The sternum is *medial* to the ribs
Lateral	Towards the side of the body	The person was placed in the left *lateral* position
Proximal	Nearest the point of attachment	The humerus is *proximal* to the scapula
Distal	Furthermost from the point of attachment	The phalanges are *distal* to the scapula

15.1.3 The cardiovascular system

The cardiovascular system is made up of the heart, blood vessels and blood. The heart is located in the **thoracic cavity** and pumps blood around the body, carrying oxygen, hormones and nutrients to the cells and waste away from the cells. The nervous system automatically controls an area of the heart that triggers each pump of the heart muscle, known as the heartbeat. Chemicals in the blood such as potassium and sodium also control the heart rate. The heartbeat is felt as a pulse in the large blood vessels, particularly where the vessels lie between soft tissue and bone, such as in the wrist. The average heart rate for an adult is between 60 and 90 beats per minute.

NORMAL STRUCTURE AND FUNCTION

The heart is a muscle about the size of a clenched fist (see Figure 15.4). It comprises four chambers: two upper chambers called atria and two lower chambers called **ventricles**. Valves separate the atria and the ventricles on each side of the heart. The septum separates the left and right sides of the heart. The heart is supported by the pericardium, which is attached to adjacent structures such as the diaphragm. The heart has three layers:

- endocardium—the innermost layer
- myocardium—the middle layer, which is made up of muscle
- epicardium—the outermost layer.

Blood from the body enters the heart through the right atrium from veins known as the superior (uppermost) and inferior (lower) vena cava. The blood moves to the right ventricle where it is pumped to the lungs through the

FIGURE 15.4 The heart showing the chambers and main blood vessels

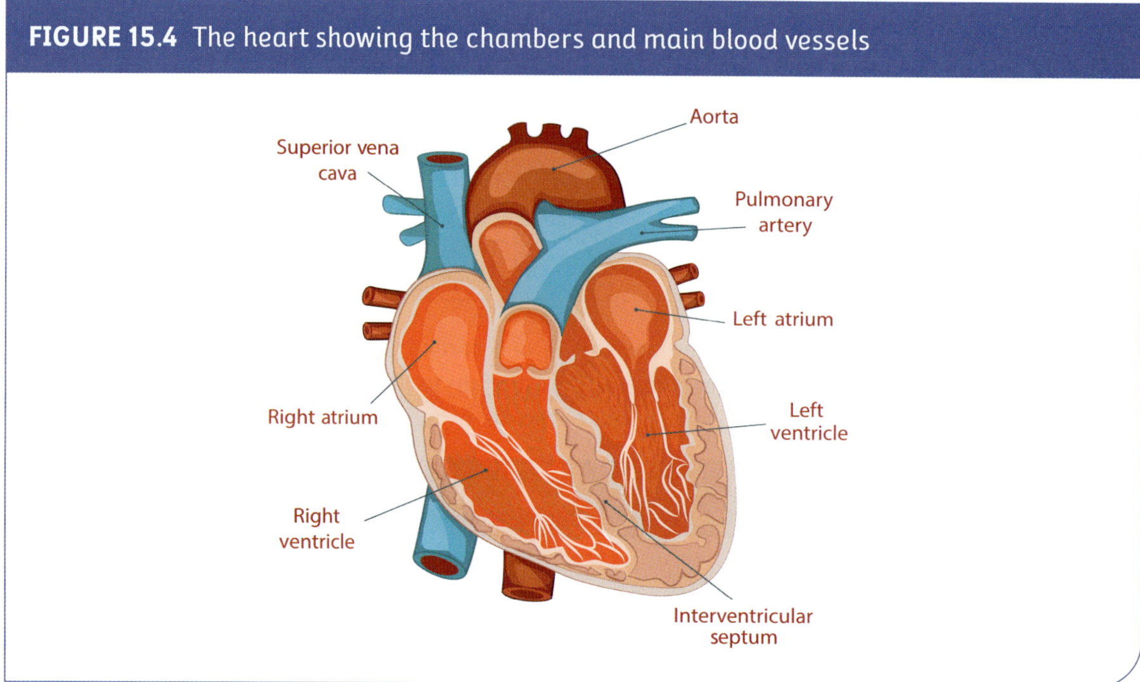

Source: okili77/Shutterstock

pulmonary arteries. In the lungs, the blood picks up oxygen and then returns to the left side of the heart through the pulmonary veins. It moves from the left atrium to the left ventricle where it is pumped to the body.

Blood vessels are a series of connected, hollow tubes that transport blood around the body. There are three types of blood vessels:

- *Arteries* carry blood containing oxygen away from the heart to the organs. The smallest arteries are called arterioles.
- *Veins* carry blood containing wastes such as carbon dioxide to the heart. Veins contain valves that keep the blood moving towards the heart. The smallest veins are called venules.
- *Capillaries* are microscopic vessels that connect arterioles and venules. Capillaries are only one cell thick, allowing for the movement of gases, nutrients and waste across their membranes.

Blood is a thick fluid that transports oxygen, hormones and nutrients to all cells in the body. The cells use these materials to produce energy, creating carbon dioxide and other substances. Carbon dioxide is transported in the blood to the lungs and is exhaled as waste. The other substances are removed from the body in sweat, urine and faeces. Blood is comprised of red cells, white cells and platelets that float in a liquid known as plasma:

- Red blood cells (erythrocytes) carry oxygen on a substance called haemoglobin.
- White blood cells (leucocytes) fight infection.
- Platelets (thrombocytes) contain substances that control clotting when there is an injury.

The force with which the blood is pumped to and from the heart is known as **blood pressure**.

MAINTAINING HEALTHY FUNCTIONING OF THE CARDIOVASCULAR SYSTEM

To ensure the healthy functioning of the cardiovascular system, the following risk factors should be avoided or managed:

- a family history of heart disease
- obesity

- a sedentary lifestyle
- poor nutrition
- high blood pressure (hypertension)
- poor sleep patterns
- depression
- substance abuse
- smoking.

REPORTING CHANGES TO THE CARDIOVASCULAR SYSTEM

Changes in the cardiovascular system that should be reported immediately include:

- changes in vital signs—that is, pulse rate, strength and rhythm; blood pressure and oxygen levels
- breathlessness
- changes to skin colour—that is, the presence of a bluish tinge to the lips, feet and hands
- changes to the temperature of the skin—feelings of coldness
- loss of balance due to dizziness
- fatigue
- confusion, slurred speech, and numbness in the face and limbs
- pain in the chest
- pain in the left arm
- swollen feet
- changes in the level of consciousness.

15.1.4 The respiratory system

The respiratory system is made up of the nasal cavities, throat, larynx, trachea, bronchus and bronchioles, alveoli, lungs, diaphragm, and the muscles between the ribs (see Figure 15.5). The respiratory system works with the heart to deliver oxygen to cells and to remove carbon dioxide. This exchange of gases is known as respiration. Breathing in (inhalation) and breathing out (exhalation) are automatically controlled by the nervous system and by the presence of chemicals in the blood.

NORMAL STRUCTURE AND FUNCTION

Air enters the nose and is filtered by tiny hairs and mucus that line the surface of the nose. The nose is also responsible for our sense of smell.

The throat or pharynx is divided into the nasopharynx and oropharynx. Both air and food pass through the pharynx; air passes into the larynx and food to the oesophagus. The larynx contains the vocal cords that vibrate as inhaled air moves over them. The vibration causes the sounds we make when we speak, sing and cough. The larynx changes the pitch of sound and assists swallowing.

The trachea is a hollow tube made of cartilage which provides support. The trachea transports moistened air from the larynx to the lungs. Just as in the nose, tiny hairs and mucus line the trachea and remove dust and other particles from the air before it goes to the lungs.

The trachea divides into the left and right bronchus, allowing for the passage of air into the left and right lungs. The bronchi branch into small tubes called bronchioles that divide even further into tiny sacs known as **alveoli**, where gas exchange takes place. Oxygen passes through the alveoli from the air to the bloodstream at the same time as carbon dioxide passes through the alveoli from the bloodstream to the exhaled air.

The lungs take up most of the thoracic cavity and are protected by the ribs. They are separated from the abdominal cavity by a thick band of muscle known as the diaphragm. During inhalation the diaphragm pushes down and the muscles between the ribs push upwards, expanding the chest cavity. During exhalation,

FIGURE 15.5 The respiratory system

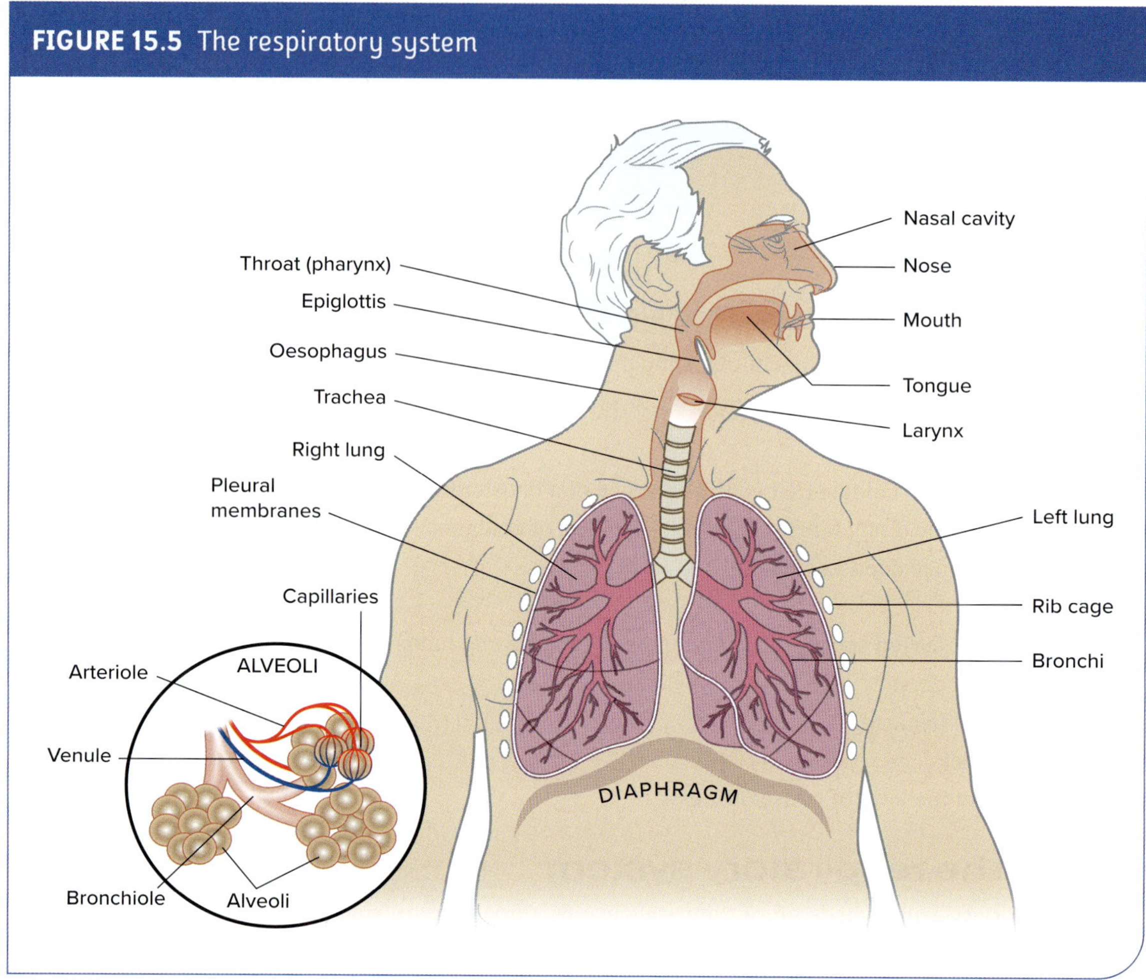

the diaphragm and the muscles relax and return to their normal position. The normal respiratory rate for an adult is between 12 and 20 breaths per minute. One breath is made up of both inhalation and exhalation.

MAINTAINING HEALTHY FUNCTIONING OF THE RESPIRATORY SYSTEM

To ensure the healthy functioning of the respiratory system, the following risk factors should be avoided or managed:

- smoking
- substance abuse
- exposure to pollutants.

Exposure to any or all of these hazards places an individual at greater risk of infections, chronic illness (e.g. chronic obstructive pulmonary disease) and cancer. Avoiding these risks will contribute to maintaining healthy functioning of the respiratory system, along with:

- maintaining a healthy diet and fluid intake
- avoiding situations where the risk of infection is increased
- achieving adequate rest and sleep
- practising good personal hygiene, especially hand washing.

REPORTING CHANGES TO THE RESPIRATORY SYSTEM

Changes to the respiratory system that should be reported immediately include signs of an infection such as a raised temperature, chills and feeling hot, watery eyes, a runny nose, sneezing and coughing. Other changes that should be reported are dyspnoea (difficulty breathing), wheezing, a rapid respiratory rate, fatigue, loss of appetite, pain in the chest on inhalation, vomiting, and changes to skin colour.

15.1.5 The muscular system

The muscular system is responsible for moving bones and the internal organs, stabilising joints, providing support to the skeleton and generating heat. Muscles contract and relax due to impulses from the nervous system and the movement of chemicals along the muscle fibres. By the time a person reaches 80 years of age, up to 50 per cent of their muscle mass is lost.

NORMAL STRUCTURE AND FUNCTION

There are three types of muscles in the body (see also Figure 15.6):

- *Cardiac muscle* is in the heart and is responsible for the heartbeat, for contracting and relaxing, and for pumping blood to different parts of the body. It is an involuntary muscle, meaning it works automatically.
- *Smooth muscle* is in the hollow organs of the body such as the digestive tract and the blood vessels. Like cardiac muscle, smooth muscle is involuntary. Smooth muscles move in a wave-like motion known as peristalsis that helps move substances such as food through the intestines.
- *Skeletal muscle* is attached to bones by tendons and supports movement, working in groups to pull the bone into a different position (see Figure 15.7). Skeletal muscle is voluntary, meaning that the muscles move when we want them to. Tendons are bands of dense tissue that connect muscles to bones.

FIGURE 15.6 The three types of muscle in the human body

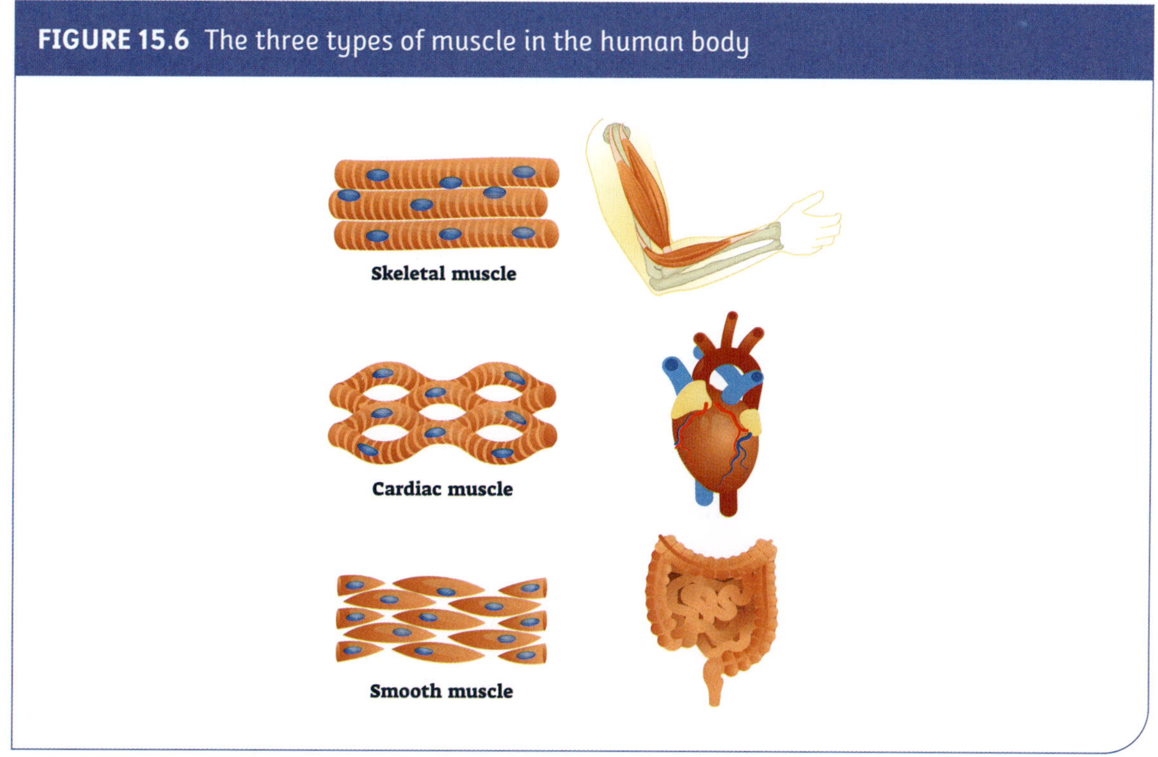

Source: VectorMine/Shutterstock

FIGURE 15.7 Muscles moving the forearm

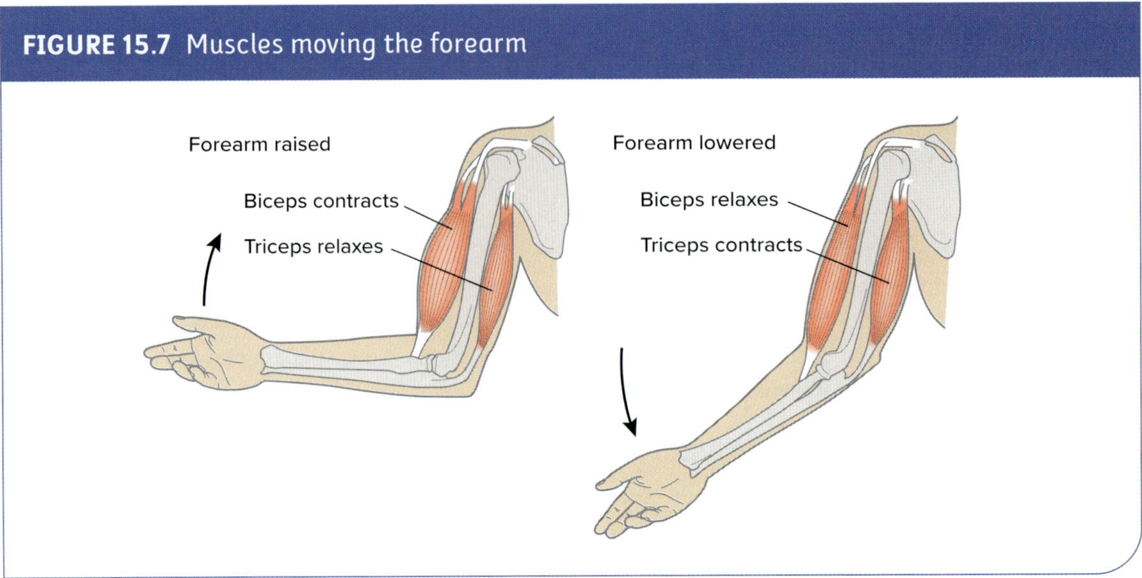

MAINTAINING HEALTHY FUNCTIONING OF THE MUSCULAR SYSTEM

To ensure the healthy functioning of the muscular system, the following risk factors should be avoided or managed:

- poor nutrition, such as insufficient protein and iron in the diet
- substance abuse
- a sedentary lifestyle with little exercise
- repeated overuse or strain, resulting in chronic problems such as lower back pain.

REPORTING CHANGES TO THE MUSCULAR SYSTEM

Changes to the normal function of muscles that should be reported immediately include:

- pain and swelling, especially on movement
- loss of function
- decrease in function of the joints.

15.1.6 The skeletal system

The skeletal system is made up of bones, joints, ligaments and cartilage. Bones vary in size from large, such as the femur in the leg, to very small, such as the ossicles in the ears. The bones of the body are illustrated in Figure 15.8.

NORMAL STRUCTURE AND FUNCTION

Bone is made up of hard, dense and flexible tissue that provides a framework for the body. Bones protect vital organs; for example, the skull protects the brain and the ribs protect the lungs. Bone stores calcium and phosphorus, and the centre of bone contains fat cells and tissue for manufacturing blood cells. Bones have different shapes, including:

- long (e.g. the femur in the upper leg)
- short (e.g. the radius in the arm)

FIGURE 15.8 The larger bones of the body

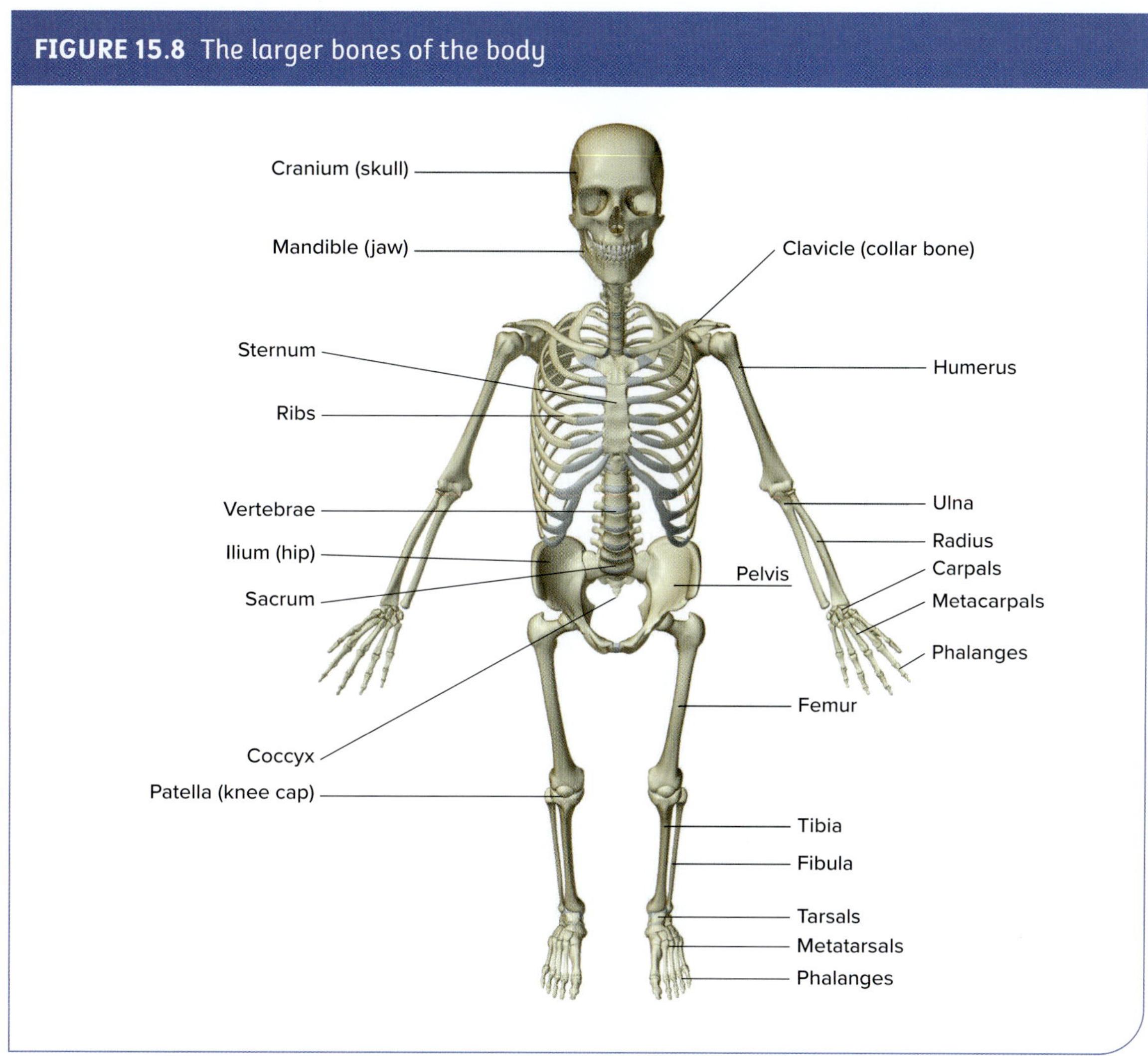

Source: MedicalRF.com

- flat (e.g. the skull)
- irregular (e.g. the vertebrae in the spinal column).

A joint is an area where two or more bones meet; it allows for the flexible and fluid movement of the body. There are three structural classifications of joints in the human body:

- Fibrous (immovable)—contain very firm fibres that maintain the bone's shape, such as the joints in the skull and semi-movable joints such as the ribs.
- Cartilaginous (semi-movable)—contain cartilage, such as the pads between the spinal bones.
- Synovial (movable)—contain synovial fluid that lubricates the joint and allows more movement, such as the top of the neck (pivot joint), knee (hinge joint) and hip (ball-and-socket joint).

Joints are held together by connective tissue called ligaments. Dislocation of a joint occurs when the ligaments move too far apart or are overstretched.

Cartilage is tough connective tissue that is softer and more flexible than bone. Cartilage is found in many places in the body and gives shape to structures such as the nose and ears.

MAINTAINING HEALTHY FUNCTIONING OF THE SKELETAL SYSTEM

To ensure the healthy functioning of the skeletal system, the following risk factors should be avoided or managed:

- a lack of vitamin D and of calcium
- exposure to heavy metals
- substance abuse
- a sedentary lifestyle
- poor nutrition and fluid intake
- medications that affect the integrity of the bones
- low oestrogen
- falls.

REPORTING CHANGES TO THE SKELETAL SYSTEM

Changes to the normal function of the skeletal system that should be reported immediately include:

- pain, tenderness and swelling over a joint or bone
- loss of alignment
- decreased movement or joint function.

15.1.7 The digestive system

The digestive (gastrointestinal) system is made up of the organs and accessory organs that ingest and digest food, absorb nutrients and eliminate waste (see Figure 15.9).

NORMAL STRUCTURE AND FUNCTION

The following are the main structures of the digestive tract:

- *Mouth:* Food is ingested in the mouth and the teeth and saliva break it down into smaller pieces, called a bolus. Enzymes in the saliva begin to act on carbohydrates in the food.
- *Oesophagus:* The oesophagus is a hollow tube that is parallel to the trachea, extending from the pharynx to the stomach. The smooth muscles of the oesophagus contract and squeeze the bolus towards the stomach.
- *Stomach:* The stomach is a small sac where the bolus is churned and combined with gastric enzymes, resulting in a thick substance called chyme. Chyme remains in the stomach for approximately three hours and is gradually released into the small intestine.
- *Small intestine:* Chyme continues to break down in the small intestine and nutrients are absorbed. Enzymes excreted by the pancreas and the small intestine contribute to digestion at this stage, allowing for the passage of water, glucose, salts, vitamins and minerals into the bloodstream through the intestinal walls, from where they are carried to the cells.
- *Large intestine:* Chyme and waste (faeces) move to the large intestine where some water is absorbed. The remainder is stored until the urge to defecate occurs. Defecation is the expulsion of faeces and is controlled by muscles and nerves in the rectum and anus.

The accessory organs are the organs that aid **digestion**:

- The salivary glands are glands in the mouth that secrete saliva. Saliva moistens and softens food and begins the process of digestion.
- The liver's functions include the regulation of blood sugar, the formation of bile, the breakdown of fats and toxins, and the storage of vitamins and iron.
- The gall bladder stores and secretes bile, which aids the process of fat digestion and assist the absorption of the fat-soluble vitamins A, D, E and K.
- The pancreas secretes enzymes that are necessary for digestion. It also secretes insulin and glucagon, which are essential for the regulation of blood glucose levels in the blood.

FIGURE 15.9 The digestive system

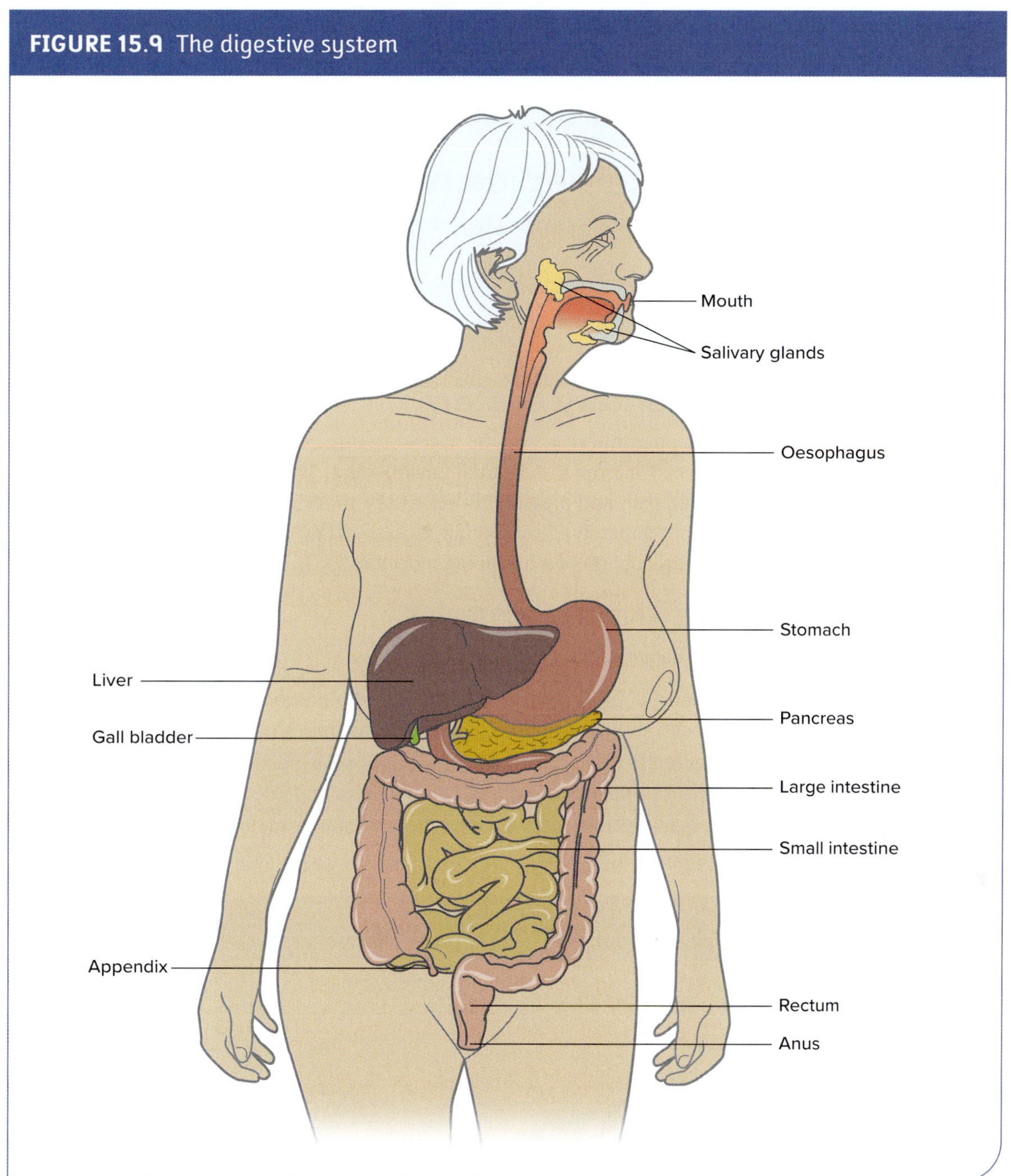

MAINTAINING HEALTHY FUNCTIONING OF THE DIGESTIVE SYSTEM

Healthy functioning of the digestive system is important in maintaining digestion, the absorption of nutrients and the **elimination** of waste. Risk factors that may cause damage to the digestive system include:

- the ingestion of toxins, including excessive alcohol
- exposure to heavy metals
- stress
- infections such as hepatitis
- chronic conditions such as Crohn's disease

- persistent constipation
- malnutrition or undernutrition
- dehydration
- inadequate oral hygiene.

REPORTING CHANGES TO THE DIGESTIVE SYSTEM

Changes to the normal function of the digestive system that should be reported immediately include:

- excessive vomiting or diarrhoea
- the inability to defecate
- bleeding from the bowel.

15.1.8 The integumentary system

The integumentary system is made up of the skin, and the accessory organs: hair, nails and glands. It is the largest organ of the body and protects it from the external environment. The skin secretes waste products via sweat; it senses touch, vibration, pain and pressure; it begins the process of forming vitamin D; and it helps the body maintain a constant temperature, preventing excessive fluid loss. The colour of the skin is determined by genetics and by the production of a hormone, melanin.

NORMAL STRUCTURE AND FUNCTION

The skin has three layers (see also Figure 15.10):

- The *epidermis* is the outermost layer. It is thin and contains no blood vessels and few nerve endings. Oxygen and nutrients diffuse into the lower epidermis from the dermis.
- The *dermis* is the inner layer and contains blood vessels, nerves, sweat glands, oil glands and hair roots. The dermis is made up of dense connective tissue and elastic fibres that give the skin its flexibility.
- The *subcutaneous layer* is made up of fatty tissue that protects and insulates deeper tissue and organs. The subcutaneous layer anchors the skin to underlying structures.

FIGURE 15.10 Human skin

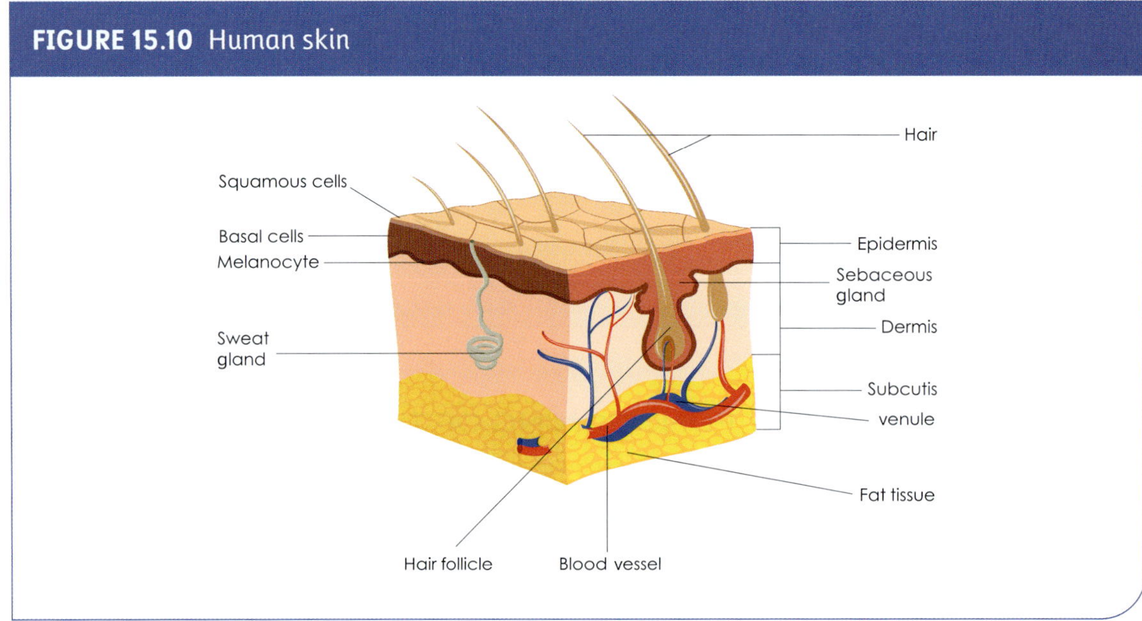

Source: stockshoppe/Shutterstock

The accessory organs of the skin are the hair, nails and glands. Hair is made up of epithelial cells that contain a protein, keratin. Hair growth is influenced by testosterone and oestrogen, and the colour of hair is controlled by melanin. Hair has different functions according to its location on the body; for example, the eyelashes and eyebrows protect the eyes from dust and sweat. Nails are made up of epithelial cells that contain keratin. They protect the ends of the fingers and toes from injury. The skin contains two types of glands: the sebaceous glands and the sweat glands. The sebaceous glands secrete an oily substance known as sebum that lubricates and protects the skin. The sweat glands secrete water and some salts and are important in maintaining body temperature.

MAINTAINING HEALTHY FUNCTIONING OF THE INTEGUMENTARY SYSTEM

Healthy functioning of the integumentary system is maintained by good skin care and hygiene. Irritants such as urine and faeces should be removed immediately, as they damage the skin. Lying or sitting in the same position for long periods undermines the skin's layers and can result in injuries and wounds. To ensure the healthy functioning of the integumentary system, the following risk factors should be avoided or managed:

- friction
- exposure to ultraviolet (UV) light
- poor nutrition and fluid intake
- substance abuse
- medications that undermine the integrity of the skin.

Healthy skin can be maintained by diet and by personal care measures such as using warm water to bathe, applying moisturiser after bathing and hand washing, patting instead of rubbing the skin dry, and using products that don't contain alcohol. Avoiding extreme temperature changes and sun exposure is also important.

REPORTING CHANGES TO THE INTEGUMENTARY SYSTEM

Changes to the skin's normal condition or its integrity should be reported immediately. These changes include:

- variations in moles or freckles
- general appearance, texture and colour
- a wound that is slow to heal
- bruising or blisters
- pressure injuries.

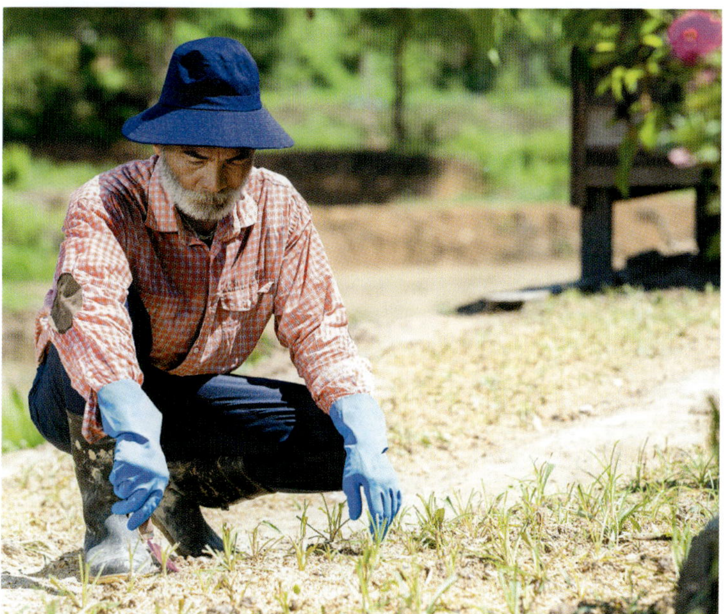

M2020/Shutterstock

Reduce exposure to UV by wearing a broad-brimmed hat and collared shirt

15.1.9 The endocrine system

The endocrine system contains glands that secrete chemicals called hormones into the bloodstream. Hormone levels are adjusted by the central nervous system and a mechanism called *negative feedback* and control numerous functions in the body, including growth and reproduction.

NORMAL STRUCTURE AND FUNCTION

Glands are situated throughout the body. The major glands of the endocrine system, their locations and the main hormones they excrete are shown in Figure 15.11 and listed in Table 15.4.

FIGURE 15.11 The endocrine system

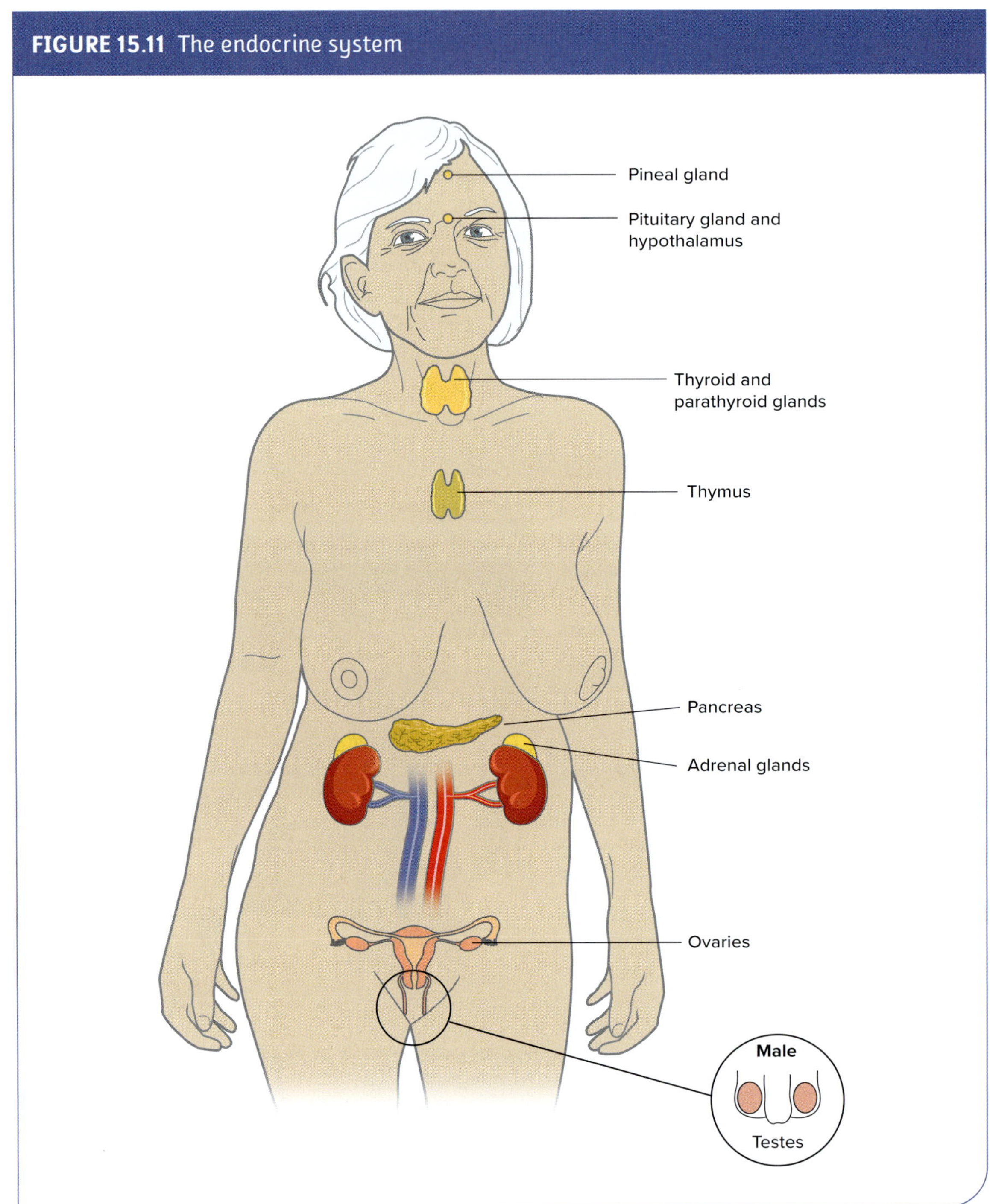

TABLE 15.4 The major glands of the endocrine system

Gland	Location	Main hormone and effect
Pituitary	In the brain	A variety of hormones that affect the production of other hormones in the body
Pineal	In the brain	Melatonin, which affects sleep and reproductive cycles
Thyroid	In the neck near the larynx	Thyroxine, which affects metabolism
Parathyroid	Within the thyroid capsule	Calcitonin, which affects calcium levels
Adrenals	On top of the kidneys	Adrenaline, which affects our response to stress
Pancreas	In the abdominal cavity behind and slightly to the left of the stomach	Insulin, which affects the level of glucose in the blood
Thymus	In the thoracic cavity behind the sternum	Thymosin, which affects immunity
Testes (male)	Below the penis	Testosterone, which affects reproduction
Ovaries (female)	In the pelvic cavity	Oestrogen, which affects reproduction

MAINTAINING HEALTHY FUNCTIONING OF THE ENDOCRINE SYSTEM

Healthy functioning of the endocrine system is necessary to ensure that the secretion of hormones maintains a balance among all body systems. This is known as homeostasis. To ensure the healthy functioning of the endocrine system, the following risk factors should be avoided or managed:

- substance abuse
- exposure to chemicals
- poor nutrition
- medications
- excessive stress
- a family history
- obesity
- high blood pressure
- a sedentary lifestyle.

REPORTING CHANGES TO THE ENDOCRINE SYSTEM

The endocrine system is usually unaffected by ageing and remains well balanced throughout life unless disease affects one of the glands. The most common disease of the endocrine system is diabetes, which affects the pancreas. Changes that should be reported that may indicate diabetes include:

- increased thirst
- fatigue
- blurred vision
- “fruity” breath
- leg cramps
- frequent urination
- excessive eating.

15.1.10 The urinary system

The urinary (or renal) system is made up of the kidneys, ureters, bladder and the urethra (see Figure 15.12). The urinary system filters the blood, regulates blood volume by determining the amount of water excreted, and regulates blood pressure, contributing to homeostasis.

FIGURE 15.12 The urinary system

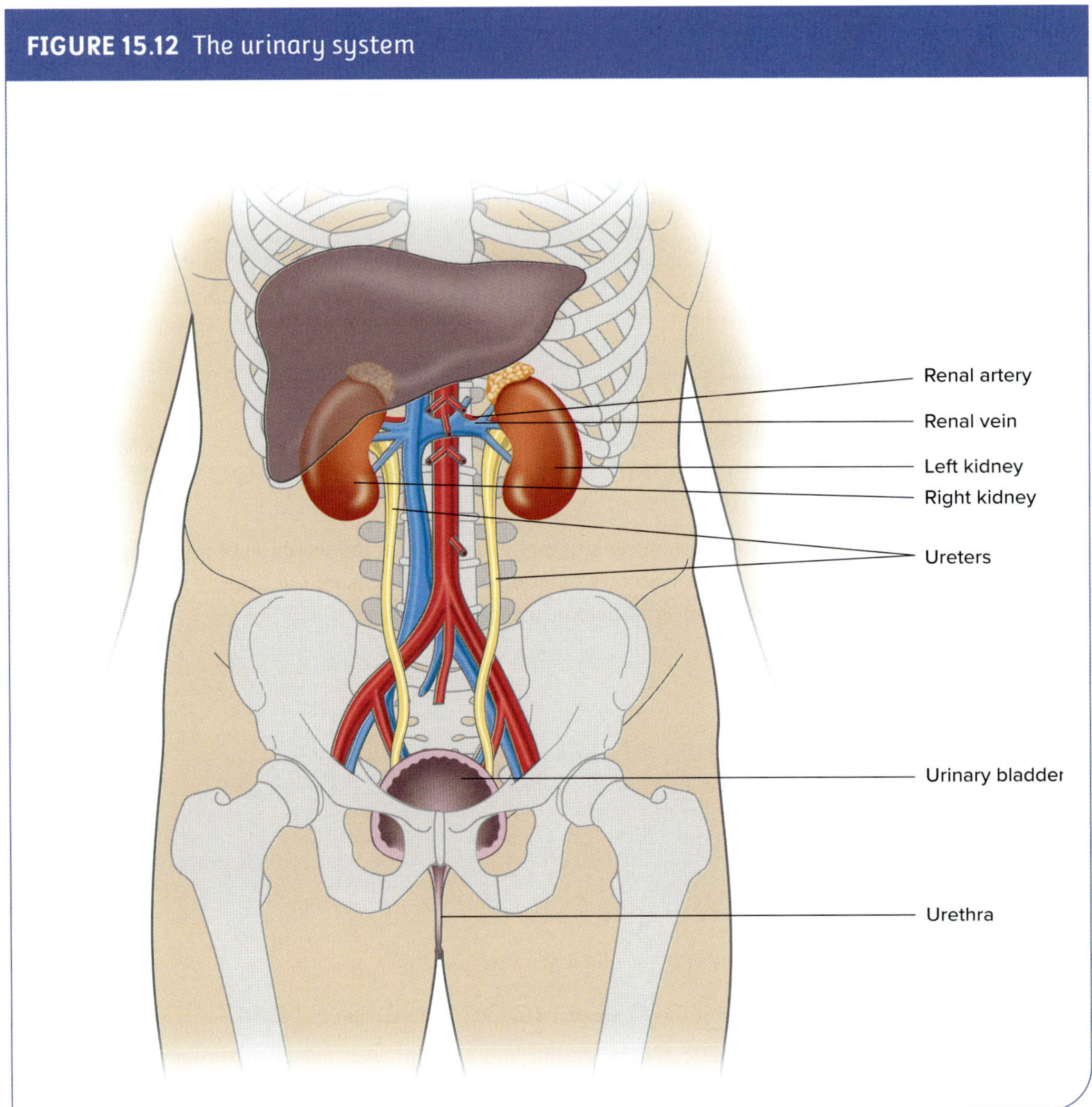

NORMAL STRUCTURE AND FUNCTION

The two kidneys are located high in the abdominal cavity, posterior to the lungs, the liver and the spleen, and are protected by the ribs. The cells in the kidneys–nephrons–filter the blood, reabsorb nutrients, and secrete chemicals and salts in waste known as urine.

The ureters extend from each kidney to the bladder. Urine produced by the kidneys flows from the kidneys where it is stored in the bladder. The bladder is a hollow sac located in the abdominopelvic cavity. The average volume of the bladder is 300–450 mL; at approximately 250 mL, nerve impulses send messages to the brain that it is time for the bladder to empty. Sphincter muscles around the bladder and the urethra hold and control the release of urine.

In males, the urethra is approximately 20 cm long and has the dual function of transporting urine from the bladder and semen from the posterior of the testicles. In females, the urethra is approximately 4 cm long. The opening of the urethra in males is on the tip of the penis; in females, it is in front of the vagina and between the labia minora.

MAINTAINING HEALTHY FUNCTIONING OF THE URINARY SYSTEM

Healthy functioning of the urinary system is important in maintaining the elimination of wastes from the body and maintaining fluid and chemical balance. To ensure the healthy functioning of the urinary system, the following risk factors should be avoided or managed:

- a family history of kidney disease
- structural problems such as a "dropped" kidney
- diseases such as diabetes and hypertension
- recurrent infections
- injury
- medications
- substance abuse.

Strategies to prevent infection and inflammation of tissues include:

- maintaining hydration
- treating vaginal infections promptly
- practising good hygiene—after voiding and/or a bowel movement, wiping from the front to the back of the perineal area (i.e. from the urethra towards the anus) to avoid transferring material from the anus to the vagina and/or urethra
- emptying the bladder immediately after intercourse
- emptying the bladder regularly.

REPORTING CHANGES TO THE URINARY SYSTEM

Changes to the functioning of the urinary system that should be reported include:

- a general feeling of being unwell
- a fever
- changes to the urine—odour, colour, clarity, volume
- changes to the frequency and urgency of urination (passing urine)
- back pain
- abdominal pain
- blood in the urine
- confusion (a common sign in an older person).

15.1.11 The nervous system and the senses

The nervous system is made up of the brain, the spinal cord and the nerves. It is responsible for the special senses: hearing, balance, vision, taste and smell, and for the general senses: touch, pain, temperature, position and pressure. There are two main divisions in the nervous system: the central nervous system (CNS) and the peripheral nervous system (PNS) (see Figure 15.13). The nervous system has three functions.

- **Sensory function**—receiving information from the senses.
- Interpretive function—processing this information.
- **Motor function**—transmitting this information throughout the body.

FIGURE 15.13 The nervous system

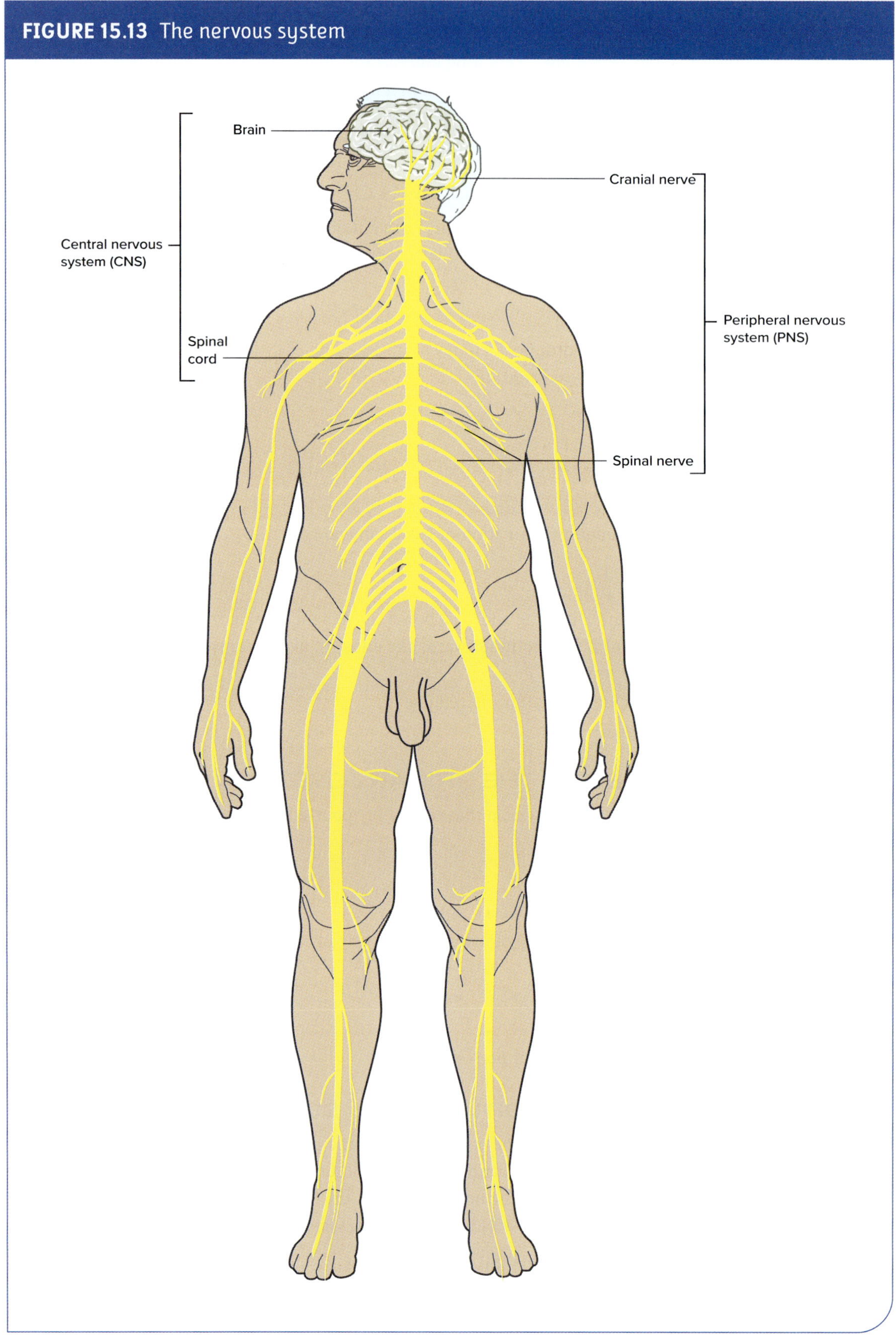

NORMAL STRUCTURE AND FUNCTION OF THE NERVOUS SYSTEM

THE CENTRAL NERVOUS SYSTEM

The brain is encased in the bones of the skull and controls all systems of the body. The brain consists of three main areas:

- The *cerebrum* is the largest part of the brain. It is responsible for conscious thought, voluntary muscle movement, the senses and complex thought processes. The cerebrum is divided into two hemispheres (left and right). Each hemisphere is divided into lobes, which are responsible for various functions, such as walking, speaking and hearing.
- The *cerebellum* is located at the back and base of the brain. The cerebellum controls and coordinates voluntary muscle movement and helps maintain balance and muscle tone.
- The *brain stem* is located at the front of the cerebellum, at the base of the brain, and is connected to the spinal cord (see Figure 15.14). The structures within the brain stem relay information between the brain and the spinal cord and are responsible for involuntary functions such as breathing, digestion, the heartbeat and blood pressure.

The spinal cord lies in a canal surrounded by vertebrae. Two types of spinal nerves enter and leave the spinal cord between the vertebrae: the sensory nerves carry information from the body to the brain, and motor nerves carry information from the brain to the body.

FIGURE 15.14 The brain

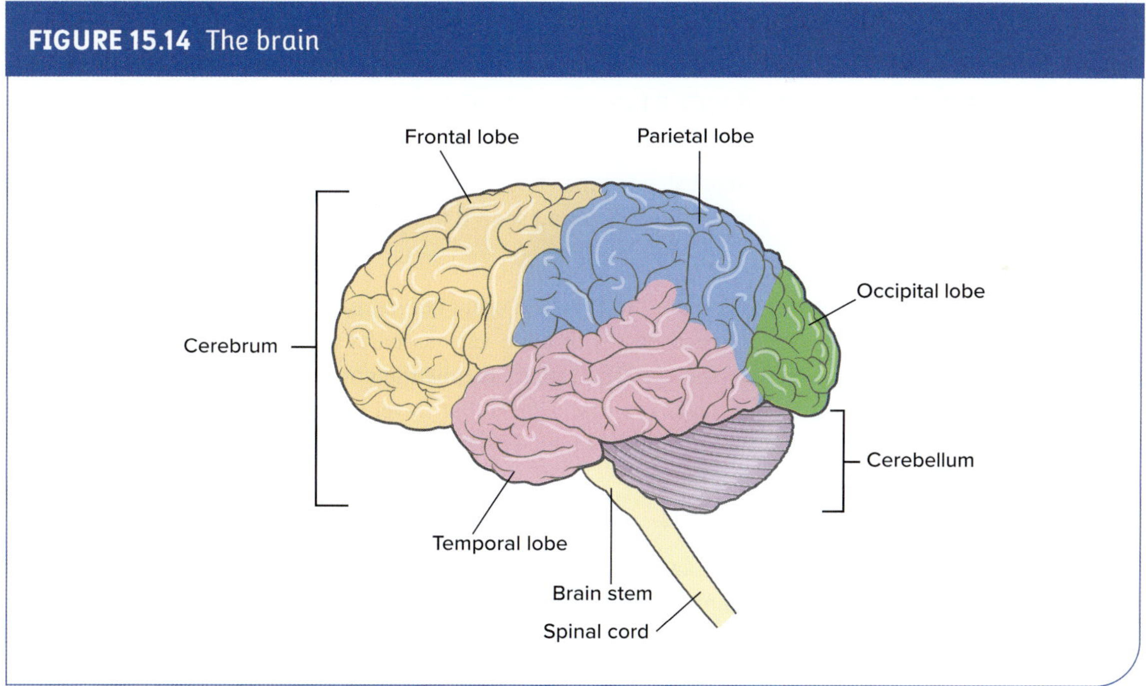

THE PERIPHERAL NERVOUS SYSTEM

The peripheral nervous system contains the nerves that lie outside the central nervous system (see Figure 15.13). There are three sets of nerves:

- The first set controls voluntary muscle movement.
- The second set controls automatic functions such as the heart rate and digestion.
- The third set receives messages from the senses and sends this information to the brain.

Nerves are made up of cell fibres called neurons. Chemicals send messages along nerves and are transferred in milliseconds. The endocrine system works with the nervous system to convey messages to the brain and throughout the body.

MAINTAINING HEALTHY FUNCTIONING OF THE NERVOUS SYSTEM

As the nervous system controls all body functions, maintaining healthy functioning of the nervous system is essential to maintaining the health of the whole body. To ensure the healthy functioning of the nervous system, the following risk factors should be avoided or managed:

- substance abuse
- exposure to toxins
- hereditary factors
- hypertension
- poor diet
- stress
- depression.

REPORTING CHANGES TO THE NERVOUS SYSTEM

Changes to the functioning of the nervous system that should be reported include:

- altered sensation
- loss of balance
- changes to speech or vision
- changes to movement and mobility
- altered mood.

NORMAL STRUCTURE AND FUNCTION OF THE SPECIAL SENSES

The special senses include vision, hearing, balance, smell and taste and function in specific areas of the body. The senses receive information from the environment and send it to the brain for interpretation.

VISION

The main structures responsible for vision are the eyes, the optic nerves and the visual cortex of the brain. The eyes receive light from an object which passes through various parts of the eye, including the pupil, lens and retina, which is at the back of the eye. The retina absorbs the colours and light properties of the projected image and converts these messages to nerve signals that travel to the brain via the optic nerve to be interpreted by the visual cortex at the back of the brain. The eyebrows, eyelashes, eyelids, conjunctiva and tear ducts are the accessory structures of the eye.

HEARING AND BALANCE

The structures of hearing and balance are the ears, auditory nerve and auditory cortex of the brain. The ear receives sounds that travel through the ear to the eardrum, which vibrates and passes these vibrations into the cavity of the inner ear. Vibrations are sent as messages via the auditory nerve to the brain where sound is interpreted. The inner ear also contains tiny organs that detect head movement and gravity and thereby our sense of balance.

SMELL

At the top of the nasal cavity are receptors that detect chemicals in the air and send messages to the brain for interpretation as particular smells. The sense of smell is closely linked to the sense of taste, and both smell and taste stimulate the appetite and the flow of digestive juices.

TASTE

There are five primary taste sensations: sweet, salty, sour, bitter and savoury. The receptors for taste are found in papillae on the tongue, within the oral cavity and in the upper two-thirds of the oesophagus. Microscopic hairs on the tongue send messages about the flavour of food to the brain, where different tastes are perceived.

THE GENERAL SENSES

The **general senses** include touch, pain, temperature, position and pressure. Receptors (nerve endings) for the general senses are located throughout the body in the skin, muscles and most organs.

MAINTAINING HEALTHY FUNCTIONING OF THE SENSES

To ensure the healthy functioning of the senses, the following risk factors should be avoided or managed:

- hereditary factors
- long-term exposure to strong UV light
- pollutants
- diseases such as diabetes and infections such as meningitis
- medications
- trauma and injury infection
- burns.

REPORTING CHANGES TO THE SENSES

Changes to the functioning of the special senses that should be reported include:

- any changes to vision
- hearing loss, loss of balance
- tinnitus (ringing in the ears)
- changes to taste and smell
- signs of infection, such as discharge from the eyes, ears or nose; swelling or redness in the eyes; pain in the eyes or ears.

Changes to the functioning of the general senses that should be reported include:

- decreased sensation in the skin
- reduced responsiveness to temperature and pressure
- pain
- damage to the skin.

15.1.12 The lymphatic and immune systems

The lymphatic system is made up of a series of vessels, nodes, capillaries, ducts and organs throughout the body. It is important for draining excess fluid from the tissues, assisting with fat absorption, and fighting against infection and disease. The immune system is a set of defences that includes various barriers and reactions to the presence of harmful microorganisms and disease-causing cells. The lymphatic and immune systems work together to protect the body from disease and illness.

NORMAL STRUCTURE AND FUNCTION OF THE LYMPHATIC SYSTEM

The main structures of the lymphatic system are the spleen, lymph nodes and vessels, thymus and tonsils (see Figure 15.15). The lymphatic system contains lymph and lymphocytes.

- The spleen is in the abdomen near the pancreas and acts as a filter for the blood.
- Lymph nodes and vessels are in various parts of the body, such as in the groin and the abdomen. The nodes filter microorganisms and abnormal cells such as cancer. The vessels contain lymph and run throughout the body adjacent to the blood vessels, transporting excess fluid from the tissues to the general circulation and assisting with fat absorption.

FIGURE 15.15 The lymphatic system

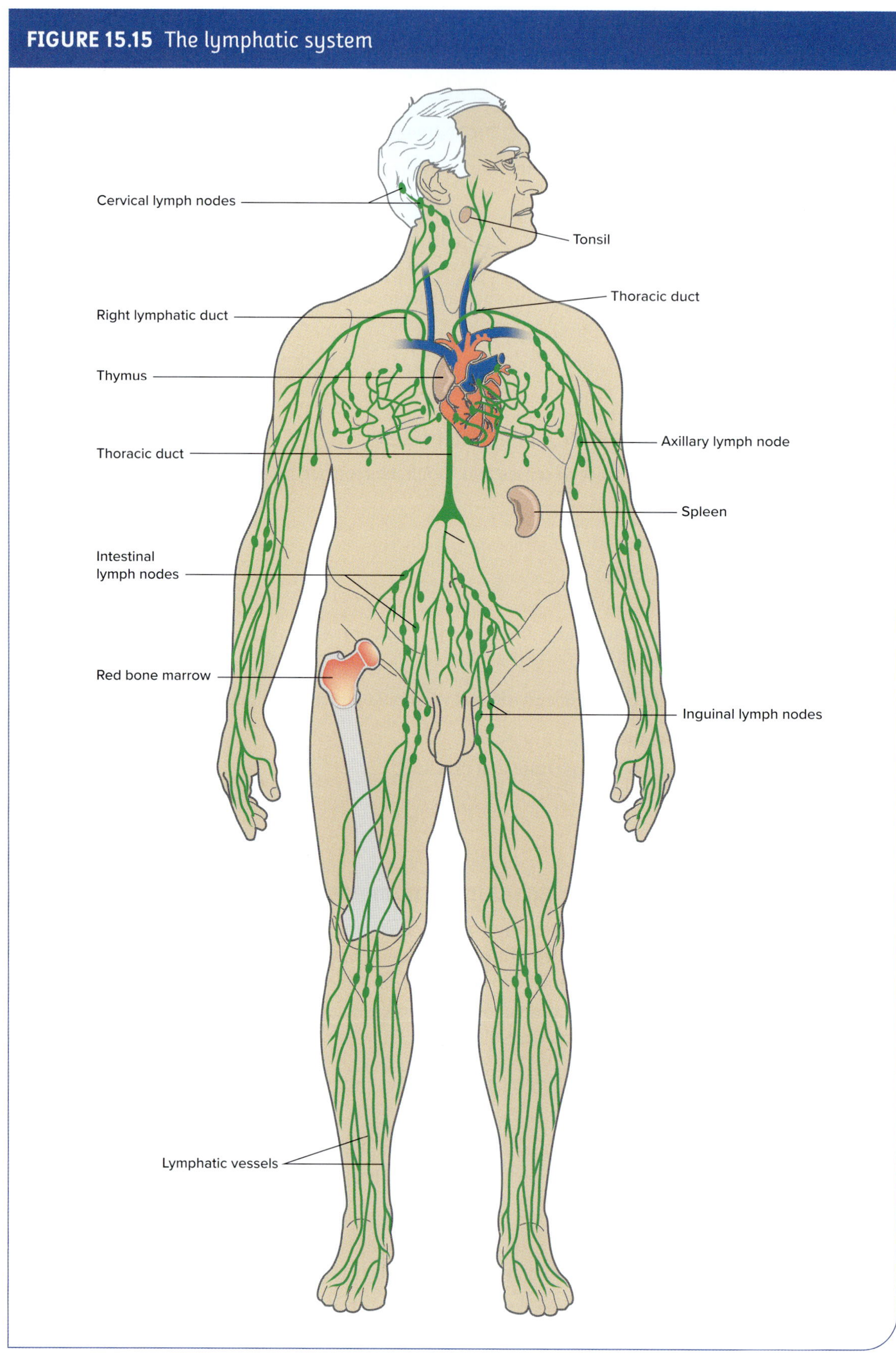

- Lymph is a fluid-like plasma that travels through the lymph nodes, ducts and vessels adjacent to the blood vessels. Lymph contains lymphocytes that are produced in the bone marrow and are important for fighting infection.
- The thymus is in the thoracic cavity and produces certain lymphocytes that fight infection.
- The tonsils are in the throat and contain white cells that fight infection.

NORMAL STRUCTURE AND FUNCTION OF THE IMMUNE SYSTEM

The immune system is made up of three barriers and reactions that protect the body against microorganisms and disease. These are best understood as lines of defence and include the following:

- The presence of barriers:
    - mechanical barriers, such as intact mucous membranes and skin
    - chemical barriers, such as tears and saliva
    - reflexes such as coughing.
- The body's response to invading microorganisms such as the actions of cells that ingest bacteria, the process of inflammation and the presence of a fever.
- The action of lymphocytes and antibodies that act directly on invading microorganisms and provide the body with **immunity**, which is the body's ability to defend itself against disease and infection.

MAINTAINING HEALTHY FUNCTIONING OF THE LYMPHATIC AND IMMUNE SYSTEMS

To ensure the healthy functioning of the lymphatic and immune systems, the following risk factors should be avoided or managed:

- exposure to radiation, smoking and chemicals
- burns
- infection
- medications
- trauma and injury.

REPORTING CHANGES TO THE LYMPHATIC AND IMMUNE SYSTEMS

Changes to the functioning of the lymphatic and immune systems that should be reported include:

- any excessive swelling (e.g. in the hands and feet)
- recurrent infections
- wounds that are slow to heal.

15.1.13 The reproductive system

The reproductive system becomes active at puberty in response to the production of hormones that determine the processes of reproduction, the development of secondary sex characteristics and the expression of sexuality.

NORMAL STRUCTURE AND FUNCTION OF THE FEMALE REPRODUCTIVE SYSTEM

The female reproductive system is in the pelvic cavity (see Figure 15.16). The main structures of the female reproductive system include the following:

- Internal organs and tissues:
    - The female egg cells (ovum) are formed in the ovaries and are released in response to the hormones oestrogen and progesterone. This is known as ovulation.

FIGURE 15.16 The male and female reproductive systems

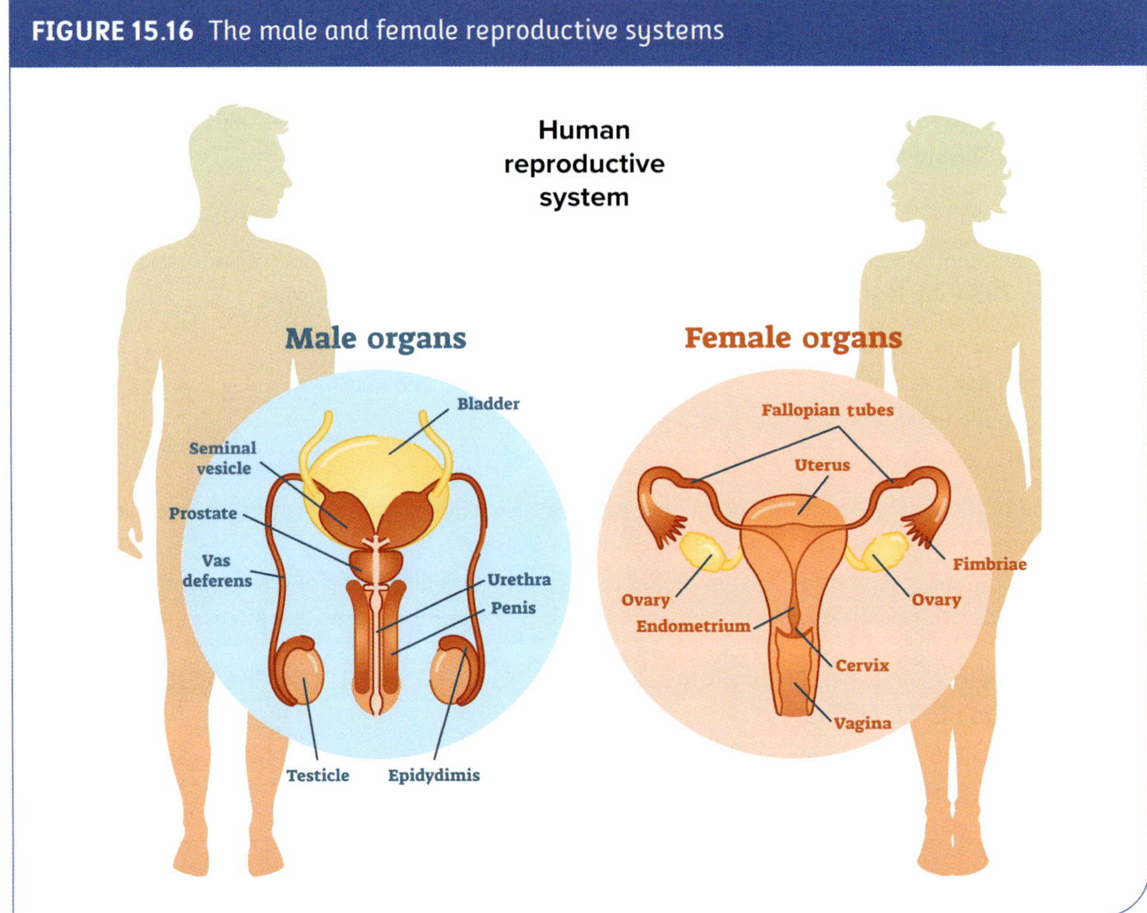

Source: normaals/123RF

- The fallopian tube transports the ovum to the uterus. Conception usually occurs in the fallopian tube.
- The uterus is a hollow organ, the lining of which sheds each month in response to the presence of hormones. This is known as menstruation. A fertilised ovum embeds in the lining of the uterus, which expands to allow for the development, growth and birth of the foetus. If fertilisation doesn't take place, the ovum passes through the uterus.
- The cervix is the opening between the uterus and the vagina.
- The vagina is a tube that extends from the cervix to the perineum. The vaginal opening lies between the urethra and the anus.

- The breasts are secondary female sex organs and increase in size and change shape at puberty due to hormonal changes. The breasts contain glands that produce milk to feed and nourish a baby.
- External organs and tissues:
    - mons pubis
    - clitoris
    - urethra
    - vagina
    - labia.

NORMAL STRUCTURE AND FUNCTION OF THE MALE REPRODUCTIVE SYSTEM

The male reproductive system is in the pelvic cavity (see Figure 15.16). The main structures of the male reproductive system include the following:

- Internal organs and tissues:
  - The testes are two egg-shaped organs that contain sperm and the cells that produce testosterone.
  - The urethra is a tube that transports both urine and semen.
  - The prostate gland surrounds the urethra and secretes a fluid that enhances the movement of sperm.
  - The vas deferens is a duct that transfers sperm to the urethra.
  - Erectile tissue surrounds the urethra and engorges with blood to maintain an erection.
- External organs and tissues:
  - The penis is the organ of reproduction and urination.
  - The prepuce or foreskin is a layer of skin covering the glans penis at the head of the penis.
  - The glans penis is the cap-shaped end of the penis.

MAINTAINING HEALTHY FUNCTIONING OF THE REPRODUCTIVE SYSTEM

To ensure the healthy functioning of the reproductive system in males and females, the following risk factors should be avoided or managed:

- hereditary factors
- exposure to heavy metals
- radiation
- infections, including sexually transmitted infections
- substance abuse
- pathological conditions such as fibroids and prostatic hypertrophy
- some medications
- trauma.

REPORTING CHANGES TO THE REPRODUCTIVE SYSTEM

Changes in females to report include:

- changes to breast tissue–shape, size, skin thickening or dimpling
- breast pain
- discharge from the nipple
- vaginal discharge
- vaginal bleeding
- changes to the external genitalia, including the presence of lesions and changes in the colour of the mucosa.

Changes in males to report include:

- changes to the patterns of urination
- painful ejaculation
- decrease in libido
- reduced ability to achieve or maintain an erection
- lower back pain
- persistent urinary tract infections.

WORKPLACE SCENARIO

The interdependence of the human body

Al, who has cardiovascular disease, sometimes finds it difficult to breathe, especially while in the shower. One morning while assisting Al in the shower, care worker Huong notices that Al is bluish around the lips. He is also breathing rapidly and says he feels dizzy. Huong stops the shower and assists Al to a chair outside the bathroom while asking a colleague to get the team leader, Sony. Sony helps Al to apply an oxygen mask, turns the oxygen on low and takes his pulse, respirations and blood pressure, and his oxygen saturations. When Al's breathing returns to normal, Sony checks his pulse and blood pressure again and asks Huong to continue with Al's personal care. Huong knows that Al has cardiovascular disease and later asks Sony why Al was bluish around the lips as well as dizzy. Sony explains that even though the cardiovascular system transports blood, it is dependent on the respiratory system to supply oxygen to the red blood cells carried in the blood. When the heart isn't working properly, oxygen cannot get to the cells as efficiently. This affects the brain (making Al feel dizzy), the tissues (making Al's lips bluish) and the lungs (making Al breathe rapidly to try to make up for a lack oxygen). Sony thanks Huong for reporting the incident and asks her to add the information to Al's records.

CHECK YOUR UNDERSTANDING

1. List four changes to the cardiovascular system that should be reported immediately.
2. What are three changes to the respiratory system that need to be reported immediately?
3. What is the muscular system responsible for?
4. List four changes to the functioning of the urinary system that should be reported immediately.
5. The nervous system is the control centre of the body. What are three changes to the nervous system that should be reported immediately?

15.2 RECOGNISING AND PROMOTING WAYS TO SUPPORT HEALTHY FUNCTIONING OF THE BODY

15.2.1 Healthy functioning

Healthy functioning of the body is dependent on several factors and in general include a balanced diet, physical exercise and activity, social engagement, and managing risk factors such as poor nutrition, exposure to toxins, substance abuse, a sedentary lifestyle, obesity, chronic disease, infections and trauma. Managing stress, getting sufficient and regular sleep, managing pain and the impact of normal changes in the body related to ageing are also important in maintaining **health**. The diagnosis, treatment and management of disease and illness, plus consideration of social factors such as income, adequate and stable housing, connections to family and friends, and intimacy, support healthy functioning as well, especially into old age.

HOMEOSTASIS

Homeostasis is a term used to describe the way in which the body maintains a stable internal environment. Homeostasis is an active and constant process whereby the body systems work together enabling the body to respond to stresses and adapt to changes in the environment, both internal and external. When the ability of the body to maintain homeostasis is disturbed or disrupted, illness and disease can occur.

There are many examples of homeostasis: when the body temperature increases and shivering commences, the body is trying to lower the temperature and bring it back to normal by dilating the blood vessels to get rid of excess heat; when blood glucose rises, the pancreas releases more insulin to bring blood glucose back to normal.

DISEASE PROCESSES

There are numerous causes of disease, including hereditary factors, lifestyle, injury and trauma, infection, the environment, degenerative factors and abnormal cell growth. Ageing results in changes to the body that increase the risk of and/or the severity of certain conditions. These are summarised in Table 15.5.

TABLE 15.5 Factors that cause a condition, a disease or an illness

Factor	The process	Examples
Heredity	A malformed gene is inherited from the parents	Huntington's chorea Cystic fibrosis
Lifestyle	Lifestyle choices place a person at risk of developing a disease (e.g. smoking and obesity)	Cardiovascular disease Diabetes type 2
Trauma	An accident or injury occurs	Psychological: post-traumatic stress disorder Physical: spinal damage, leading to tetraplegia
Infection	Disease-causing microorganisms are transmitted between people, between species or from one part of the body to another	Pneumonia COVID-19 Dengue fever Thrush
Environment	The person is exposed to toxins in the environment, such as lead and asbestos	Liver disease Lung disease
Degeneration	Parts of the body change and function is lost over time	Osteoarthritis
Abnormal cell changes	Cells are damaged and grow at an abnormal rate, sometimes spreading elsewhere in the body	Lung cancer (spreads or metastasises to the brain)
Ageing	Cells throughout the body may change or deteriorate	The ability to see objects at close distance deteriorates The older body cannot automatically control blood pressure as effectively

PAIN AND DISCOMFORT

Pain is an unpleasant sensation and is often described as aching, stabbing, throbbing or burning. The way in which a person perceives pain depends on several factors, including its cause, their prior experience of pain, their culture and expectations, anxiety level, and the type and level of support available during episodes of pain.

Pain may be associated with a disease or a condition, and has both physical and psychological components, ranging in severity from mild to severe. Pain may be acute (short term) or chronic (long term) or acute on chronic–that is, a sudden, short-term pain that occurs amid chronic pain. The effects of pain include:

- reduced function
- loss of sleep

- anxiety
- reduced appetite
- depression
- social isolation
- loss of independence and self-esteem.

ASSESSING PAIN

Assessing a person's experience and level of pain is difficult. Common signs and symptoms of pain include:

- changes in facial expression
- changes in posture
- moaning
- pale, clammy skin
- restlessness
- crying
- flinching
- reluctance or inability to move
- shallow breathing.

There are several pain assessment tools, such as the Numerical Rating Scale, the Faces Rating Scale and the Abbey Pain Scale (used for people with dementia). Each tool aims to identify various aspects of pain: its character, intensity, location, onset, duration and causes, and its impact on the person. No matter what tool is used, the care worker needs to obtain sufficient information by both observation and questioning, and report this information to the registered nurse or supervisor.

PAIN MANAGEMENT

Well-managed pain contributes to a person's overall health and sense of wellbeing and improves their quality of life by improving sleep and activity levels plus appetite and ability to engage with others.

Medications that provide pain relief are known as analgesics and provide the most common and consistent pain relief. The specific type of analgesic prescribed will depend on the various aspects of pain the person is experiencing, what other medications they are taking, and whether they are at risk of having side effects or an adverse reaction to the medication.

The care worker can use various alternative management strategies, such as the following, to assist a person to manage their pain:

- Have a calm manner.
- Avoid rushing the person as they attempt to move or to mobilise.
- Observe and report the person for activities or times of day that change their level of pain.
- Assist the person to reposition.
- Use cold/heat packs or warm baths to alleviate pain and promote comfort according to facility policy.
- Provide emotional support.

Other management strategies include:

- massage
- pet therapy

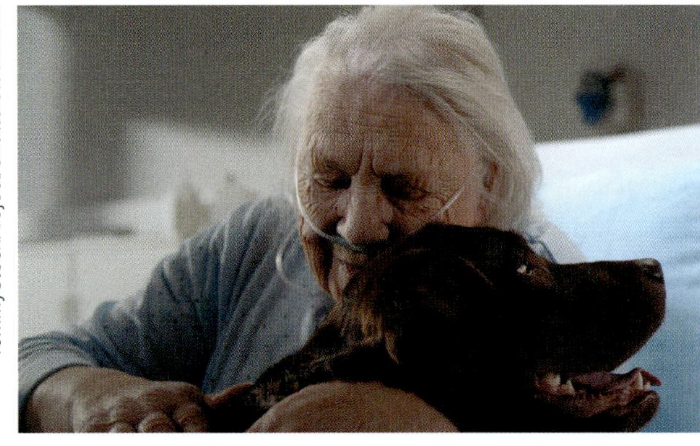
TommyStockProject/Shutterstock.com

Pet therapy can be used as a pain management strategy

- music therapy
- hydrotherapy
- acupuncture
- physiotherapy.

15.2.2 Factors that contribute to health

Many strategies contribute to healthy functioning. Some of these have been mentioned previously in this chapter and are related to lifestyle choices such as avoiding substance abuse and smoking. Others require active decision making and engagement and include practising good oral and personal hygiene, having adequate exercise and movement, eating nutritious meals, ensuring sufficient comfort, rest and sleep, and undertaking measures to prevent infection.

ORAL HYGIENE

Oral hygiene and dental care are important for a person's sense of wellbeing and to prevent infection. Poor oral health contributes to bad breath, bleeding gums and loss of teeth, lowering the person's self-esteem as well as contributing to poor nutrition. Bacteria in the mouth can increase rapidly, causing tooth decay and inflammation of the gums. Plaque can enter the airways and bloodstream, leading to pneumonia; infections in the heart, kidneys and digestive tract; and lowered overall immunity.

PERSONAL HYGIENE

Personal hygiene is important for comfort, health and safety and includes showering, bathing and grooming. Showering removes bacteria, prevents body odour, stimulates the circulation, and mobilises joints and muscles. For most people, showering and grooming are part of their daily routine, adding to their self-esteem and sense of wellbeing. Many factors impact on the person's hygiene and grooming practices, including cultural and religious practices, their level of independence, whether the use of assistive devices is necessary, and their personal choices regarding the timing and frequency of showering/bathing and grooming.

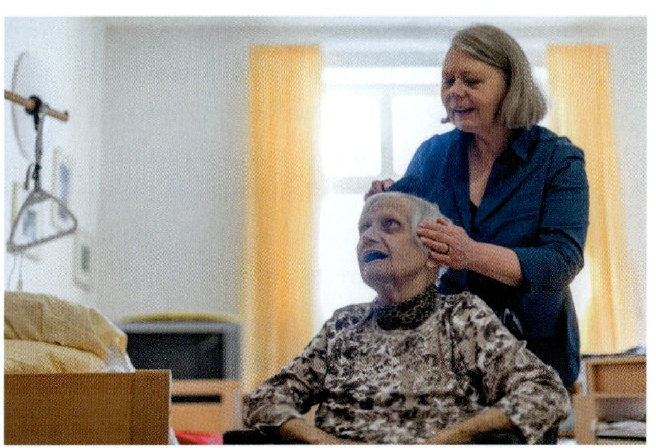

Westend61/Oliver Marquardt/Image Source

Personal hygiene is important for comfort, health and safety

EXERCISE AND MOVEMENT

Exercise and movement are important for maintaining health and for preventing several illnesses and diseases. Everyday physical activity, varying in intensity, is an ideal and builds strength, maintains balance, helps to prevent falls and has a positive impact on the nervous system and the cardiovascular system, among others. Regular physical activity enhances digestion and promotes wellbeing. Exercise contributes to bone health and better sleep patterns and can provide an opportunity for social interaction.

NUTRITION

A balanced diet is important because the body requires a variety of nutrients to maintain healthy functioning. A balanced diet includes varying amounts of carbohydrates, protein, fats, vitamins, minerals and water. Salt, sugar, saturated and trans fats, and alcohol should be limited, while water is needed to support digestion and urinary function. As a person ages, they require increased calcium and vitamin D to prevent osteopenia and osteoporosis. Weight should be managed to prevent the pain that accompanies arthritis. Overall, eating should be enjoyable and can improve mood.

ADEQUATE REST

Comfort, rest and sleep are essential to maintain healthy functioning.

- Comfort is a state of wellbeing due to an absence of physical and psychological pain.
- Rest is a state of feeling relaxed and calm.
- **Sleep** is a specific state that occurs on a cyclical basis and is necessary for repair and regeneration in various body systems, including the nervous and integumentary systems. When a person is comfortable and rested, their quality of life improves, as does their ability to participate in activities. Fatigue and pain significantly and negatively impact a person's energy, motivation and mental health. Sleep is promoted by practising a sleep routine, by being comfortable and rested, and by being free from distractions and from pain.

PREVENTING INFECTION

Older adults are more susceptible to infection as they have lowered immunity. In both a personal environment and in residential aged care, the following measures are necessary to prevent the spread of infection:

- Regularly wash and dry the hands.
- Employ "respiratory" or "cough etiquette" (see Chapter 16) by coughing into the elbow, disposing of single-use tissues and washing the hands.
- Use gloves when cleaning surfaces.
- Maintain a clean and tidy environment.
- Maintain good personal hygiene.
- Dispose of wastes appropriately.
- Store and prepare food safely.
- Access medical advice in the event of an infection.
- Maintain immunisations against contagious diseases.
- Avoid overuse of antibiotics.

15.2.3 Communicating information about health

Communications skills–verbal, non-verbal, written and digital–are critical to performing work safely and providing excellent care and support. Communicating with a person in our care requires us to understand their needs and preferences and to focus on them, as an individual. It also requires the care worker to understand the body and what changes should be observed and reported, how and to whom. Accurate documentation ensures the person's best interests are addressed in all areas.

COMMUNICATING WITH THE OLDER PERSON

When discussing a person's health, it is necessary to consider:

- your role and scope of practice
- professional boundaries
- your lines of reporting
- clarity and accuracy
- minimising the use of jargon
- active listening
- showing empathy
- providing feedback
- confidentiality and privacy.

Information should be kept simple and clear, and concerns should be discussed with the supervisor. The use of concrete examples such as "Where is the pain?", "Is your skin itchy?" and "Do you feel sick in the stomach?" can be useful. It is important to listen to all of a person's concerns, as well as to those of their carer and family, both to convey respect and empathy and to avoid missing something critical.

CULTURAL AWARENESS IN COMMUNICATION

Cultural awareness in communication requires care staff to be sensitive to the differences between cultures. Some of these differences include:

- language
- interpretations of pain
- the level of family involvement in a decision
- variations in diet and beliefs about illness and treatment.

Taking these differences into account may assist in identifying specific health and care issues and contribute to accurate reporting.

COMMUNICATING WITH COLLEAGUES AND SUPERVISORS

Communicating with colleagues and supervisors involves being able to accurately interpret and follow instructions and to work together as a team. Standards, guidelines, policies and procedures must be understood in order to fulfil work roles and responsibilities and to meet compliance requirements. Asking questions clarifies issues and ensures everyone knows what is expected of them. Communication should be respectful and consider professional boundaries and appropriate workplace behaviour.

15.2.4 Recording health information

Most organisations use computerised records and care staff log-in to record information. Records can take several forms, including the care plan, test results, checklists, medical practitioner notes, allied health team notes and funding information. Some items will be standardised, depending on the size of the organisation, and some will be specific to the person and to the staff.

Accurate documentation should:

- be concise, clear and progressive
- include information about observations and assessments, care and outcomes, plus risks and changes to health and behaviour
- meet legal requirements.

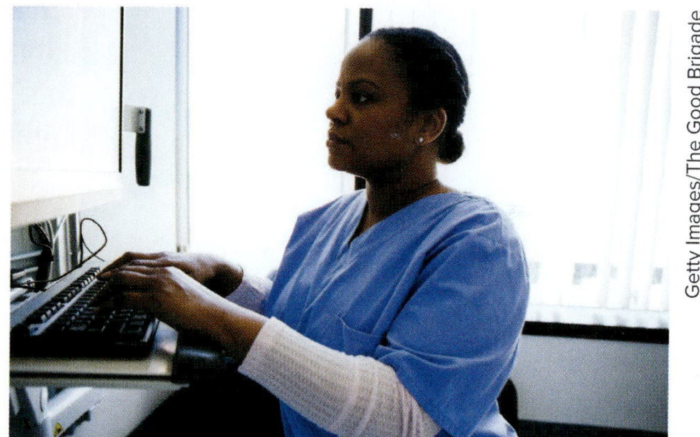

Getty Images/The Good Brigade

Most organisations use computerised records to record information

Other computerised systems include the facility's incident management system and the provider portal (via My Aged Care).

15.2.5 Processes and resources to support health

In addition to changes that should be reported to support a person to maintain their health, observations of various processes are required, including body temperature, fluid balance, blood pressure and elimination. All these observations require specialised equipment and are recorded on specific forms and checklists.

BODY TEMPERATURE

Body temperature normally ranges between 36.0 and 37.2 degrees Celsius. The body has natural mechanisms for regulating temperature, including shivering (where blood vessels constrict to reduce heat loss) and sweating (where blood vessels dilate to increase heat loss). Body temperature increases in the presence of an infection as the body fights microorganisms by initiating an immune response, making the internal environment less favourable to the invading microorganisms. Occasionally body temperature will rise above 40 degrees Celsius, which can result in seizures and delirium.

HYDRATION AND DEHYDRATION: FLUID BALANCE

The balance of fluid in the body (**hydration**) should remain constant, otherwise dehydration or overhydration will occur, disrupting the movement of fluids and electrolytes throughout the body and resulting in confusion and/or changes to the heart rhythm. The average intake of fluid per day is 2400 mL and the main regulator of fluid intake is thirst. The average output of water per day is 2500 mL and occurs via the kidneys, the skin, the digestive tract and the lungs. Dehydration is not uncommon and can occur because of vomiting, diarrhoea and excessive sweating, such as occurs in a fever. A fluid balance chart is a record of a person's daily fluid input and output.

BLOOD PRESSURE

Blood pressure is the force exerted by the blood against the walls of the arteries when the heart contracts. Normal blood pressure is 120/80 mmHg and maintaining normal blood pressure is very important to the overall health of the body. When blood pressure is too low, blood flow to vital organs decreases, potentially compromising their function. When blood pressure is too high, the blood vessels may burst, leading to a stroke and resulting in loss of functions such as speech and movement. Persistently high blood pressure is known as hypertension and can result in damage to the kidneys, resulting in a loss of function and damage to the retina, leading to loss of vision. Together with temperature, blood pressure is one of the "vital signs" and both observations are recorded on a specific chart, often with the respiratory rate and the percentage of oxygen in the blood.

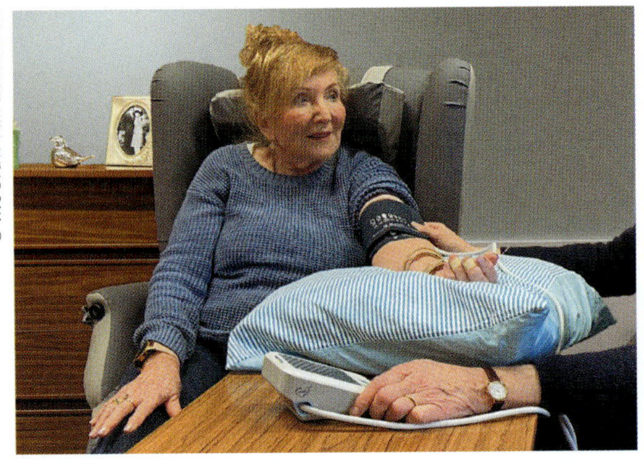

Blood pressure observations should be recorded on a specific chart

ELIMINATION

Elimination is the process by which wastes in the form of faeces are expelled from the rectum via the anus. Faeces are composed of non-digestible food residue or fibre, electrolytes and water; they form a stool or bowel movement, accumulating in the large intestine and moving to the rectum, to be expelled via the anus. The urge to defecate occurs via messages sent by nerves within the sphincter muscles. Faeces that remain in the large intestine for too long lose water and become dry and hard, resulting in constipation. Rapid movement of faeces through the large intestine allows insufficient time for the reabsorption of water and results in diarrhoea. Both constipation and diarrhoea are uncomfortable and often painful and may require medications to resolve. Any loss of control of bowel movements is known as incontinence and may be caused by poor mobility, low fluid intake, low fibre intake, nerve damage or medications. Bowel movements should be observed and recorded each day specifically on a bowel chart. The observations on a bowel chart include the frequency, colour and consistency of faeces, which indicate healthy functioning or a need for further observation, assessment and intervention.

RESOURCES

Information about promoting and maintaining health is available through My Aged Care and organisations such as COTA (Council of the Ageing), Dementia Australia, the Department of Veterans Affairs, and the federal and state health departments. General practitioners (GPs) can refer a person over the age of 65 who is subject to complex health problems and may be at risk of poor health outcomes to a specialist geriatrician, who will conduct health assessments and provide a report to the referring GP who will manage their treatment. GPs can also support individuals with chronic diseases by preparing a Chronic Disease Management Plan and Team Care Arrangements specific to the person's needs. Both these assessments are funded by Medicare. In residential aged care facilities, people can access similar resources, as well as those provided by the organisation, such as exercise classes, physiotherapy, diversional therapy, and support for people with dementia and their carers.

WORKPLACE SCENARIO

Maintaining health

Fran has diabetes and is struggling to maintain a healthy weight. She is reluctant to exercise and recently has had an increase in blood glucose levels. Her partner, Joy, is concerned about Fran's health and has asked care staff for advice and support. At a team meeting, the supervisor Sally shares Joy's concerns about Fran's health and asks team members Ceza, Mary, Penny and Olga to share what can be done to encourage Fran to maintain her health.

Ceza says that she encourages Fran to practise good personal hygiene, with particular attention to her feet, to prevent damage to the skin and the possibility of infection.

Mary explains the risk factors associated with diabetes, which include damage to blood vessels that can lead to loss of vision and kidney disease, loss of sensation and chronic wounds. She is concerned that Fran has a small blister on her left heel and says she will reassess it in the morning.

Penny outlines an activity program for Fran and says she has asked Joy to be involved. Fran enjoys looking at flowers, so Penny has devised a walking program that follows a particular route around the facility. Penny has organised another mobility frame for Fran that is safer for negotiating concrete paths.

Olga has discussed Fran's food preferences and revised her diet, considering her love of sweets and dislike of red meat. Olga explains that it is important for Fran to eat what she enjoys and says she will speak to the kitchen staff about the importance of regular meals and sufficient daily protein. She also says that in her plan she will allow for dark chocolate and one piece of fruit per day, plus 1 glass of wine with dinner.

CHECK YOUR UNDERSTANDING

1. What general risks compromise the healthy functioning of the body?
2. William is susceptible to developing infections. What steps would you take to prevent him from getting an infection?
3. What is important when you are communicating with a person in your care about their health?
4. Nina is from Turkey. When you take her to the bathroom, she tells you she has pain in her abdomen. The GP visits and requests that Nina remove her clothes so that he can examine her abdomen. Due to her modesty, Nina refuses. What would you do to support Nina in this situation?
5. What are the common signs and symptoms of pain?

SUMMARY

- The human body is comprised of many complex and interconnected elements. Changes occur throughout the life span because of the ageing process and factors such as illness and disease, the use of medications, exposure to risk factors, and lifestyle choices.
- Body systems are groups of organs that perform a particular function, such as the digestive system. Eleven systems work together to maintain healthy functioning.
- The cardiovascular system contains the heart, blood vessels and blood. Its function is to transport blood to all parts of the body, deliver oxygen and nutrients to cells, and transport waste such as carbon dioxide and salts to the lungs and kidneys. Changes to be reported include breathlessness, and changes to pulse, blood pressure and skin colour.
- The respiratory system contains the nasal and oral cavities, trachea, bronchi, lungs and alveoli. Its function is to transport oxygen and waste to and from the lungs. Changes to be reported include difficulty breathing, increased or decreased respiratory rate, and coughing.
- The muscular system is comprised of three types of muscle: skeletal (allows movement of bones), smooth (allows movement within cavities and organs) and cardiac (allows the heart to pump blood). It also contains the tendons, which connect muscles to bones. Changes to be reported include pain and changes to mobility.
- The skeletal system consists of bones and joints. Its function is to allow movement, protect internal organs, produce blood cells and store calcium. Changes to be reported include deformity of a limb and pain.
- The digestive system contains the mouth, oesophagus, stomach, small and large intestines, rectum and anus. Its function is to ingest and digest food, absorb nutrients and eliminate waste. The system's accessory organs include the liver, gall bladder and pancreas, which excrete substances that aid digestion. Changes to be reported include nausea, vomiting, constipation, diarrhoea and loss of appetite.
- The integumentary system is comprised of the skin, hair and nails. The skin has three layers: epidermis, dermis and subcutaneous layer. Its function is to protect the body against changes in the environment and to regulate body temperature. Changes to be reported include loss of skin integrity, wounds and excessive dryness.
- The endocrine system comprises the glands and the hormones they excrete. Its function is to control and regulate complex functions in the body. Changes to be reported include signs of metabolic variations such as excessive fatigue, unexplained weight gain or loss, excessive thirst, and changes in appetite.
- The urinary system contains the kidneys, ureters, bladder and urethra. Its function is to excrete waste in the form of urine and to regulate fluid and electrolyte levels in the body. Changes to be reported include alterations in the pattern of urination, pain or swelling in the feet, and signs of infection.
- The nervous system consists of the brain, spinal cord and nerves. Its function is to receive messages from the environment via the senses, to interpret and integrate these messages, and to send messages to the glands, muscles and organs. Changes to be reported include alterations to consciousness, confusion, and loss of limb function.
- The five special senses include vision, hearing, balance, smell and taste. The general senses are made up of touch, pain, temperature, position and pressure. The function of all the senses is to send messages from the environment to the brain. Changes to be reported include any loss of vision and hearing.
- The lymphatic system contains lymph and the lymph glands and vessels, plus the lymphocytes. Its function is to regulate the movement of fluid between tissues and the circulatory system and to contribute to fighting infection. The immune system comprises mechanisms that defend the body against disease. Changes to be reported include swelling in the hands and feet, and infection.
- The female reproductive system consists of the ovaries, fallopian tubes, uterus, cervix, vagina, clitoris, labia and breasts. The male reproductive system comprises the testes, urethra, prostate, epididymis, vas deferens, penis and

scrotum. The function of the reproductive system is reproduction and the expression of sexuality. Changes to be reported include unexplained discharge, lumps and changes to the breast and testicular tissue, and inability by a male to pass urine.

- Maintaining the healthy functioning of the body generally involves managing risks that affect most systems, such as hereditary factors, exposure to toxins, substance abuse, the side effects of medications, and trauma.
- As a person ages, it is important to understand and manage age-related changes in the body, and to manage and treat illness, by accessing resources in the health system. It is also necessary to consider the social factors that impact an older person's health, such as housing, income, connection to family and friends, and intimacy.

REVIEW QUESTIONS

15.1 Name three types of cells.

15.2 What organs are found within the abdominopelvic cavity?

15.3 How would you, as a care worker, promote healthy skin?

15.4 Name four processes involved in maintaining healthy body function.

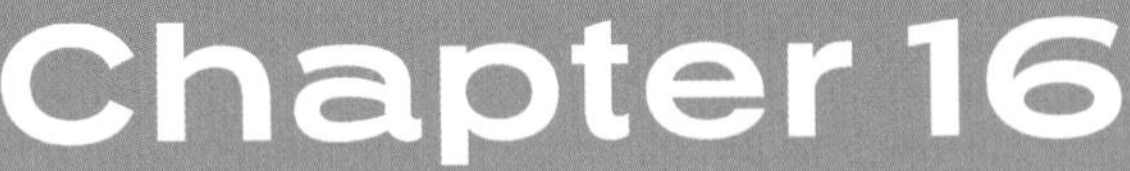

Preventing and controlling infection

LEARNING OBJECTIVES

16.1 Understand standard and transmission-based precautions

16.2 Identify infection hazards and risks

16.3 Manage risks associated with specific hazards

INTRODUCTION

INFECTION PREVENTION AND CONTROL are vital components of the safe provision of support to older people within aged care services. Older people are more likely to experience poor outcomes from infection due to the ageing process and the presence of chronic disease. The risk of infection also increases for older people who reside in a residential aged care facility (RACF) because the transmission risk is higher among communal living environments.

All staff working within government-subsidised aged care services are required to follow infection control and prevention policies and procedures. Care workers can prevent infection and minimise the serious outcomes of infection in the workplace by implementing safe work practices such as standard precautions and, when necessary, transmission-based precautions.

Knowledge of the transmission process of infection is important for developing a solid foundation of practice that includes the identification of the hazards and risks that are associated with infection. Risk minimisation is at the core of infection control and prevention strategies that aim to minimise the risk of infection for older people. Infection control and prevention practices not only protect older people from illnesses; they protect staff, too.

INDUSTRY IN FOCUS

National COVID-19 Aged Care Plan

Infection control and prevention is not a new concept to aged care services. Infection control education is among the mandatory topics in the annual training of RACF staff. RACFs have been following the advice of the government with regards to outbreaks of gastroenteritis and influenza for many years. The global COVID-19 pandemic, however, has presented many challenges to community and residential aged care services around the world. Older people are more likely to experience catastrophic health outcomes or death when they become infected with COVID. Even when vaccinated, older people will struggle to fight COVID due to their ageing immune system and the presence of one or more chronic diseases.

The Commonwealth government of Australia, in collaboration with the state and territory governments and peak industry bodies from the aged care, health and infection control sectors, has developed a *National COVID-19 Aged Care Plan,* at the time of writing in its 7th edition. The plan complements other COVID-19 response protocols and activities around the country and aims to expediate an emergency response to COVID-19 in aged care in a smooth and coordinated manner. The four areas of focus in the plan comprise:

- prevention
- preparedness
- response
- recovery.

The plan maps out the roles and responsibilities for actions under each area of focus. While the Commonwealth and state and territory governments have separate responsibilities, they also have shared responsibilities under the plan. These include ensuring access to personal protective equipment, reporting and surveillance of cases, activation of a surge workforce if needed, and other liaison responsibilities.

Aged care providers have specific responsibilities under the four focal points. They include adhering to the Aged Care Quality Standards, ensuring they have a management plan for COVID that can be activated immediately, working closely with the local Public Health Unit, and maintaining ongoing communication and liaison with all relevant government departments. In addition, aged care providers are required to provide consumers who have experienced and survived COVID-19 with access to government-sponsored opportunities for reablement and healing activities.

The key principles of the plan include:

- the concept of personal dignity, regardless of age
- the right of the older person to have the same protection from COVID as any other person
- the right of the older person to have their mental health and wellbeing maintained
- the right of the older person to have access to the same emergency and medical treatment as other people during the COVID pandemic
- the right of the older person and their family to be provided with information about COVID and the pandemic, and with available supports
- the right of the older person to receive quality care and service delivery according to the Charter of Aged Care Rights
- the right of the aged care workforce who support older people to be respected and supported.

The *National COVID-19 Aged Care Plan* is accessible on the Department of Health and Aged Care website: https://www.health.gov.au/resources/publications.

16.1 STANDARD AND TRANSMISSION-BASED PRECAUTIONS

16.1.1 Standard precautions

Standard precautions are practices that health workers put into place every day at work. Standard precautions are practised within aged care services and in all health settings such as hospitals. The aim of standard precautions is to prevent the transmission of infection between people. They are implemented on a continual basis, whether infection is known to be present or not. The implementation of standard precautions minimises the risk of infection being transmitted between multiple, frail people and health workers. Standard precautions are evidence-based practices that aim to prevent infection and include:

- hand hygiene
- appropriate use of personal protective equipment
- respiratory hygiene, including cough etiquette
- appropriate waste disposal
- sharps disposal and sharps management, including safe use of sharps
- aseptic technique
- routine cleaning and disinfection of the environment
- safe cleaning and reprocessing of reusable medical equipment (including sanitising, disinfecting and sterilising)
- safe linen handling.

Care workers have a duty of care to do everything reasonably practicable to prevent foreseeable harm to the people in their care. The implementation of standard precautions will ensure that workers' duty of care requirements are met.

HAND HYGIENE

Microorganisms are the agents that cause infection and illness among people, and they need a way to get from one person to another (**transmission**). Many microorganisms are transferred between people by touch, and our hands can spread infection to others and even to ourselves. Pathogens such as bacteria and viruses can remain alive and active on surfaces like bedside lockers, door handles and the equipment workers rely on to do their job.

It is essential that care workers wash their hands properly and frequently in order to eliminate pathogens on their hands. Working within aged care services may involve providing support to multiple older people within a shift or another given time frame, and high-contact work practices such as personal care can increase the risk of infection transmission among service users.

Hand hygiene includes effective handwashing procedures that will minimise transmission of pathogens from the hands of the worker and prevent infection from spreading, and includes washing hands with liquid soap and water and using an alcohol hand rub. When the hands are visibly dirty, liquid soap and water should be used. Alcohol hand rub can be used in clinical settings when hands are visibly clean.

PRACTICE POINT

Any alcohol hand rub must contain at least 70 per cent alcohol to be effective. When used several times, the hands may develop a "tacky" feel about them. In this instance, handwashing with liquid soap and water is helpful.

Figures 16.1 and 16.2 demonstrate the steps for effective handwashing using liquid soap or alcohol hand rub, according to the World Health Organization (WHO). When performed correctly, hand hygiene can prevent the cross-contamination of contact microorganisms that cause severe illness in older people. The correct handwashing technique is important to ensure that all parts of the hand, including the fingertips and nails, are clean. Areas most missed in handwashing include the thumb and the fingertips; therefore, it is important to become familiar with the correct technique to ensure that handwashing is effective. The WHO advocates that the process for washing hands with soap and water should take around 30–40 seconds, while hand hygiene with alcohol rub should take around 30 seconds.

Hands should be washed frequently and at prescribed times when working with older people. Care workers who provide support to people in their own home should also attend to hand hygiene in the same manner as those who provide support in an RACF.

Hand hygiene should occur:

- at the start and end of every work shift
- before and after a break
- before and after eating
- before and after smoking
- before and after using the bathroom.

The Australian Commission on Safety and Quality in Health Care and the National Hand Hygiene Initiative have developed the poster "5 Moments for Hand Hygiene" (see Figure 16.3), an Australian approach to the key moments for hand hygiene based on the WHO "My 5 Moments for Hand Hygiene". The "5 Moments" aims to reduce the spread of infectious material between a care worker, the person they are providing care to and the environment in which care is provided. The poster is a good reminder for care workers as to when they should be attending to hand hygiene. The "5 Moments" guidelines are used in many health-care settings, including aged care. In the context of the illustration, "HCW" refers to health-care worker and "patient" refers to the older person who receives aged care services.

HAND CARE

Some microorganisms can find their way into the body via open areas such as wounds, cuts, and even broken and dry skin. Frequent handwashing with antimicrobial substances can leave the hands red and irritated at times, causing dermatitis. Hand care involves self-care practices that ensure the hands are looked after to prevent infection and irritation. These practices include:

- using a daily moisturiser, with a neutral pH, on the hands
- covering any cuts or other open areas according to the workplace policy
- checking the hands at the commencement of work for cuts and open areas
- informing the workplace of skin irritation of the hands
- seeking medical advice for skin irritations on the hands
- not wearing rings and wrist jewellery to work
- keeping fingernails short and clean.

Long fingernails, rings and wrist jewellery (including wristwatches) not only harbour microorganisms, but also pose a risk of injury to older people. Frail skin can be damaged easily, and skin tears are the acute injury of the aged. Skin tears can ulcerate and can easily become infected.

FIGURE 16.1 WHO "How to Handwash?" guidelines

How to Handwash?

WASH HANDS WHEN VISIBLY SOILED! OTHERWISE, USE HANDRUB

Duration of the entire procedure: 40-60 seconds

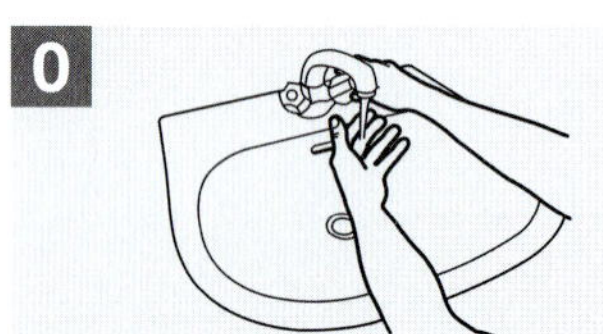

0 Wet hands with water;

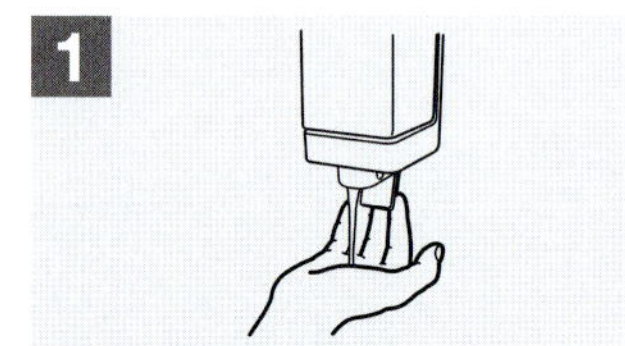

1 Apply enough soap to cover all hand surfaces;

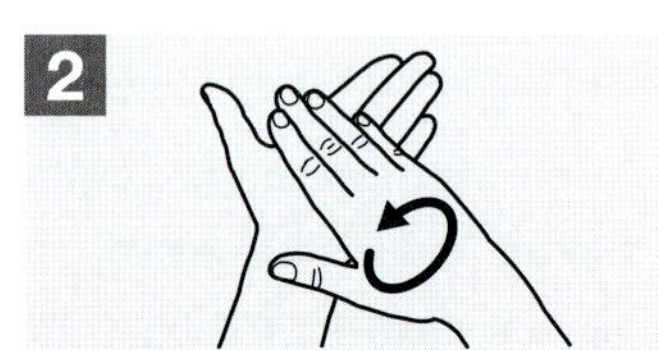

2 Rub hands palm to palm;

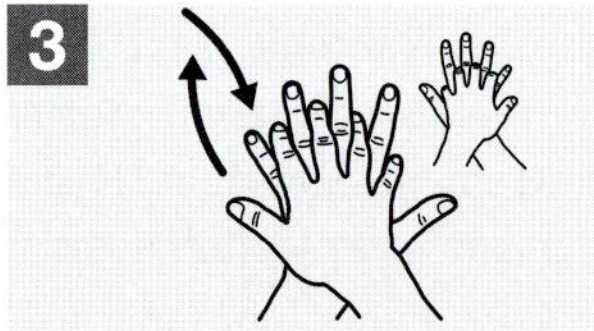

3 Right palm over left dorsum with interlaced fingers and vice versa;

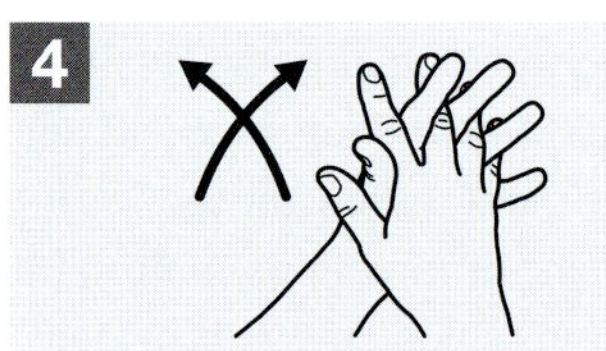

4 Palm to palm with fingers interlaced;

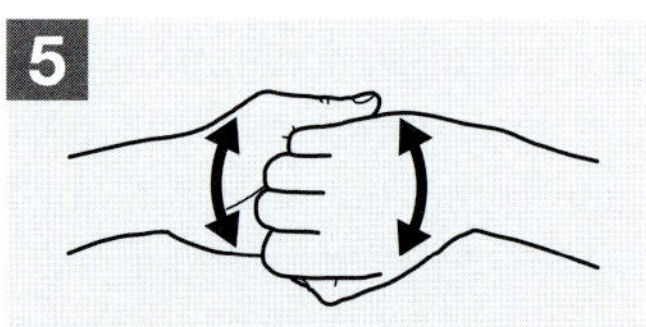

5 Backs of fingers to opposing palms with fingers interlocked;

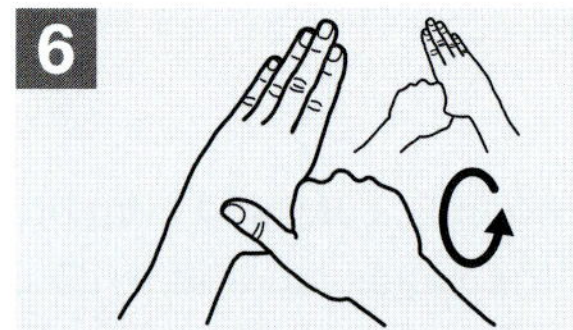

6 Rotational rubbing of left thumb clasped in right palm and vice versa;

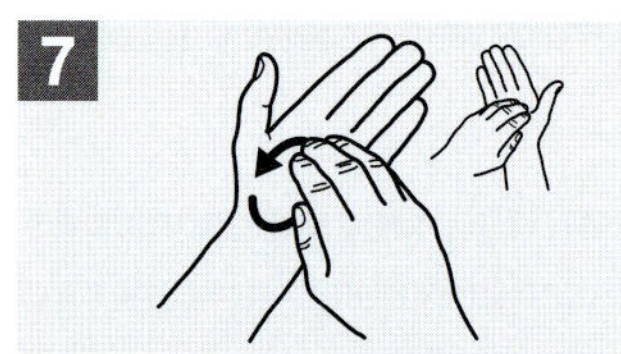

7 Rotational rubbing, backwards and forwards with clasped fingers of right hand in left palm and vice versa;

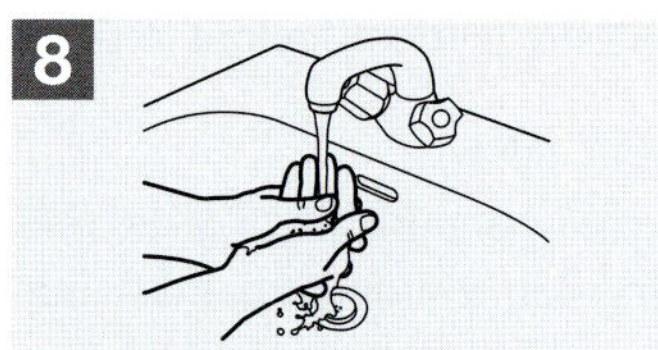

8 Rinse hands with water;

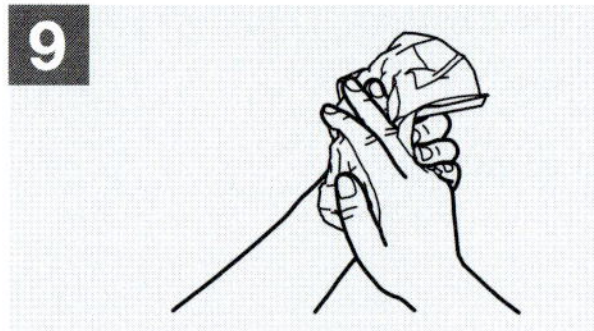

9 Dry hands thoroughly with a single use towel;

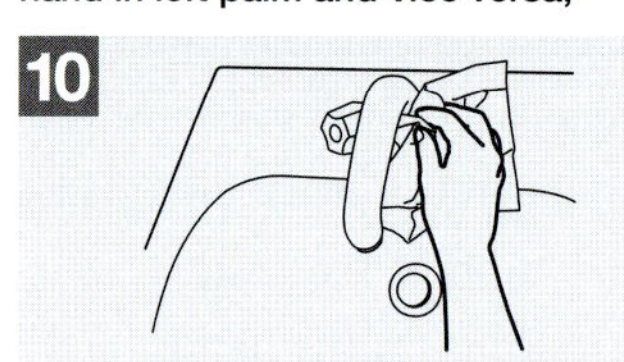

10 Use towel to turn off faucet;

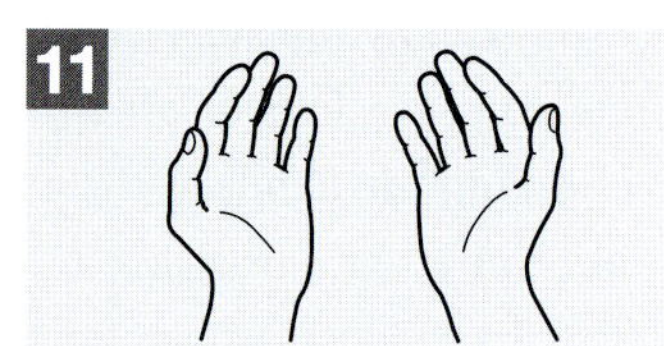

11 Your hands are now safe.

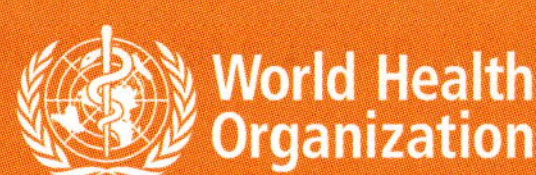

World Health Organization

Patient Safety

A World Alliance for Safer Health Care

SAVE LIVES

Clean **Your** Hands

WHO acknowledges the Hôpitaux Universitaires de Genève (HUG), in particular the members of the Infection Control Programme, for their active participation in developing this material.

May 2009

Source: Reproduced from https://www.who.int/teams/integrated-health-services/infection-prevention-control/hand-hygiene/training-tools © 2009 WHO

FIGURE 16.2 WHO "How to Handrub?" guidelines

How to Handrub?

RUB HANDS FOR HAND HYGIENE! WASH HANDS WHEN VISIBLY SOILED

Duration of the entire procedure: 20-30 seconds

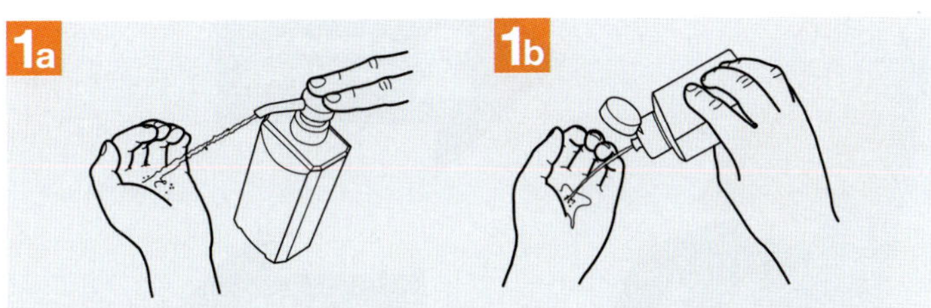

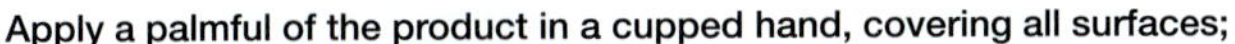

Apply a palmful of the product in a cupped hand, covering all surfaces;

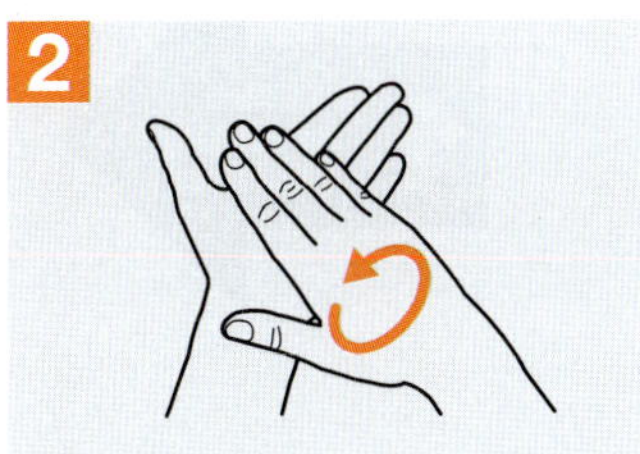

Rub hands palm to palm;

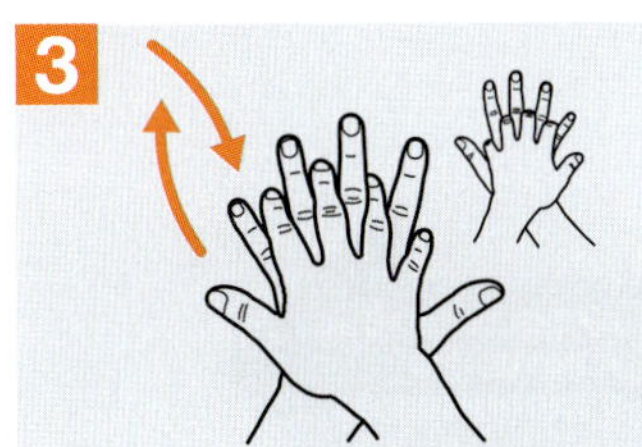

Right palm over left dorsum with interlaced fingers and vice versa;

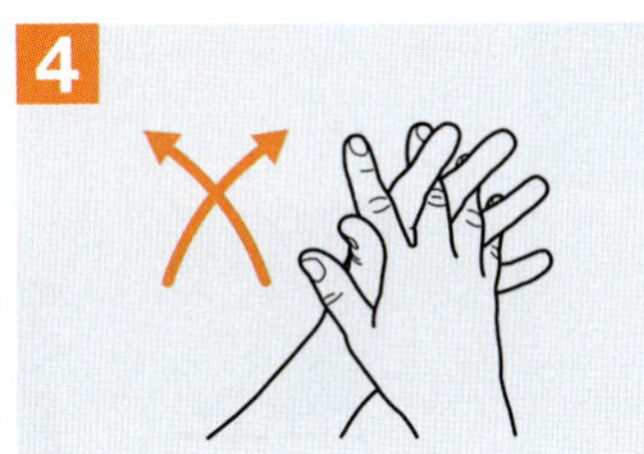

Palm to palm with fingers interlaced;

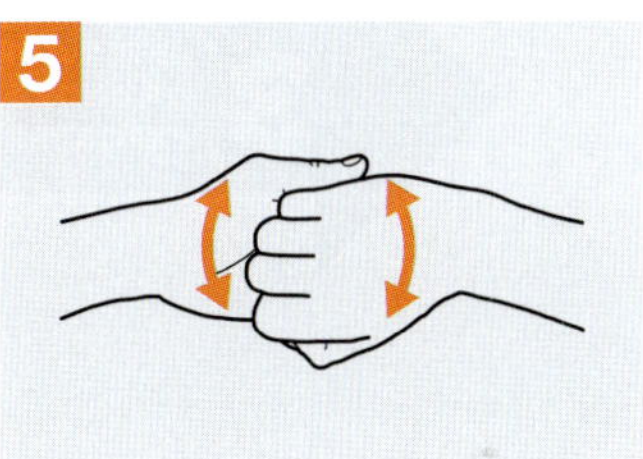

Backs of fingers to opposing palms with fingers interlocked;

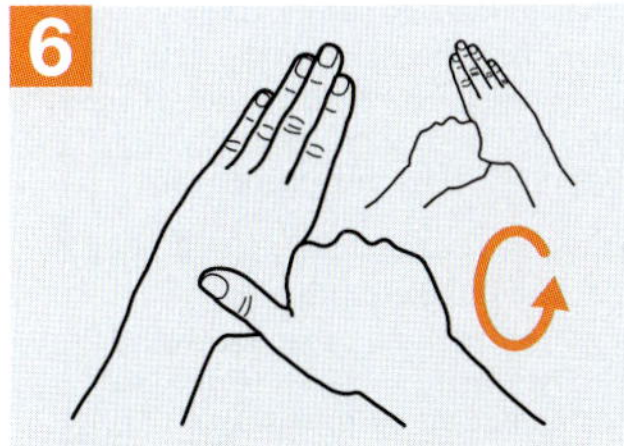

Rotational rubbing of left thumb clasped in right palm and vice versa;

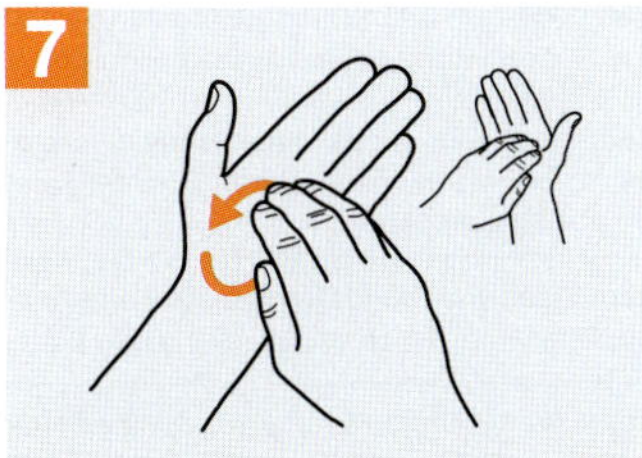

Rotational rubbing, backwards and forwards with clasped fingers of right hand in left palm and vice versa;

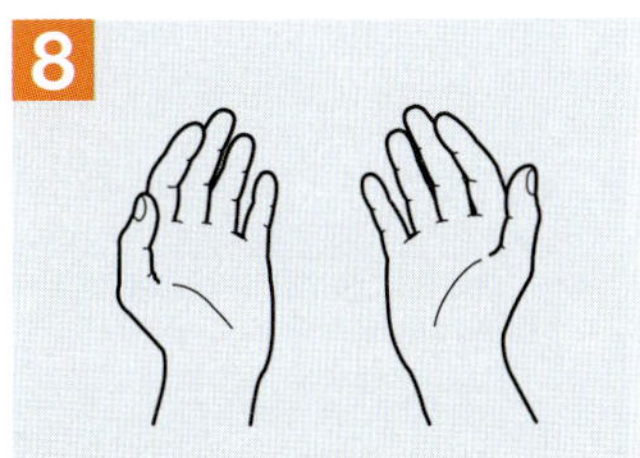

Once dry, your hands are safe.

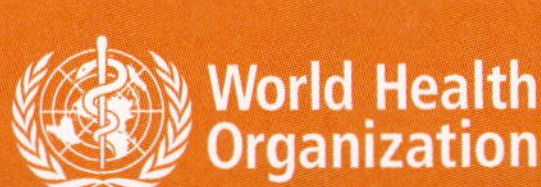

Patient Safety

A World Alliance for Safer Health Care

SAVE LIVES

Clean **Your** Hands

WHO acknowledges the Hôpitaux Universitaires de Genève (HUG), in particular the members of the Infection Control Programme, for their active participation in developing this material.

May 2009

Source: Reproduced from https://www.who.int/teams/integrated-health-services/infection-prevention-control/hand-hygiene/training-tools © 2009 WHO

FIGURE 16.3 "5 Moments for Hand Hygiene"

5 Moments for HAND HYGIENE

Ambulatory care settings

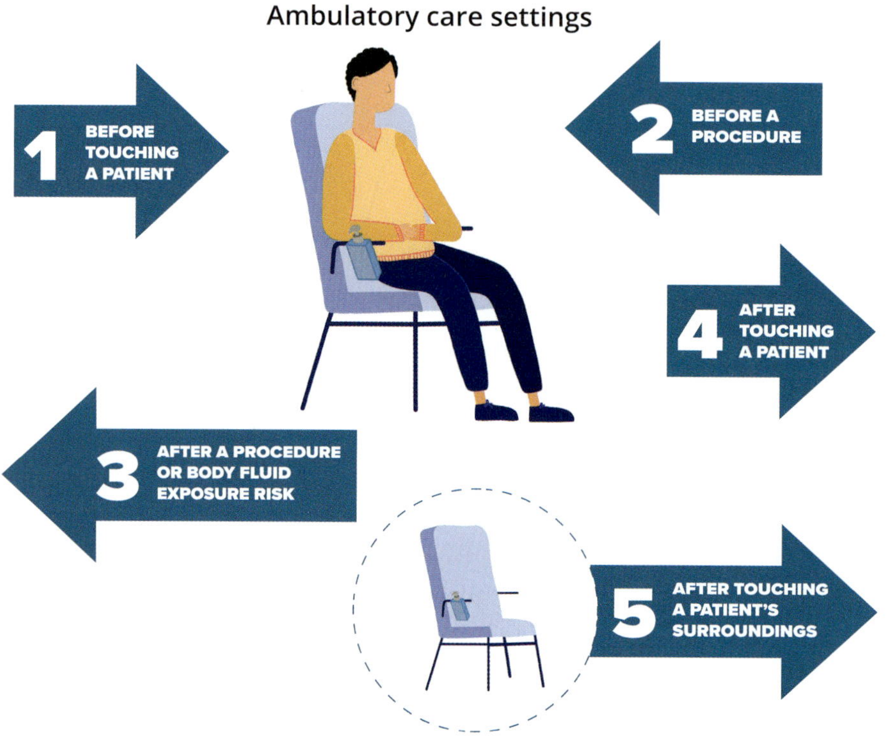

1	BEFORE TOUCHING A PATIENT	**When:** Clean your hands before touching a patient and their immediate surroundings. **Why:** To protect the patient against acquiring harmful germs from the hands of the HCW.
2	BEFORE A PROCEDURE	**When:** Clean your hands immediately before a procedure. **Why:** To protect the patient from harmful germs (including their own) from entering their body during a procedure.
3	AFTER A PROCEDURE OR BODY FLUID EXPOSURE RISK	**When:** Clean your hands immediately after a procedure or body fluid exposure risk. **Why:** To protect the HCW and the healthcare surroundings from harmful patient germs.
4	AFTER TOUCHING A PATIENT	**When:** Clean your hands after touching a patient and their immediate surroundings. **Why:** To protect the HCW and the healthcare surroundings from harmful patient germs.
5	AFTER TOUCHING A PATIENT'S SURROUNDINGS	**When:** Clean your hands after touching any objects in a patient's surroundings when the patient has not been touched. **Why:** To protect the HCW and the healthcare surroundings from harmful patient germs.

This poster is based on the World Health Organization's My 5 Moments for Hand Hygiene approach, which defines the key moments when healthcare workers should perform hand hygiene.

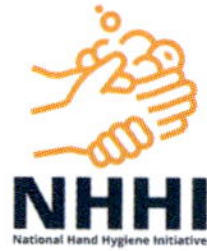

AUSTRALIAN COMMISSION ON SAFETY AND QUALITY IN HEALTH CARE

Source: Reproduced with permission from "5 moments for hand hygiene poster–ambulatory care settings. Poster 2", developed by the Australian Commission on Safety and Quality in Health Care (ACSQHC). Sydney: ACSQHC, 2022.

PRACTICE POINT

At the start of your shift, check your hands for open areas such as cuts and abrasions. If you can't see them, using alcohol hand rub will surely alert you to an open area! Remember that pathogens are microscopic and even the smallest of cuts can provide a portal of entry for infection into your body. Cover all open areas with an occlusive film dressing, which is waterproof and will keep out bugs. Check your organisation's policy to determine the required dressing to protect your hands.

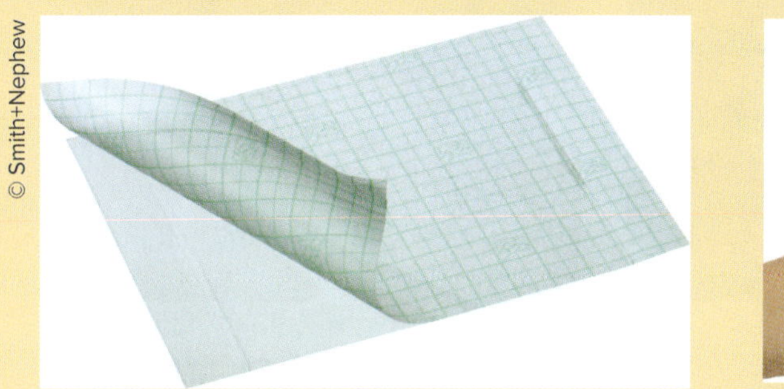

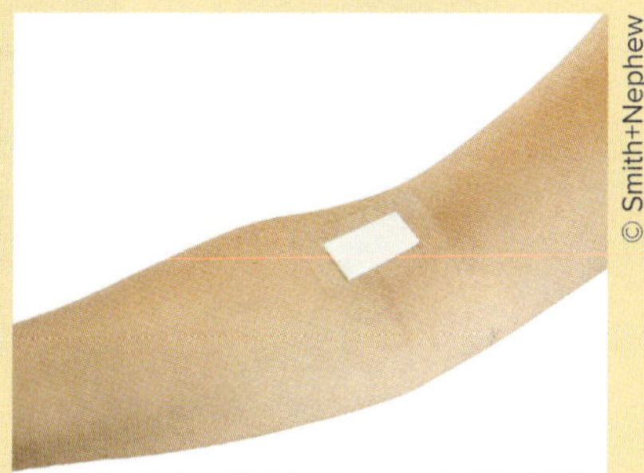

Occlusive film dressing is waterproof and will keep out bugs

PERSONAL PROTECTIVE EQUIPMENT

Another important component of standard precautions is the use of personal protective equipment (PPE). All organisations have policies and procedures that provide guidance on the appropriate use of PPE. All PPE used in aged care services must be used in accordance with the task that requires infection prevention and control, and consideration must be given to the type of PPE to be used based on the likelihood of splashes and splatters of body fluids or hazardous substances. The following PPE is used in aged care services:

- *Gloves:* Gloves are used when contact with the person's body fluids is a possibility. Sterile gloves are used for aseptic procedures such as complex wound care.
- *Eye protection:* Goggles, safety glasses and face shields are used if there is a risk of splashing of body fluids, such as when emptying a catheter bag. Prescription glasses are not classed as PPE unless they have been specifically made as PPE.
- *Gowns and waterproof aprons:* These are worn to prevent the clothing becoming contaminated with microorganisms such as gastroenteritis and splashes of body fluids. Gowns are single use. Full body gowns are required for transmission-based precautions.
- *Masks:* Different types of masks are worn according to the situation, which is guided by the workplace. Most masks used for infection prevention and control are surgical masks; however, where there is a likely high risk of SARS-CoV-2 transmission (COVID-19), the use of a fitted mask such as the P2/N95 respirator is recommended. Surgical masks are single use only and must be changed between tasks when working with multiple people. They must not be worn around the neck for convenience; and if they become wet, they must be discarded and replaced immediately.
- *Enclosed shoes:* All health-care workers, including aged care workers, benefit from wearing comfortable and enclosed leather shoes to protect the feet from dropped items that pose a risk of harm, such as used sharps.

Figure 16.4 demonstrates the correct use of PPE for different transmission types.

FIGURE 16.4 A visual guide to the application of PPE

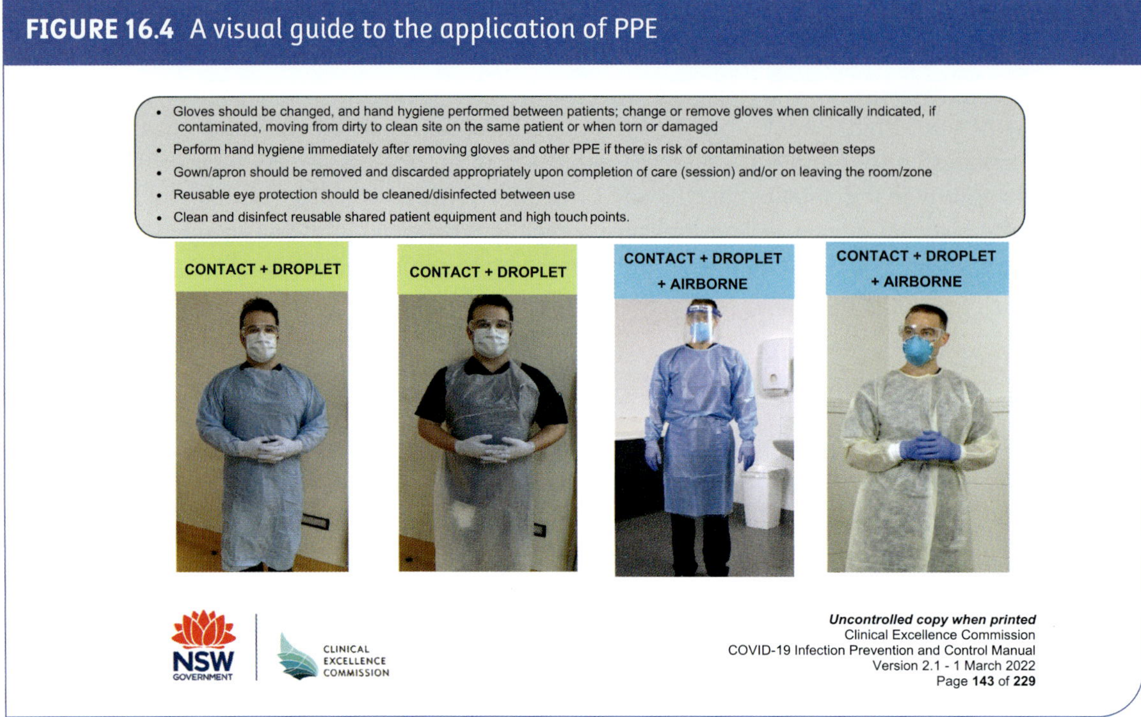

Source: Clinical Excellence Commission, 2022, *Covid-19 Infection Prevention and Control Manual Version 2.1,* Appendix 4B, Sydney, Australia: Clinical Excellence Commission

PRACTICE POINT

Wearing gloves does not negate the need to handwash; in fact, handwashing should occur before and after wearing gloves. Ensure that hands are dry before wearing gloves, as damp hands attract microorganisms and can cause skin irritation.

Gloves are single use and must not be reused for multiple procedures. Replace damaged gloves immediately.

DONNING AND DOFFING

A specific procedure must occur when putting on (donning) and removing (doffing) PPE, in order to minimise transmission of infection. Figures 16.5 and 16.6 illustrate how to don and doff PPE correctly.

16.1.2 Transmission-based precautions

Transmission-based precautions are extra infection control and prevention practices that are implemented when standard precautions may not by themselves prevent transmission. The type of transmission-based precautions used will depend on the microorganism and the way it is transmitted (the mode of transmission). Infectious agents may be spread through contact, droplet and air-borne modes of transmission. Transmission-based precautions may be implemented for one person, and they are also used in an outbreak of an infectious agent within an RACF. Each organisation will have policies and procedures to provide guidance on the

FIGURE 16.5 The sequence for putting on (donning) PPE

AUSTRALIAN COMMISSION
ON SAFETY AND QUALITY IN HEALTH CARE

Table 5: Sequence for putting on personal protective equipment

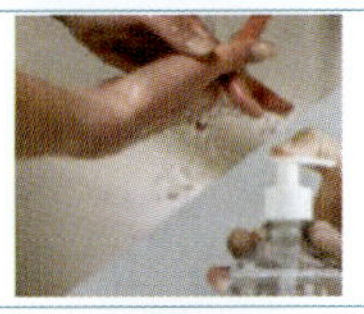	1. Perform hand hygiene
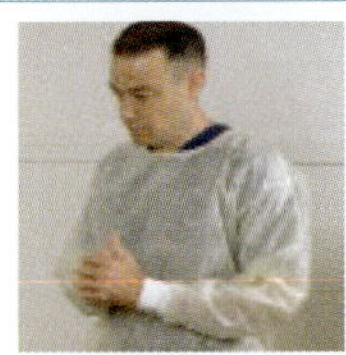	2. Put on gown • Fully cover torso from neck to knees, wrap around the back • Fasten at the back of the neck and waist
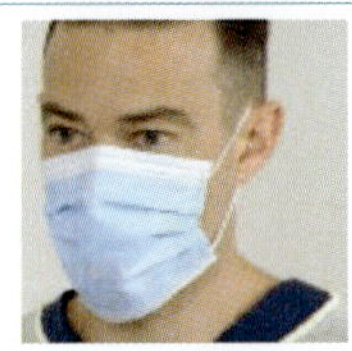	3. Put on mask • Secure ties or elastic bands at the middle of head and neck
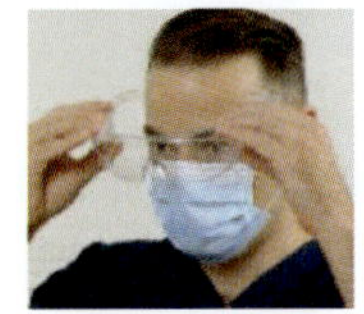	4. Put on protective eyewear • Place over face and eyes and adjust to fit
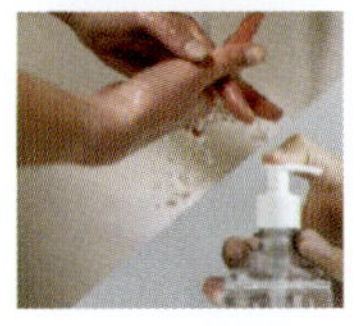	5. Perform hand hygiene
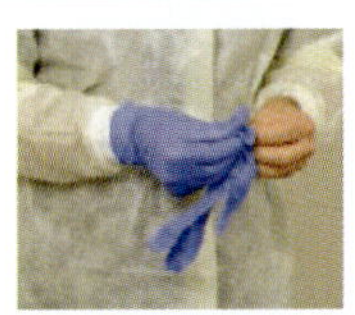	6. Put on gloves • Extend to cover wrists of gown

Source: Australian Commission on Safety and Quality in Health Care, *Infection Prevention and Control Workbook*, 2019, p. 8.

implementation of transmission-based precautions in the relevant context against the infectious agent. Transmission-based precautions include:

- increased use of PPE such as long-sleeved gowns, surgical masks, eye protection and gloves
- increased surveillance of hand hygiene
- isolation of infectious people into a single room (if possible) and the placement of a PPE station outside their door

FIGURE 16.6 The sequence for removing (doffing) PPE

AUSTRALIAN COMMISSION ON SAFETY AND QUALITY IN HEALTH CARE

Table 6: Sequence for removing personal protective equipment

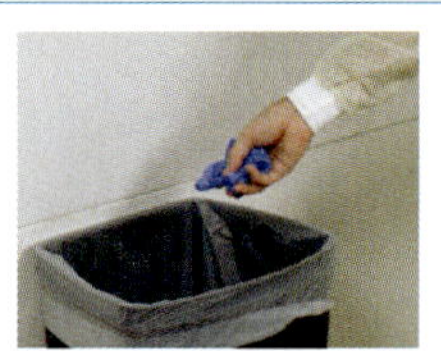	1. Remove and dispose of gloves
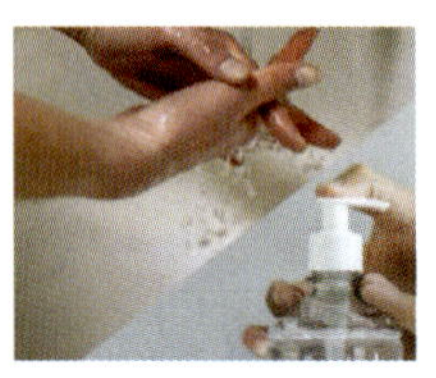	2. Perform hand hygiene
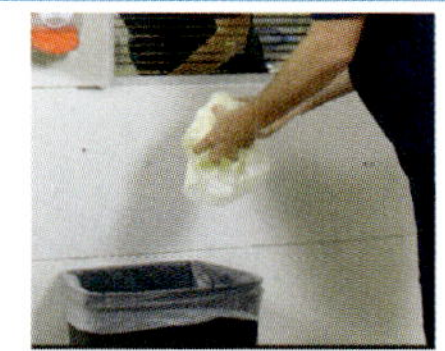	3. Remove and dispose of gown
Alternatively gloves and gown can be removed as one step. Then perform hand hygiene	
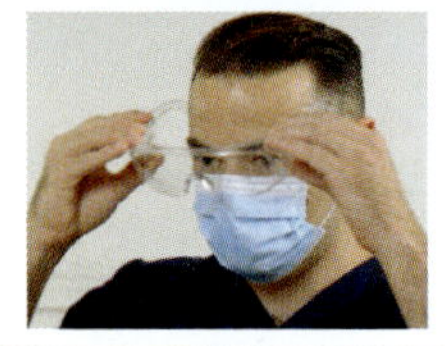	4. Remove protective eyewear
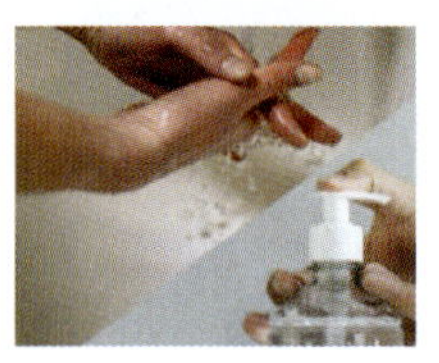	5. Perform hand hygiene
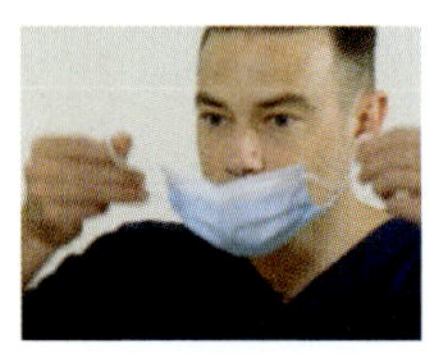	6. Remove mask and dispose of mask
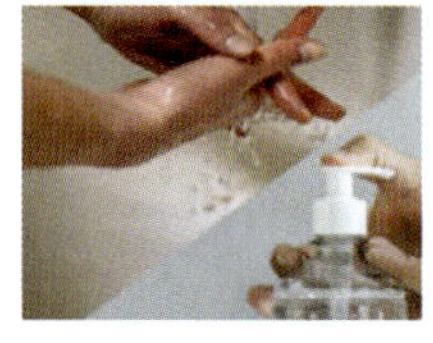	7. Perform hand hygiene

Source: Australian Commission on Safety and Quality in Health Care, *Infection Prevention and Control Workbook*, 2019, p. 11.

- minimisation of staff rotation to affected areas
- provision of person-dedicated equipment
- increased cleaning protocols.

Outbreak interventions include the use of standard and transmission-based precautions, as well as:

- outbreak coordination by an infection control lead/coordinator
- contact with the Public Health Unit to report cases
- signage to alert staff, visitors and contractors
- careful staff rotation
- increased cleaning protocols
- restricting visitors
- careful cohorting when single rooms are unavailable
- ongoing risk management and monitoring of the outbreak.

16.1.3 Respiratory hygiene and cough etiquette

Many infectious agents are transmitted between people through coughing and sneezing. Droplet and airborne infections such as influenza and COVID-19 are easily passed on from one person to another when someone sneezes or coughs without covering their mouth. Cough etiquette involves coughing or sneezing into the elbow, followed by hand hygiene; or coughing or sneezing into a tissue, discarding the tissue into a bin and attending to hand hygiene. Figure 16.7 demonstrates the correct cough etiquette.

One of the responsibilities of all workers who work with older people is to monitor their own health. A worker who is unwell should stay at home and not go to work. It is always a better option to work with reduced staff than to risk older people becoming extremely unwell with an infection that was preventable.

16.1.4 Environmental cleaning procedures

Microorganisms can contaminate the environment. Routine cleaning is an important part of risk management processes for infection control and prevention, and ensures the workplace is hygienic.

Different cleaning procedures are required for different areas and activities. They involve the use of disinfectants and other chemicals that are approved by the Therapeutic Goods Administration (TGA). All chemicals must be used according to the manufacturer's instructions.

Routine surface cleaning includes cleaning of surfaces that have high contact such as door handles, bed frames and sinks. However, the routine cleaning of equipment used for the support of older people, such as lifting devices and wheelchairs, may be the responsibility of nurses and care workers. The organisation will have policies and procedures to ensure that correct cleaning procedures occur within the facility.

Care workers who provide support to people who live in the community will have different cleaning responsibilities than those who work in an RACF. Working within the person's home may include cleaning duties, and a home-care organisation will have specific guidelines and procedures around cleaning tasks and chemical use in order to minimise the risk of harm to the person and to the staff member. These procedures may include information about the safe use of equipment such as vacuums to prevent a manual handling injury and the safe use of chemicals.

Within an RACF, a colour coding system may be in place for reusable cleaning equipment, to minimise the risk of cross-infection. For example, a mop and bucket that is yellow is used to mop up urine, but a mop and bucket that is blue is used to mop general areas such as bedrooms. Table 16.1 illustrates a colour coding system that is frequently used in RACFs to minimise the risks of cross-infection.

Many facilities have an environmental schedule that allocates specific cleaning tasks at specific times, and that directs staff on the required frequency of the cleaning processes. Environmental cleaning is an important part of standard precautions, but it also has a key role in transmission-based precautions. Specific procedures

FIGURE 16.7 Correct cough etiquette

Cough etiquette

Cover your cough

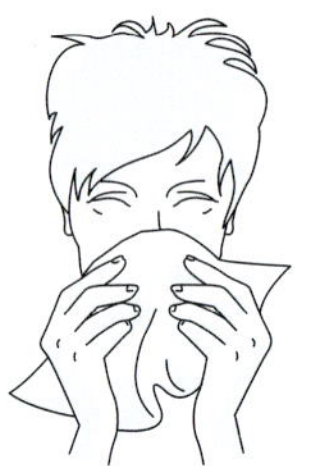

- When coughing or sneezing, use a tissue to cover your nose and mouth
- Dispose of the tissue afterwards
- If you don't have a tissue, cough or sneeze into your elbow.

Wash your hands

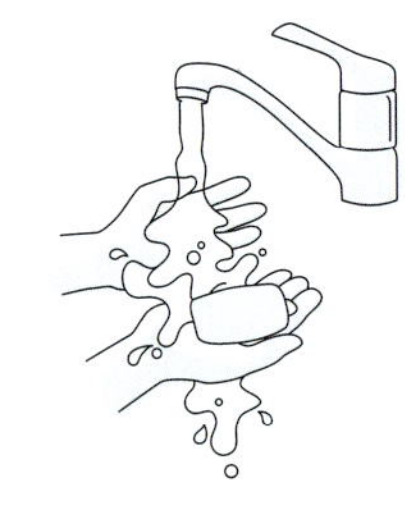

- After coughing, sneezing or blowing your nose, wash your hands with soap and water
- Use alcohol-based hand cleansers if you do not have access to soap and water

Remember hand washing is the single most effective way to reduce the spread of germs that cause respiratory disease.

Anyone with signs and symptoms of a respiratory infection, regardless of the cause, should be instructed to cover their nose/mouth when coughing or sneezing; use tissues to contain respiratory secretions; dispose of tissues in the nearest waste receptacle after use; and wash their hands afterwards.

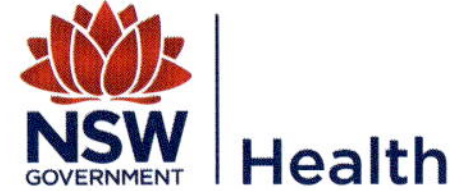

Source: (NSW Health:2014) © State of New South Wales NSW Ministry of Health. For current information go to www.health.nsw.gov.au. CC BY 4.0 https://creativecommons.org/licenses/by/4.0/

TABLE 16.1 An example of a colour coding system for environmental cleaning in an RACF

Colour	Classification
Blue	General cleaning (bedrooms, communal living areas, etc.)
Green	Food handling and food service areas
Red	Bathrooms, toilets and amenities
Yellow	Biohazards; infectious areas

are necessary during an outbreak or when a person is known to have an infection that is transmissible to others. One such procedure is the two-step clean, which involves either:

- cleaning surfaces with a neutral detergent followed by a hospital-grade disinfectant (TGA approved) or
- cleaning with a combined product of detergent and disinfectant (TGA approved).

The disinfectant must be hospital grade with activity against viruses. The two-step process may be used in outbreaks, including a COVID-19 outbreak, in RACFs.

All cleaning personnel must wear appropriate PPE when entering a person's room, or home if applicable, and follow the correct procedure for putting on and removing the PPE. Hand hygiene is essential for all staff working with older people regardless of the job description they hold.

16.1.5 Handling food

Infection can occur when contaminated food is consumed. Older people can lose valuable hydration when infected with microorganisms that cause vomiting and diarrhoea.

Food safety is essential in the prevention of infection, and specific practices must occur routinely to minimise risk of food contamination and cross-contamination between people. These practices include ensuring that:

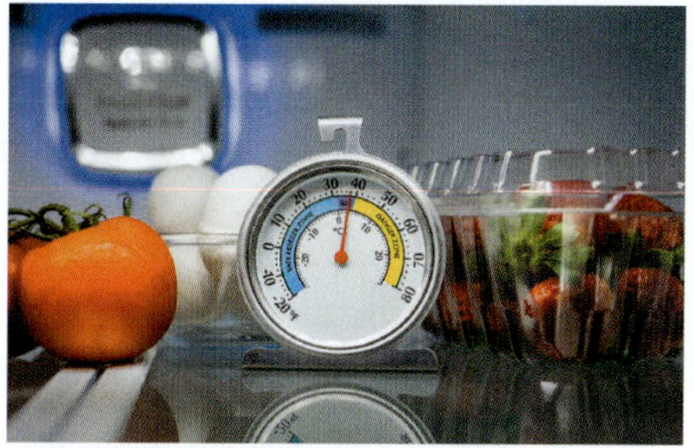

Refrigerated food requires temperature management using a thermometer

- all food preparation areas are cleaned according to the organisation's policies and procedures
- hand hygiene is practised by all staff involved in food handling
- colour-coded chopping boards are used to prevent cross-contamination
- PPE is worn appropriately (gloves, hair and beard nets, aprons, shoe covers)
- food is stored, prepared and consumed at the correct temperature.

One of the Food Safety Standards of the Food Standards Australia New Zealand (FSANZ) is Standard 13.3.1, "Food Safety Programs for Food Service to Vulnerable Persons". The standard states that all aged care facilities must have a food safety program for the people who use the service that includes auditing and monitoring the program to ensure the risk of food-borne illness is minimised.

Food-borne illnesses such as **gastroenteritis** and **salmonella** poisoning can occur when food is not refrigerated, stored, thawed, prepared or heated correctly. A strict code of food safety, the Australia New Zealand Food Standards Code, ensures that aged care services and other organisations are compliant with the FSANZ standards. The food safety program within aged care facilities may also include information for carers and families about the safety requirements of the food they bring from home for their loved one to consume.

16.1.6 Handling linen

In the context of aged care services, linen includes bath towels and face washers, sheets, blankets and other bed linen, and the person's clothing. Clean linen and soiled linen must not be stored in close proximity, due to the risk of cross-contamination. Linen and textiles can harbour microorganisms, which can be readily spread through touch and by air-borne transmission routes. The management of dirty linen under the standard precautions is to use different-coloured linen bags to hold soiled linen. To prevent the transmission of infection from contaminated linen, care workers should consider the following:

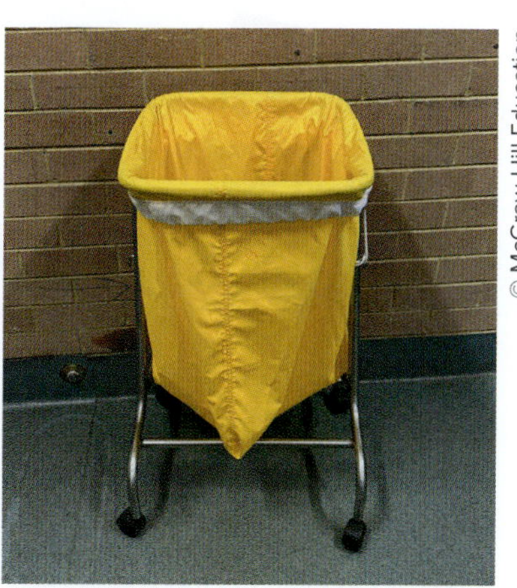

Yellow linen bag for contaminated linen

- Place soiled linen (contaminated with blood, vomit, faeces) into a dedicated linen bag at the site of generation (e.g. the bedside).
- Don't carry soiled linen.

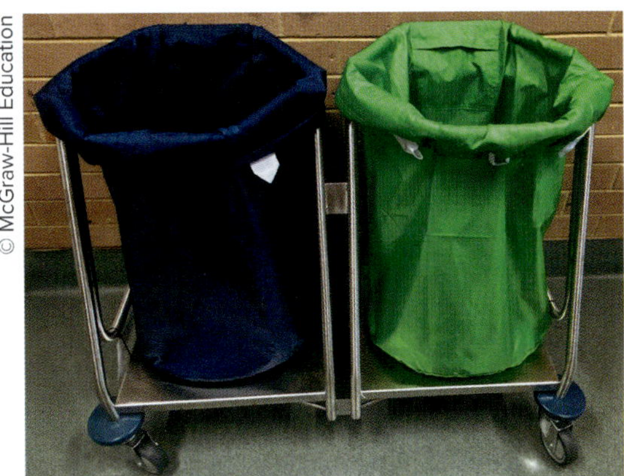

Linen bags in a linen skip

- Wear PPE appropriate to the task. Always wear gloves when body fluids are involved.
- Don't carry clean linen against the body.
- Place soiled linen into an alginate bag or leak-proof bag in the first instance.
- Don't hose or rinse off any solid matter from linen.
- Don't leave soiled and contaminated linen on furniture, the floor or in a corridor at any time.
- Don't shake linen, as this can release microorganisms into the air for others to breathe in.
- Don't drop used sharps (such as used syringes and razors) into linen bags.

Follow the organisation's policies and procedures for handling linen. Remember that microorganisms can also be present on your uniform, so be sure to shower and change when you get home, and to wash your uniform as soon as possible.

16.1.7 Handling contaminated waste

Waste management is an important aspect of infection control and prevention within aged care services. Waste includes all items and materials that are deemed unwanted. Within aged care services, some types of waste can be hazardous and increase the risk of infection. In RACFs, waste is categorised into general waste, clinical and biological waste, and cytotoxic waste. Colour codes for waste categories minimise the risk of contamination by ensuring that waste with a higher risk of causing infection is easily recognised and managed. The colour codes for waste types are as follows:

- *White, blue* or *black* waste bags and receptacles are for general waste that doesn't contain contaminated items. General waste includes the by-products of everyday work activities; however, it may contain microorganisms.
- *Yellow* waste bags and receptacles are for biological and contaminated waste. This type of waste includes items that carry a high risk of infection and contamination, such as blood and other body fluids, human tissue, and products used for procedures (such as used wound dressings). The yellow bag has a black biological hazard symbol printed on it and the words "CLINICAL WASTE" to alert people to the risks within.
- *Purple* bags are allocated to the waste that contains cytotoxic material. Someone may take cytotoxic medication to treat, for example, some types of cancer. The prefix "cyto" refers to cells and "toxic" means danger. This medication attacks cancer cells; however, good cells can be harmed in the process. If a person is taking these medications, their body fluids are also potentially cytotoxic, and care workers and nurses must always wear the designated "purple" gloves when providing care where body fluids are involved. Waste such as soiled incontinence pads must also be discarded in a purple waste bag. The purple bag has a white symbol of a cell and the words "CYTOTOXIC WASTE", to alert workers to the danger within.

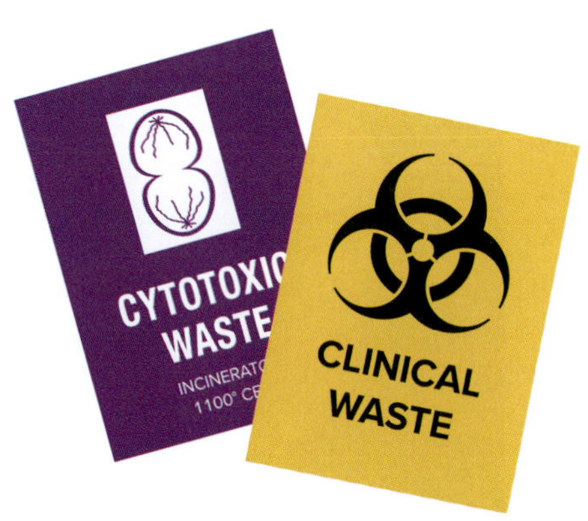

Designated colours for specific types of waste are used in the aged care sector, including the purple cytotoxic waste bag and the yellow clinical waste bag

The colour system for waste is universal and may also be used in the home care sector. All care workers, regardless of their place of employment, must have a solid understanding of infection control and prevention processes.

Residential aged care facilities have a utility room that is used to minimise risk of infection. The utility room is used to clean contaminated items such as urinals and bedpans, to discard body fluids such as catheter bags, and to house the contaminated waste bin. Utility rooms are used frequently by many staff, and so hand hygiene should occur after exiting the room.

SHARPS

Sharps are objects that are used in the provision of clinical and personal care. As such, they can transmit infection from one person to another. Blood-borne diseases such as HIV and hepatitis C can be transmitted from one person to another via blood contact. All used sharps such as used needles, scalpels, stitch cutters, syringes with needles, and razors must be disposed of safely into a sharps container under the Australian Standards. Sharps containers may also be used in the in-home care environment for people who require injections for medical purposes.

In an aged care facility, sharps containers are collected by an authorised waste collection company for incineration when they are full. Full sharps containers used by people in the community can be taken to a community sharps disposal facility. Sharps containers are available in many sizes.

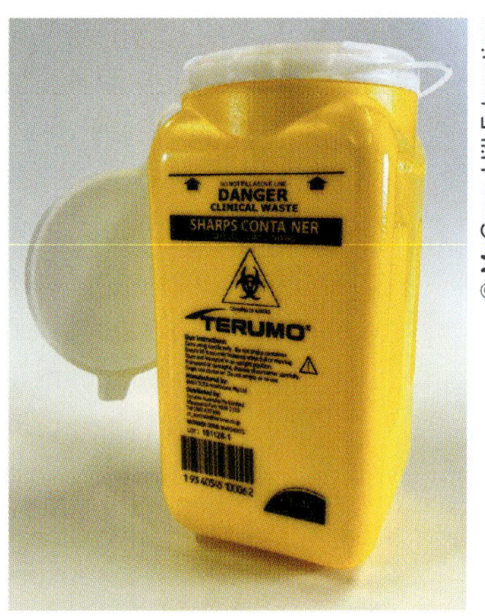

Small sharps disposal container with a biohazard symbol and a written warning on the front

PRACTICE POINT

To minimise the risk of a sharps injury, avoid passing the sharp from hand to hand and never recap needles. Use a puncture-proof tray to carry the sharp to the person and place the used sharp into the sharps container immediately after use.

MANAGING A SPILL

Spills of blood and other infectious material require specific management to prevent possible cross-contamination of harmful microorganisms. All aged care services have protocols for handling spills in the workplace. The prompt management of spills includes donning gloves and other necessary PPE and using absorbent disposable paper to clean the spill once it has been confined. All used absorbent paper should be placed into the correct waste container. The area of the spill can then be cleaned with detergent. A TGA-approved disinfectant compatible with the substance in the spill may be used if warranted, based on assessment of risk (NHMRC 2019). All aged care providers have spill kits in specified areas of the work environment.

16.1.8 Equipment

All equipment must be kept clean when not in use. The cleaning procedure for equipment will vary, depending on the equipment type and how frequently it is used. All health-care organisations have the responsibility of risk minimisation in regard to infection control and prevention, including the management of the reprocessing procedures for equipment that is not disposable. Equipment can be reprocessed at different levels, and policies and procedures will exist in the workplace that guide the cleaning or reprocessing activities.

- *Cleaning:* Equipment that is used generally within the organisation may be cleaned with soapy water or using a damp dusting procedure. Items that are generally cleaned in this way include wheelchairs and hydraulic lifter frames. The slings used for lifters should ideally belong to the individual and be washed in the washing machine. Individual equipment and shared equipment such as nebulisers and automatic blood pressure machines might also be cleaned with warm water with a neutral detergent. The model of cleaning for medical and personal care equipment changes when infection is suspected or known, and transmission-based precautions are implemented.

- *Disinfection:* Disinfection of equipment is required when the risk of infection is high, such as during an outbreak of an infectious agent such as gastroenteritis. Many organisations require equipment to be cleaned with hot soapy water first, followed by a disinfection process. All disinfectants used must be approved by the TGA. Disinfection of equipment such as nebulisers and other medical equipment is important in the prevention of infection during an outbreak.
- *Sterilisation:* Some equipment will carry a very high transmission risk of infection–for example, non-disposable used medical items such as wound care scalpels, scissors and forceps. This type of equipment must be reprocessed using one of the several available sterilisation processes. Organisations may perform sterilisation of equipment onsite or outsource the reprocessing of contaminated equipment from an external sterilisation service. An alternative may include the purchase of pre-sterilised single-use items.

The manner in which the reprocessing of reusable medical equipment occurs must meet the criteria within the standard on preventing and controlling infections as part of the broader National Safety and Quality Health Service Standards (NSQHS). All policies and procedures around the cleaning processes of equipment should be available for staff to access.

When handling and cleaning equipment, workers must wear the PPE appropriate to the task. It is important to remember that PPE is only one aspect of infection control and prevention; other components of standard and transmission-based precautions are also essential in order to protect yourself and others in the workplace.

WORKPLACE SCENARIO

"5 Moments for Hand Hygiene"

Amelia has arrived at Mrs Black's home to help her with her blood glucose testing and her medications. Amelia knocks on the door and is greeted by Mrs Black, who asks her to retrieve her blood glucose machine from the bathroom. After retrieving the blood glucose machine from the bathroom, Amelia sets about preparing to test Mrs Black's blood glucose. She uses alcohol rub, as she is *about to* perform a procedure. She dons disposable gloves and proceeds to test Mrs Black's blood glucose. *After the procedure,* Amelia disposes of her gloves and performs hand hygiene again, according to the "5 Moments for Hand Hygiene".

Amelia packs up the machine and returns it to the bathroom at the request of Mrs Black, then quickly helps her put on her cardigan. *Before* assisting Mrs Black with taking her medications for the day, Amelia washes her hands again.

Before leaving Mrs Black's home, she packs away Mrs Black's laundry and arranges her newspapers and magazines so that it is easy for her to access them. On her way out of the house, she uses alcohol rub one more time as she has been *in contact with Mrs Black's surroundings*, even though she hasn't made any physical contact with her since giving Mrs Black her medications earlier in the visit. Amelia is satisfied that she has correctly performed the "5 Moments for Hand Hygiene", knowing that infection prevention is always better than infection control.

CHECK YOUR UNDERSTANDING

1. What is the aim of standard precautions?
2. List four practices within standard precautions that care workers perform in the workplace.
3. When should you attend to hand hygiene, according to the "5 Moments for Hand Hygiene"?
4. What are transmission-based precautions?
5. How should used sharps be disposed of?

16.2 IDENTIFYING INFECTION HAZARDS AND RISKS

16.2.1 Infection hazards

THE BASIS OF INFECTION

Infection occurs when a harmful microorganism enters the body (the host), reproduces and causes a reaction in the body. A microorganism that causes infection is known as a **pathogen.** Not all microorganisms are harmful. Many microorganisms live happily in and on the body within their own environment. However, harmful microorganisms challenge the immune system when they release toxins and other inflammatory substances.

The body's ability to fight an infection will depend on several factors, such as the:

- type of pathogen (virulence)
- host's immune system abilities and general health status
- location of the pathogen
- effectiveness of antibiotics and other prescribed treatments.

Some pathogens don't cause serious harm; however, others are serious and life-threatening. Unfortunately, many pathogens are resistant to treatment and medical science continues to search for new and effective treatments.

Colonisation occurs when microorganisms and pathogens live on or in the body without causing infection. Pathogens that colonise an area can become harmful as an infection if the environment changes. For example, the pathogen *Staphylococcus aureus* can exist harmlessly on the skin of some people; however, it becomes a serious and challenging infection in open wounds.

Some infections can result in disease, causing a decline in the host's general health and wellbeing. The diseases caused by pathogens can be short-lived or have long-term health effects. For example, the varicella-zoster virus that causes chickenpox can stay in the body long after the initial infection has resolved. The virus remains in a dormant state within nerves and can reactivate at a later time as shingles.

There are various types of pathogens that cause infection, and they differ from each other in the way they act on, or in, the body. Table 16.2 describes the groups of pathogens that cause infection.

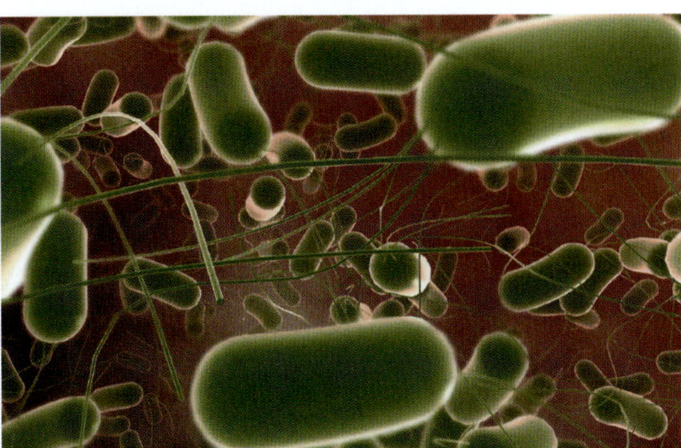

MedicalRF.com

Salmonella (rod-shaped bacteria) can cause food poisoning if food is not refrigerated, stored, thawed, prepared or heated correctly

TABLE 16.2 Types of pathogens and their characteristics

Type	Characteristics	Example
Bacteria	• A single-celled organism. • Found in and on all living creatures. • There are trillions of bacteria in the world. • Some good bacteria can destroy bad bacteria. • Can survive in extremely harsh conditions. • Need food, moisture, warmth and time to survive. • Three main shapes: — spherical (known as cocci) — rod-shaped (known as bacilli) — spiral (known as spirilli). • Bacterial infections can cause debilitating and life-threatening diseases such as tuberculosis, typhoid and cholera. • Bacterial infections are treated with antibiotics; however, many types of bacteria are becoming resistant to the effectiveness of antibiotics. • A bacterial spore is a spore or spore-like structure produced by bacteria. They can survive unfavourable conditions. Some can spread poisonous chemicals (e.g. the spores of tetanus can survive in the soil for years). Not all bacteria have spores.	• Some respiratory infections • Otitis media (ear infection) • Pneumonia • Urinary tract infection • Food poisoning • Conjunctivitis (eye infection) • Skin infections
Fungi	• Fungi include yeasts and moulds. • Fungi absorb nutrients from the surrounding environment. • Can be a single-celled organism (such as yeast) or huge multicellular organisms. • The feet have the most fungi of the body. • Fungi can release spores that can be inhaled into the lungs and can be life-threatening to people with impaired immune systems. • Fungi can reproduce in the top layers of the skin. • Antifungal treatment is required to manage fungal infections.	• Tinea • Ringworm • Candidiasis • Histoplasmosis
Prions	• A prion is a protein and is not a living microorganism. • Prions that change their shape can cause infection, affecting the structure of the brain and the nervous system. • Abnormal, or rogue, prions cause the body's cells to behave differently. • Cause degenerative brain diseases.	• Creutzfeldt Jacob disease (CJD) • Bovine spongiform encephalopathy (BSE) (mad cow disease} • Some types of dementia have been linked to prion deformity
Viruses	• Contain genetic information and are protected by protein and lipids (fats). • Viruses enter the cell and replicate themselves by releasing genetic information or code. • Antibiotics are ineffective against viruses. • Antiviral medication is helpful with symptoms of some viruses. Some can increase the host's immune response and others can prevent reproduction of the virus.	• Common cold (rhinovirus; adenovirus) • Influenza • HIV • Varicella • Hepatitis • COVID-19 • H1N1 (swine flu)

THE CHAIN OF INFECTION

The process by which an infection is shared between people (hosts) can be described as the chain of infection. The chain has six links, and each link facilitates the cross-contamination of infection from one person to another. The aim is for care workers and other health practitioners to break the chain to prevent the cross-contamination process from moving forward. There are six links in the chain of infection (see also Figure 16.8):

1. *Infectious agent (pathogen):* The pathogen causes harm, such as a virus or bacteria.
2. *Reservoir (the environment of the pathogen):* A reservoir for pathogens can include other people, a dirty linen skip, a waste bag, contaminated food, unwashed hands.
3. *Portal of exit from the reservoir:* Pathogens can exit the reservoir when an infected person coughs or sneezes into the air, through vomiting and diarrhoea, and by touching, shaking linen, overfilling linen bags, using incorrect waste management procedures, and poor food-handling techniques.
4. *Mode of transmission:* The mode of transmission is the way the pathogen gets to another person. The mode can be indirect or direct. For example, gastroenteritis can be spread from person to person by touch when hands aren't washed correctly.
5. *Portal of entry:* Pathogens need to find a way into or onto another host. Portals of entry include non-intact skin, the mucous membranes (eyes, mouth), the respiratory system, the digestive system (eating and drinking) and the genitourinary tract.
6. *Susceptible host:* Pathogens thrive when the host has a vulnerable immune defence, such as an invasive medical device (e.g. an indwelling catheter). The type of pathogen also affects how the host can use natural immune defences to prevent the infection.

FIGURE 16.8 Chain of infection

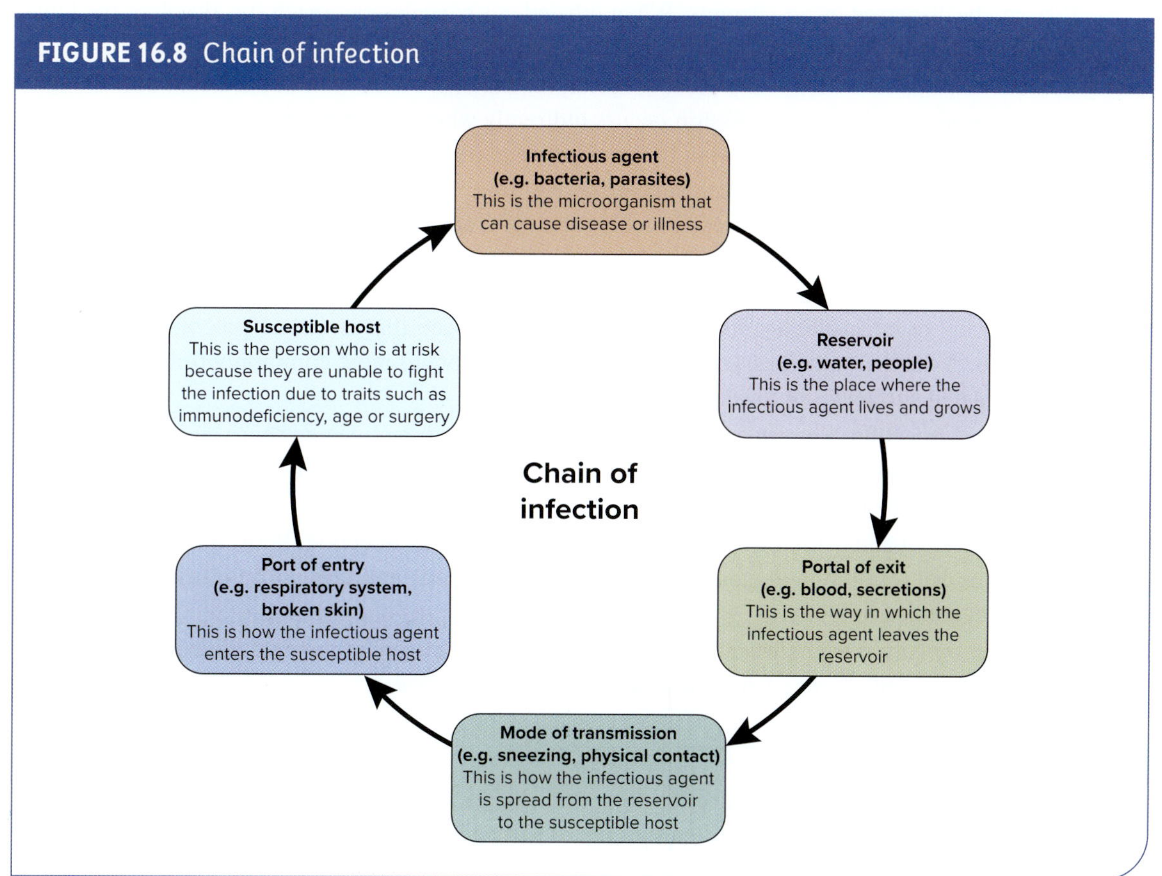

Source: Adapted from https://www.cdc.gov/csels/dsepd/ss1978/lesson1/section10.html#:~:text=More%20specifically%2C%20transmission%20occurs%20when,called%20the%20chain%20of%20infection

Standard and transmission-based precautions are designed to break the chain of infection. Effective handwashing is a critical component in preventing the cross-contamination of infection among older people.

MODES OF TRANSMISSION

The mode of transmission is the way pathogens spread between people. The main modes of transmission include contact, droplet and air-borne transmission. The process of the transmission of pathogens can be direct or indirect.

DIRECT TRANSMISSION

Direct transmission of infection occurs from human-to-human contact of infected blood or body fluids (such as through intercourse, kissing, handshaking). Direct transmission can also occur between mother and her unborn baby via the placenta.

Droplet transmission is also classed as direct transmission. When an infected person sneezes or coughs, droplets can be sprayed before falling to the ground or other surfaces. Droplets can be inhaled by another person, who then becomes the host. Speaking and laughing can also infect other people via droplet transmission if people are in close proximity to each other.

INDIRECT TRANSMISSION

Infectious pathogens can be spread indirectly through the air and other mechanisms, including contact. Indirect transmission involves the following:

- *Air-borne transmission:* Air particles are much smaller and finer than droplets and can remain suspended in the air for a longer period of time. Infected air particles can also travel distances as they can be dispersed by air currents. When inhaled, air particles can reach the alveoli of the lungs and cause diseases such as tuberculosis and measles.
- *Contact transmission:* One of the most common modes of transmission in aged care and health services, contact transmission occurs indirectly when surfaces, objects and hands are contaminated. Pathogens remain on the surfaces (e.g. door handles) for another person to touch. Many infectious microorganisms are spread from person to person through touching contaminated objects and surfaces. Touching the eyes, nose and mouth after touching contaminated objects can provide the pathogen with a portal of entry into the body. Effective handwashing and environmental cleaning are essential strategies for preventing the contact transmission of infectious agents. An example of a pathogen that is spread via contact is norovirus. Norovirus is a form of gastroenteritis and is spread most commonly through contaminated surfaces and unwashed hands.
- *Inoculation:* Infection can result when the skin is pierced with an infected sharp such as a used needle. People can also become infectious when a clinical procedure involving inoculation is performed incorrectly.
- *Ingestion:* Eating and drinking contaminated food can result in infection. Poor food-handling techniques can result in food poisoning. Some pathogens such as *E-coli* can be transmitted via food that is not cooked properly.
- *Vector transmission:* Occurs when insects transmit infectious agents to people. Examples include mosquito-borne infections such as Ross River fever and malaria.

SIGNS AND SYMPTOMS OF INFECTION

When the immune system is fighting infection, common signs and symptoms of infection may be present. The signs and symptoms displayed depend on the type of pathogen and the capacity of the person's immune system to fight the infection.

Local infection occurs when a specific area of the body shows signs of infection. For example, the signs and symptoms of a local infection of a wound include:

- redness of the skin surrounding the wound
- swelling of the tissue around the edge of the wound
- possible pus production within the wound
- noticeable heat in the skin that surrounds the wound
- pain.

Localised infection can rapidly develop into a systemic infection if the person develops sepsis (blood poisoning). Systemic infection occurs when pathogens are present in the blood and multiple body systems are affected. An example of a systemic infection is influenza, because the whole body is affected. Systemic infection requires rigorous treatments and often involves sepsis.

Signs of systemic infection in older people may include:

- lethargy
- loss of appetite
- fever
- delirium (sudden onset of confusion regardless of cognitive abilities)
- fluctuating levels of consciousness
- **cellulitis**.

Any sign of infection, whether localised or systemic, must be reported to the registered nurse (RN) or the supervisor immediately. Always document your observations according to your organisation's policies and procedures.

PRACTICE POINT

Immunosenescence is the term that describes age-related decline in the function of the immune system. The ageing process and the presence of chronic disease can challenge the older person to fight infection well. Because of this, older people may not show the obvious signs of infection, including a fever. It may take them longer to develop a high temperature, if at all. Don't rely on the thermometer for an indication that the person is unwell. Often, changes in mental state and the ability to perform basic tasks may be the only indicator that an older person is acutely unwell with infection.

COMMON INFECTIOUS DISEASES AMONG OLDER PEOPLE

Older people are just as likely to experience the same infections as everyone else; however, there are some common infectious diseases that prevail among older people who use aged care services, predominantly in RACFs. Table 16.3 describes some of the common infectious disease that older people may experience.

16.2.2 Responsibilities associated with infection control

In the context of aged care services, infection control and prevention are the responsibility of all workers, as well as the people using the service and visitors to the service. How infection control and prevention issues are managed by the service is governed by legislation and industry guidelines, on the basis of which organisational policies and procedures are developed and implemented.

TABLE 16.3 Common infectious diseases among older people

Infectious disease	Characteristics
COVID-19	• COVID-19 is a viral infection (coronavirus). • COVID-19 is the disease caused by SARS-CoV-2 (emerged in 2019). • Ongoing global pandemic of COVID-19 as at 2022. • Outcomes for vulnerable people are poor. Death or long-term illness often results. • Spread by contact, droplet and air-borne transmission (direct and indirect transmission). • Outbreaks in RACFs require specific management as per government instructions.
Gastroenteritis	• A contagious viral infection that affects the digestive system. • Several strains; norovirus is the most prevalent among older people in RACFs. • Symptoms include abdominal cramping, nausea, vomiting and diarrhoea. • Spread by direct and indirect transmission including contact transmission and eating and drinking contaminated food and water. • Outcomes can include death due to severe dehydration, electrolyte depletion and metabolic acidosis. • Outbreaks require lockdown of facility and the implementation of outbreak protocols.
Influenza	• A contagious viral infection that affects the respiratory system. • Can be mild to severe. • Symptoms include fever (or lack of), chills, muscle aches, cough, congestion, runny nose, headaches and fatigue. • Spread by direct and indirect transmission through contact, droplet and air-borne transmission. • Outcomes are often poor for older people. • Outbreaks require lockdown of facility and the implementation of outbreak protocols.
Methicillin-resistant *Staphylococcus aureus* (MRSA)	• *Staphylococcus aureus* is a bacterium that many people carry on the skin and in the nose. • Staph bacteria that are resistant to methicillin and other antibiotics are called MRSA. • Known as staph or golden staph. • Staph doesn't belong in the body, such as in wounds or in the lungs. • Staph can cause localised infections such as boils, or systemic infections that affect the bones, lungs and other organs. • Spread through direct and indirect contact transmission. • Outcomes can include ongoing infections, amputations, sepsis, pneumonia and death.
Pseudomonas	• Pseudomonas is a bacterium found in soil and water. • Can cause infection to any part of the body, usually mild in healthy adults. • *Pseudomonas aeruginosa* is a strain of Pseudomonas that causes septicaemia and pneumonia. • Infections can be fatal for older people. • Spread by exposure to contaminated soil and water and via direct and indirect contact transmission.
Vancomycin-resistant enterococci (VRE)	• A bacterial infection that is resistant to an important antibiotic called vancomycin. • Enterococci are bacteria found in the intestine and vagina; also found environmentally in water and soil. They can cause infection for **immunosuppressed** people. • Common infections caused by enterococci include urine infections, septicaemia and wound infections. • Spread by direct and indirect contact transmission.

LEGISLATION

The two important pieces of Commonwealth legislation that provide governance on infection control and prevention matters in aged care are the *Aged Care Act 1997* and the *Work Health and Safety Act 2011* (WHS Act). Other important legislation that relates to infection control and prevention are the *Biosecurity Act 2015* and the *Public Health Act 2010,* which was followed by the *Public Health Amendment (Review) Act 2017.*

As is the case with other types of legislation, the states and territories also have their own public health legislation for infection prevention and control.

DEPARTMENTAL GUIDELINES

Information for health-care settings, including aged care, is available from state, territory and other government departments. Organisations in the private sector may be commissioned to work for the government to provide specific guidance and information about particular issues.

The Australian Commission on Safety and Quality in Healthcare (ACSQH) works collaboratively with the government, health professionals and health-care workers, patients and health organisations to improve the safety of health practices and ensure positive health outcomes for people who are provided with a health-related service. This applies to aged care services. The ACSQH has developed the National Safety and Quality Health Service (NSQHS) Standards to provide a cohesive approach to care delivery. One of these is the 2021 Preventing and Controlling Infections Standard, which is aimed at supporting health-care organisations to manage infection control and prevention and respond appropriately to outbreaks.

The ACSQH has also worked collaboratively with the National Health and Medical Research Council (NHMRC) to produce the *Australian Guidelines for the Prevention and Control of Infection in Healthcare* (2019). These guidelines provide a framework for organisations to implement a risk-based approach for managing infection control and prevention. Valuable information provided in the guidelines includes:

- standard and transmission-based precautions
- correct use of PPE
- environmental cleaning/disinfection management
- spills management
- antimicrobial resistance
- hand hygiene
- sharps management.

In 2008, the ACSQH developed the National Hand Hygiene Initiative (NHHI) to promote the prevention and reduction of infection in care settings. All health service organisations must have a hand hygiene program as stated in the NSQHS Standards.

FACILITIES AND SERVICES

Part of the accreditation requirements for RACFs is to manage infection risks according to the Age Care Act requirements. The Aged Care Quality and Safety Commission (the Commission) is the governing body that oversees the compliance of all government-subsidised aged care services, including compliance with the Aged Care Quality Standards (the Standards).

The eight standards often overlap to ensure a contextual continuum of care. Standard 3, "Personal Care and Clinical Care", is most relevant to infection control and prevention. The Commission requires RACFs to demonstrate that they have "a dedicated clinical staff member responsible to support the design, implementation and continuous improvement of infection prevention and control policies, procedures and practices". The Commission also ensures that aged care services adopt standard and transmission-based precautions within the workplace, and it provides those services with education and training relevant to infection control and prevention.

All aged care facilities must identify and respond to incidents of high-risk infection and outbreaks of high-risk infection according to the WHS Act, other jurisdictional requirements and the Commission. Policies and procedures that support all aspects of infection control and prevention must be available to staff, visitors and the Commission on request.

STAFF

As a work health and safety (WHS) requirement, all staff, including care workers, are responsible for managing infection control and prevention in the workplace. Workers are supported by the workplace to understand the requirements for working safely through the provision of guidance and information, education and training, and policies and procedures.

In the context of infection control and prevention, care workers have a responsibility to:

- comply with workplace policies and procedures
- follow the person's care plan to determine infection control and prevention strategies
- comply with safe work practices
- identify and report when an older person is unwell
- use PPE appropriate to the task
- participate in workplace education and training
- follow policies and procedures
- stay home if sick
- report breaches of work practice (such as staff who don't use PPE)
- document infection control matters according to organisational requirements
- use standard precautions at all times
- use transmission-based precautions as instructed by the workplace.

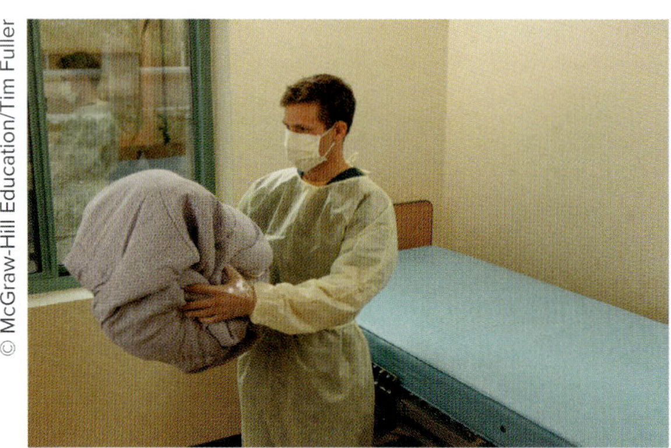

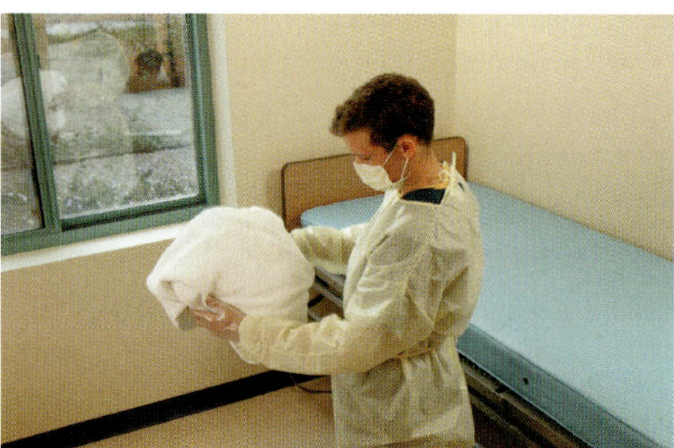

Carry contaminated linen away from the body to avoid cross-contamination

16.2.3 Risk management

Infection control and prevention are primarily a safety issue and, as such, require a risk minimisation approach. A hazard is something that has a risk of harm associated with it. In the context of infection control and prevention, hazards that carry the risk of infection to others may include:

- blood and body fluids
- actions of infected people, such as coughing, sneezing, laughing and yelling
- used sharps
- contaminated linen

- contaminated surfaces and equipment
- infectious workers and visitors
- living in a communal environment or shared room.

When hazards are identified, they must be reported to management as soon as possible so that strategies to contain the infectious agent and prevent cross-contamination can be implemented immediately.

FACTORS THAT PLACE A PERSON AT RISK OF INFECTION

All people are prone to experience infection; however, some people have minimal signs and symptoms of infection, while others have life-threatening experiences. The key function of a person's immune system is to enable them to fight infection. Anything that reduces the immune system's ability to function at its optimal level will increase the risk of severe infection. Table 16.4 describes some factors that place a person at risk of infection.

TABLE 16.4 Factors that place a person at risk of infection

Risk factor	Description	Risk management strategies
Age	The ageing process affects all body systems, including the immune system. T-cells are fighter cells that attack "bad" cells and remember them, so they fight them harder the next time. We have fewer T-cells as we age, and this can decrease the efficiency of vaccines. We all age differently. Immune cells don't communicate well with each other, so we can have a delayed response to infection and healing.	The ageing process affects individuals differently and is influenced by many factors, including the health and wellbeing of the person. Healthy ageing practices, such as getting good sleep, eating and drinking well, and exercising, may improve the way we respond to illness. Specific protocols and practices around infection control and prevention must be followed by workers who look after the vulnerable aged, including correct hand hygiene practices and following standard and transmission-based precautions in the workplace.
Medication	The side effects of some medications affect the immune system, such as those that are used to treat asthma, arthritis and inflammatory bowel disease (corticosteroids). Some medications that are used to treat autoimmune diseases can also decrease the immune system. These medications are called immunosuppressant.	Medications are important for management of diseases, but their side effects can be debilitating. Staff must be aware of the immune-suppressing drugs that older people take and ensure that practices for infection control and prevention take place in the context of providing support for the person. The person's care plan should reflect their risk of infection if they take immunosuppressants. Medications should also be reviewed by medical practitioners and pharmacists on a regular basis.
Invasive medical devices	Clinical evidence suggests that people with an invasive medical device have a higher risk of infection than those who don't. An invasive device is one that enters the body (e.g. a urinary catheter).	Any older person who has an invasive medical device should have a care plan that directs the care requirements for the device. Infection control and prevention will be a component of this plan. Care workers should always observe the site of the invasive device for signs of irritation and infection and report their observations to the RN or the supervisor to be followed up.

(Continues)

TABLE 16.4 Factors that place a person at risk of infection (continued)

Risk factor	Description	Risk management strategies
Chronic disease and autoimmune disease	Chronic disease can affect the immune system and increase the severity of illness. Some chronic diseases engage the immune system constantly and create an ongoing inflammatory response. **Autoimmune** disease can cause the body's immune system to fight itself, thereby destroying valuable immune cells. Cell reproduction can be affected by illness and age.	Older people with an ageing immune system may also be compromised with one or more chronic diseases that affect their ability to cope with infection. Older people with chronic disease should have access to chronic disease management practices and interventions to ensure they are in the best possible health considering their disease. Care plans should document the chronic disease and the strategies that can be implemented to ensure optimal management of the disease.
Environment	The environment is a risk factor for infection. • People in RACFs live in a communal environment where they may share a room with another person, gather with others for meals in a dining area and spend time in common areas. • Health workers are at risk of infection because of the nature of the work they do. They can be exposed to infection when providing support to older people. • Hazards exist in the work environment (sharps, contaminated linen and waste, etc.). • Outbreaks occur in RACFs. • There are also issues in the global environment, such as the coronavirus pandemic.	The hazards and risks of infection in the environment can be mitigated with the infection control and prevention practices that are stipulated in the organisation's policies and procedures. When staff all follow the procedures, infection risk is minimised. Staff who do the wrong thing (e.g. come to work when they are sick) create opportunities for infection to proliferate in the environment. Follow procedures for standard precautions at all times to minimise risk of harm to others. Outbreaks require a specific response that is coordinated and pre-planned. Care workers must follow the instruction of infection control leads or coordinators in the event of an outbreak.

16.2.4 Documentation of risk

Documentation is a critical component of effective infection control and prevention. All activities and incidents that are identified as an infection risk must be reported immediately to the RN or the supervisor. An RACF will have at least one infection prevention and control (IPC) lead, who is a designated person who oversees infection control and prevention in the organisation. As a care worker in an RACF, you may be required to report directly to the IPC lead about your concerns regarding risk of infection in the workplace.

Any report must be followed by clear documentation. A hazard report may be used to document a possible risk of infection in the workplace, or an incident report may also be used. For example, if an older person residing in an RACF refuses to have their chronic leg ulcers covered with a dressing and they continue to mingle with other older people in common areas, the care worker should report their concerns to the RN or supervisor and document the incident. The incident needs to be managed appropriately to eliminate the risk of infection.

Other methods of documentation that are used in the context of infection control and prevention include:

- the person's progress notes or case notes (to keep an ongoing record of infection-related information that is relevant to the person)
- written instructions from the RN or the medical practitioner regarding treatments for infection
- lists of names of people who have infections in an outbreak
- contacts of people who have infections (to allow for tracing and communication)

- handover and hospital transfer forms
- medication charts
- minutes of infection control and prevention meetings
- care plans of older people who have, or are at risk of having, an infection.

Documentation in the aged care setting is essential to ensure a continuum of care and unbroken communication among the care team.

16.2.5 Control measures to minimise risk

When infection risks are identified, ways to eliminate or control the risk must be implemented. Using the hierarchy of controls for infection control and prevention is an effective mechanism for reducing risk. It is important to determine the likelihood of the risk occurring and how severe the harm from the risk might be. In the context of aged care services, any risk of infection has a high likelihood of occurrence in older people, based on age and chronic disease. The severity of harm from infection can be catastrophic, and even fatal, for older people based on their decreased ability to fight infection, the presence of chronic disease and high multiple medication use. For those living in a communal environment, the risk of infection is higher.

Control measures are ways to minimise risk. In regard to infection risks, they may include:

- using PPE
- following standard precautions
- isolating infected people where possible
- rostering staff appropriately
- ensuring a hand hygiene protocol is in place
- implementing transmission-based precautions as appropriate
- ensuring policies and procedures are current and are followed by all staff
- requiring all visitors to sign in and out of the premises
- ensuring that lockdown of facilities occurs in a timely manner when an outbreak occurs
- using signage and other methods of communication to inform people of risks
- liaising with other organisations such as the Aged Care Quality and Safety Commission, the Public Health Units and other government supports.

The ultimate control is to eliminate the hazard, therefore eliminating the risk. This can be difficult with infections in a facility where many people live and work. Any control measures that are implemented must be monitored and evaluated for effectiveness to ensure a process of improving practices related to infection control and prevention.

WORKPLACE SCENARIO

Roles and responsibilities of workers in relation to infection control

Sienna, a care worker, is woken early by her alarm. Her head hurts, and she feels like she might vomit. She was up during the night with stomach cramps, she remembers. She is due to start work at 7 am at the community residential aged care facility but doesn't feel well enough to go to work. If she cannot work, however, her team won't have enough members of staff.

(Continues)

Sienna feels guilty for not being well enough to go to work and support her team and the people she cares for. However, she realises that part of her role and responsibility is to keep the people at the facility safe. She calls her supervisor and reports that she is unwell, knowing that she is doing the right thing to prevent others becoming unwell should she be contagious. Having fewer staff for the shift is better than putting older people at risk of infection and putting the facility into lockdown.

CHECK YOUR UNDERSTANDING

1. What are the six links of the chain of infection?
2. List three signs of systemic infection in an older person.
3. List four infectious diseases that older people may experience.
4. What are five responsibilities of a care worker with regards to infection control and prevention in the workplace?

16.3 MANAGING RISKS ASSOCIATED WITH SPECIFIC HAZARDS

Some hazards have higher risks than others. As a care worker, you need to understand what the protocols in your workplace are for managing specific hazards and their associated risks.

16.3.1 Accidental exposure

Sometimes, care workers may be exposed to a hazard directly. In the context of infection control and prevention, workers may be exposed to the blood and/or body fluids of an older person they support. Specific protocols regarding exposure management will provide information and guidance regarding the required actions that must occur when an accidental exposure occurs in the workplace.

If accidently exposed to blood or body fluids, the worker should (where applicable):

- safely remove contaminated clothing
- wash the affected area well with warm, soapy running water
- if inoculated with a contaminated sharp, ensure the sharp is discarded safely
- if eyes have been splattered, rinse the eyes thoroughly with eyes open
- if the mouth has been splattered, spit it out; rinse the mouth with water several times and spit out after each rinse
- inform the RN or supervisor immediately and follow policies and procedures
- go to the doctor or the nearest emergency department as soon as possible.

All instances of accidental exposure to blood and body fluids in the workplace that involve staff are a WHS issue and must be reported using an incident form/report. Always follow organisational policies and procedures regarding accidental exposure.

16.3.2 Wound management

Current clinical practice for wound management advocates infection control and prevention principles. Many multi-resistant organisms such as MRSA and VRE can infect wounds, and careful management is necessary to prevent cross-contamination.

Wound management practices are designed to minimise the risk of infection by incorporating aseptic technique, single-use equipment, the use of modern dressings that don't require frequent handling, and specific cleaning processes, including waste disposal. In an RACF, wound care occurs in the person's room to minimise infection. **Aseptic** technique is a procedure used by nurses that aims to keep the procedure as clean as possible. It involves using a trolley that has been cleaned with disinfectant, a specific hand hygiene protocol and the use of sterile equipment. The packages of equipment (such as a dressing pack) are opened in a specific manner so as not to contaminate the sterile area that the nurse creates. Sterile gloves are worn, and at no time during the procedure does the sterile area become contaminated. Aseptic technique is used for wound care, catheterisations, suturing and other clinical procedures that may be performed by the nurse or the medical practitioner. After the procedure, the used equipment is discarded into the clinical waste bin, more hand hygiene occurs, and the trolley is once again disinfected.

16.3.3 Outbreak management

An outbreak of an infectious agent such as gastroenteritis or influenza can be declared in an RACF when two or more people have signs and symptoms of the illness. If the infectious agent is extremely virulent, such as COVID-19, one person with signs and symptoms is enough to declare an outbreak. It is important to note that a COVID-19 outbreak may be handled differently than another type of outbreak. During an outbreak, an RACF will initiate its outbreak plan. Depending on the infectious agent involved, the plan may include:

- locking down the facility and restricting visitors and external services
- ongoing communications with the local Public Health Unit
- implementing transmission-based precautions such as full PPE (long-sleeved gowns, face shields, etc.)
- rostering staff to ensure that exposure to other staff is limited
- liaising with supports such as the Commission and other government-based health organisations (e.g. pathology and health departments)
- having the ICP lead act as a key coordinator
- posting signage to keep people informed of risks, such as "Stop" and "Do Not Enter" signs, even when an outbreak isn't occurring, and to convey everyday messages for work health and safety (e.g. signs that encourage people to wash their hands or that show how to wash their hands)
- screening, monitoring and testing of residents and staff
- collecting specimens and swabs
- communicating with relatives and carers of residents about the outbreak, and ensuring that communication is ongoing between residents and their loved ones
- keeping residents informed of the situation
- maintaining detailed documentation.

The government has information available to support RACFs on outbreak management for gastroenteritis and influenza. In the context of COVID-19 a number of publications are available to support the aged care sector. The *National COVID-19 Aged Care Plan* is a government publication that describes the national approach to preparing for and responding to COVID-19 in RACFs and home-based aged care services. The plan provides information and guidance about COVID-19 and results from a recommendation by the Royal Commission into Aged Care Quality and Safety in 2020.

The Communicable Diseases Network Australia has also developed national guidelines that are available to residential aged care service providers. Titled *COVID-19 Outbreaks in Residential Care Facilities,* the guidelines are designed to provide best practice information to facilities, staff and consumers about COVID-19 management.

The Aged Care Quality and Safety Commission also has guidance available regarding COVID-19 outbreaks in RACFs. *Outbreak Management Planning in Aged Care* provides practical information to providers of residential aged care services about developing and implementing an outbreak plan for COVID-19 within their facility.

16.3.4 Notifiable diseases

Australia's states and territories have public health legislation that requires the notification of some infectious diseases to their Public Health Units. The reporting requirements include mandatory reporting from hospitals, aged care facilities, other health organisations and some health professionals. These reports are de-identified and collated by the Australian Government Department of Health and Aged Care for data collation in the National Notifiable Diseases Surveillance System (NNDSS). Some of these notifiable diseases include:

- botulism
- campylobacteriosis
- chickenpox
- cholera
- hepatitis A, B, C and E
- human coronavirus with pandemic potential
- listeriosis
- Middle East respiratory syndrome coronavirus (also known as MERS-CoV)
- pertussis
- pneumococcal disease
- salmonellosis
- severe acute respiratory syndrome (also known as SARS)
- shingles.

The Department of Health and Aged Care website lists all nationally notifiable diseases classified by type (see https://www.health.gov.au).

16.3.5 Immunisation

Immunisation is one of the fundamental protective mechanisms we have for preventing and fighting infection. Vaccines tell the body how to recognise a disease, and if the immunised person does become infected, their body will be able to recognise it, combat it and prevent it from causing immediate complications. Immunisation can also prevent the development of long-term complications that may be associated with the disease. The more people who are immunised against a disease, the less chance the disease has of spreading. This is called herd immunity and is very important for population health.

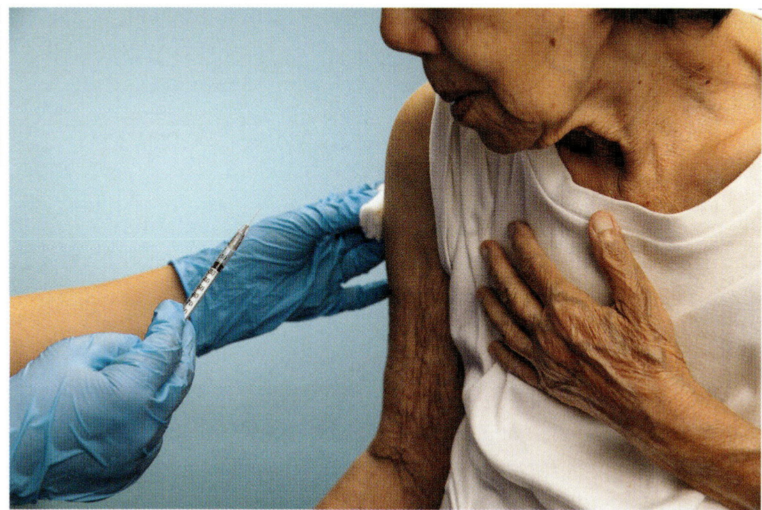

Toa55/Shutterstock

The more people who are immunised against a disease, the less chance the disease has of spreading

Nurses have been receiving vaccinations as a requirement of their role for many years, not only to protect themselves from infectious diseases but also to protect their patients. It is mandatory for all workers in aged care services in Australia to be vaccinated against influenza and COVID-19. Older people are vulnerable to catastrophic outcomes such as severe illness and death as a result of influenza, COVID-19 or other diseases. Even if the older person is vaccinated, they may still succumb to infection if they have underlying health conditions, so it is important that exposure to infectious disease doesn't come from the staff who provide their care. These immunisations protect staff, too.

Working with older people requires staff to be vaccinated as an infection control and prevention measure. Being vaccinated is also one of the key responsibilities for working with vulnerable people.

16.3.6 Clean and contaminated zones

Another strategy for minimising contamination in the RACF is the practice of designating zones as clean or contaminated. Clean zones are areas where non-contaminated items are kept. These areas may include storage rooms, linen rooms or trolleys, and medication rooms. Sterile and clinical equipment may have their own dedicated room. It is important that clean work areas are not contaminated with infectious, or potentially infectious, microorganisms.

Contaminated zones are areas that are known to have a high risk of infectious, or potentially infectious, microorganisms. These areas include the utility room, soiled linen areas and waste areas. Another example of a contaminated zone is the room of an older person who is known to have a transmissible infection. The person will be isolated in their room, and all necessary equipment such as nebulisers and blood pressure machines will be contaminated. Therefore, if possible, it is best practice to keep dedicated equipment in the person's room. A PPE station will be set up at the door of the person's room, and anyone who is required to enter the room will don and doff PPE. The room and equipment will undergo more frequent cleaning under the transmission-based precautions protocol. Where possible, work from clean areas first before working in contaminated areas.

All workers are in close proximity to several people throughout their shift, and it is essential, therefore, that we take personal responsibility for practising standard and transmission-based precautions to prevent older people in our care from becoming sick. Breaking the chain of infection can be as simple as washing your hands often and well.

WORKPLACE SCENARIO

Outbreak management

Bryce is a care worker at The Ferns RACF. Most of the time, he works night shifts. When he receives his handover report tonight, he learns that Mr Lords had complained of stomach pain during the afternoon. During the night, Mr Lords experiences an episode of vomiting and complains of abdominal cramping and headache. Bryce reports the incident to the RN, and he makes sure to use PPE and correct hand hygiene procedures when assisting Mr Lords to get changed. Around dawn, Mrs James, who resides in a shared room down the corridor, starts experiencing vomiting and diarrhoea.

Bryce knows that two or more cases of vomiting or diarrhoea within a 24-hour period mean the facility is probably experiencing a gastroenteritis outbreak. The RN sets up a PPE station at the doors of both affected residents and instructs Bryce to use transmission-based precautions for the rest of his shift. Common areas such as the dining and TV areas are closed off, and the facility's outbreak plan is launched, including an immediate lockdown.

The infection control coordinator is notified and proceeds to commence coordinating the outbreak, including notifying the Public Health Unit about the infectious cases.

CHECK YOUR UNDERSTANDING

1. After an accidental exposure to blood or body fluid, a worker follows organisational policies and procedures to manage the exposure. What documentation is required when an accidental exposure occurs?
2. What are five things that may occur in the event of an outbreak of an infectious agent in an RACF?
3. Why is it important for aged care staff to be vaccinated against influenza and COVID-19?
4. Why do aged care facilities need to have designated clean and contaminated zones?
5. What is the difference between a clean zone and a contaminated zone?

SUMMARY

- Standard precautions and transmission-based precautions are practices that aged care workers follow to minimise the risks associated with infection prevention and control.
- Hand hygiene is one of the most effective ways to break the chain of infection and is a gold standard practice to prevent cross-contamination of pathogens between people. The "5 Moments for Hand Hygiene" is a useful guide for knowing when to attend to hand hygiene at work.
- Infection control hazards in the workplace are managed using the hierarchy of control. Effective control measures can minimise the risk of infection in the workplace and keep older people safe.
- All facilities must have an outbreak management plan that is ready to be deployed at any given time. Community aged care services also need to have a plan of action for managing community outbreaks of infectious agents.

REVIEW QUESTIONS

16.1 What is "hand care", and why is it important?
16.2 Identify hazards associated with body fluids that are a risk to care workers.
16.3 How do you control the risks associated with these hazards?
16.4 What factors place an older person at higher risk of contracting an infection?

BIBLIOGRAPHY

Aged Care Quality and Safety Commission, *Quality Standards*, 18 March 2021, https://www.agedcarequality.gov.au/providers/standards, accessed 22 December 2021.

Australian Commission on Safety and Quality in Health Care (ACSQHC), *Infection Prevention and Control Workbook*, ACSQHC, Sydney, 2019.

Australian Government, Department of Health, *Updated National COVID-19 Aged Care Plan*, 7th edition, 2020, https://www.health.gov.au/sites/default/files/documents/2020/12/updated-national-covid-19-aged-care-plan-7th-edition_2.pdf, accessed 22 December 2021.

Clinical Excellence Commission (CEC), *COVID-19 Infection Prevention and Control Manual for Acute and Non-Acute Healthcare Settings*, CEC, Sydney, 2021.

Communicable Diseases Network Australia, *COVID-19 Outbreaks in Residential Care Facilities*, National Guidelines for the Prevention, Control and Public Health Management of COVID-19 Outbreaks in Residential Care Facilities in Australia, last updated 15 February 2022.

Infection Control Expert Group, *Guidance on the Use of Personal Protective Equipment (PPE) for Health Care Workers in the Context of COVID-19*, 2021, https://www.health.gov.au/sites/default/files/documents/2021/06/guidance-on-the-use-of-personal-protective-equipment-ppe-for-health-care-workers-in-the-context-of-covid-19.pdf, accessed 22 December 2021.

National Health and Medical Research Council (NHMRC), *Clinical Educators' Guide: Australian Guidelines for the Prevention and Control of Infection in Healthcare*, NHMRC, Sydney, 2019.

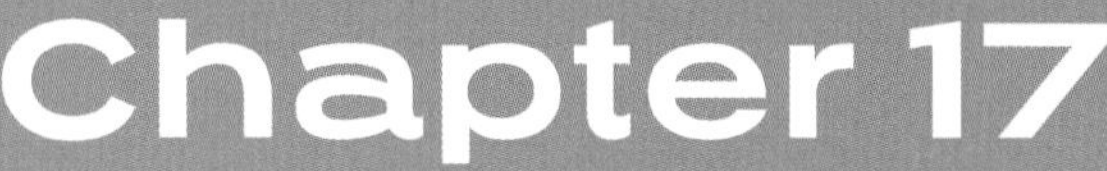

Chapter 17

Assisting with medications

LEARNING OBJECTIVES

17.1 Prepare to assist with medications

17.2 Support the individual with medications

17.3 Handle contingencies

17.4 Follow required procedures and methods of documentation

INTRODUCTION

MEDICATIONS (DRUGS) ARE USED TO treat, alleviate, diagnose, cure, enhance and manage many health issues. For example, vaccines prevent the spread of diseases such as influenza, and medicines such as paracetamol provide pain relief.

Medication use is far more common in older people than in younger populations. As we age, we are more likely to experience chronic disease and health conditions such as hypertension and diabetes. Treatment for these conditions and other health issues will include prescribed medications, non-prescription medications and, possibly, complementary medicines.

There are several health professionals involved in medication support, each with their own scope of practice and legal requirements. As a care worker providing support for older people, you may be required to assist the people you care for with their medication. To do this in a legal and ethical manner, you need to ensure you have received the appropriate training in medication assistance, and the organisation you work for must support you in this role with relevant organisational policies and procedures. You will need to have a sound understanding of these procedures and policies and maintain your knowledge and skill base surrounding medication assistance. You will also need to know how to manage contingencies, such as when a person refuses to take a medication.

INDUSTRY IN FOCUS

Legislation and regulations relevant to the administration of medications in aged care

Medication use in Australia is regulated by a complex web of laws and guidelines. There is no major law that governs medicine use in isolation. Instead, multiple laws and regulations are necessary to address the many legal issues that medicines and other poisons present to the safety and wellbeing of all Australians. While Australia is governed as a whole by the Commonwealth Government, each state and territory government is permitted to pass its own laws. This means that while Commonwealth legislation exists governing medication use by all Australians, each state and territory will also have its own specific laws around medication use that are applicable to people living and visiting in those jurisdictions.

While the various state and territory medication laws are unique to their jurisdiction, they all address how medicines are to be used safely. They state how medicines are prescribed and administered, and by whom, how they are provided and how they are stored. The following state and territory laws are relevant to medicines, drugs and other poisons:

- Northern Territory: *Medicines, Poisons and Therapeutic Goods Act 2012*
- Victoria: *Drugs, Poisons and Controlled Substances Act 1981*
- Western Australia: *Medicines and Poisons Act 2014*
- South Australia: *Controlled Substances Act 1984*
- New South Wales: *Poisons and Therapeutic Goods Act 1966*
- Queensland: *Medicines and Poisons Act 2019*
- Australian Capital Territory: *Medicines, Poisons and Therapeutic Goods Act 2008*
- Tasmania: *Poisons Act 1971*.

The use of medicines in Australia is regulated by the Therapeutic Goods Administration (TGA) under the guidance of the *Therapeutic Goods Act 1989* (Cth). This law regulates how medicines are imported and exported, and how they are manufactured and supplied for use in Australia. The TGA monitors and evaluates reported adverse drug events from medicines used in Australia and is also responsible for the labelling, advertising and availability of medicines. Prescription and non-prescription medications are placed into the Australian Register of Therapeutic Goods (ARTG) to ensure a national list of medicines approved for use in the country.

The safety of medication use relies on the ability of health professionals such as medical specialists, doctors and nurses to practise ethically and legally. The role of the health professional in medication use is a very important one that requires qualified practices including correct clinical assessment for the needs of medication, safe prescribing, safe dispensing, safe administration, and ongoing professional standards of risk minimisation regarding medications. Health professionals are regulated by national boards that support the Health Practitioner Regulation National Law. This law ensures that health professionals are registered and accredited to practise. Examples of national boards include the Medical Board of Australia and the Nursing and Midwifery Board of Australia. The agency that oversees the registration and accreditation of health professionals is the Australian Health Practitioner Regulation Agency (AHPRA).

There are other laws that are applicable to the use of medicines in Australia, such as those that apply to criminal law and common law. The best way a care worker can work within the legal and ethical boundaries of medication support is to follow the policies and procedures of their workplace. Most importantly, if a care worker is in doubt about any aspect of medication support, they should seek clarification from the registered nurse (RN) or their supervisor in the first instance.

17.1 PREPARING TO ASSIST WITH MEDICATIONS

17.1.1 Legislation and guidelines

There are many laws that regulate the aged care industry. Legislation exists to provide laws and guidance that enable workplace processes to occur in a safe manner, either at a Commonwealth level or a state/territory level. Legislation is regulated by codes of practice, guidelines and policies.

In Australia, medications are regulated by the **Therapeutic Goods Administration (TGA)** under the legislation of the *Therapeutic Goods Act 1989*. The TGA is responsible for the safety and quality of medications, as well as of medical devices. It also regulates prescription and non-prescription medications and approves medicines for use in Australia. Other responsibilities of the TGA include managing how medicines are labelled and stored. Once approved, medications and other drugs are placed on the Australian Register of Therapeutic Goods. Legislation that relates to medication support includes the *Aged Care Act 1997,* the *Disability Discrimination Act 1992,* the *Work Health and Safety Act 2011,* the *Privacy Act 1988* and the *Poisons Act 1971.* These Acts are all Commonwealth legislation. Each state and territory has its own more specific laws relating to medications.

The Aged Care Quality Standards (the Quality Standards) provide government-funded aged care services with a framework for working legally and ethically. The Quality Standards apply to residential aged care facilities (RACFs) and community aged care services and provide information to ensure that organisations are compliant with providing safe and quality care to older people. Application of these eight standards ensures that all aspects of wellbeing for an older person receiving services can be addressed. In particular, Standard 3, "Personal Care and Clinical Care", supports safe medication management.

17.1.2 Workplace policies

Organisations that provide support to people with their medication management have policies and procedures that have been developed in alignment with legislation in order to be compliant and to minimise risk of harm to staff and to the people they support. The regulation of medication management in the aged care sector is present in a compliance framework that reflects the Quality Standards, the quality indicator program and quality care principles.

The National Medicines Policy has the objective of managing medicines in Australia in a way that promotes health and economic outcomes as a collaborative effort between the Commonwealth, state and territory governments and the health industry. The *Guiding Principles for Medication Management in Residential Aged Care Facilities* and the *Guiding Principles of Medication Management in the Community* are publications that aim to ensure the safe and effective use of medications in the aged care industry. Both publications are representative of the National Medicines Policy. Procedures that you may find in the workplace that stem from these publications include the organisation's medication advisory committee, pharmacist-led medication reviews for people using the service, and more stringent processes for medication incident reporting.

17.1.3 Medications

HOW DO MEDICATIONS WORK?

Medications have an important role in the health and wellbeing of individuals and are designed to have an intended effect in the body. These intentions include the alleviation of symptoms such as nausea and pain, the elimination of infection-based illnesses, immune support during cancer treatments and the management of chronic conditions.

Medications work in the body through a process of absorption, distribution, metabolism and elimination. In other words, the chemicals in the medication make their way to the cells in the body via the bloodstream where they will make something happen, or block something from happening, within those cells.

Most medications are eliminated from the body in the urine. Not all medications follow this process, however, as some will work at the intended site of administration. For example, the medication in a puffer is inhaled into the lungs, where it will take effect; likewise, a dose of antacid that is swallowed will work in the stomach. Some medications are eliminated through sweat, breathing, breast milk and saliva.

TYPES OF MEDICATIONS

The three types of medications available to consumers include prescription medications, non-prescription medications and complementary medicines.

PRESCRIPTION MEDICATIONS

Prescription medications are those ordered by a doctor or other health practitioner who has prescribing rights in Australia. Prescriptions are written instructions for medications and are decided by the practitioner based on a medical or other consultation. Prescriptions, also known as scripts, are taken to a pharmacist to be dispensed. Prescriptions state the medication name, the amount to be taken or used, and the time when it should be taken or used. Prescription medication is highly regulated by the TGA, due to the risks attached to the medication and the potential for it to be misused by people in the community.

NON-PRESCRIPTION MEDICATIONS

Non-prescription medications are also known as over-the-counter (OTC) medications. They are available without a prescription and an individual can purchase them at pharmacies, supermarkets or other places of general purchases, such as service stations. However, some are only available at a pharmacy with a pharmacist consultation, based on the level of risk associated with them. Non-prescription medications are also regulated, where some are registered and others are listed with the TGA–for example, medication used to treat hay fever.

COMPLEMENTARY MEDICINES

These medications don't require a prescription from a doctor and are available for people to purchase off the shelf, from an alternative health practitioner or from a compounding pharmacy. Complementary medicines include products such as vitamins and minerals, traditional herbal remedies, Chinese medicines and nutritional supplements. While these types of medication have not necessarily been clinically proven as effective, there is evidence that some of them can cause adverse effects when taken with prescribed medications. While many of these medications are regulated by the TGA, there are also some that are not. Many people view complementary medicines as harmless; however, some unintended effects of these medications can cause serious health problems for older people. For example, St John's wort can influence the effectiveness of important prescription medications such as some antidepressants and blood thinners like warfarin.

PRACTICE POINT

As a care worker assisting older people with their medications, you have a duty of care to report your concerns about medication use to your supervisor or RN. For example, the person may tell you that they have started to use Ayurvedic (traditional Indian) medicines for pain relief. Of course, the person has the absolute right to do so; however, it is important that they and their doctor have the opportunity to discuss possible risks associated with using prescribed and complementary medications simultaneously. It is not within your role to give advice about medication; however, you can facilitate the opportunity for discussion by reporting to the RN or your supervisor.

FORMS OF MEDICATION

Medication is used in many varieties, and the same medication may be available in more than one form. Forms of medication are considered when they are first prescribed by the medical practitioner or recommended by the pharmacist. Table 17.1 illustrates common forms of medication used in Australia.

TABLE 17.1 Common forms of medication used in Australia

Image	Form	Description	Example
	Lotion/cream	Cream-based medication that is rubbed into the skin.	Antifungal cream for a fungal infection, such as Tinaderm or Canesten. Calamine lotion for pruritus.
	Ointment	Thicker than creams; a greasy substance with less absorption; tends to work on affected area of application.	Barrier creams to prevent excoriation of the skin, such as Calmoseptine and Sudocrem. Advantan for eczema. Antibiotic ointment to treat infections such as conjunctivitis (eye infection), for example Chlorsig.
	Transdermal patches	A patch that adheres to the skin and contains a slow release of medication that is absorbed into the bloodstream.	Pain relief: Norspan. Heart: Transiderm Nitro. Quit smoking: Nicabate.
	Capsules	Powdered, granule or liquid medication dose encapsulated in a gelatinous cover that can be hard or soft and is designed to be swallowed whole.	Antibiotics such as amoxicillin and cefalexin. Medications such as ergocalciferol (vitamin D).
	Caplets	A tablet that is shaped smoothly like a capsule to assist swallowing.	Cold and flu caplets, vitamins, Panadol caplets.
	Tablets	Medication that is compressed into a hard shape. Can be crushable or not crushable, depending on the medication type.	Crushable: Panadol. Not crushable: Nurofen.
	Syrup/elixir/suspension	Syrup: Liquid medication that contains dose per mL. Doesn't need to be shaken. Prescribed dose is measured into measure cup or syringe. Suspension: Liquid medication that is thicker than syrups or elixirs. Contains microgranules of medication in a thick liquid. The bottle must be shaken to distribute medication in bottle for correct dosage when measured.	Cough elixirs, some vitamins. Anticonvulsant medication: Epilim. Pain relief: Panadol syrup. Antibiotics such as amoxcillin and cefalexin.

TABLE 17.1 Common forms of medication used in Australia (continued)

Image	Form	Description	Example
	Drops	Medication that is instilled into the eyes or the ears using a dropper.	Liquifilm Tears eye drops; Soframycin ear drops for infection.
	Powder	Powdered medication that can be applied to skin or mixed if it is to be taken internally.	Macrogel powder mixed with water for constipation: Movicol. Antifungal powder applied to the skin for tinea.
	Wafer	Medication that is compressed into a wafer that is dissolved almost immediately in the mouth. Fast-acting medication.	Nausea and vomiting: Zofran. Antipsychotic: Zyprexa.
	Injection	Can be intravenous (IV), intramuscular (IM) or subcutaneous (SC).	Preloaded insulin pens are a subcutaneous injection. Care workers are not authorised to administer IV, IM or other SC injections.
	Suppository	A bullet-shaped medication that is designed to be inserted into the rectum where it is absorbed into the bloodstream for effect.	Glycerine suppositories for constipation. Pain and fever: Panadol suppositories.
	Pessary	A small tablet-shaped medication that is designed to be inserted with an applicator into the vagina.	Pessaries may be used to deliver antifungal medication to treat infection or other medications for women, such as hormone-based drugs.
	Inhaler	A device that is also known as a puffer, in which a dose of medication is inhaled into the lungs. The medication can be powder or aerosol.	Asthma: Ventolin. Corticosteroids for lung disease: Pulmicort.

(Continues)

TABLE 17.1 Common forms of medication used in Australia (continued)

Image	Form	Description	Example
	Nebule	A nebule contains a dose of liquid medication that is converted into a mist for inhalation when used in a nebuliser.	Salbutamol for asthma; corticosteroids for lung disease.
	Lozenge	A medicated form of tablet that is designed to dissolve slowly in the mouth to lubricate and soothe the throat.	Cold and flu lozenges, antibacterial and anti-inflammatory lozenges such as Difflam, Strepsils. Quit smoking aid: Nicorette lozenges.
	Gargle	Medication that is diluted to gargle; aimed at treating the pharynx and oral cavity.	Povidone-iodine and anti-inflammatory sore throat gargles such as Betadine throat gargle.
	Gel	Water-based cream that leaves a film on the skin that can relieve itching and pain. Easy to spread and often self-drying.	Anti-inflammatory gel such as Voltaren gel.

Lozenges, Svetlana Lukienko/Shutterstock. All other images © McGraw-Hill Education

MEDICATION ROUTES

The way a medication is administered can have a direct impact on its effectiveness. The route of administration refers to the way the medication gets into the body. Routes of administration include the following:

- *Oral:* Medication is swallowed (includes liquids, tablets, caplets and capsules). Oral medication may be required to be taken with or without food, as instructed by the pharmacist, as some medications are designed to be absorbed more slowly than others. Some people will need to have tablets crushed, for various reasons–for example, they may have dysphagia (swallowing problems due to dementia or having had a stroke)–and it is the prescribing doctor or the pharmacist who can advise if crushing is necessary. Not all tablets can be crushed, and the doctor or pharmacist will need to provide a liquid alternative. Tablets that have a scoring mark on them can be crushed; tablets that are unscored and have a hard (enteric) coating cannot be crushed, as they are designed to be absorbed into the bloodstream slowly. For example, paracetamol tablets and caplets can be crushed; however, ibuprofen must not be crushed as it can cause damage to the lining of the stomach.
- *Sublingual and buccal:* Medication is dissolved under the tongue (sublingual) or in the mouth (buccal). These medications are absorbed very quickly for a rapid action.

- *Instilled:* Medication is instilled into the eye or the ear, and often consists of drops or sprays.
- *Intranasal:* Medication is inhaled into the nasal cavity (the nose).
- *Topical:* Medication is applied to the skin (e.g. creams and transdermal patches). Sometimes called cutaneous and transdermal routes of administration.
- *Rectal:* Medication is inserted into the rectum (e.g. suppositories and enemas). As this is an invasive procedure, care workers are generally not authorised to administer medications rectally.
- *Vaginal:* Medication is inserted into the vagina with an applicator. This is also an invasive procedure and is not included in the role of a care worker.
- *Inhalation:* Medications are breathed in or inhaled into the body. These include nebulised medications, inhalers and puffers used with or without spacers.
- *Injection:* Medication can be inserted into the body via injections. Intravenous injections (IV) are injected directly into the vein for an immediate effect. Intramuscular (IM) injections are delivered by injection into the muscle. Both methods are not practised by care workers as they are nurse-only procedures. Subcutaneous (SC) injections are medications that are delivered into the subcutaneous or fat layer of the skin. These include preloaded insulin pens which appropriately trained and delegated care workers can perform if supported by training and workplace policy.
- *Enteral feeding tubes:* Medications can be administered to the stomach via feeding tubes; however, this is a procedure that carries significant risk of adverse events for the person with the tube, including aspiration. An appropriately qualified nurse or other health professional can administer medications via feeding tubes; however, this skill is not within the scope of practice of the care worker when assisting people with medications.

CLASSIFICATION OF MEDICATIONS

Medications are classified into groups based on their intended action in the body, and there are many types of medication in any one group. Generally, most medications are grouped into one classification. However, a medication may be categorised into more than one group, depending on its therapeutic properties (or uses) (Table 17.2).

MEDICATION NAMES

Every medication has a generic name and a brand name. The generic name is the name of the active ingredients and compounds that have the intended action. Medications can be sold by their generic name. The brand name is given to the medication by the pharmaceutical organisation that markets it. There are many different names for the same medication available for purchase by the consumer. For example, paracetamol is a generic name of the brand names that include Panadol and Panamax.

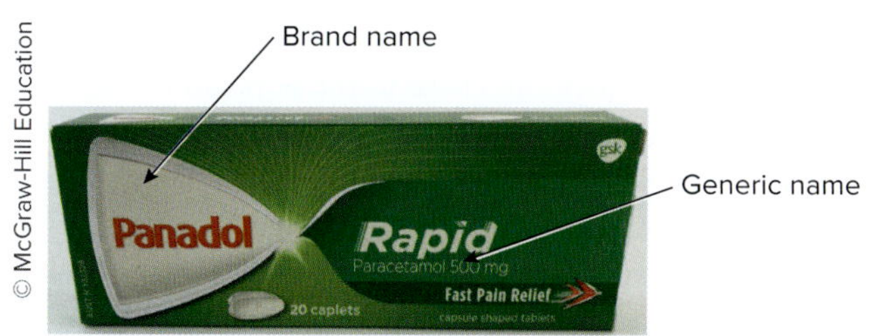

Every medication has a generic name and a brand name

Many doctors and nurse practitioners will prescribe medications by their generic name and the pharmacist may ask the person if they would like to purchase the brand or generic medication. Both work the same way, but the price the person pays may be different. Generic brand medications have the same active ingredients and dose as branded medications and are required to meet the same safety standards in Australia as branded medications under the TGA.

When assisting a person with their medication, you will need to be aware that the medication supplied to them may be either generic or brand medication and at any time be subject to change from one to the other.

TABLE 17.2 Classification of medications

Medication group	Action
Analgesic—narcotic	Treats acute pain and severe chronic pain
Analgesic—simple	Relieves mild to moderate pain
Antacid	Minimises acidity in the gut that causes **reflux** symptoms
Antibiotic	Combats infection
Anticoagulant	Thins the blood
Anticonvulsant	Manages epilepsy and mood disorders
Antidepressant	Treats depressive and anxiety disorders
Antihypertensive	Lowers blood pressure
Anti-inflammatory	Reduces inflammation
Antipsychotic	Affects the brain to change behaviours
Aperient	Mild laxative to prevent and manage constipation
Bronchodilator	Aerosol and inhalation that opens the **bronchi** in the lungs to support gas exchange
Diuretic	Manages excess fluid within the body that threatens organ function
Expectorant, mucolytic, decongestant	Treats and manages cough and cold symptoms
Hypnotic/sedative	Treats acute anxiety; also used prior to medical procedures
Hypoglycaemic	Alters blood glucose levels
Laxative	Encourages bowel evacuation of faeces
Muscle relaxant	Relaxes muscles (e.g. to relax tremors to enable movement)
Vaccine	Protects against infections such as influenza and whooping cough
Vasodilator	Opens up blood vessels to decrease work by the heart

SCHEDULING OF MEDICINES AND POISONS

In Australia, all medications and other poisons are classified due to their level of **toxicity** and the potential harm they can cause to the population. Medications and other poisons are grouped into a schedule, based on the characteristics they share.

The legislation that governs the scheduling of medicines and poisons is the Poisons Standard, June 2021, which is also known as the Standard for the Uniform Scheduling of Medicines and Poisons (SUSMP) No. 33. This national classification system for identifying medicine and poisons schedules also reflects how these substances are regulated in Australia by state and territory legislation.

The schedules are shown in Table 17.3. The schedules most relevant to assisting people with their medication within the care worker's scope of practice are Schedules 2, 3, 4 and 8.

Schedules 2 and 3 medications include those that may be purchased at the supermarket or pharmacy (such as aspirin, antihistamines and laxatives). Schedule 4 medications are those that are prescribed by a doctor and dispensed from a pharmacist and are labelled "Prescription Only Medicine". Some Schedule 4 (S4) drugs have a risk of misuse and dependency and are called S4D drugs. These drugs have prescription restrictions and require an RN and a second appropriately trained worker to dispense. These drugs are accountable, and each dose is recorded in the drug register. Examples of S4D drugs include diazepam and tramadol. Schedule 8 (S8) drugs are controlled drugs that are also accountable and are also dispensed by an RN and witnessed by an appropriately trained worker. S8 drugs also have prescription restrictions due to their potential for misuse and addiction. S8 medications include narcotics such as morphine and codeine. Oxycodone is another example of an S8 drug.

TABLE 17.3 Schedules of medications

Schedule number	Schedule description
1	Not currently in use
2	Pharmacy Medicine
3	Pharmacy Only Medicine
4	Prescription Only Medicine or Prescription Animal Remedy
5	Caution
6	Poison
7	Dangerous Poison
8	Controlled Drug
9	Prohibited Substance
10	Substances of such danger to health as to warrant prohibition of sale, supply and use

Source: https://www.tga.gov.au/scheduling-basics.

STORAGE OF MEDICATIONS

Under the law, all medications within an RACF and other residential living organisations are to be stored in a way that not only protects the integrity of the medication, but also keeps people safe from harm. Medication can cause harm to vulnerable people when it is accessible and not secured safely.

PRACTICE POINT

In an RACF, all Schedule 8 medications require two people to administer: one person (the RN) to administer and one person (a trained care worker) to witness the person take the medication.

After applying the correct checking procedure, always accompany the RN to the person being given the medication to witness the administration process. This is a legal obligation. Remember: you have signed the Drug Register to indicate that you have witnessed the person actually take the medication.

All medication must be stored in a locked room when it is not being accessed by an RN or trained worker. This room will contain the medication trolley that is used for medication rounds within a facility, or a locked cupboard to contain medications that are not in immediate use. Sometimes this room is referred to as the consultation room or the procedure room, depending on the organisation. In the RACF, the medication trolley is used to transport medication during medication rounds such as those that occur at breakfast, lunch and dinner. The trolley is lockable and must never be left unattended.

Schedule 4D and Schedule 8 drugs are required by law to be locked in a purpose-built drug safe. This safe is attached to an internal fixture within the locked room. The RN in charge of the shift has responsibility for the keys to the safe and therefore is responsible for accounting for the contents of the safe on that shift. The safe is only opened in the presence of a trained witness for the purpose of drug administration, for signing in further supply of drugs or for counting the balance of drugs stored there.

People living at home also need to store their medications in a manner that is safe and that will protect the medications from damage. While some people in the community may use a blister pack for their pills, many

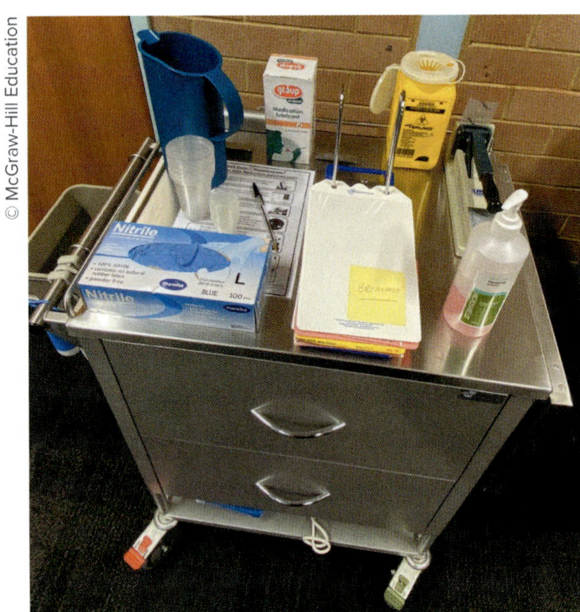

A medication trolley

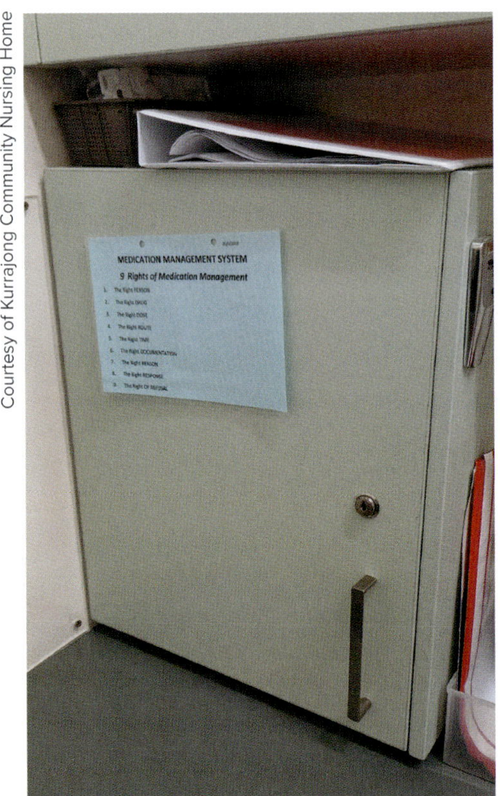

A lockable safe for S4D and S8 drugs

will use the original packaging of the medication from the pharmacy. Many medications have pharmacy placed alert stickers on the packaging that outline how the medication should be stored–for example, "Keep in refrigerator".

Some considerations about safe storage of medications in the person's home may include:

- Keep out of reach of children and pets.
- Follow manufacturer or pharmacy instructions about storage.
- Don't place medications next to food in the refrigerator.
- Keep medications out of direct sunlight.
- Keep medications in a dry place, away from damp.
- Store medications in a separate container and place, away from other people's medications.
- Don't store medications that have expired. Return them to the pharmacy for safe disposal.

Correct storage of medications is important for preventing damage to the chemical components of the drug. The environment where the medication is stored can cause changes within the medication that can make it less effective or make the person unwell. Sunlight, excessive heat and dampness can affect the medication's chemical structure. Some medications are stored in the refrigerator and others in a dark, dry environment such as a cupboard. The manufacturer of the medication will provide written instructions about how it should be stored.

THE EFFECTS OF MEDICATION

Medications have both wanted and unwanted effects for the person using them. These effects include therapeutic effects, side effects and adverse effects.

THERAPEUTIC EFFECTS

The therapeutic effect of medication refers to its ability to do the job it was meant to do. The therapeutic effect of analgesia is to reduce or eliminate pain, and the therapeutic effect of antibiotics is to support the body's immune system to fight infection by destroying bacteria or preventing bacteria from multiplying. The therapeutic level of medication refers to the amount of the medication in the blood that is needed to have the desired effect. This outcome is affected by age and the decrease of body fat, body fluid, gastrointestinal tract function, and liver and kidney function.

SIDE EFFECTS

A side effect is an unwanted or unintended effect that a person may experience from a medication. Side effects can be mild, but some can be severe. All medications, including OTC and complementary medications, will have side effects. Many side effects are common and pass after a short time. These may include a dry mouth, constipation, nausea and tiredness. Some side effects are severe and may cause significant health-related issues, such as depression and anxiety, suicidal ideation, changes to sex drive, weight gain or loss, and changes to the heart rhythm (arrythmia). Side effects can occur regardless of the dose of medication.

ADVERSE DRUG REACTIONS

An adverse drug reaction is where harm occurs to a person as a result of taking the drug at normal and recommended doses. In some people, their body doesn't process the medication as expected and they may experience a reaction as a result. An example of an adverse drug response is an allergic reaction with or without **anaphylaxis**, such as a rash caused by penicillin. In the older population, an adverse drug reaction may include experiencing delirium from the side effects of multiple medications.

ADVERSE DRUG EVENTS

An adverse drug event results when harm occurs from the drug use and includes overdose, taking incorrect doses, drug-to-drug interactions and the early discontinuation of a drug that should be ceased over time. When an older person takes four or more medications, known as polypharmacy, the risk of adverse events is increased. Some medications interfere with other medications to cause an adverse outcome, such as dizziness that can lead to a fall. Drug-to-drug interactions can have serious outcomes for the older population. In the older population, an adverse drug event may include suffering a fractured hip or a head injury as a result of delirium or a fall from the adverse drug reaction.

SENTINEL EVENTS

A sentinel event is an adverse event that impacts the safety of a person receiving support. These events are avoidable and often result in the serious harm or death of a person. All sentinel events are reportable to the Australian Commission on Safety and Quality in Health Care. An example of a sentinel event that is relevant to assisting people with their medication includes medication error resulting in harm or death.

CONSUMER INFORMATION

Information about prescription and some non-prescription medications is available to consumers in the form of Consumer Medicine Information (CMI) documents. These small brochures or leaflets of information are available at pharmacies, online and within the packaging of most medications. The pharmaceutical company that produces the medication is responsible for providing this consumer information. CMIs are designed to improve awareness about the correct and safe use of medications and include information such as:

- side effects
- dosage and what to do in the event of overdose
- the intended effects of the medication
- warnings and precautions
- storage of the medication.

CMIs are updated when the medication changes or when new information about it becomes available. Therefore, all CMIs state the date when the information was last updated. CMIs can be a valuable source of information not only for consumers, but also for care workers.

LABELLING AND PACKAGING

Medication labels and packaging provide important information about the contents within. Labelling and packaging of medications in Australia is regulated by the TGA, which made significant changes to the requirements of information to be presented on packaging and labelling in 2020. Information found on packaging and labelling of medication will include:

- the generic and trade names of the medication
- the amount of medication
- the active ingredient of the medication and how much active ingredient is present in each dose
- expiry date
- warnings about the medication
- storage information
- use of the medication (if not prescribed)
- directions for use (if not prescribed)
- batch number and Australian Register of Therapeutic Goods (ARTG) number.

PHARMACY LABELS

A pharmacy label is placed on the medication packaging by the pharmacist when prescribed medication is dispensed or processed. The pharmacist uses information provided on the prescription from the doctor. This information includes the generic and trade names of the medication, the prescribing doctor's details and the date of the prescription. Directions for use and dosages are also included. Specific warnings and instructions, such as "Take directly after meals" or "Keep out of direct sunlight", may also be included. Importantly, the name of the person for whom the medication is intended is also on the pharmacy label.

Pharmacy labels play a very important role in minimising medication errors and incidents, and in providing valuable information to support workers when assisting people with medication.

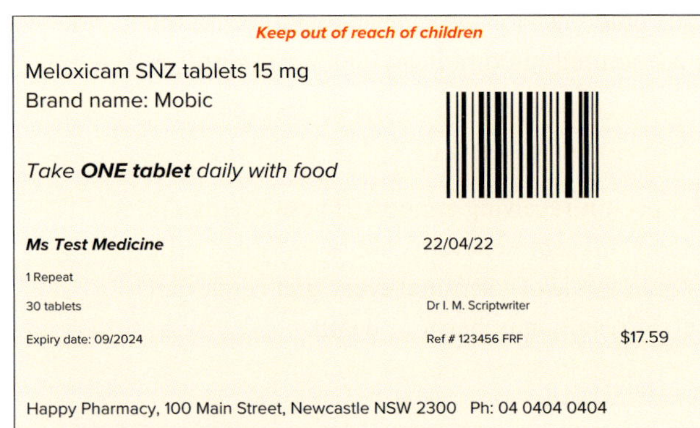

Example of a pharmacy label

DOSE ADMINISTRATION AIDS

Dose administration aids (DAAs) are types of packaging that organise multiple tablets and capsules according to the times they are to be taken. People may benefit from a DAA if they are required to take multiple medications at different times of day and may risk missing medications or double dosing from the original packaging. These aids are not ideal for everyone, as dexterity, good vision and cognition are all required to safely use a DAA.

Commonly used DAAs include blister packs, sachet systems and dosette boxes.

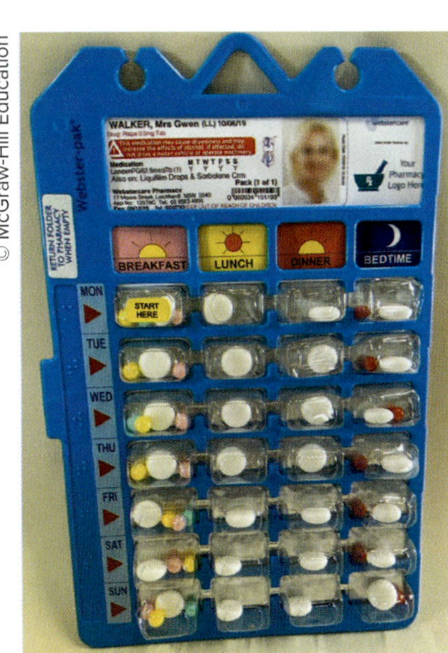

A blister pack

BLISTER PACKS

Blister packs contain multiple doses of medication, often with supply for one week. Each dose is sealed in a plastic blister or bubble to protect the tablets and is packed for specific times of the day, such as breakfast, lunch and dinner. The person pushes the medication out of the appropriate blister, based on the day and the time the medication is needed. For example, if they take four tablets at breakfast time, they will push out four blisters, as each medication is packed separately.

Blister packs are prepared by a pharmacist and may contain prescribed and pharmacy medications. Each pack has an identification label prepared by the pharmacist that also includes the name and dose of each medication, often printed on the reverse side of the package label. The sheet of "blisters" is most often held within a hard, coloured plastic frame, although some aged care organisations are supplied the packs without the frame. It is obvious when a blister pack has been tampered with.

It is important to note that blister packs used by people in the community will look different from those used by people who reside in an RACF. Community dwellers usually have all their medications in one, or maybe two, packs, while people in an RACF may have packs specifically designed for separate times of the day.

SACHET SYSTEMS

Sachet systems are comprised of pharmacy-prepared sachets that contain multiple doses of medication within one sachet. Unlike blister packs, where each medication is packed in a separate blister, sachets contain all the medications required at the time. For example, if a person takes four tablets at breakfast time, all of these tablets will be in the one sachet. The sachets required for the day are presented in a roll, in chronological order, and are usually placed within a purpose-designed receptacle. Each sachet is labelled with the person's name, the date, and the name and dose of the medications within it. Some brands will include a descriptor of each tablet. Sachets are tamper evident.

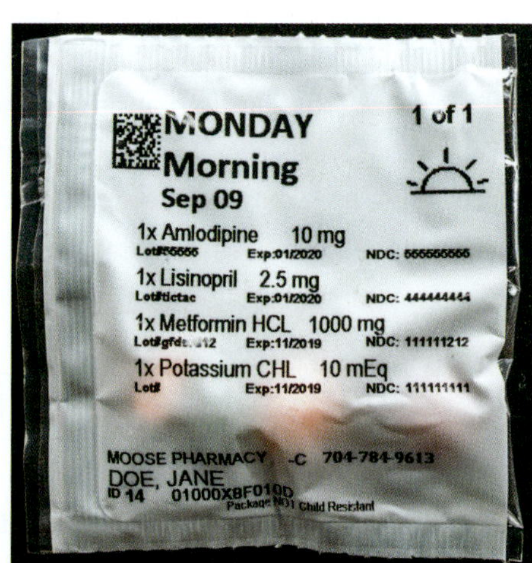

Courtesy of Moose Pharmacy

A sachet system

DOSETTE BOXES

Dosette boxes are also known as medication compartment boxes and are available for purchase at pharmacies and supermarkets. People who manage their own medication and some health professionals will fill these boxes with medication. Dosette boxes are available in many styles and sizes and are designed to sort medications into doses and times. It is important to remember to follow your organisation's policies and procedures when assisting someone with medications from a dosette box. Ultimately, you don't have any information about the contents of the box and your scope of practice doesn't include packing the person's medications into a dosette box. People who require a support worker to assist them with their medication may benefit from a blister pack or sachet system, as these methods of medication organisation provide risk management processes. It is difficult to determine whether a dosette box has been tampered with.

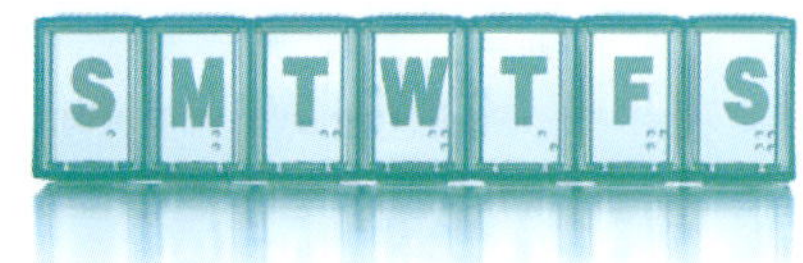

© McGraw-Hill Education

A dosette box

WORKPLACE SCENARIO

What to do when someone has an adverse reaction to a medication

Bibi works at a residential aged care facility and is responsible for assisting residents with their medication management. One of the people she supports is Mrs Dodd, who has been prescribed penicillin for a chest infection and had her first dose at lunchtime. When Bibi goes to assist Mrs Dodd with her evening dose of antibiotics, she notices that Mrs Dodd has a rash on her arms, face and neck. On further examination, she sees the rash is also present over Mrs Dodd's chest and back. Mrs Dodd complains that her chest feels "a little tight" and her throat is "feeling scratchy". Bibi doesn't give her any further medication and instead asks a colleague to call the RN for immediate assistance. Bibi stays with Mrs Dodd until the RN calls for an ambulance, as Mrs Dodd has signs of a pending anaphylaxis.

CHECK YOUR UNDERSTANDING

1. What are the three types of medication that a person might be using?
2. Complete the table.

Medication classification (group)	Action	Medication examples
Anticoagulant		warfarin, clopidogrel, aspirin
	Lowers blood pressure	ramipril, amlodipine
	Mild laxatives to prevent and manage constipation	bisacodyl, docusate sodium
Diuretic		furosemide, amiloride, spironolactone

3. What are the two names used to refer to any medication?
4. What types of valuable information can be found on a pharmacy label?
5. Give an example of a dose administration aid.

17.2 SUPPORTING THE INDIVIDUAL WITH MEDICATION

As a care worker providing assistance with medication, you will need to be aware of how you can support the individual in a way that respects their autonomy and rights while ensuring their safety. You can provide support to people with their medications in their own home, in a day-care program, in respite care and in RACFs. Every person has their own preferences and needs when it comes to taking their medication, which are documented in their care plan or medication profile.

When assisting a person with their medication, you need to be aware of the following:

- Do they like to take pills one at a time or multiple pills at a time?
- Do they have problems swallowing?
- Do you have instruction from a health professional to crush medications?
- What type of fluids does the person prefer to swallow medication with?
- Do they have a particular routine for taking medications?
- How much of the medication process can they do independently?
- Do they have a medical or psychological condition that affects their ability to take medication safely and on time?

PRACTICE POINT

When assisting a person with their medications, remember at all times that you are accountable for your actions. Follow procedures regarding individual support for medications and always be safety conscious when assisting with medication management.

Medications must never be left at the person's bedside, or in any unattended manner, at any time. Vulnerable people, such as those with dementia or visiting children, may take the medication that is left unattended. This in turn may have serious outcomes for the safety and wellbeing of the person.

Most importantly, if you observe that the care plan doesn't reflect the person's preferences, needs or capabilities, it is your duty of care to report your observations to the supervisor or RN.

17.2.1 Roles and responsibilities in medication management

Safe and effective medication management involves the expertise and skills of several professionals and health workers. The individual for whom the medication is required also plays a key role in this process. The following people have a role in safe and effective medication management.

PRESCRIBER

Medications are prescribed by a person with the authority to do so. This is a medical practitioner or specialist, and sometimes a nurse practitioner. Medical practitioners are regulated by the AHPRA. Medical practitioners have a responsibility to prescribe medication based on the therapeutic needs of the person. It is the scope of practice of medical practitioners to determine what these needs may be, through the clinical consultation process. Doctors are required to follow prescribing rules that contribute to safe medication use. Most prescriptions are computer generated; however, some prescriptions or orders may be handwritten. It is the prescribing practitioner's responsibility to ensure that any communication regarding medications is written in a clear and concise way that is easily interpreted by the reader.

PHARMACIST

The role of the pharmacist in medication management is not only to dispense medications according to the doctor's prescriptions, but also to support safe medication use by providing information and advice about the medications. The pharmacist is responsible for the correct labelling information and for ensuring the person has adequate information about the medication's side effects and warnings.

REGISTERED NURSE

Registered nurses are health professionals with a tertiary degree and are registered with the Nursing and Midwifery Board of Australia (NMBA). RNs must meet specific standards as set out by the NMBA to maintain the right to practise in Australia and are regulated by the AHPRA.

Within a residential aged care facility, RNs are responsible for the safe management of medication. This includes using clinical judgement and best nursing practices, in a collaborative manner, to make decisions about medications. These decisions may include when to withhold medication, when a higher or more frequent dose is necessary, if side effects of a medication are outweighing its benefits, and when more medication may need to be given. RNs will liaise with other health professionals such as doctors and pharmacists to ensure medication management is safe and effective for all people they represent. RNs are also responsible for the accountability and administration of S4D and S8 drugs.

ENROLLED NURSE

The enrolled nurse (EN) has completed an 18-month diploma course in nursing at TAFE and works under the delegation and supervision of the RN. Enrolled nurses can administer medications, other than S4D and S8 drugs, unless organisational policies state differently. Like RNs, ENs are registered with the NMBA and regulated by the AHPRA. In many organisations that provide care and support for older people, ENs may play a vital role in leadership and management processes, and offer support to care workers with regards to policies and procedures relating to medication administration and assistance. ENs may also be required to liaise with other health professionals such as doctors and pharmacists in order to ensure safe medication management.

TEAM LEADER

A team leader (TL) is a worker who has most likely completed a Certificate IV level qualification in ageing, disability or community services. This role is a supervisory one, and the TL may be responsible for other staff within a given time frame, such as a work shift. The TL can assist with medications, and often in the RACF environment they can administer insulin according to the organisation's policies and procedures. An RN must be accessible for any necessary support and supervision for insulin administration. The TL will report any discrepancies with medication assistance to the RN or the EN, including (but not limited to) if:

- prescriptions need renewing
- medication is refused
- a person appears unwell or has observable problems when they are assisted with medications
- blood glucose levels are abnormal
- a medication is out of stock
- errors are made regarding medication.

CARE WORKER

The care worker plays a significant role in medication support. Under the guidance of the organisational policies and procedures and the delegation of RNs, care workers can assist people with some of their medications. This assistance doesn't include invasive procedures such as injections, or suppository and pessary insertion, and care workers are generally not permitted to give medications via feeding tubes. It is the responsibility of care workers to work within their scope of practice when assisting people with medications, and you can do this by working within your qualification and knowledge base, under the supervision of others, and by following the relevant policies and procedures in the workplace. Care workers work under the supervision of an RN, an EN or a TL and are responsible for reporting to their supervisor any issues that may arise with medication support. These issues include (but are not limited to):

- Medication is expired.
- The person refuses their medication.
- The person looks or behaves differently.
- Medication is missing or dropped.
- Medication is given to the wrong person.
- The wrong dose of medication is given.

Care workers can assist a person with taking the following medications:

- tablets, capsules and other solid medication from a blister pack or sachet that has been packaged by a pharmacist
- medications that have a pharmacy label (with relevant information and instructions on it), including:
  - tablets, capsules and other solid medication to be taken orally from an original medication package
  - liquid medication
  - eye drops and eye ointments
  - ear drops
  - creams and lotions
  - inhalers and other puffers
  - nebulised medication
  - some transdermal medicated patches
  - intranasal medication.

The organisation you work for will have a specific policy relating to what you can and cannot do regarding supporting a person to take their medications, regardless of your qualification. This policy will often be similar between organisations in the industry; however, some organisations may have different expectations about medication management. Job descriptions also detail the role of the care worker in medication assistance. A care worker who is trained in medication support doesn't have the right to assist with medications unless the organisation supports them to do so.

Always follow the organisation's policy and take instruction from supervisors such as the RN or EN, the TL or another person in the supervisory role. Asking for clarification about any instruction is important, too, as this is a direct way to minimise risks with medication support.

EMPLOYER

The organisation that provides support to people with their medication as a service is responsible for ensuring that relevant laws are implemented throughout policies and procedures in the workplace. Employers provide education and supervision to staff who are providing medication support and have other important systems in place to monitor compliance and industry regulation around medication management. These systems include reporting systems, quality improvement systems and risk management frameworks. Safe medication management is supported by the Quality Standards.

A quality improvement system that many RACFs implement to support safe medication management is the medication advisory committee (MAC). The aim of this committee is to monitor and review the policies, procedures and practices of medication management within the organisation, including medication incident report reviews. The MAC can re-evaluate procedures to improve safety outcomes for people residing in the organisation by minimising the risks of harm that are directly related to medication use.

The organisation's policies and procedures around medication support will specify the tasks that are within the care worker's scope of practice, and the expectations the organisation has of employees who assist people with medications.

THE INDIVIDUAL

The individual for whom the medication is prescribed also has responsibilities for the safe and effective use of medicines. The person has the responsibility to take their prescribed medication as they previously consented to do, and it is also important that they report any problems they are experiencing with the medication. The individual also has the right to refuse the medication.

People who live in their own home may require less support with their medication than people who live in an RACF. They will have similar responsibilities to manage their medication; however, they will likely be responsible for replenishing their own prescriptions and for informing the doctor if they have problems with their medication, such as side effects. In the RACF, health workers are often the people who notify the person's doctor of medication issues, and the facility has a service contract with a local pharmacy for the ongoing replenishment of medications on behalf of the individuals in their care.

A NOTE ON DELEGATION

Delegation is the term used to describe the process by which an RN delegates a particular task to another person. Delegation is a process that is part of the decision-making framework for nursing and midwifery, under the guidance of the NMBA. An RN can delegate tasks to care workers if the RN deems the worker to be competent in the task, if the organisation under which the task is performed has in place policies and procedures that support the delegation, and if the worker is confident and understands their accountability in performing the task. RNs are accountable for the worker performing the task and must be available to supervise or support that worker.

17.2.2 Infection prevention and control

Infection prevention and control is the term given to the processes and practices that health workers implement to minimise the spread of infection from one person to another in the workplace. Older people and other vulnerable populations are more susceptible to long-term illness and death from infection. The ageing process reduces the body's ability to fight infection effectively as the immune system experiences a reduction of important cells that are responsible for a robust immune response.

When assisting people with their medication, it is extremely important to follow both standard and transmission-based precautions to prevent and minimise infection.

STANDARD PRECAUTIONS

Using standard precautions when supporting older people with their medication is important to prevent and control infection and is part of your duty of care as a care worker. Standard precautions can be implemented in any work environment you may work in to support older people, such as respite care, a day centre program, an RACF or on the person's own home.

With regards to medications:

- Wash hands with hand soap and water, or use an alcohol-based hand gel, before and after any medication support procedure.
- Handle tablets and other medications using the non-touch method. At no time touch the person's medication directly with your hand.
- Place tablets directly into a receptacle, such as a medication cup, or onto a small plate, or sometimes into the hand of the older person. This will vary between workplace environments, but the non-touch method will not.
- Use personal protective equipment (PPE) appropriate to medications. Gloves are usually only required to be worn if the medication has a warning about skin contamination that can be harmful for those for whom the medication is not prescribed (such as cytotoxic drugs). Some organisations prefer workers to wear gloves when they are administering eye drops, as the eyes are very sensitive and prone to infections such as conjunctivitis. Wear gloves when applying topical creams to the person.
- Dispose of medications, and waste associated with medication support, correctly and safely.
- Clean surfaces and equipment (trolley surfaces, nebulisers, etc.) correctly, during and after use.
- Dispose of sharps into a sharps container.

TRANSMISSION-BASED PRECAUTIONS

Transmission-based precautions are extra safeguards that are implemented when a person is known to have an infection such as influenza or gastroenteritis. They include precautions such as the following:

- increased use of PPE that includes full-length, long-sleeved disposable gown face mask, eye protection (glasses/goggles)
- increased handwashing regimen
- changes to duration and time of cleaning (surfaces, equipment and rooms)
- implementation of facility lockdown processes when appropriate
- reporting and monitoring of specific known infections such as gastroenteritis, influenza and COVID-19
- changes in practices such as staff allocation and isolation care
- change of waste disposal systems to minimise handling of infectious substances
- dirty linen management to minimise handling of soiled and contaminated linen.

In the event you are required to assist a person with medication, and they are known to have an infection such as influenza or gastroenteritis, you will need to follow the organisation's policies and procedures regarding barrier or isolation nursing practices. The type of infection the person has will dictate what type of PPE to wear. Transmission-based precautions are implemented in addition to standard precautions.

17.2.3 Observations and changes in the individual's health

One of the key responsibilities that falls within the scope of practice of a care worker is to report any concerns and observations about the person's health. As a care worker, you may be the first person to notice changes in an older person's health and therefore you have a critical role in the health and wellbeing of those older people you support. Health professionals and supervisors need to be informed of your observations so they can be addressed promptly and correctly.

When providing support to an older person, regardless of the environment, you will notice when something doesn't seem right about how the person looks or behaves. There are a multitude of observations that you might make about the person; however, there are some very important observations that relate to the person's ability to take their medications safely. Table 17.4 presents some of these observations.

All health workers have a duty of care to do everything practicable to prevent or minimise foreseeable harm. In the event a worker fails to do this through an act of omission, such as not reporting their observations about the person's health, they can be regarded as breaching their duty of care. In this case, if observations are not reported and the person suffers harm, the worker may be seen as negligent through breaching their duty of care and possibly face litigation.

WORKPLACE SCENARIO

Scope of practice

Grant has worked as a care worker for a community care service provider for two years. He is part-way through his qualification that will enable him to assist with medications, as his organisation doesn't allow staff to assist with medications if they don't hold the qualification. Grant assists people in their home and is scheduled to help Jeff with his morning shower. When Grant arrives, Jeff tells him he doesn't feel well and asks Grant to give him his insulin injection. Grant politely declines, explaining to Jeff that he isn't trained to give injections, but says he will contact the RN immediately to get some help for him.

CHECK YOUR UNDERSTANDING

1. What document can provide information that enables you to support the individual in a way that respects their autonomy and rights while ensuring their safety?
2. How can care workers ensure they are working within their scope of practice?
3. What are examples of standard precautions that are put into place for medication management?
4. One of the key responsibilities that falls within the scope of practice of a care worker is to report any concerns and observations about a person's health. What are some observations about a person that may concern you?

17.3 HANDLING CONTINGENCIES

A contingency is something that might occur that could have a negative outcome or result. Despite policies, procedures and practices, contingencies may and do occur when assisting people with their medication. When a contingency occurs, it is important that you know how to handle the situation.

TABLE 17.4 Observations that require reporting and documentation

Observations	Possible problem	Associated risks	Actions	Outcomes
The person doesn't appear to swallow properly. Drooling; reluctance to swallow; pooling liquids in the mouth; coughing. The person has slurred speech.	• Dysphagia (difficulty swallowing) • Stroke • Any change to **neurological** abilities • The person may be diabetic and be experiencing hypoglycaemia (low blood glucose level).	• Choking • Aspiration with chest infection or pneumonia. • Death	• Apply first aid if the person's airway is compromised or they have a known condition that can be addressed (such as hypoglycaemia). • Notify the RN or supervisor immediately and follow instructions. • Don't continue with medications assistance or offer fluids or food. • Document according to the organisation's policy.	• The person will be reviewed by a doctor, who will refer them to a speech pathologist to assess their swallow reflex. • The speech pathologist will determine the appropriate course of action, which may include more tests, diet modification and sometimes artificial feeding.
The person appears confused, or more confused than is normal for them. They may or may not **hallucinate**.	• Delirium is a sudden onset of confusion over hours and days that results from infections, pain and other issues. Medications can cause delirium.	• Risk of injury or harm due to lack of insight into safety. • **Sepsis** due to overwhelming infection. • Death	• Don't give medications. • Don't argue with the person or tell them they are confused. Their experience is very real to them in the moment. • Report observations to the RN or supervisor immediately and follow instructions. • Document according to the organisation's policy.	• The person will be assessed for a clinical cause of the delirium, such as a urinary infection. • The person will be assessed by their doctor, who will address any physical cause such as infection and may also review the person's medication.
The person has changes to their balance or has experienced falls and near misses.	• The person may be experiencing hypotension (low blood pressure) due to an illness or medication. They may experience a drug to drug interaction if they take multiple medications, or may experience unintended effects of a particular drug.	• The risk of falls is very high in older people who take multiple medications. • Falls can have catastrophic and life-changing outcomes for older people. • Risks include loss of independence due to injury, or death.	• Report observations to the RN or supervisor immediately and follow instructions. • Follow procedures for supporting a person who has fallen, or almost fallen, and document incident reports and notes as per policy.	• The person will be reviewed by the doctor, who may refer them to a physiotherapist for a mobility assessment. • The person's medication will be reviewed as a potential causative factor for the hypotension, along with other observations such as blood pressure measurements and urinalysis.

There are many reasons that a contingent event can occur when assisting with medication and it is essential that all these events are managed safely and transparently. All organisations have procedures that guide workers on the processes to follow in the event an incident occurs. The person's immediate safety and wellbeing is the primary issue, and all contingent events are required to be reported to the RN or supervisor. As part of the reporting process, you may be required to complete an incident report to document the event. Incident reports not only provide a record of the event but are also used in quality improvement processes to minimise risk in safe medication management. Reports can identify why the event may have occurred. At no stage should the report be an immediate disciplinary issue. When things don't go to plan, you have a duty of care to report the incident and document it accordingly.

Reasons that medication assistance may not go to plan that relate to the care worker include lack of concentration, being disrupted by other staff during medication assistance, leaving medications unattended, inexperience and work-related stress (such as being short-staffed). Reasons for incidents that relate to the person being assisted with medications include the behaviour of the person at the time (delirium or intrusive behaviour), refusal, incomplete ingestion or ejected medication.

17.3.1 Incidents related to medication assistance

OVERDOSE

A person may take too much medication when they take it themselves—for example, they forget they have taken the initial dose and then take another—or the care worker or nurse gives them too much of the medication. This can happen when the worker is distracted from the task at hand or doesn't follow the correct procedures for safe medication support.

In the event of overdose, first observe the person for immediate physical symptoms such as chest pain and changes to breathing. Apply first aid and call for immediate assistance. If this occurs when you are working in the person's home, apply first aid and call an ambulance on 000, and follow their instructions. Report the incident to the RN or supervisor as soon as it is safe to do so. Document the event according to the organisation's policy.

UNDERDOSE

Underdose occurs when the person has an insufficient amount of the medication to have the intended (therapeutic) effect. This may be more obvious by the way the person looks and the things they tell you. If a person is prescribed regular pain medication (analgesia) and you observe that they are in pain, it is possible the analgesia needs to be reviewed by the doctor. This outcome likely depends on you and your ability to report your observations to the RN or supervisor, to facilitate a doctor visit. Remember to document your observations.

Underdosing can also occur when the person refuses medications regularly. In this case, they may benefit from a discussion with the RN or their doctor. Underdosing also results when the care worker or nurse misinterprets the instructions for the medication.

MISSED MEDICATIONS

When a person misses a dose of medication, the effect of the medication in the body changes. The more doses that are missed, the more significant are the changes that occur. The intended effect of the medication is achieved by the prescribed dose and time of dosage, and changes to the prescription will affect the intended outcomes. Often, missed medication doses are obvious when they are in a blister pack, and this should be reported to the RN or supervisor. The person may self-administer their medications and missed doses might signal that the person is struggling to do so. If possible, try to determine why the medication was missed, as often it is the care worker or nurse who hasn't administered the medication for a reason, and they may have inadvertently neglected to document the reasons.

INCORRECT TIME

Medication that is given at the incorrect time can have negative outcomes for the person taking it. Time is an important component of a prescription as the availability of the medication in the bloodstream needs to be at a level whereby the chemicals can achieve the desired effect. Just like missed medication, medications given at the incorrect time can result in underdosing or overdosing and can have serious implications for the person's health and wellbeing. Some groups of medications are designed to be taken at certain times to be effective; for example, some need to be taken with food and others without food. This has a direct impact on how the body absorbs the medication. Other medications are designed to be taken at certain times of the day, such as sleeping tablets and other sedatives. If a sedative is given to a person at 5 pm instead of the prescribed time of 8 pm, the intended effect will be brought forward to a time when the person may be at risk—for example, of falling if they are drowsy before going to bed—or they may be awake and alert in the early hours.

INCORRECT ROUTE

Medications are prescribed to be taken a certain way. The route of administration is the way the medication is accessed by the body and includes (but is not limited to) the oral, intranasal, topical and rectal routes. The route prescribed by the doctor reflects how the medication is absorbed and distributed in the body in order to work effectively. When a medication is administered via the incorrect route, the person may experience an adverse reaction that requires first aid and medical assistance. In the event an incorrect route is used for medication, the first thing to address is the immediate first aid needs of the person and then call for assistance. This may be the RN or supervisor, or an ambulance on 000. Ensure the appropriate documentation is completed.

INCORRECT PERSON

Another contingent event when assisting with medication is when the wrong person receives or takes the medication that is intended for someone else. Reasons for this occurring include a distracted or inexperienced care worker or nurse, unattended medication that is accessed by someone else, or the person takes medication that has been labelled incorrectly by the pharmacy. As with other contingent events, address the immediate first aid needs of the person, including calling an ambulance on 000 if their breathing is affected or they experience an anaphylaxis. Report to the RN or the supervisor at the earliest opportunity and follow their instructions, including documenting the incident.

17.3.2 Other issues

REFUSING MEDICATION

The people you support have the right to refuse to take their medication, and there are several reasons they may do this. Some people may not like the taste of the medication or find it difficult to swallow, while others may not like the effects of the medication. For example, fluid tablets (diuretics) are prescribed to remove excess fluid from the body by increasing the production of urine. Many people who are prescribed diuretics refuse to take them at times, especially if they are going out somewhere, for fear of needing to use the toilet in a hurry or of having an incontinence episode in public. In these situations, it is important to identify why the person is refusing their medication and to report these concerns to the RN or supervisor so the individual can be provided with accurate information about their medications, including the possible consequences of refusing them.

People with dementia and other conditions that affect cognition may refuse medication frequently. They may not understand what the medication is, or what it is for, and they may think you are trying to harm or poison them. People with cognitive decline may misinterpret your intentions, so it is essential when you approach them that you aren't intrusive or loud and that you use gestures to assist communication. When a person with changes in their cognition refuses medication, try again a few minutes later.

Remember: people with dementia and other issues that affect their decision making have the right to refuse their medication. They should be encouraged, but not coerced, to take it.

CHOKING AND VOMITING

There are times during the medication assistance process when the person may have an unexpected response to taking medication. They may experience choking and/or vomiting as a result of incorrect ingestion of the medication, which can be related to a change in their physical health status. Medical events such as stroke can affect the person's swallow reflex and may result in choking and aspiration. A person may also choke or vomit if they are encouraged to swallow the tablets whole when their care plan clearly states they are required to have medications crushed and mixed with thickened fluid. It is essential to be aware of the person's care plan or medication management plan in order to understand how best to assist them with as little risk as possible.

In the event the person is choking, stop assisting with medication immediately and provide any first aid or other assistance that is required. Report the incident to the RN or supervisor and ensure that you document the event. If the person vomits during the medication assistance process, stop what you are doing and attend to their immediate care needs. Don't give further or repeat doses of medication, as the person may be experiencing a side effect or may have already absorbed some of the medication. Again, report and document the incident.

EJECTION OF MEDICATION AND INCOMPLETE INGESTION

Sometimes, the person may spit out the medication, and this may be intentional or non-intentional. The reasons a person may eject medications from their mouth include an unacceptable taste of the medication, a coughing or sneezing episode, or a distressed behaviour. In any case, when this occurs it is important to stop the medication assistance process and not give the person another dose of the medication they ejected. The medication may have been partly ingested and may have had time to be absorbed in the bloodstream while in the mouth. Further doses may cause toxicity or another adverse effect that can cause harm to the person. Report to the RN or supervisor and discard the ejected medication safely. Document the incident according to policy.

WORKPLACE SCENARIO

When a person refuses to take their medication

Riku is a care worker at a day respite centre for older people. Part of his role is to ensure that the participants at the centre receive the assistance they need with their lunchtime medication. He has noticed that Mr Ross, who is a regular participant at the centre, appears withdrawn and doesn't want to participate in any activities. When Riku approaches Mr Ross to ask him if he is ready to have his midday pills, Mr Ross becomes animated and yells at Riku: "I will not take those tablets! You're trying to poison me! You're a spy, aren't you?" Riku suspects that Mr Ross may be experiencing a delirium as he appears unusually confused and delusional. Riku doesn't give the medication but instead reports his observations to his supervisor, so that Mr Ross can get the help he needs. Riku also documents the incident in Mr Ross's notes and completes an incident form. Rather than sign the medication chart, Riku places an "R" for "Refuse". Further investigations by Mr Ross's health-care team reveal that he had a urinary tract infection that triggered his confusion, which was reversed when antibiotic therapy was completed.

CHECK YOUR UNDERSTANDING

1. List three reasons why a medication contingency may occur that is related to the care worker.
2. How should a care worker respond to a medication error?
3. Why is it important to give medications at the correct time?
4. List three reasons that medication may be taken by the incorrect person.

17.4 FOLLOWING REQUIRED PROCEDURES AND METHODS OF DOCUMENTATION

Assisting a person with their medication involves procedures and specific methods of documentation that are considered best practice within the aged care industry and are also required to comply with relevant legislation. All procedures and documentation that an aged care provider implements are designed to minimise the risk of adverse events associated with medications and to optimise the safety of the medication management process. Care workers can find information and instructions about the relevant procedures and documentation expectations from sources such as the person's care plan, the policies and procedures of the workplace, and through clarification from the RN or supervisor.

17.4.1 Preparing to assist a person with their medication

The process of assisting a person to take their medication safely involves procedures and checks to ensure risk is minimised as much as possible. Prior to assisting a person with medication, it is important to check that they are capable of taking it. Using observation skills, consider if the person appears their usual well self. If your observations indicate that they are unwell, don't proceed with the medication support. Instead, report your concerns to the RN or supervisor and follow their instructions.

Before commencing medication support, ensure that you have the authority to proceed with assisting the person. In other words, does your policy enable you to assist with medications?

PRIVACY, DIGNITY AND CONSENT

Part of any procedure that you may assist with when caring for people is to ensure that their dignity is respected. We all have a different definition of dignity as it applies to us as individuals. Some people may be comfortable taking medication in the presence of others, such as in a dining area, while others may prefer to take medications in a more private environment, such as their room. Dignity is a concept that supports the individual's preferences in all aspects of service delivery.

Privacy doesn't only apply to the environment, but also to the person's health and medical information. Policies exist that direct how a person's sensitive information is handled by the organisation and the staff who represent it. Under the concept of duty of care, all staff are required to support the person's right to privacy. It is a breach of your duty of care to disclose, with their consent, information about someone's medical condition and the medication they are prescribed. Disclosure can only occur under specific circumstances.

Always ask the person for consent before assisting them with their medication. This gives them the opportunity to prepare to take their medication or to refuse it.

POSITIONING

To facilitate safe medication assistance, it is necessary to consider the correct positioning of the person to minimise risk. Consider the medication the person requires, and once they have given consent and their privacy needs have been met, ensure you support them to position themselves correctly. When assisting with oral medications, the person should be sitting in an upright position to prevent choking and aspiration. Don't give oral medications to a person who is lying down or is reclined. Correct positioning is also important for the safe delivery of medications, such as eye drops, nebulised medications, topical treatments and inhalers.

CHECKS THAT APPLY TO ALL MEDICATIONS

Once consent is obtained and the person is positioned comfortably, remind yourself of the safe procedures you can put in place by thinking, "I need to give the *RIGHT PERSON* the *RIGHT MEDICATION.* I need to give that person the *RIGHT DOSE* at the *RIGHT TIME,* and I will give it via the *RIGHT ROUTE.* After this, I will attend to the *RIGHT DOCUMENTATION.*" The 6 Rs provide a safety risk management check that can be applied every time you assist a person with their medications. The 6 Rs involve:

- Is it the *RIGHT PERSON?* Confirm the identity of the person for whom the medication is prescribed by asking for their name. Don't ask if their name is "Mrs Smith"; instead, say "Can you tell me your name, please?" Someone with a cognitive decline may answer "Yes" to the first question even if they are not "Mrs Smith". The correct identity of the person can also be confirmed by their photograph, which is present on their medication chart, and also on the blister pack (although a photograph is not always available). The person's name is also present on the medication chart and the pharmacy label on the medication.
- Is it the *RIGHT MEDICATION?* Regardless of whether the person takes one medication or multiple medications, it is extremely important to check that they are about to use the correct one. Medications are often prescribed and dispensed in either the brand name or the generic name, and this can cause confusion. Both the brand and generic names should appear on the medication and the medication chart or profile.

  Most blister packs have identification of the contents on the back of the pack that includes the name of the medication and sometimes what it is used for. The reasons that the person may receive the wrong medication include pharmacy error, prescriber error, medication chart error, and the human error of the individual who is assisting the person. Always check the name of the medication on the pharmacy label against the name of the medication on the medication chart or profile. If they don't match, don't proceed and report the inconsistency to the RN or supervisor immediately.
- Is it the *RIGHT DOSE?* Along with the medication name, the prescribed dose is also found on the medication and the medication chart or profile. The dose isn't the amount of the medication in each tablet or patch, etc. The dose is the amount of the medication the doctor has prescribed for the person, and it is stated clearly on the medication chart and most often on the pharmacy label.
- Is it the *RIGHT TIME?* Medications are prescribed to be given at a specific time in order to work effectively in the body, and documented times are to be adhered to. The time the medication is to be taken or applied is found on the medication chart or medication profile, and on the pharmacy label.
- Is it the *RIGHT ROUTE?* It is important that medication is taken the correct way, or via the right way into the body, and this information is on the medication chart or profile and the pharmacy label. This check is important to prevent harm to the individual.
- Is it the *RIGHT DOCUMENTATION*? After medication has been administered, you are required to sign the medication chart (or other signatory document) to indicate that you have assisted the person to take their medication safely. Remember: some medication charts are electronic and when you log into and use an electronic medication system, your passcode is your signature. Never share your passcode, because you are accountable for any documentation or lack of documentation when it is used.

Don't sign off on medication administration before or during medication assistance, as a problem may arise that doesn't allow for the medication to be taken. In this case, you will have another medication incident because you have signed off on something that didn't occur.

EXPIRED MEDICATION

All medications have an expiry date after which they are not to be used. Expiry dates exist to ensure people are not using medicines that can effectively make them very unwell because, over time, the chemical composition changes. Factors such as light and heat can affect the life of medications. The expiry date must always be checked before the administration of any medicine. Expiry dates will be different for the various forms of medications. Out-of-date medicines should be returned to the pharmacist for safe disposal.

17.4.2 Equipment

The correct equipment is an important component in the provision of safe medication support. Any equipment used that is not disposable must be cleaned according to the organisation's standard precautions practices. Policies and procedures related to infection prevention and control will provide information about the cleaning processes for equipment used in medication support and administration.

The type of equipment available will depend on the work environment, as it is not appropriate to use some equipment in the person's home that may be used in the RACF. Remember that in a facility, multiple people are supported with their medications from a medication trolley during a medication round, while in the community setting, a single person may need support with medication.

Table 17.5 illustrates common items of equipment used for safe medication assistance.

TABLE 17.5 Equipment used for medication support

Equipment	Description	Purpose
	Alcohol-based hand gel or rub	Hand hygiene should be carried out before, during and after medication assistance. The care worker uses alcohol hand gel after assisting a person and before assisting the next person with medications within a facility.
	Disposable syringe	Used to measure liquids accurately. Also used to assist with the administration of oral liquid medications when the need is based on assessment and is documented in the person's care plan or medication plan. Consent from the person is required to use oral syringes for medication administration purposes.
	Thickened fluids or medication lubricant	To assist the person with swallowing oral medications. Thickened fluids act as a medium for crushed medications to be swallowed safely. Note that the thickened fluid must be compatible for use with medications, as some cannot be used with medications.
	Garbage receptacle	For general waste such as used tissues and gloves.

TABLE 17.5 Equipment used for medication support (continued)

Equipment	Description	Purpose
	Gloves	For use when assisting with eye medications, topical medications and medications that can cause harm if exposed to the skin.
	Nebuliser	An electrical machine that forces high-pressure air into a nebuliser mask to change liquid medication into aerosol medication in order to be inhaled into the lungs.
	Note pad and pen	Information that needs to be passed onto the RN or supervisor is noted during medication rounds (e.g. information such as a person refusing their medication, expired or out-of-stock medication, etc.).
	Medicine measure cups	Cups used to measure liquid medication; also used to collect multiple medications from blister packs for presentation to the individual.
	Pill crusher	Designed to crush tablets. There are various styles on the market; however, they all perform relatively the same. Some are handheld devices, while others are fixed to the top of the medication trolley. Some organisations use the traditional mortar and pestle for grinding medications.
	Pill cutter/divider	A small plastic device with an inbuilt blade for cutting scored tablets into halves.
	Plastic spoons	To support the use of thickened fluids and crushed medication.
	Sharps container	A yellow puncture-proof container marked with the safety sign "Biohazard" for the disposal of sharps.
	Water carafe and cups	To contain and dispense water to assist with swallowing medications. Also useful for mixing some powdered medications as per instructions (e.g. Movicol).

Gloves, Burlingham/Shutterstock; notepad and pen, IhorL/Shutterstock; all other images © McGraw-Hill Education

Apart from ensuring that all equipment used for assisting with medications is cleaned or disposed of according to policy, it is a professional courtesy to ensure the medication trolley is restocked and cleaned ready for use by the next person.

17.4.3 Procedure

PROCESSES FOR ASSISTING THE PERSON WITH THEIR MEDICATIONS

Before participating in any medication procedure, always ask yourself the following questions:

- Do I have the authority to proceed? Am I trained to assist with medications and does my organisation allow me to do so?
- Do I have the appropriate delegation from the RN to assist with medications?
- Am I working within my scope of practice?
- Are there any risks or reasons that I should not proceed?
- Do I understand the medication and its safe use?

Table 17.6 outlines processes for assisting the person with their medications.

TABLE 17.6 Processes for assisting the person with their medications

Prior to assisting the person with administration of medication	
Step	*Process*
1	Read the person's medication care plan or profile to understand the relevant information for the safe administration of medication. Clarify any information you don't understand with the RN or supervisor.
2	Greet the person and observe for signs that medication assistance should proceed.
3	Inform the person that you would like to assist them with their medication and gain their consent to do so. Ensure privacy.
4	Attend to hand hygiene and prepare medications and necessary equipment.
5	Take the medication trolley or package to the person's bedside or chairside. Assist the person into a comfortable position relevant to the medication that is to be administered.
Assisting the person with administration of medications	
Step	*Process*
6	Attend to hand hygiene.
7	Identify that you have the RIGHT PERSON by asking them to tell you their name, and check that the photo on the chart matches the person and the name on the pharmacy label is the person's name.
8	Read the medication chart to determine you have the RIGHT MEDICATION and that you are administering the RIGHT DOSE at the RIGHT TIME. Check for any special instructions relevant to the medication and check the RIGHT ROUTE on the chart. Compare the medication itself to the information on the chart. Do they match?
9	Check the expiry date on the medication and the integrity of the medication. Don't proceed if the medication has expired or appears to be damaged.
10	Explain the procedure to the person and have appropriate fluids at the ready.
11	Once all checks have been performed, prepare the medication and assist the person to use it according to the information in their plans, and the correct administration procedures relevant to each type of medication.

TABLE 17.6 Processes for assisting the person with their medications (continued)

Specific administration procedures for medications (after steps 1–11)	
Medication type	*Process*
Tablets and capsules	*Blister pack:* Check the tablets in each blister match the medication name and dose on the medication chart. Count them and check the medication names on the back of the blister pack. Push the tablets out of the blister using your thumb, into a medication cup or other clean holding place of the person's preference. *Bottles and boxes:* After the necessary checks, shake the bottle gently and extract the required amount into the lid of the bottle, then tip into medication cup. Check dose against the label. Tablets in foil palettes from a box are pushed outwards, similar to a blister pack. Don't touch tablets with your hands at any point in the administration process.
Liquids	Follow instructions on the bottle, such as "shake well". Holding the bottle with the pharmacy label away from you, so as not to spill medication on the label, pour the required dose into a medication measure cup at eye level. Place the measure cup on a level surface and check the dose is accurate. Don't tip excess liquid medication back into the bottle; discard excess as per policy. Wipe the bottle clean of any spillage and return to original storage place.
Eye drops and eye ointment	*Eye drops:* Assist the person to position themselves with their head back. Using gloved hands, ask the person to look upwards and outwards while you pouch the bottom eyelid. Instil one drop at a time into the eye, using a tissue to dab any trickles on the person's face. Use a fresh tissue for each eye. Wait a few minutes between medications if the person has more than one type of eye drops. *Eye ointment:* Assist the person to position themselves with their head back. Using gloved hands, ask the person to look upwards and outwards while you pouch the bottom eyelid. Discard a small amount of ointment from the tube prior to use to minimise infection. Squeeze a ribbon of ointment from one corner of the inner bottom eyelid to the other. Ask the person to close and roll their eye to encourage a covering of the ointment over the eye.
Ear drops	Assist the person to position themselves comfortably and ask them to tilt their head to the side. Gently hold the upper ear upwards and outwards and instil the drops as prescribed. Encourage the person to stay in the position for a few minutes.
Inhaler (aerosol)	*Without spacer:* Assist the person into a sitting/upright position. The inner cannister can be removed from the casing to check the expiry date and medication name. Replace the cannister and shake well. Ask the person to place the mouthpiece between their lips and tilt their head back slightly. Tell the person that on the count of three you will depress the cannister to administer one puff of medication. Remind them to keep their tongue down and hold their breath for around 5–10 seconds. Wait approximately 20 seconds between puffs if more than one puff is prescribed. Encourage the person to rinse their mouth after administration. *With spacer:* Assemble the inhaler and spacer. Ask the person to place the mouthpiece of the spacer between their lips. Depress the inhaler and ask the person to take 3 or 4 deep breaths. Repeat this process if more than one puff is required. Don't depress multiple puffs into the spacer at once. Encourage the person to rinse their mouth after administration. Disassemble and clean the spacer as per protocol.
Nebuliser	Assist the person into a comfortable upright sitting position. Attach the nebuliser to the electrical outlet and switch the power on, ensuring the nebuliser is on a flat and firm surface, not a bed. Don't cover the nebuliser when in use, as this may pose a fire hazard as the machine heats. Assemble the nebuliser mask to the medication chamber and the tubing from the chamber to the nebuliser. Unscrew the medication chamber and place the pre-dosed nebule of medication into the chamber and close it. Apply the person's own mask to their face and explain the procedure. Switch the nebuliser on. When misting has stopped, turn the nebuliser off and remove the person's mask. Ensure their face is dry and they are comfortable before you leave. Cleanse the mask and tubing as per protocol, and pack away the nebuliser. Some medications will require you to apply a damp facecloth over the person's eyes to prevent irritation. Always check instructions prior to proceeding.

(Continues)

TABLE 17.6 Processes for assisting the person with their medications (continued)

<table>
<tr><td>Topical creams</td><td>Ensure privacy and that the person is positioned comfortably. Don gloves and remove the cap from the tube. Discard a small amount of the cream or ointment from the tube. Apply the correct amount of the cream to your gloved finger (use the size of the tube to indicate how much to use if the medication chart isn't specific). Apply the cream to the affected area and gently rub into the skin. Replace cap without using contaminated fingers. Remove gloves.</td></tr>
<tr><td>Transdermal patch</td><td>Ensure privacy and that the person is positioned comfortably. Check the expiry date and the name of the medication on the single unit outer package of the patch. Don gloves. Peel off backing of patch and apply to clean, dry and scar-free skin. Don't apply to skin that is open, has burns or is hairy. Patches are most often applied on the upper back, shoulder or upper chest area. Check medication chart to ensure you are applying onto the correct area of skin according to the daily site rotation. Hold the patch in place for around 20–30 seconds, ensuring the entire patch is in touch with the skin.</td></tr>
<tr><td>Preloaded insulin pen</td><td>Obtain a blood glucose level (BGL) prior to administration and report to the RN. Confirm with the RN that you have authority to proceed with insulin administration. If the BGL is within the documented parameters for the person and the RN has given authority to proceed, you can prepare the person and provide them with privacy.
Two trained health workers are required to administer insulin: one to administer (wearing gloves) and one to witness. The procedure is as follows:
• Both workers will check the pen is the correct one and contains the correct insulin.
• Both workers will check the expiry date.
• You can then place the insulin cartridge into the insulin pen.
• Gently tilt the pen back and forth to mix (long-acting insulin). Don't shake it.
• Ensure a new needle is attached to the pen every time it is used.
• Dial the pen to number 2 (2 units) on the dial, remove the protective sheath from the needle, and press the end of the pen to eject the small amount of insulin into the air or tissue (air shot). Place the pen into a puncture-proof tray.
• Both workers will now check the medication order for the 6Rs and check the dose again.
• Pick up the pen and dial up the required amount of insulin. Confirm the dose with the second worker who is witnessing the procedure.
• Administer the insulin by placing the needle directly into the skin of the abdomen and holding the pen in place. Press the release button at the end of the pen to eject the insulin into the person's body. Usually, a count of 10 is sufficient time. Remove the pen and immediately discard the needle safely into an approved sharps container. Remove gloves.
• Both workers sign the medication chart to indicate that the insulin has been administered.
It is important to remember that insulin injections are given into subcutaneous, or fatty, tissue such as the abdomen. The site of injection should be rotated each time the person is injected.</td></tr>
<tr><td colspan="2">During the process of assisting the person with administration of medication</td></tr>
<tr><td>Step</td><td>Process</td></tr>
<tr><td>12</td><td>Assist the person to use the medication according to their needs (e.g. one tablet at a time, crushed with thickened fluid, etc.).</td></tr>
<tr><td>13</td><td>Observe the person for any difficulties they may have using the medication (e.g. swallowing problems), and act appropriately.</td></tr>
<tr><td>14</td><td>Ensure the medication has been taken correctly (e.g. the tablets are ingested).</td></tr>
</table>

TABLE 17.6 Processes for assisting the person with their medications (continued)

After the medication administration process	
Step	*Process*
15	Ensure the person is comfortable.
16	RIGHT DOCUMENTATION: Sign the medication chart immediately after the medication has been taken or applied.
17	Observe the person for any immediate reactions or non-intended effects of the medication and report them accordingly.
18	Dispose of waste correctly.
19	Attend to hand hygiene.
20	Clean and restock any equipment.
21	Attend to any other documentation.

Assisting people with medications is an important role of the qualified care worker. It is essential to stay focused and to avoid interruptions from others when assisting with medications, as a lack of concentration is a common contributor to medication errors. Always ask the RN or supervisor for clarification of any aspect of the medication assistance process that is unclear. It is always better to be cautious if you are uncertain. Remember that organisational policies and procedures are also in place to assist you to assist others safely.

17.4.4 Documentation medication terminology

Medical terminology is useful as a universal language in health care to enable a shared understanding of health- and medical-related information, with little ambiguity. Medical terminology has a Latin background from medical history, and specific terminology is used to define medication-related words and meanings. Table 17.7 illustrates some common medical terminology that you will need to learn within your role as a care worker who assists with medication. The majority of the terms are found on prescriptions or in client medical notes.

TABLE 17.7 Common terminology used in medication management

Terminology	Meaning
Frequency or time	
Mane	Morning—usually breakfast time
Nocte	Evening—usually 8 pm
qd; d	Daily
bd; bid	Twice a day
tds; tid	Three times a day
qid	Four times a day
q4h	Every four hours
prn (pro re nata)	As necessary (with a prescription)
stat	Give immediately
ac	Before meals
pc	After meals
Measurements	
unit	Unit of insulin
mL	millilitre
mg	milligram

(Continues)

TABLE 17.7 Common terminology used in medication management (continued)

Terminology	Meaning
Measurements (continued)	
mcg	microgram
gm	gram
neb	nebule
Routes of administration	
po	Orally, by mouth
gutt	Eye drops
b.e	Both eyes
top	Topically
bilateral	Both sides
PR	Per rectum
PV	Per vagina
IM	Intramuscular
SC; SUBCUT	Subcutaneous
IV	Intravenous
NEB	Nebuliser
INH	Inhaler
NG	Nasogastric tube
PEG	Percutaneous enteral gastroscopy tube
SL; SUBLING	Under the tongue

It is important to remember that doctors may have personal preferences for the terminology they use, and many medication errors that have caused injury or death to people of all ages have been directly related to misinterpretation of terminology. A key aim of the National Residential Medication Chart (NRMC) is to minimise this occurrence by implementing terminology that is clear, concise and more in line with modern medicine and health care. In the event you don't understand the terminology used, or the instructions are vaguely written, don't give the medication. Report to the RN or supervisor for clarification of terminology or the written instruction.

MEDICATION CHARTS

The prescription instructions for a medication are known as "doctor's orders", and a medication chart is a document that states necessary information about the person's medication regime. The chart is a legal document that has printed prescription instructions about each medication the person takes, although more commonly in RACFs the doctor may handwrite prescriptions onto the medication chart. Any handwritten doctor's order must be written legibly in order to prevent a medication error. Never give medications from an order you cannot decipher, as the risk of harm to the person is very high if the order is misinterpreted. Always refer any poorly written instructions to the RN or supervisor so it can be rectified.

Medication charts have different names in the community sector, including medication profile, medication signature sheet and medication plan. Regardless, medication charts include:

- the person's name and address/ID number
- any allergies
- the doctor's name
- medication name; dose; time to be given; route to be administered
- special instructions (such as crush or do not crush)
- tabled spaces for dates, times and signatures.

The format of medication charts is variable within the aged care industry. Some charts consist of a single sheet of paper and others are more detailed booklets that cover other aspects of medication support. A uniform and standardised medication chart such as the NRMC may minimise medications errors.

The Australian Commission on Safety and Quality in Health Care (ACSQHC) is an organisation that works closely with the Commonwealth, state and territory governments and all public and private health-care facilities to ensure that health-care provision in Australia is standardised to prevent risk of harm to individuals. One of the projects of the National Safety and Quality Health Service (NSQHS) is the National Residential Medication Chart for use in RACFs. The NRMC is designed to minimise medication incidents and to increase safety for the people living in RACFs.

It is not mandatory for aged care providers to implement the NRMC; however, government funding can assist providers to transition to the NRMC. The NRMC is available as a paper-based chart or an electronic chart. The following examples of the components of medication charts are taken from the ACSQHC's *National Residential Medication Chart User Guide for Nursing and Care Staff* (ACSQHC 2014).

Figure 17.1 illustrates the medication management details of the person, including photo identification. You may note that this part of the NRMC also has a tabled "considerations" box that provides specific information about the person's needs.

FIGURE 17.1 National Residential Medication Chart: medication management details

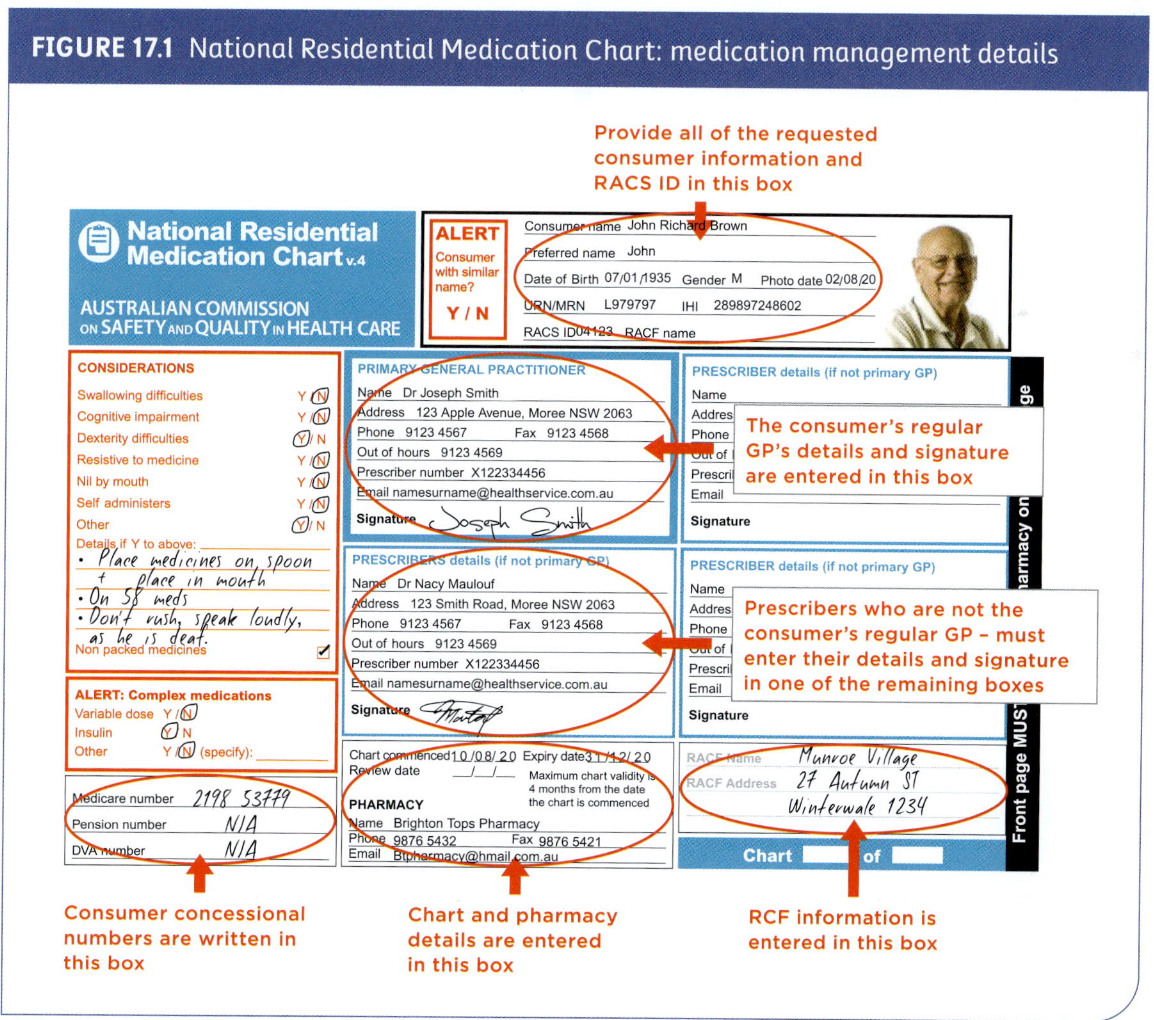

Source: Reproduced with permission from National Residential Medication, developed by the Australian Commission on Safety and Quality in Health Care (ACSQHC). Sydney: ACSQHC, 2021.

FIGURE 17.2 National Residential Medication Chart: prescription orders

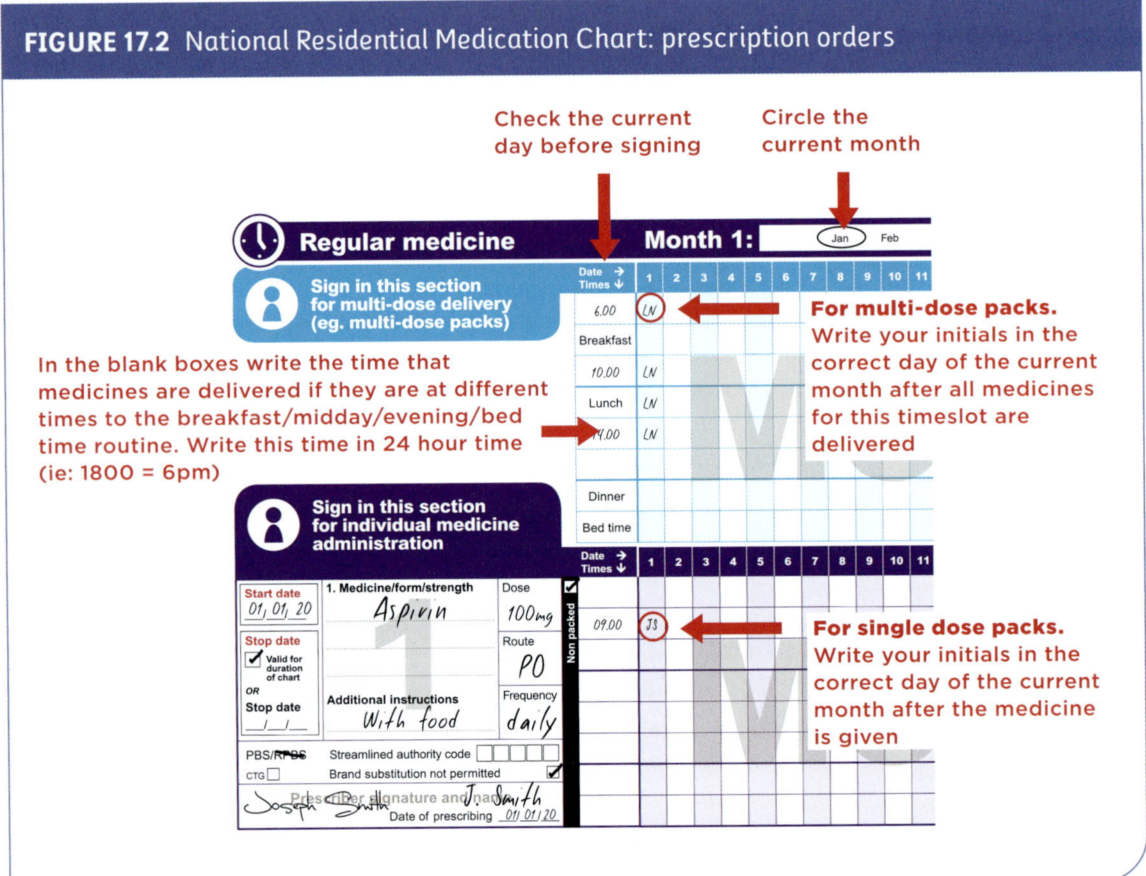

Source: Reproduced with permission from National Residential Medication, developed by the Australian Commission on Safety and Quality in Health Care (ACSQHC). Sydney: ACSQHC, 2021.

Figure 17.2 illustrates how to document and sign the medication chart. It also demonstrates the prescription orders that include the medication name, the dose to be given, the time to be given and the administration route.

ELECTRONIC MEDICATION MANAGEMENT SYSTEMS

While some organisations use paper medication charts, many use electronic medication management systems. These systems reduce the risk of medication incidents as a result of the alerts and alarms that are built into the system. The electronic medication administration record is the digital version of the paper-based medication chart. RACFs are more likely to use electronic medication management systems due to the large number of people who require assistance with medications.

ABBREVIATIONS

The medication chart will have a small table of abbreviations that must be used to identify when something occurs that can impede the medication process. These abbreviations are commonly used to ensure that a continuum of understanding occurs among all health workers regarding the person's medication. Figure 17.3 is an example.

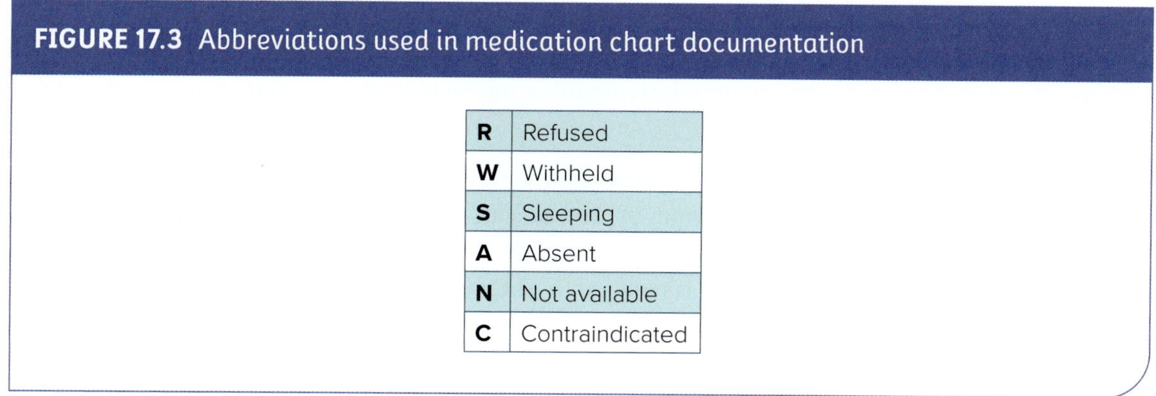

R	Refused
W	Withheld
S	Sleeping
A	Absent
N	Not available
C	Contraindicated

FIGURE 17.3 Abbreviations used in medication chart documentation

The relevant abbreviation is noted on the medication chart. For example, if you are asked by the RN to withhold a medication from a person because the person is required to have a blood test, you will write "W" and initial the chart. The reason for a medication to be withheld must be clinically based and documented. The RN can instruct a medication to be withheld; however, it is not in the scope of practice of the care worker to independently withhold medications.

Figure 17.4 provides an excellent example from the NRMC of information that is designed to ensure everyone is using the medication chart effectively and minimising risk.

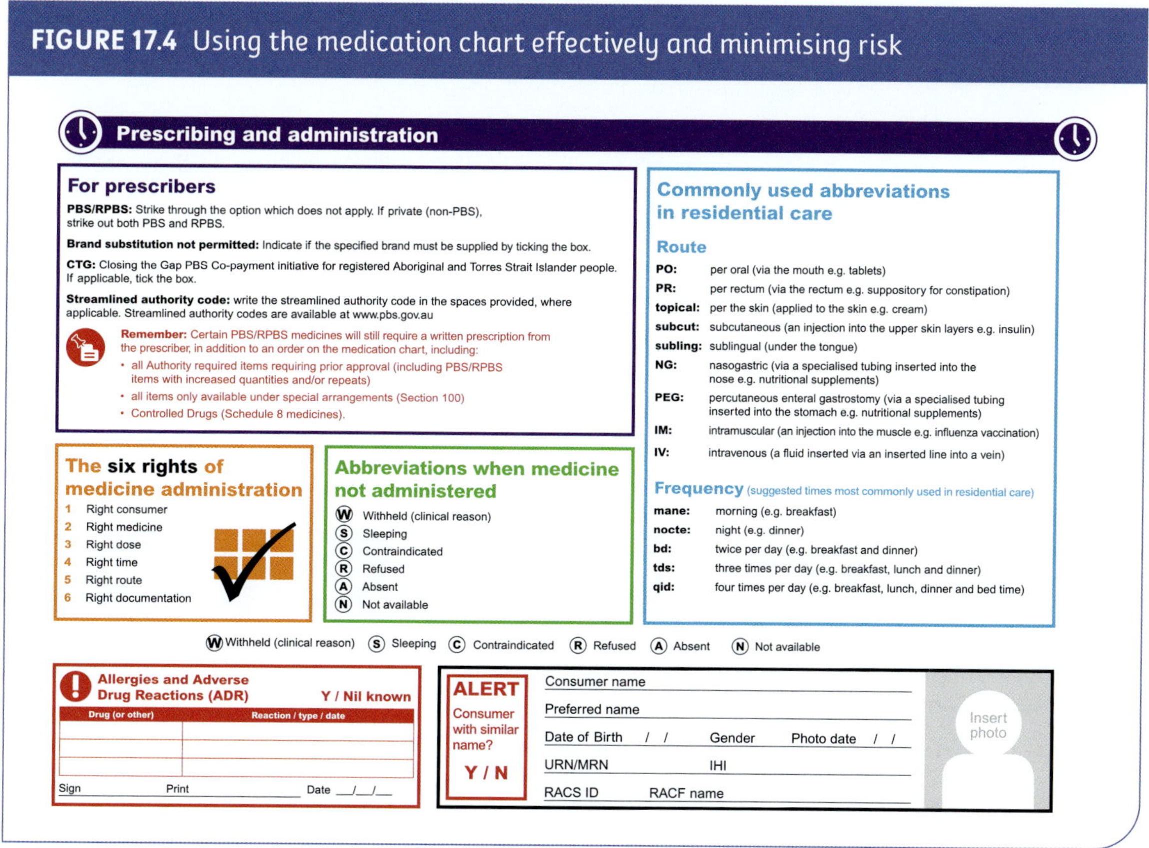

Prescribing and administration

For prescribers

PBS/RPBS: Strike through the option which does not apply. If private (non-PBS), strike out both PBS and RPBS.

Brand substitution not permitted: Indicate if the specified brand must be supplied by ticking the box.

CTG: Closing the Gap PBS Co-payment initiative for registered Aboriginal and Torres Strait Islander people. If applicable, tick the box.

Streamlined authority code: write the streamlined authority code in the spaces provided, where applicable. Streamlined authority codes are available at www.pbs.gov.au

Remember: Certain PBS/RPBS medicines will still require a written prescription from the prescriber, in addition to an order on the medication chart, including:

- all Authority required items requiring prior approval (including PBS/RPBS items with increased quantities and/or repeats)
- all items only available under special arrangements (Section 100)
- Controlled Drugs (Schedule 8 medicines).

Commonly used abbreviations in residential care

Route

PO:	per oral (via the mouth e.g. tablets)
PR:	per rectum (via the rectum e.g. suppository for constipation)
topical:	per the skin (applied to the skin e.g. cream)
subcut:	subcutaneous (an injection into the upper skin layers e.g. insulin)
subling:	sublingual (under the tongue)
NG:	nasogastric (via a specialised tubing inserted into the nose e.g. nutritional supplements)
PEG:	percutaneous enteral gastrostomy (via a specialised tubing inserted into the stomach e.g. nutritional supplements)
IM:	intramuscular (an injection into the muscle e.g. influenza vaccination)
IV:	intravenous (a fluid inserted via an inserted line into a vein)

Frequency (suggested times most commonly used in residential care)

mane:	morning (e.g. breakfast)
nocte:	night (e.g. dinner)
bd:	twice per day (e.g. breakfast and dinner)
tds:	three times per day (e.g. breakfast, lunch and dinner)
qid:	four times per day (e.g. breakfast, lunch, dinner and bed time)

The six rights of medicine administration

1. Right consumer
2. Right medicine
3. Right dose
4. Right time
5. Right route
6. Right documentation

Abbreviations when medicine not administered

- (W) Withheld (clinical reason)
- (S) Sleeping
- (C) Contraindicated
- (R) Refused
- (A) Absent
- (N) Not available

(W) Withheld (clinical reason) (S) Sleeping (C) Contraindicated (R) Refused (A) Absent (N) Not available

Allergies and Adverse Drug Reactions (ADR) Y / Nil known

Drug (or other)	Reaction / type / date

Sign Print Date __/__/__

ALERT Consumer with similar name? **Y / N**

Consumer name

Preferred name

Date of Birth / / Gender Photo date / /

URN/MRN IHI

RACS ID RACF name

Insert photo

FIGURE 17.4 Using the medication chart effectively and minimising risk

Source: Reproduced with permission from National Residential Medication, developed by the Australian Commission on Safety and Quality in Health Care (ACSQHC). Sydney: ACSQHC, 2021.

DOCUMENTATION OF ERRORS AND OTHER EVENTS

All contingent events are first and foremost reported to the RN or supervisor, or sometimes to the emergency services. When relevant and appropriate interventions to the incident have occurred, it is important to document the event using the following:

- *Progress notes or case notes:* A daily record of all events is kept in the person's file.
- *Handover report:* To ensure a continuum of care, all staff who support the person must be informed of any contingent event and any relevant instructions.
- *Hospital transfer form:* If the person is required to be transferred to the hospital as a result of a contingent event, clear information about the incident must be documented on a hospital transfer form or similar form.
- *Incident report:* An incident report is a form that documents the details of a contingent event. As a legal document, incident forms are a work health and safety requirement of the organisation. Information included in an incident report includes the person's details, the worker's details, the date and time of the event, a detailed description of the event, and the actions taken at the time the event occurred. Incident reports are used to record an incident; however, they are also used to monitor medication safety processes and to identify processes that can be improved.

WORKPLACE SCENARIO

Checking medications

Yana is required to assist eight people with their morning medications. The morning shift is short-staffed and the two colleagues she is working with aren't familiar with the facility's routine, as they are from a nursing agency. Yana finds herself distracted many times while assisting with medications, as she answers questions from the staff, and is rushing to complete the medication assistance so that she can start on the other morning tasks. The last two people she assists with medications are Mrs Robson and Mr Robinson. Just as Mr Robinson is about to take his pills that Yana had dispensed from a blister pack, he says: "Hang on a minute. Since when do I take an orange capsule?" Yana's heart skips a beat as she realises she has given Mrs Robson the medication meant for Mr Robinson. She is angry with herself for not having checked the 6 Rs.

CHECK YOUR UNDERSTANDING

1. What are the 6 Rs?
2. Why should expired medication not be used?
3. How can the person's identity be checked to ensure you have the right person?
4. List three questions you can ask yourself before you start medication assistance that ensures you are working within your scope of practice.
5. How many workers are required to assist with a preloaded insulin pen?

SUMMARY

- Medication assistance in aged care services is regulated by a range of laws and regulations under the Commonwealth, state and territory governments.
- Always work within your scope of practice when assisting people with their medications.
- Report any concerns you may have about a person's wellbeing to the RN or supervisor.
- Ensure that all safety checks are performed when assisting a person with medications.
- Follow policies and procedures for medication management, infection control, waste disposal and correct documentation procedures.

REVIEW QUESTIONS

17.1 How do medications work?

17.2 As a care worker, what is your role when preparing to assist a person with their medications?

17.3 What rights does the person being assisted to take their medication have?

17.4 **(a)** List the relevant checks (6 Rs) that must be performed when assisting a person with their medication.

(b) List the specific checks that should be made in relation to the following:

Tablets:

Cream:

Eye drops:

17.5. Outline how the care worker should respond to a medication error.

BIBLIOGRAPHY

Australian Commission on Safety and Quality in Health Care (ACSQHC), *National Residential Medication Chart User Guide for Nursing and Care Staff*, ACSQHC, Sydney, 2014, https://www.safetyandquality.gov.au/our-work/medication-safety/national-residential-medication-chart, accessed 16 December 2021.

Australian Government, Department of Health, *Consumer Medicines Information* (CMI), August 2020, https://www.tga.gov.au/consumer-medicines-information-cmi, accessed 16 December 2021.

Australian Government, Department of Health, *Grant to Support Residential Aged Care Facilities to Upgrade to an Electronic National Residential Medication Chart*, https://www.pbs.gov.au/info/news/2021/07/grant-to-support-residential-aged-care-facilities-to-upgrade, accessed 16 December 2021.

Australian Government, Department of Health, *Guiding Principle 8: Storage of Medicines*, https://www1.health.gov.au/internet/publications/publishing.nsf/Content/nmp-guide-medmgt-jul06-contents~nmp-guide-medmgt-jul06-guidepr8, accessed 16 December 2021.

Australian Government, Department of Health, *Improved Medicine Labels*, https://www.tga.gov.au/sites/default/files/poster-improved-medicine-labels-1.pdf, accessed 16 December 2021.

Australian Government, Department of Health, *Labelling and Packaging*, https://www.tga.gov.au/labelling-packaging, accessed 16 December 2021.

Australian Government, Department of Health, *Medicines and TGA Classifications*, https://www.tga.gov.au/medicines-and-tga-classifications, accessed 2 December 2021.

Australian Government, Department of Health, *Prescription Medicines Overview*, https://www.tga.gov.au/prescription-medicines-overview, accessed 15 December 2021.

Australian Government, Department of Health, *What's on My Medicine Label?*, https://www.tga.gov.au/whats-my-medicine-label, accessed 16 December 2021.

Elliott, R.A. "Appropriate use of dose administration aids", *Australian Prescriber* 37, 2014, pp. 46–50. DOI: 10.18773/austprescr.2014.020.

Health Direct, *Generic vs Brand-Name Medicines*, https://www.healthdirect.gov.au/generic-medicines-vs-brand-name-medicines, accessed 16 December 2021.

Health Direct, *Scheduling of Medicines and Poisons*, https://www.healthdirect.gov.au/scheduling-of-medicines-and-poisons, accessed 16 December 2021.

HealthinAging.org, *Medications Work Differently in Older Adults*, https://www.healthinaging.org/medications-older-adults/medications-work-differently-older-adults, accessed 15 December 2021.

Home Caring, *Swallowing Assessments*, https://www.homecaring.com.au/swallowing-assessments/, accessed 16 December 2021.

NSW Health, *List of Substances in Appendix D of the Poisons and Therapeutic Goods Regulation 2008*, https://www.health.nsw.gov.au/pharmaceutical/Pages/sch4d.aspx#bookmark1, accessed 16 December 2021.

NSW Health, *Residential Care Facilities*, https://www.health.nsw.gov.au/pharmaceutical/Pages/residential-care-facilities.aspx, accessed 16 December 2021.

NSW Health, *Storage of a Schedule 8 Medicine (Drug of Addiction) Requiring Refrigeration*, https://www.health.nsw.gov.au/pharmaceutical/Pages/refrigeration-s8s.aspx, accessed 16 December 2021.

Patra, K.P. & De Jesus, O., *Sentinel Event*, StatPearls Publishing, 2021, https://www.ncbi.nlm.nih.gov/books/NBK564388/, accessed 15 December 2021.

Vaughan, G., "The Australian drug regulatory system", *Australian Prescriber* 18, 1995, pp. 69–71. DOI: 10.18773/austprescr.1995.068.

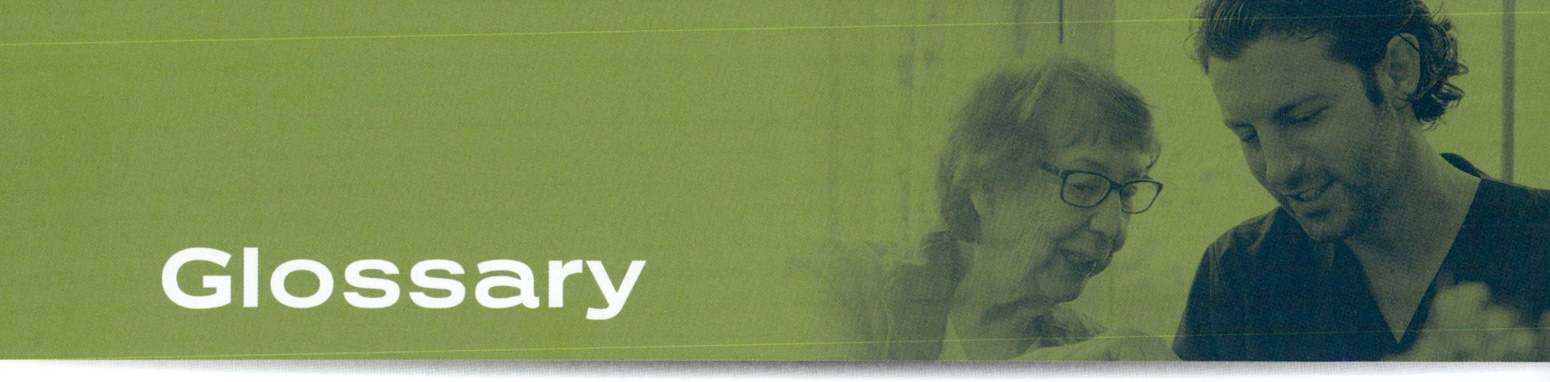

Glossary

A

ABC approach acronym for antecedents, behaviour and consequence; this approach suggests that by avoiding triggers, consequences are limited

abuse mistreatment of a person physically, socially, emotionally, religiously, culturally or financially

active listening being attentive, understanding what the person is saying, responding, reflecting on and retaining the information given

activities of daily living (ADLs) those activities that an individual does every day to ensure health and wellbeing, including personal hygiene activities, eating and drinking, and using the toilet

advance care directive a legal document that advises the wishes, values, and expected care and intervention the person wants should they become incapacitated and unable to make decisions for themselves in the future; also known as a living will

advance care plan a care plan developed in relation to the advance care directive, formulated ahead of time so that the entire multidisciplinary team are informed

Aged Care Assessment Team (ACAT) the team responsible for assessing a person's eligibility for a government-subsidised home package or residential aged care services

Aged Care Diversity Framework seeks to embed diversity in the design and delivery of aged care and to support action to address perceived or actual barriers to consumers accessing safe, equitable and quality aged care, while enabling consumers and carers to be partners in the process

Aged Care Funding Instrument (ACFI) an assessment process that determines the level of support a person living in residential care needs. The higher the care needs, the more government funding the provider is entitled to

ageism a form of discrimination based on a person's chronological age

agnosia the inability to recognise things and to know how to use them

alveoli small, sac-like structures in the lungs where carbon dioxide and oxygen are exchanged

Alzheimer's disease (AD) the most common and most frequently diagnosed dementia in Australia; AD is a progressive neurological disease where the person exhibits signs and symptoms of memory loss, forgetfulness and lack of personal care of varying degrees

anaemia a reduction of red blood cells in the blood, resulting in a decrease of available oxygen in the body; anaemia causes paleness and tiredness and can lead to falls

anaphylaxis a severe allergic reaction that is triggered by an allergen, causing a hypersensitive reaction in the body that can threaten loss of life

apathy a lack of interest or concern

apraxia the inability to sequence tasks or to complete a task from beginning to end

arrythmia an irregular heartbeat

aseptic a technique health professionals use to perform a procedure using a sterile field of equipment that is free from contamination

asexual having an absent or minimal sexual attraction to others or in sexual activities

aspiration in the context of eating, aspiration is the process of inhaling food or fluids into the airway

assertive communication being firm, but fair, when communicating

ataxia changes to balance or coordination

auditing the process of an official inspection by the Aged Care Quality and Safety Commission to ensure the organisation can demonstrate compliance requirements

Australian National Aged Care Classification (AN-ACC) an assessment process that determines the level of support a person living in residential care needs; the higher the care needs, the more government funding the provider is entitled to

autoimmune relates to diseases and conditions that cause the immune system to attack normal substances that are found in the body

autonomy self-governance; making choices and decisions without being influenced by others

B

bariatric related to the treatment for obesity

behavioural and psychological symptoms of dementia (BPSD) behaviours that cause distress or harm in any way to another person; also known as behaviours of concern, challenging behaviours or distressed behaviours

bias inclination or prejudice for or against one person or group, especially in a way considered to be unfair

blood pressure the measurement of the force of the blood against the walls of the arteries

bronchi the airways of the lungs

C

care plan a document describing the needs, interventions and goals for the support of an individual, based on assessment and information sharing

care worker a person who provides aged care services to older people who receive government-funded services, under the instruction of a registered nurse, team leader or supervisor; the care worker works for an aged care service and holds a qualification to do so

carer a spouse, family member, friend or neighbour who supports those people who are frail, aged, have a disability or are chronically ill

Carer Gateway carers can access supports such as in-person counselling, peer support and emergency respite from Carer Gateway service providers

Carers Australia represents carers of people with a disability, mental illness or chronic condition or those who are frail or aged; it provides information, support, education, training, counselling, advice and referral to services that can assist carers in their caring role

cartilage tough connective tissue that supports joints

catastrophic reactions reactions where the person with dementia overreacts to a stimulus

cell the basic unit of life

cellulitis a bacterial skin infection that can become severe if left untreated and may threaten life

clarify presenting information in different ways or asking questions to make sure the message is understood

coercive approach forcing someone to do what we want

collaboration involves the coming together of different people with different skills and knowledge to reach a common goal

Commonwealth Home Support Programme (CHSP) provides support to people at home with activities of daily living that include meal provision, domestic activities (such as cleaning), general home maintenance, home modification, transport, and some nursing and allied health services

communication the process of sending and receiving a message; it involves interaction between the participants

communication hierarchy flow of information up, down and across the levels of an organisation

comorbidities the existence of more than one medical condition or disease

compliance following the rules and regulations that are necessary to be a provider of aged care services that are funded by the government

confidentiality an ethical expectation; often a person (and sometimes their family members and friends) will, in conversation with care workers, talk about their private life, their aspirations and their past experiences. It will generally be assumed that these conversations are confidential; that is, they are not for sharing with others, such as work colleagues or people outside the work organisation

conflict resolution the process of coming to an amicable agreement after a disagreement

confrontation opposing people or groups who have a difference of opinion and can disagree in a heated manner

constraints barriers to or restrictions on something, such as effective communication

consultation a key element of the WHS process; requires a two-way exchange of information about WHS issues between managers and workers

consumer-directed care (CDC) a government initiative that promotes autonomy of choice when a person is eligible for in-home care; the person determines how their package of care is delivered and by whom

continuous improvement the ongoing improvement of services where regular evaluation leads to improved practices over time

Cornell Scale for Depression in Dementia (CSDD) a scale used to score a person's symptoms indicating depression

Creutzfeldt-Jakob disease (CJD) a rare and fatal degenerative disease of the brain; one of a group of diseases known as the transmissible spongiform encephalopathies

cultural awareness the ability to reflect on and be aware of our own cultural values, beliefs and perceptions

cultural competence the ability to understand, communicate and interact effectively with a diverse range of people from different cultures and backgrounds

cultural safety when an environment is safe and supportive for people and doesn't expose them to assault, challenge or denial of their identity, needs and wants

culturally and linguistically diverse (CALD) Australia's population includes many people who were born overseas, have a parent who was born overseas or speak a variety of languages; together, these groups of people are known as CALD populations

culture set of customs, traditions and values of a society or community, ethnic group or nation; attitudes, beliefs, customs, language, arts, food preferences, family connections, expectations of the world, concepts of time, and so on, are all bound up in culture

curative care the care provided to a person which aims to extend their life span by diagnosing a health problem and implementing active treatment to cure their illness, thereby resolving their health problem

D

death doula acts as a companion, advocate and educator for the dying and their families; commonly gives the dying person the opportunity to die at home, if that is their wish

delirium a set of signs and symptoms that occur suddenly, including confusion, disorientation and agitation

dementia an extremely challenging neurological condition affecting many people worldwide; it is described as being a group of symptoms that indicate interruption in memory, thinking, communication and judgement

depression a mood disorder causing constant feelings of sadness, worthlessness and loss of interest

digestion the breakdown of food so that nutrients can be absorbed by the body

digital media a form of media that uses electronic devices to distribute information

discrimination unjust or prejudicial treatment of different categories of people, especially on the grounds of race, age, sex or disability

diversity understanding that each individual is unique and recognising our individual differences; these can be along the dimensions of race, ethnicity, gender, sexual orientation, socioeconomic status, age, physical abilities, religious beliefs, political beliefs or other ideologies

duty of care the responsibility to do no harm; in relation to WHS, everyone has a responsibility to ensure that all people in the workplace are safe

dysphagia any difficulty in swallowing that can occur at any point during the swallowing process

dystonia a complex condition that is characterised by abnormal spasms or contractions of muscles

E

effective communication communication that has been heard, understood and acted upon

elimination the removal of waste from the body

empowerment being in control of one's rights and living life according to one's own expectations; people can be empowered through actions or processes of others that help to optimise self-esteem and confidence

end-of-life care care delivered at the end stage of life, which could be weeks, days or hours; also known as terminal care

ethically to work in a manner that does not cause harm to others

euthanasia also known as voluntary assisted dying, where legal access to medications that will assist dying at a particular time and place is made possible

explicit in no uncertain terms; without doubt; obvious

exploitation taking advantage of an individual for personal gain

F

faeces waste that is eliminated from the body via the anus

feedback receiving information back about information that was sent

food security the term used to describe the situation whereby a person doesn't have access to nutritious or healthy food on a regular basis

frontotemporal lobe dementia (FTLD) affects the frontal and/or temporal regions of the brain; FTLD occurs over several years and is progressive and degenerative in nature; also known as frontotemporal lobar degeneration or Pick's disease

G

gait the pattern of walking

gangrenous tissue of the body that is lacking blood supply and is dying

gaslighting a type of emotional manipulation of a person by another that results in the person doubting their reality and state of mind

gastroenteritis any infection of the gastrointestinal tract that causes symptoms of diarrhoea, vomiting, fever and headache; can be viral or bacterial

general senses senses of touch, pain, temperature, position and pressure

H

hallucinate to see, smell, taste or feel things that others cannot

hazard something, including behaviour, that has the potential to cause injury, illness or death

hazard identification a process of observing and identifying hazards

health an overall state of wellbeing

health and safety representative (HSR) person voted for by the workplace to act on their behalf on WHS matters with management

holistic the consideration of all factors of a person's health domains (physical, psychological, sexual, social, spiritual, cultural)

Home Care Packages (HCP) Program offers four levels of home care packages, based on need; higher support is offered than with the CHSP

homeostasis a state of steadiness of the systems and processes in the body

Huntington's disease an inherited degenerative, neurological disorder caused by a single gene abnormality of chromosome 4

hydration sufficient fluids to meet the body's needs

hypertension the condition of having high blood pressure

I

immunity the ability of the body to defend itself against disease

immunosuppressed a weak immune system and a decreased ability to fight infection; can be caused by illness, disease, some medications and age

implicit something that is understood but is not obvious or stated clearly; suggestive

in situ in the original or appropriate place

inclusion when a diverse range of people (e.g. of different ages, cultural backgrounds, genders) feel valued and respected, have access to opportunities and resources, and can contribute their perspectives and talents to improve their organisation

inclusivity the term used to describe access to all aspects of living in a society that is diverse, regardless of age and stereotype; inclusivity supports the concept that all people have the same human rights and therefore should not have varied access to opportunities in life

industry terminology particular words, phrases and acronyms used and understood by a particular industry

instrumental activities of daily living (IADLs) those activities that an individual does frequently to ensure aspects of taking care of themself and their home, including shopping, using the phone, paying bills

intersex describes a person who is born with neither a wholly male nor a wholly female anatomy

ISBAR tool an acronym used as a prompt for communication during handover and written reports

L

legally to work in alignment with the expectations of the legal system and to abide by legal obligations within a work role

Lewy body dementia (LBD) or dementia with Lewy bodies a rapidly progressive and degenerative cognitive disease where abnormal round structures form in the neurons in several areas in the brain, causing death of the neurons

LGBTQIA+ acronym for lesbian, gay, bisexual, transgender, questioning, intersex and asexual and other sexual identities not listed

life-limiting illness any illness that restricts, limits or cuts short a person's abilities, and where death is a direct consequence of the illness

living will a legal document that advises the wishes, values, and expected care and intervention the person wants should they become incapacitated and unable to make decisions for themselves in the future; also known as an advance care directive

M

manual handling physical work that puts the body at risk of injury through actions such as pushing, pulling, lifting and twisting

message information sent in the form of words (in speech or writing) and/or other signs and symbols

morbidity the presence of one or more chronic diseases or health conditions that contribute to a state of physical vulnerability

mortality related to death

motivational interviewing a counselling method that motivates a person to make a change by drawing on their strengths and valuing their contributions

motor function the movement of voluntary muscles throughout the body

multiculturalism public endorsement and recognition of cultural diversity; it means a national community defines its national identity not in ethnic or racial terms, but in terms that can include immigrants

My Aged Care the Australian government's starting point on a person and their carer's aged care journey; the government-funded services needed could range from help at home or short-term care, to access to aged care homes

myopathy a condition or disease that involves voluntary movement of muscles

N

neglect mistreatment or omission of treatment and care

neurological pertaining to the nervous system (brain and spinal cord)

non-verbal communication includes body movements and posture, eye contact, appearance, facial expressions and sign language

O

objective language language that is free from emotion and opinion; facts only

P

palliative care care given to improve quality of life for those with a life-threatening illness; the goal is to prevent or treat pain and other problems as early as possible, and the care addresses the person as whole, not just their illness

Parkinson's disease a progressive neurological condition that alters the level of dopamine to the extent that movement, balance and coordination are affected

pathogen a microorganism that causes disease

perineum the area between the anus and the genitals

perpetrator the abuser; the person causing harm to the older person through abusive methods

perseveration repetition over and over of actions, stories, questions and behaviours

person conducting a business or undertaking (PCBU) often the employer or business owner

person-centred care a way of thinking and doing things that sees the people using health and aged care services as equal partners in planning, developing and monitoring care to ensure it meets their needs

personhood focuses on the status of being an individual person with individual physical, mental, cognitive, social, emotional, religious, cultural and financial characteristics, likes, dislikes, needs and wants

policy a document that states *what* needs to be done and *why* it needs to be done

polypharmacy the use of multiple medications

power of attorney the legal responsibility for managing another person's financial matters; often held by a family member or someone in a position of trust

privacy principles the legal obligations describing what organisations must do when they collect, hold, use and disclose health information

procedure a document that states *how* a policy will be carried out

professional development the process of developing skills and knowledge relevant to a worker's roles and in alignment with industry best practice

progress notes daily notes that keep a continual record of the person's issues and relevant happenings; includes actions and pending actions; also known as case notes

psychosocial aspects of a person that relates to their behaviour, thoughts and social contexts

pureed food food items that have been blended to create a texture that minimises the risk of choking or aspiration; pureed foods are often used for safe eating with dysphagia

R

receiver the person who is listening and receiving the information

reflux a condition whereby stomach acid backs up into the oesophagus due to the oesophageal sphincter failing to relax at the correct time

residential aged care facility (RACF) a facility that provides support for people who can no longer live independently in their own home

restrictive practice any practice that inhibits an individual's freedom of movement or rights

rights-based approach an approach to providing services that focuses on the person's rights and recognises their autonomy

risk the possibility that injury, illness or death could occur when exposed to a hazard; it refers to the likelihood and severity of harm caused

risk management a systematic way of looking at workplace risks and finding solutions

S

sacrum the bone between the hips, located on the buttock; a flat, triangle-shaped area at the base of the spine

saliva fluid produced in the mouth by salivary glands; also known as spit

salmonella a bacterial disease caused by contaminated water or food

sanctions penalties that are imposed on a government-funded aged care provider, such as withdrawal of funding for a period of time, when compliance is not met and there is the risk of harm to consumers

scope of practice the boundaries by which a person can work according to their qualifications and job description

self-care recognising your own needs and taking whatever action is required to care for yourself physically, emotionally, culturally, religiously, spiritually, socially and financially

self-determination the right of the person to set and pursue goals that are unique to their quality of life

sender the person who is relaying the message to others

sensory function receiving information through our senses to be interpreted by the brain

sepsis an overwhelming response to infection by the body that can cause release of chemicals that may result in organ failure and death

Serious Incident Response Scheme (SIRS) implemented to identify and report reportable incidents and those related to abuse of older people

service information information in the form of policies and procedures, employment contracts, service contracts, care plans, audit outcomes, budgets, funding, and codes of conduct

sleep a specific state of consciousness that occurs on a cyclical basis

stereotype a widely held view or opinion about something or a group of people

stereotyping the process of judging individuals on the basis of what you consider to be their cultural affiliation; gender, sexual and racial stereotypes are often denigrating and unkind

stress a very individual state described as anything that causes an interruption to a person's activities of daily living, including physically, mentally, socially, emotionally, religiously, culturally, spiritually, sexually or financially

substitute decision maker a person who has been appointed to make decisions on behalf of the person who is unable to make them

sundowning behaviour associated with dementia where the person with dementia becomes agitated, restless, anxious, confused and disorientated, and goes wandering, in the late afternoon and early evening

T

terminal care care delivered at the end stage of life, which could be weeks, days or hours; also known as end-of-life care

Therapeutic Goods Administration (TGA) the government agency that regulates medication and medical devices in Australia

thoracic cavity chest cavity

toxicity the amount of a substance that can cause harm due to its poisonous state

transmission the passing on of an infectious agent (e.g. influenza transmission can occur between a care worker and the person they are caring for)

trauma a deeply distressing or disturbing experience

traumatic an experience that is very distressing

U

unilateral one-sided

V

v+i+p+s (VIPS) Valuing, Individuality, Person-centred perspective and Social aspect

vascular dementia a dementia occurring due to circulation problems whereby blood flow and oxygen supply to the brain are interrupted; also known as multi-infarct dementia

ventricles the two lower chambers of the heart

verbal communication communication through language, written or spoken; the use of words to get a message across

voluntary assisted dying where legal access to medications that will assist dying at a particular time and place is made possible; also known as euthanasia

W

Wernicke-Korsakoff syndrome a dementia type attributed to excessive alcohol intake over a prolonged period of time

work health and safety (WHS) legislation legislation based on the principle of duty of care that employers and workers have to protect the health, safety and welfare of themselves and others in the workplace

written communication the sending of messages or instructions in writing

Y

younger onset dementia (YOD) a set of signs and symptoms detected earlier in life than expected and which interferes with a younger person's activities of daily living sooner than when detected in an older person

Index

A

B

C

D

E

F

Q

R

S